Ben Cao Gang Mu Dictionary

Volume Two

Ben Cao Gang Mu Dictionary

Volume Two

Geographical and Administrative Designations

Hua Linfu, Paul D. Buell, and
Paul U. Unschuld

A Volume of the
Ben Cao Gang Mu Dictionary Project

Paul U. Unschuld, General Editor

University of California Press

University of California Press, one of the most distinguished university presses in the United States, enriches lives around the world by advancing scholarship in the humanities, social sciences, and natural sciences. Its activities are supported by the UC Press Foundation and by philanthropic contributions from individuals and institutions. For more information, visit www.ucpress.edu.

University of California Press
Oakland, California

Library of Congress Cataloging-in-Publication Data

Ben cao gang mu dictionary / edited by Zhang Zhibin, Paul U. Unschuld.

volumes cm

Includes bibliographical references.

Contents: Volume 1. Chinese historical illness terminology.—Volume 2. Geographical and Administrative Designations.

ISBN 978-0-520-29196-6 (cloth : alk. paper)—ISBN 978-0-520-96555-3 (ebook)

1. Li, Shizhen, 1518-1593. Ben cao gang mu. 2. Medicine, Chinese—History—16th century. 3. Medicine, Chinese—Dictionaries. 4. Materia medica, Vegetable—China. I. Zhang, Zhibin, 1953– editor. II. Unschuld, Paul U. (Paul Ulrich), 1943– editor. III. Title: Dictionary of the Ben cao gang mu.

RS180.C5B45 2015

615.3 210951—dc23

2014018742

Manufactured in the United States of America

25 24 23 22 21 20 19 18 17 16

10 9 8 7 6 5 4 3 2 1

CONTENTS

Acknowledgments

The research leading to the preparation of this volume of the *Ben cao gang mu Dictionary* was financed by Stiftung Volkswagenwerk. The institutional framework enabling us to pursue this project was the Horst-Goertz-Stiftungsinstitut, Charité-Universitätsmedizin Berlin, funded by the Horst-Goertz-Foundation from 2006 through 2013. Martin Huber, Klaus Neugebauer and David Dornier, as well as the Chinese Broad Group Yuan da 遠大, generously provided us with additional support to continue our work into 2016 and complete the compilation of this volume. Prof. Hua Linfu 華林甫 of the Institute of Qing History of Renmin University of China laid the foundations to the present volume by researching and documenting all Chinese data required. He was assisted by his four postgraduates Gao Maobing 高茂兵, Li Cheng 李誠, Huai Qian 懷倩 and Zhang Min 張敏. Prof. Zheng Jinsheng 鄭金生, former head of the Research Institute for the History of Medicine and Medical Literature of the China Academy of Chinese Medical Sciences, and Ulrike Unschuld helped to prepare the numbered list of pharmaceutical substances in Appendix A. Siglinde Mooney assisted in technical matters. Christine Hu gave the manuscript its final layout. I am most grateful to all these individuals and institutions for their belief in this project and their conceptual as well as financial support.

Paul U. Unschuld
Berlin, March 2016

I. INTRODUCTION

1. The *Ben cao gang mu* Project

This is the second volume of a project aiming at providing better access to the *Ben cao gang mu* (*BCGM*) 本草綱目, China's great encyclopedia of pharmaceutical lore, first published in 1593 and designated a UNESCO world cultural heritage text in 2012. In addition to the current volume, which focuses on verifying and localizing 2,158 geographical and administrative designations in the *BCGM*, three additional volumes will complete the *Ben cao gang mu Dictionary*. They include the first volume, published in 2015, on Chinese historical illness terminology, and a forthcoming third volume identifying all book titles and authors named in the *BCGM*. A fourth volume will offer a historical survey of the identifications of all pharmaceutical substances mentioned in the *BCGM*.

The *Ben cao gang mu* was composed over more than three decades from perhaps 1547 until 1580. Li Shizhen 李時珍 (1508–1593), who turned to his family tradition of medicine after failing the imperial exams required for entering the civil service, is traditionally named its sole author. In his preface, he mentions assistance provided by several family members but, presumably, it came from a team extending beyond his immediate household. No details, though, are available on the team's possible size.

Li Shizhen and his coworkers excerpted data from the rich pharmaceutical literature of the previous 1,500 years and numerous other literary sources.[1] In addition, Li Shizhen included pharmaceutical knowledge he had obtained from practitioners and other contemporary sources during his travels throughout the Chinese empire.

All geographical and administrative designations quoted from more ancient texts were left uncommented and frequently were no longer applicable to administrative reality during the sixteenth century. Hence, even Li Shizhen and his coworkers in

1 Paul U. Unschuld, *Medicine in China. A History of Pharmaceutics*. (Berkeley: University of California Press, 1976).

many instances may not have known the exact location referred to by a more ancient place name or administrative structure. This is even truer for today's readers of the *BCGM*. In fact, the value of the *BCGM* for providing reliable hints regarding the occurrence of certain herbal material with specific therapeutic effects is severely limited by the absence of verification and localization of the ancient place names specifying their geographical origins. The present volume of the *Ben cao gang mu Dictionary* will change this offering clarity as to where an herb, mineral, or animal was said to have been grown, gathered, or simply used.

2. Scope and Purpose of the Dictionary

The present dictionary comprises all the purely geographical and associated administrative names mentioned in the *BCGM*. Most are straightforward, easily established place names that usually applied only for a given period, even if the periods in question could be quite long. A particular focus of the dictionary is the multitude of abbreviations used in the text, as for example, Jiang dong 江東, "East of the Yang zi River." Although these are usually general regional designations, they are extremely important in terms of the ways that the Chinese of Li Shizhen's time and before viewed their country and its parts. Some abbreviations may have been quite obsolete by the time the *BCGM* was compiled, even if they were traditional. This is particularly true of names recalling the old states of pre-Qin China.

Each name in the dictionary is fully explained and expanded where appropriate and cross-referenced where necessary. Appendix C at the end of this volume provides a listing of all the 2,158 headings of the dictionary in alphabetical sequence. This index allows the user to determine quickly what is in the dictionary and what is not. This feature is, among other things, intended to aid those using the dictionary for general purposes not necessarily associated with the *Ben cao gang mu* alone.

The purpose of this volume of the dictionary is to provide a general reference work for all the geographical material in the *BCGM* and help to conveniently determine precisely what area the *BCGM* is referring to in its textual discussions and in terms of specific pharmaceutically relevant items. These are in every case associated with specific places and administrations. To make it still easier to use, the old place names and administrative units, looked at historically to begin with, are usually localized in terms of the modern administrative geography of China.

Altogether the *BCGM* lists 2,463 place names.[2] This number includes 1,139 names of administrative divisions, 270 names of mountains and mountain ranges, 213 names of geographic regions, 108 names referring to "Western territories" and the "South

2 For the numerical data presented in this Introduction and a more detailed analysis of the numerical distribution of place names and administrative divisions in the *Ben cao gang mu*, see Hua Linfu 华林甫, *Ben cao gang mu* shi di ba shuo 本草纲目》释地八说, in *Di li* 地理, *Geography* 3(2013): 110–18. All quantitative statements concerning the *BCGM* are based on the following edition: Li Shizhen 李时珍, *Ben cao gang mu* 本草纲目, edited by Liu Hengru 刘衡如, 2nd ed. (Bei jing 北京: Ren min wei sheng chu ban she 人民卫生出版社, 2004).

Sea", 86 names of rivers, lakes, ponds and marshlands, 60 names referring to places created by fantasy or known from tradition only, 60 general regional references, 58 names referring to settlements of minority nations, 43 names of ancient cities no longer extant, 38 names of ancient countries no longer extant, 30 names erroneously ascribed to places, 20 names of small towns, and 20 names that cannot be identified and require further research. In addition, more than two hundred names refer to temples, harbors, mills, springs, cities, wells, relay stations, imperial tombs, palace parks, royal palaces, salt works, mountain passes, gardens, tea plantations, government and military commands, sandbanks, islands, and traffic routes. Proportionally, 46.2 percent of the designations refer to regional administrative divisions, 14.5 percent to geographical areas. The geographical regions most often named in connection with the production or use of certain pharmaceutical drugs are, first, Ling nan 岭南 with 163 appearances, then Jiang nan 江南 with 151 appearances.[3] The Nan hai 南海 is mentioned 124 times; the "South" as such, Nan 南, appears 108 times. In contrast, the "North" as such, Bei 北, appears 71 times. The region Jiang dong 江东 is mentioned 104 times. That is, virtually all place names that appear in the *Ben cao gang mu* more than one hundred times are located in the South. Apparently, this is the region where most of the pharmaceutical data gathered by Li Shizhen and his team originated. Also, Shu 蜀 is named 89 times, Shu zhong 蜀中 is mentioned 54 times, Guang 廣 61 times, Guang zhou 廣州 appears 54 times, Wu 吴 60 times, Min 闽 and Chu 楚 both appear 53 times, and Jiang Huai 江淮is named 55 times. These locations are located south of the Huai he 淮河 river, which is further evidence of a preponderance of the association of Chinese *materia medica* with southerly regions.

3. The Chinese Geographical World View

The places and administrative units of the present dictionary (both the Chinese places and units and the place and administrative names from Central Asia and points south and west) reflect Chinese geographical tradition and the Chinese worldview. In particular, they reflect how this tradition and perspective have changed over time. Please note in this respect that any single area may have had multiple names over the course of time. This is particularly true for Central Asian, Western, and Southeast Asian as well as Indian Ocean place names. Names may also have different transliterations in Chinese characters, often reflecting the differing pronunciations of Chinese characters over time. These differences are noted in the entries below.

In ancient times, the Chinese landscape was often charged with a mythology, as for example in the so-called "Tribute of Yu 禹" (*Yu gong* 禹貢), one of the most ancient Chinese attempts to describe China as a whole, which is referred to repeatedly in the present dictionary. Not only was most of ancient China associated with considerable mythology, but also government and thus administrative geography was likewise quite different from what would come later. Shang 商 and Western Zhou 周 had a system stressing personal delegation of authority in association with

3 For an identification of these place names, see the respective entries in the main section of this dictionary.

land holding, and such held lands often became states, sometimes quite independent, existing at various levels. Some of these states were quite small and some, for example, the Chu 楚 of later Zhou times, quite large. Although the "Tribute of Yu" does attempt to delineate larger, purely regional units—its nine *zhou* 州—this delineation was largely fictional and the situation was dominated by the patriarchally ruled state, usually designated as *guo* 國, a character meaning, semantically, a region or even a "state" in a boundary.

As China's "feudal" order broke down, the Zhou 周 monarch became little more than a titular national ruler confined to a small domain. Not only did the Chinese states become independent but, increasingly, the way that they attempted to rule changed drastically. Personal connections continued to exist alongside new state subunits that were bureaucratically managed. That is, they were ruled not by lords but by regular officials appointed by the central authority: the first mandarins. A focal point of this development, which actually started elsewhere, was the state of Qin, later founder of the first Chinese imperial dynasty and thus of great importance for subsequent history. The basic pattern of government established then persists today.

Qin, following the example of a number of its neighbors, divided its own and newly conquered territories into "appendages," their names written in various ways, all of which had, by the time of the writing of *BCGM* long been superseded by *xian* 縣, a term we translate as "county" in this dictionary, following a broad convention established in the Western literature. Qin also established what are probably the first effective regional units in Chinese history, commanderies, *jun* 郡, the translation being another convention of the Western literature. Under Qin, the *jun* were mostly larger groupings in newly conquered areas, gradually including all of China except for the original Qin state. The system of jun, commanderies, flourished during the eras of Qin, Han, Wei, Jing, and the Southern and Northern Dyanasties. It ended in 758, during the Tang. That is, at the time the *BCGM* was compiled, the commanderies had already been abolished for more than seven hundred years. Based on the medical literature quoted, the *BCGM* lists more than 223 commanderies for the simple reason that these names were still used by subsequent authors. The identification of commanderies requires an exact knowledge of their seats of administration and administered territory. Even one incorrect rendering of a commandery's name makes this task all the more difficult. For example, the commandery Bao han 枹罕 was listed in the *BCGM* erroneously as Bao han 抱罕. The commandery Bo hai 勃海 was mistakenly given as Bo hai 渤海.

4. Some General Remarks on the History of Chinese Administration

The subsequent history of China's administration is complicated, each dynasty having its own preferences. *Xian* and *jun* long persisted, as did their importance, the former into the present day and under Han, for example. Han also created its own regional and even local units, as did subsequent dynasties, as the need arose.

Under subsequent dynasties, these local units gradually became a hodgepodge of conflicting authority, to the point where individual parts of the government had their own special administrative units. This was true under Tang, for example, primarily late Tang, when indirect rule was the pattern rather than the exception due to the ruling house's loss of direct influence over taxpayers and direct control of tax revenues. In the case of Tang, such things as monopolies were used to tap revenue in place of direct taxation, giving rise to a unique period in Chinese administrative history.

Hence, while a given administrative unit may be considered to have existed from early Tang to late Tang, for example, reality was often altogether different. Users need to take this into consideration in using the dictionary entries. Under Yuan, there was also a marked difference between administrative terminology and reality thanks to the Mongolian organizational reality behind the Chinese-style terminology widely adopted by the dynasty.

Despite the clear need for effective hierarchical authority from the center to a provincial unit and then on down, greatly simplifying the ability of the central government to govern, it was nearly a thousand years after Qin-Han that provincial level units appeared, as can be seen from the discussion below. Notably, during this entire period (and during Li Shizhen's time), old-style states continued to exist alongside more centralized administrative units.

This was partly due to nostalgia as well as to the problem that progressively larger dynastic clans created for dynasties. In Ming times, holdings of nonruling members of the dynasty became more and more significant and developed into a source of considerable weakness, since more and more territory was removed from the direct purview of the Ming central government. This was a problem under Yuan as well, when all members of the ruling house and many people associated with it, for example, through marriage had rights to appanages or revenue from these, administered in their name by the imperial authority or the qanate authority, i.e. Yuan China.

Something that must always be taken into consideration is that the administrative geography of the *BCGM* generally reflects that of the sources quoted, no matter how obsolete they were by its time. Although the *BCGM* does occasionally attempt to modernize terminology or refers to a place by a very broad, regional generalization, place and administrative references are generally those of a particular source, and reflect the era when the source was produced.

Even the *BCGM's* generalizations often are period-connected. Many, however, are simply regional collectives. Some such entries assume truly large proportions, almost as if the authors of the *BCGM* gave up trying to be specific. The dictionary entries for Wu 吳, mentioned 60 times in the *BCGM*, and Nan fang 南方, mentioned 124 times, are examples of these voluminous groupings.

5. A Brief Survey of the History of Chinese Administrative Geography

Some generalizations may be made regarding place names and administrative units mentioned in the *BCGM*.

China's most ancient administrative geography was highly disunified and dissimilar, varying considerably from one part of China to the other. For much of pre-Qin history, each state had its own traditions. However, at the national level the state, *guo*, was an important identity, and the old state names continued to be used to designate regions through Li Shizhen's time, long after the states themselves had become dead letters except as pseudo-feudalistic structures, in theory the state domains of princes. In this connection, some of the "states" represent a Chinese façade covering a non-Chinese reality, as for example in the terminology of the various Yue 越 (written various ways), Viet, entities. The problem is that ancient Chinese texts were usually not all that ancient and reflected later eras when such places had begun to be Chinese or were already clearly Chinese.

5.1. The County

Concurrent with the old "feudal" structure of early China some "new" units that emerged after the fifth century BCE were also present, reflecting an attempt to organize territory locally based on bureaucratic (and not feudal) links to the center. The major legacy of this effort is the *xian* 縣, here universally translated "county," a term written a single way today but that appeared in many variants with the basic meaning of an appendage, in this case of the central government, although sometimes of other local units as well. *Xian* still exist today and represent a major vestige of the most ancient times in China. Since Qin times, *xian* have continued to be more or less the same size, unlike some other units. They usually centered about a *xian* city, most often with the same name as the *xian*. In recent premodern times, they were the seat of the county magistrate. The *xian*, counties, constituted the lowest level of administrative divisions. Hence they appear in the *BCGM* most often. During the *wan li* 萬曆 reign period of the Ming (1572–1620), there were a total of 1,169 counties. The *BCGM* mentions 331, or almost a third of them. Many are easily identifiable. For example, in *juan* 10, in the description of *she huang* 蛇黄, an iron ore, the text states: "In Guang xi 廣西, Ping nan 平南 county, there exists a mountain ridge with *she huang*. In the ninth month, the locals dig seven to eight *chi* 尺 deep and obtain *she huang* there. Large specimens resemble chicken eggs. Small ones are of the size of marbles/shots. The color is purple." Ping nan 平南 is the name of a county established in 633 under Tang. Its seat of administration was in present-day Ping nan county. More difficult are those where over time or at the same time identical county names were given to different territories. These require more intensive research. An example is Dong yang 东阳 county. One Dong yang county was established during the Qin. Its seat of administration was in present-day Dong yang cheng 東陽城, located thirty-three kilometers southeast of Xu yi 盱眙 county in Jiang su 江蘇. It was abolished under Southern Dynasties' Chen

陳. A second Dong yang county was established under the Tang 唐, in 686. Its seat of administration was in present-day Dong yang city in Zhe jiang 浙江 In 1988, it became a city with county rank.

In some instances the name of a county is well known, but its administrative rank remains unclear. An example is Chen liu 陳留. This may be a reference to a commandery, but could also be the name of a county. Chen liu county was established under Qin 秦. The seat of its administration was in present-day Chen liu town, 26 *li* southeast of Kai feng 開封 city in He nan 河南. In 1957, it was combined with Kai feng county. The commandery of Chen liu was established under Western Han 漢 in 122 BCE. The seat of administration was in present-day Chen liu county and its territory comprised an area extending from present-day Kai feng city in the west, to Ning ling 寧陵 county in the east, north to Yan jin 延津 and south to the counties of Qi 杞 and Sui 睢. Under Northern Wei 魏, the administration was moved to the present Kai feng city. In 758, the area was changed to Bian zhou 汴州. Basically, the county and the commandery were located in the same area. Other instances, in which the names are identical and the administrative ranks differ, are more difficult to identify as they refer to different regions. For example, in *BCGM juan* 52, in the text on *fu ren yue shui* 妇人月水, women's monthly period, it is said: "There are girls who at the age of twelve, thirteen years give birth to a child. As is recorded in the *Xi ji shi* 禧記室, the daughter of Su Da 蘇達, a high ranking official in Ping jiang 平江, became pregnant at the age of twelve." According to the *Nan cun chuo geng lu* 南村輟耕錄, Su Da was a Yuan 元 era official. During the Yuan era, both a Ping jiang fu 平江府 (for the term *fu*, see section 5.4 below) and a Ping jiang county, Ping jiang xian 平江縣, existed. The county had been established by Five Dynasties' Chu 楚 by changing the name of Chang jiang 昌江 county. Its seat of administration was in the present-day Ping jiang county in Hu nan 湖南. Ping jiang fu was established under Northern Song 宋 in 1113 by raising the status of Su zhou 蘇州. Its seat of administration was in present-day Su zhou city in Jiang su 江蘇. Under Yuan 元, in 1276, its name was changed to Ping jiang lu 平江路. At the beginning of Ming 明, it was changed to Su zhou fu 蘇州府. As no further evidence is available, the identification of the location Ping jiang mentioned in the *BCGM* must end here.

5.2. The Commandery

The spread of administrative units of this sort and also of *jun*, commanderies, was associated with the state of Qin and its efforts to conquer China, ultimately establishing the first unified dynasty. Qin administration was intended to be based on bureaucratic rule instead of on a "feudal" order, that is, on the old states and personal links that had hitherto dominated. The *jun* were at first largely connected with the frontiers and ranked below the *xian* but this changed over time and their military strength made them more powerful units almost to begin with. *Jun* persisted as a major administrative unit until Tang times when other, corresponding units replaced them. Unlike the *xian*, they have not lasted until the present day. It should be realized that the *jun* referred to in the sources came in various sizes and powers. Still, all were strong regional units ultimately possessing power beyond that of any county.

5.3. The Zhou

Han introduced its own administrative variants including some special regional units, among them those under special regional inspectors, *ci shi*. Later, *ci shi* became a title of aboriginal chieftains but that is not its application in this dictionary. Under Tang, the office applied often to the head of a *zhou*.

The *zhou*, using a word that is related to another *zhou* 洲, rendering the idea of an area surrounded by bodies of water such as rivers, first became important in late Han times when it emerged as a regional unit that could control large areas, including several *jun*. Following the Jin era, the number of *zhou* rose continuously. It reached several hundred during the Eastern Jin and the Sixteen Kingdoms, and the North-South Division. Following the North-South Division, more than five hundred *zhou* had been established. Three hundred *zhou* were said to exist at the time of Sui emperor Wen di. At the same time, their territorial size continuously decreased. By Tang there were 367 *zhou*. They had replaced the commandery but continued to administer several subordinate units, in this case *xian*. With the Song and Yuan period elevating more and more *zhou* to the status of *fu* and *lu*, many of the *zhou* were split and became smaller still. Many of the *zhou* mentioned in the *BCGM* had either been abolished in earlier times, or had been converted into *fu*. Examples are Ai zhou 爱州, Bi zhou 壁州, Cai zhou 蔡州, Dan zhou 丹州, E zhou 鄂州, Fang zhou 坊州, Gan zhou 赣州, Hang zhou 杭州, Bin zhou 宾州, Kai zhou 开州, Lai zhou 莱州, Meng zhou 孟州, Nan en zhou 南恩州, Pan zhou 潘州, Qi zhou 岐州, Rao zhou 饶州, Sha zhou 沙州, Tai zhou 台州, Wan zhou 万州, Xi zhou 西州, Yan zhou 严州, and Zhen zhou 真州. Also, during Ming and thereafter, *zhou* was often simply part of a place name and not a functioning administrative unit; *zhou* as administrative units had long since ceased to exist. Of the 468 *zhou* 州 mentioned in the *BCGM*, the majority no longer existed by that time. The number of defunct administrative divisions mentioned in the *BCGM* is therefore quite large.

Fortunately, most of the divisions designated as *zhou* were comparatively well-known regions, with many references in ancient literature. Hence they are easily identified. Also, even though different regions were given identical names over time, it is not difficult to identify them. We encounter difficulties when the name of a *zhou* is erroneously ascribed to a specific region. For example, in *juan* 18, the text on *He shou wu* states: "According to Tang era Regional Inspector Li Yuan 李遠: 'Those samples of *he shou wu* originating from Nan he county and in the Ling nan 嶺南 region from En zhou 恩州, Shao zhou 韶州, Chao zhou 潮州, He zhou 賀州, Guang zhou 廣州, and from Si hui 四會 county in Pang zhou 潘州, they are superior. Those originating from Qie zhou 且州, Gui zhou 桂州, Kang zhou 康州, Chun zhou 春州, Gao zhou 高州, Le zhou 勒州, and Jin xing 晋興 county in Xun zhou 循州, they are of secondary quality.'" In fact, in Chinese history a Le zhou 勒州 never existed. The *BCGM* edition by Liu Hengru 刘衡如 has correctly changed this to Qin zhou 勤州. Similarly, in *juan* 29, the text on *li* 栗 states: "In Guang zhong 廣中 there are no *li* 栗. Only in the mountains of Jin zhou 靳州 there are *shi li* 石栗. They ripen within one year. They are round like a marble. The skin is thick, and they taste like walnuts." Again, no Jin zhou 靳州 ever existed. This, too, is Qin zhou 勤州. Once the error is corrected, the identification of Qin zhou poses no problems.

5.4. The Fu

The administrative divisions identified as *fu* date from 713, the first year of the *kai yuan* reign period (713–741) of the Tang. Their number was increased during the Song and, by the beginning of the Ming, *fu* had been established all over the country. A *fu* was similar to a *zhou* but enjoyed special status because of military importance or strategic location. Like a *zhou* it could coordinate and manage several subordinate *xian* or even *zhou* under Ming. The term could in particular be applied to some garrison or command in a generic sense. For example, in the present dictionary, a *du du fu,* "area command," is mentioned which in Ming times was a major military commission. Also note *du hu fu* 都護府, "chief protection *fu* 府," which strictly speaking however, applied to alien groups. The usage is complicated and in many cases a *fu* is simply an office of some official, a headquarters and not an administrative unit at all. An important characteristic of the *fu* was direct subordination to the central authority, something that stressed the significance of the *fu* itself. During Ming times, this could mean subordination to a province as well. According to the Dynastic History of the Ming, *Ming shi* 明史, during the *wan li* reign period (1572–1620), there were a total of 159 *fu*. The *BCGM* mentions 85 *fu* that existed during Li Shizhen's time. That is, approximately one half of the *fu* mentioned in the *BCGM* existed at the time. Others had already been abolished without leaving a trace. Examples of the latter are He zhong fu 河中府, Jiang ning fu 江宁府, Jian kang fu 建康府, Jiang ling 江陵府, Ping jian fu 平江府, Shou chun fu 寿春府, Xing yuan fu 兴元府, and Zhong shan fu 中山府.

5.5. Tang 唐 Era

Medieval China largely retained Han administrative terminology except in the North, where a greater tribal presence blurred lines. In any case, later units did not always correspond to how things were organized under the Han even if the names were the same. Tang, though in many ways a continuation of China's medieval period, also introduced many changes. This was in particular due to the lingering effects of the great An lu shan 安祿山 rebellion of mid-Tang, which reduced the ability of the central authority to control local areas and their taxpayers directly. The authority shifted instead to military governors and a system of monopolies to at least secure revenue if not control territories and populations. This indirect system of rule reached its high point in the early ninth century under Emperor Xian zong 憲宗 (r. 805–820). It nearly led to a Tang restoration, a remarkable achievement.

Even before the rebellion, an important Tang innovation was the *jie du shi* 節度使, military commissioner (before Tang a supply commissioner), a powerful official assigned largely to frontier areas. The number of such officers and commands rapidly increased after the rebellion, when the *jie du shi* became largely autonomous regional authorities in the absence of other officers due to the breakdown of the central authority.

Tang also established regional circuits, *dao* 道, which originally applied to frontier areas and actually predated Tang. Tang *dao* were nearly province level and managed at first *jun* and then *zhou* and *fu*.

5.6. Song 宋*, Liao* 遼*, Jin* 金*, Yuan* 元*, and Ming* 明 *Eras*

Under Song, the *dao* became even more important and under Liao 遼, the *dao* were primarily province-level structures, closely following Song precedent but applied more specifically as the primary organizational feature of the Chinese side of the Liao empire. Still, under Song, the *lu* 路 superseded the *dao* as the main regional unit and were clusters of other units including *zhou* and *fu*. In Song times there were also *jian* 監, best thought of as industrial prefectures, that is *fu*. Previously *jian* were most significant in the administrative structure as central directorates but under late Tang in particular *jian* could be associated with special regional units including horse pastures under the *tai pu si* 太僕寺, "administration of the imperial stud."

Jin 金 mostly followed Song in administrative naming practices, and the Mongols at first used the existing terminology though their administrative units were often quite different in character. Thus the *lu* of the Mongol period was much smaller than the Song or Jin *lu* and, despite its Chinese name, was a Mongolian administrative unit, the *cölge*. This was basically a city and its hinterland, including even an oasis with a city. Even Tibet, a Mongol protectorate, had its *cölge*, the *chol-kha gsum*, "the three *cölge*" of central Tibet. Although the word does not occur in the available sources for the Mongol West, the idea was almost certainly a Turkistanian one.

Besides their *lu*, the Mongols had various other native administrative units, many existing only briefly. Typical were the various *xuan wei si* 宣慰司, pacification offices, that existed at the beginning of Qubilai's reign. In fact, such offices had little that was Chinese about them; they were Chinese covers for Mongolian local government structures, in this case occupation units, usually headed by officials with Mongolian titles such as *jarquci*, "administrator for *ulus* or patrimony affairs," or *bicigci*, an official concerned with documents. The *ulus* meant here were those of the entire Mongolian empire. Technically *bicigci* were associated with *dao*, circuits, and coordinated various local units and were responsible to the large regional *xing sheng* 行省, agency for carrying out supervision, a proto-province which we will examine more closely later. Under Ming, the *xuan wei si* was associated with chieftains and aboriginal tribes. This was a typical pattern once national offices had been reduced to little more than tribal administrations.

The *xing sheng* 行省, today's *sheng* 省, province, was, in theory, a branch of a national *zhong shu sheng* 中書省, the main executive of the central government. In fact, at the time when the *xing sheng*, a permanent regional unit (unlike the *xing sheng* of Jin, which were temporary and limited), first emerged during the era of the Mongolian empire there was no *zhong shu sheng* as such, although the term was occasionally used as a cover for what Mongolian central government there was, for example during the first years of *qan* Ögödei's reign in the 1230s.

Basically, in imperial times, the term *xing sheng* was applied to the great regional provinces of the Mongolian empire (*el* or *il*, "pacified population"), with central administration at Qaraqorum in Mongolia, established in such areas as China, which was governed from Zhong du 中都, the old Jin central capital located just south of what is now Beijing 北京; Turkistan; and later Iran.[4] Later, as the Mongolian empire expanded and broke up into successor states, further provinces were established, including in Yun nan 雲南 where a joint administration of *jarquci* and other Mongolian officers, even representatives of princes, was established, marking the beginning of the first effective control of this area by any Chinese dynasty.[5]

Later, other provinces, *xing sheng*, were established under the auspices of the Yuan dynasty, the Mongol successor state for China, and the province subsequently became a typical administrative unit, except that the terminology was changed again under the Ming. But the provincial administration commission or *bu zheng shi si* 布政使司, also *cheng xuan bu zheng shi si* 承宣布政使司, of Ming is nothing more than the Yuan *xing sheng*. In fact, the name *sheng* for modern provinces was even then in widespread popular usage. Under the Qing 清 the name even reappeared as the official name of China's provinces. It has persisted into the present day.

Ming, in addition to taking over the idea of the province from Yuan, was also unique in the many special administrations for tribal government it used, primarily in the far south. Many occur in the present dictionary and their wide use reflects a Ming concern with its southern and southwestern borderlands, as its interests in these areas increased as overseas contacts declined.

5.7. *Military Administration*

Also in the dictionary, and referring to various periods, are numerous terms for guards and armies. In many cases units so designated were actually military garrisons, at least in their origins, although many became simply place names as the distinction was lost. Xing hua jun 興化軍, Xing hua 興化army, for example, was originally an army base established in what is now Fu jian 福建 to keep the local aboriginals under control. Later it became a city and survives as such today. By contrast, *wei* 衛, guards, were always just that and the name generally disappeared with the guard.

Another military term occurring in the text is *du si* 都司. In Ming times this was often used as an abbreviation of *du zhi hui shi si* 都指揮使司, "administration of a commanding official." This was a regional military commission. Also a military office was the *du du fu* 都督府, before Ming an area command, after 1380 a high-ranking military command, one of several controlling the armies of the dynasty. Another military command under the Ming was the *an fu si* 安撫司, more properly *an fu shi si* 安撫使司, military commission, an administration designed to control and pac-

4 On this and the assumptions behind it see Paul D. Buell and Judy Kolbas, "The Ethos of State and Society in the Early Mongol Empire: From Chingiz Khan to Güyük," in *The Mongols and Post-Mongol Asia: Studies in Honour of David O. Morgan*, edited by Tim May, Journal of the Royal Asiatic Society 26, nos. 1–2 (January 2016): 43–64.

5 See the biography of the first chief of this administration: Paul D. Buell, "Saiyid Ajall (1211–1279)," in *In the Service of the Khan: Eminent Personalities of the Early Mongol-Yüan Period (1200-1300)*, edited by Igor de Rachewilty, Hok-lam Chan, Hisao Ch'i-ch'ing and Peter W. Geier (Wiesbaden: Otto Harrassowitz Verlag, 1993), 466-79.

ify troubled areas, under Tang generally referred to as *jie du shi* 節度使. Later, the office could be associated with a circuit but under Ming this office was most often associated with a chieftainship of southwestern aboriginal tribes.

Administrative units pertaining to a very local administration occur from time to time in the present dictionary. These include the *ting* 廳, a subprefecture existing between *xian* and the next-level unit, in reference to Qing, and *xiang*, first a district, township, or ward, but later, for example in the Canton area, a traditional designation without real meaning. It is rendered below simply as "subadministrative unit."

Finally, important terms in the present dictionary are certain modern descriptives occurring when traditional administrative geography is linked to modern practice. This includes the *shi* 市, usually just translated as "city," though today, the *shi* can exist at various levels and can even be independent units in the People's Republic. Since units of these kinds did not exist in Ming times or before, the additional information is added in the entries only when relevant or appropriate, as when modern differences are observed in passing. Otherwise *shi* is just translated as "city." Another term for city is *cheng* 城, originally a walled city or walled settlement, but this is usually left untranslated in place names.

6. Non-Chinese Places and Peoples

For areas outside China local names (although often the local name used in the area in question but rather what local outsiders called a place or a people) generally applied, except when China controlled the areas directly and set up administrations, in which case Chinese terms were used. The authors of the *BCGM* occasionally use these Chinese terms, usually not from their own time, but more frequently they use the local names for places, for example An xi 安息 (various writings), an older name for Persia from the name of the ruling house, including the variant An shi guo 安石國.[6]

As was the case with China's foreign trade in medicinals, foreign place names are usually associated with Central or West Asia or with Southeast Asia and points along the Indian Ocean. But more than simple geography is involved since the Central and West Asian names are, more often than not, ancient names, principally dating to Han times but also to Tang, another period of active communication with Central and West Asia. By contrast, Southeast Asian and Indian Ocean names, along with some Han names, mostly represent more recent maritime contact. Interestingly, these include names such as Aden that are very recent in Chinese knowledge, dating back only to the Zheng He voyages.

In the dictionary entries, Chinese foreign names are identified as often as possible with more widely recognized forms, for example India for Tian zhu 天竺, and Khotan for Yu dian 于闐. But sometimes it is not so simple. An xi 安息, for example, is Arsacid, the name of the ruling dynasty and not Persia *per se*. Also, we can only guess at the original meanings of many old forms, even when we know

6 Not to be confused with the perhaps homophone An xi 安西, "Pacifying the West," a Tang-era protectorate in the western regions of Turkistan.

approximately where the places they name are located or to which groups they refer. In part this may be due to the fact that many of the forms we have may constitute not the name that a people gave themselves or how a place was known to the locals, but a name applied by neighbors or even known throughout a region, perhaps not particularly correctly.

The following is another typical example of an entry of this type, for modern Samarqand, but with many variants of the name:

> **Sa ma er han** 撒馬兒罕 [2]
> Name of an ancient city in Central Asia, present-day Samarqand in Uzbekistan. Ancient Greek sources refer to it as Marcanda. Semescant is a Turkic spelling found in Yuan 元 sources. The *Shi ji* 史記, "Historical Records," the *Han shu* 漢書, "Book of Han Dynasty," the *Wei lüe* 魏略, "Account of Wei Dynasty," and the *Jin shu* 晉書, "Book of Jin Dynasty," refer to it as Kang ju 康居 territory. The *Wei shu* 魏書, "Book of Wei Dynasty," refers to it as Xi wan jin 悉萬斤. The *Xi yu ji* 西域記, "Records of Western Territories," refers to it as Sa mo jian 颯秣建, the *Jing xing ji* 經行記, "Record of [my] Experiences," refers to it as Sa mo jian 薩末鞬, and the *Xin Tang shu* 新唐書, "New Book of Tang Dynasty," refers to it as both Kang guo 康國, Kang country, and Sa mo jian 薩末鞬, identifying it as Kang ju Area Command, Kang *ju du du fu* 康居都督府. The *Liao shi* 遼史, "History of Liao Dynasty," refers to it as Xun si gan 尋思干, identifying it as He zhong fu 河中府. The *Yuan shi* 元史, "History of Yuan Dynasty," too, names it Xun si gan 尋思干, and also Xue mi si gan 薛迷思干. The *Ming shi* 明史, "History of Ming Dynasty," refers to it as Sa ma er han 撒馬兒罕, and identifies it as the ancient capital of Kang ju 康居/Kan guo 康國.

7. The Methodology of Identifying Geographical and Administrative Designations

7.1 Identical Designations, Different Meanings

The *BCGM* lists many geographical designations that have multiple meanings. A closer look at the example of Guang 廣 may illustrate the variances encountered.[7] A location named Guang appears sixty-one times in the *BCGM* (not counting combinations such as Guang dong 廣東, Guang xi 廣西, etc.). Among these sixty-one appearances, the designation Guang may refer to Liang guang 两廣, to Guang dong 廣东, to Guang zhou 廣州, to the territory administered by the regional inspector and military commissioner of Guang zhou including a region in Ling nan 嶺南 during the Tang 唐 era, and to Song 宋 era Guang nan lu 廣南路.

---

7 For more regarding the following analysis 7.1. through 7.3., see Hua Linfu, *Ben cao gang mu* shi di ba shuo.

In *BCGM juan* 9, in the text on *hua shi* 滑石, Li Shizhen is quoted: "*Hua shi* is found all over Gui lin 桂林 and in Yao dong 瑶峒." During the Ming era, Gui lin was part of Guang xi. Hence the Guang mentioned here obviously has the meaning of Liang guang.

In *juan* 44, in the text on *chang yu* 鯧魚, Li Shizhen: "*Chang* 昌 means mei 美, 'pleasant.' The name [of this fish] results from its flavor. It is said that when these fish swim in water, all the other fish follow them and consume the foam emerging from their mouths. They resemble prostitutes, *chang* 娼; hence their name. The people in Min 閩 erroneously identify them as *cang yu* 鯧魚. The people in Guang call them *gou ke shui yu* 狗瞌睡魚, 'sleepy dog fish.'" Chen Cangqi 陳藏器 (681–757) is quoted as stating: "*Chang yu* live in the Nan hai 南海." Li Shizhen then concludes: "Min and Guang are in the Nan hai." That is, the Guang here refers to Guang dong.

In *juan* 9, in the text on *shi zhong ru* 石钟乳, Su Gong 蘇恭 (died 674) is quoted with the statement: "The top quality is found in Shi xing 始興; of secondary quality are those from the *zhou* of Guang 廣, Lian 連, Tan 潭, Lang 朗, and Bang 梆." Hence the Guang mentioned here refers to Guang zhou.

In *juan* 34, in the text on *chen xiang* 沉香, Liu Xun 劉恂 (fl. 10th c.) is quoted as saying: 廣管羅州多棧香樹, "In Luo zhou, administered by Guang, there are many *zhan xiang* 棧香 trees." The Guang referred to here is the territory administered, in Tang 唐 times, by the regional inspector, *ci shi* 刺史, of Guang zhou 廣州 who was jointly military commissioner, *jing lue shi* 經略使, of the five *fu* 府 of Ling nan 嶺南. This territory encompassed much of the present province of Guang dong 廣東 and of Guang xi 廣西.

In *juan* 30, in the text on *ju* 橘, the Song 宋 author Han Yanzhi's 韓彦直 *Ju pu* 橘譜, "Manual on Tangerines," is quoted as stating: 柑橘出蘇州、台州，西出荆州，南出閩、廣、撫州，皆不如温州者爲上也, "*Gan*, 'oranges', and *ju*, 'tangerines,' come from Su zhou and Tai zhou. In the West, they come from Jing zhou. In the South, they come from Min, Guang, and Fu zhou. They are all not as good as those originating from Wen zhou." The Guang mentioned here is the Guang nan lu 廣南路 of Song times.

Similarly, Dong hai 東海, Huai nan 淮南, Jing shi 京師 and Gao li 高麗 also have five different meanings each. The designations Bei hai 北海, He dong 河東, Jiang nan 江南, Liao dong 遼東 and Shan dong 山東 each refer to four different areas. Han 漢, Chi shui 赤水, Fu jian 福建, Lan ling 蘭陵, Liang shan 梁山 and Ling ling 零陵 have three different meanings each. Bei di 北地 and Dong ting 洞庭 are examples of designations with two different meanings. Often, intensive research was required to assign these designations to the proper geographical regions and administrative divisions. Details may be learned from the respective entries in the main part of this dictionary.

7.2 Designations Quoted Erroneously in the BCGM

Often, quotes from earlier literature in the *BCGM* are unreliable. This is particularly problematic in the case of place names, given their importance for assessing the quality of pharmaceutical substances originating from specific regions.

In *juan* 8, in the text on *gu jing* 古鏡, "ancient mirrors," the *History of Song, Song shi* 宋史, is quoted with the statement: 秦寧縣耕夫得鏡，厚三寸，徑尺二寸, "In Qin ning county a peasant ploughing found a mirror. It was three inches thick and had a diameter of two inches." However, the original text in the *Song shi* states: 泰寧縣耕夫得鏡，厚三寸，徑尺有二寸. That is, the Tai ning 泰寧 county of the original text was erroneously changed to Qin ning 秦 county in the *BCGM*.

In *juan* 10, in the text on *shi dan* 石膽, Su Gong 蘇恭 is quoted as saying: 出蒲州虞卿縣東亭谷窟及薛集窟中，有塊如鷄卵者爲真, "Those originating from the Dong ting gu cave and from the Xue ji cave in Yu qing county of Pu zhou, their pieces resembling chicken eggs, they are genuine." Su Gong lived during the early Tang era. At that time in Pu zhou a Yu xiang 虞鄉 county existed but no Yu qing 虞卿 county. The close resemblance of the characters Qin 秦 and Tai 泰, as well as Xiang 鄉 and Qing 卿 may account for the erroneous quotes.

In *juan* 36, in the text on *shan zhu yu* 山茱萸, the *Ming yi bie lu,* "Further Records of Renowned Physicians," is quoted with the statement: 山茱萸生漢中山谷及琅琊、冤句、東海承縣, "*Shan zhu yu* grows in the mountain valleys of Hanzhong, and in Lang ya, Yuan ju and Cheng counties of Dong hai." Cheng xian 承縣 should be Zheng xian 氶縣. Gu Zuyu 顧祖禹 (1631–1692), in *juan* 232 of his *Du shi fang yu ji yao* 讀史方輿纪要 states: 氶讀拯，俗作承，误也, "氶 is read Zheng, but it is commonly given as Cheng 承. That is a mistake." Similarly, Yang Shou jing 楊守敬 in *juan* 7 of his *Sui shu di li zhi kao zheng* 隋書地理志考証, "The Geographical Annals of the *Book on the Sui* Reexamined," states: "Zheng xian 氶縣 was named after the Zheng river, Zheng shui 氶水... Today the local annals write the name of the county as Cheng 承. That is a mistake."

In *juan* 36, in the text on *shi nan* 石南, the *Fan shi hu ji* 范石湖集, "Fan's Collection [of Poems] from the Rock Lake," is quoted as saying: 修江出欒茶，治頭風。今南人無所謂欒茶者，豈即此物耶, "Xiu jiang produces *luan* tea. It serves to cure head wind. Nowadays the people in the South do not speak of Luan tea. How could this be this item?" However, the original text of the *Fan shi hu ji*, in *juan* 14, reads: "蛮茶出修仁，大治头风, "*Man* tea originates from Xiu ren; it is very effective in curing head wind." That is, the *BCGM* quote includes two mistakes when it writes Xiu jiang 修江 instead of Xiu ren 修仁, and *luan* 欒 tea instead of *man* 蛮 tea.

In *juan* 51, in the text on *shan zao*, the *Yong jia ji* 永嘉記 , "Yong jia Records," is quoted as saying: 安國縣有山鬼，形如人面，一脚，僅長一尺許, "In An guo county mountain demons exist with a human face. They have one leg and are only slightly over one *chi* tall." Two different books are recorded with the title *Yong jia ji*. One was compiled by Zheng Qizhi 鄭緝之 during Liu Song 劉宋. It is also documented as *Yong jia jun ji* 永嘉郡記, "Yong jia Commandery Records." The second version was compiled by Xie Lingyun 謝靈運 (385–433). The lack of listings in bibliographies suggests that it may not have been transmitted for some time. Both books are lost today. The version compiled by Zheng Qizhi was available in three editions. As the present *BCGM* quote was taken from one of these editions, the reference to an An guo county must be an error. The An guo county of Han and Wei times was located southeast of present-day An guo city in He bei 河北. The An guo county of Northern Qi 齊 and Northern Zhou 周 times was located north of present-day Xin ji 辛集 city in He bei. The An guo county of the early Five Dynasties Song time was located north of present-day Lin an 臨安 city in Zhe jiang 浙江. None of these counties was located in the region of the Yong jia 永嘉 commandery of the Six Dynasties era. If the *BCGM* had referred to An gu 安固 instead of An guo, that would have been appropriate because an An gu county had been established in 280, during the Western Jin. Its seat of administration was located in present-day Rui an 瑞安 city in Zhe jiang. In 323, during the Eastern Jin 晋, and during the Southern Dynasties, An gu county was subordinated to Yong jia commandery.

7.3 Errors Identified in Older Literature

In a section titled *zheng wu* 正误, "correction of mistakes," Li Shizhen addresses more than seventy mistakes he has identified in earlier literature. For example, in *juan* 34, in the text on *gui* 桂, Wang Haogu 王好古 (1200–1264), the author of the *Tang ye ben cao* 湯液本草, "Materia Medica of Decoctions," is quoted with a commentary on the following passage in Kou Zongshi's *Ben cao yan yi* 本草衍義, "Expanded Meaning of Materia Medica": "I do not know why [*gui*] was given the name *guan gui* 官桂." Wang Haogu then explains: "I have consulted the [*Ben cao*] *tu jing* [本草]圖經, 'Illustrated Classic of Materia Medica,' where it is stated: 今觀賓宜諸州出者佳。世人以觀字畫多, 'Nowadays, those coming from the *zhou* 州 of Guan 觀, Bin 賓 and Yi 宜 are of fine quality. Because the people considered the character *guan* 觀 to consist of too many strokes they wrote it as *guan* 官.'" To this Li Shizhen remarks: "That is wrong. The wording *jin guan* 今觀 in the [*Ben cao*] *tu jing* has the meaning of *jin shi* 今視, 'Now looking [at those *gui* from Bin zhou and Yi zhou, they are of fine quality].' There never was a Guan zhou 觀州 in the Ling nan 岭南 region. The term *guan gui* 官桂 refers to superior quality *gui* 桂 offered to officials, *guan* 官.

The quotes of earlier literature found in the *BCGM* often show discrepancies, examples of which follow.

Example 1, regarding Le ping 樂平 commandery. In *juan* 8, in the text on *yin* 銀, silver, the *Shan hai jing* 山海經, "Classic on Mountains and Seas," is quoted with the following statement: 東北樂平郡堂少山出銀甚多, "Large quantities of silver originate from Tang shao shan in Le ping commandery in the Northeast." The received text of the *Shan hai jing* does not have such a passage. Also, it is unlikely that a pre-Qin 秦 text should speak of a *jun* 郡, commandery. The Le ping commandery was established towards the end of the Eastern Han 漢 era. Hence this quote cannot have been taken from the *Shan hai jing*.

Example 2, regarding Xin yang zhou 信陽州. In *juan* 9, in the text on *tao hua shi* 桃花石, in the *Wen yuan ge si ku quan shu* 文淵閣四庫全書 edition of the *BCGM*, Su Song 蘇頌 (1020–1101) is quoted with the following statement: 今信陽州有之，形块似赤石脂、紫石英輩，采無時, "Nowadays it is available in Xin yang zhou. Its shape resembles chunks of *chi shi zhi* or *zi shi ying*. It can be gathered at any time of the year." The version edited by Liu Hengru repeats this passage as 今信州有之， that is, omitting the character *yang* 陽. This omission was explained by Liu Hengru as being based on the original text found in the *Da guan ben cao* 大

觀本草, "Materia Medica of the *Da guan* Reign Period," and the *Zheng he ben cao* 政和本草, "Materia Medica of the *Zheng he* Reign Period." The fact is, Xin zhou was established in 758, under Tang 唐. Its seat of administration was in present-day Shang rao 上饒 city in Jiang xi 江西. The seat of administration of Xin yang zhou was located in present-day Xin yang city in He nan 河南. These two areas are far apart from each other. Even more important, Xin yang county was established only as late as under Yuan 元, in the fifteenth year of the *zhi yuan* 至元 reign period, in 1278. Su Song who lived during the Northern Song cannot have known of it. While therefore it is evident that Xin zhou is the correct geographical designation, it remains unclear whether the error in the *Si ku quan shu* edition of the *BCGM* originated from the primary source used or was introduced by the *BCGM* authors.

Example 3, regarding Zhang shan 鄣山. In *juan* 10, in the text on *yu shi* 礜石, the following statement is found, quoted from Hong Mai's 洪邁 *Rong zhai sui bi* 容齋隨筆, "Casual Notes from the Studio of Tolerance": 劉表在荊州，與王粲登鄣山，見一岡不生百草, "When Liu Biao was in Jing zhou he climbed, together with Wang Can, Zhang shan mountain. There they saw a ridge where no herbs grew at all." In the *Shang hai gu ji ban* 上海古籍版 edition of the *Rong zhai sui bi*, Zhang shan mountain is written 障山 instead of 鄣山. A Zhang shan 障山 mountain is located forty *li* east of present-day An lu 安陸 city in Hu bei 湖北.

Example 4, regarding Xi shan, 錫山. In *juan* 15, in the text on *wei xian* 薇銜, Li Shizhen commentating on Li Daoyuan's 酈道元 *Shui jing zhu* 水經注, "The *Water Classic*, Annotated," writes: 魏興錫山多生薇銜草, "Many *wei xin* herbs grow on Mount Xi shan of Wei xing." The related passages in the original text in *juan* 27 of the *Shui jing zhu shu* 水經注疏 have the following wording: 魏興郡之錫縣故城北.縣有錫義山，方圓百里，形如城，四面有門 ...多生薇銜草, "It is located north of the old walled city of Xi xian in Wei xing commandery. . . in that county Mount Xi yi shan is located with a circumference of one hundred *li*. It is shaped like a walled city. Each of the four sides has a gate... Many *wei xin* herbs grow there." That is, the Xi yi shan of the original text was changed to Xi shan in the *BCGM*. There exists only one Xi yi mountain in China, located southwest of present-day Yun xi 鄖西 county in Hu bei 湖北, while there are at least seven places named Xi shan.

Example 5, regarding Shi cheng 石城. In *juan* 26, in the text on *cong* 葱, a commentary by Li Shizhen on the *Jing yan fang* 經驗方, "Recipes Based on Experience," by Zhang Congzheng 張從正 (1156 – 1228) reads: 石城尉戴堯臣，試馬損大指，血出淋漓。餘用此方，再易而痛止, "The official Dai Yaochen of Shi cheng injured his thumb while testing a horse. The thumb bled profusely. I made use of this recipe. After two applications, the pain ended." Zhang Congzheng's 張從正 biography is documented in the *History of the Jin Dynasty*, *Jin shi* 金史, in *juan* 131. The story of Dai Yaochen's injury was also related by Zhu Su 朱橚 (1361 – 1425) in his recipe collection *Pu ji fang* 普濟方, "Recipes for Encompassing Assistance," in *juan* 303, in the section Jin chuang men 金瘡門, "Injuries by Metal Objects." Here Zhang Congzheng's *Jing yan fang* is quoted too, but with a more complete wording. The related passage reads: 荊門軍點頭錄、石城鄉人戴尧臣作尉，試

馬, "Dai Yaochen was a military officer of the Jing men Army. Shi cheng was his native home."

8. Pharmaceutical Substances

The *BCGM* focuses on substances applied in pharmaceutical therapy. Its approximately nineteen hundred monographs describe, identify, and discuss a wide range of items including plants of all types, animal and human body parts and fluids, minerals, human-made objects, and, judged from hindsight, products of human fantasy. The *BCGM* regularly quotes older and contemporary sources offering information on regions, in general or specific terms, where the items in question are found, gathered, produced, or simply used. In the present dictionary, numbers representing these items are listed at the end of the majority of the entries, introduced by the words "[Place name A is] mentioned with [items X, Y, Z]." A complete listing of all these numbers is given in appendix B of the dictionary together with brief botanical, mineralogical, and zoological identifications. Comprising 1,583 items, this listing does not include all substances discussed in the *BCGM*. Rather, this is a selection meant to offer a first and preliminary idea of which items were mentioned in connection with certain geographic regions and administrative territories.

To keep this part of the dictionary simple, no distinction is made, for example, between various parts of the same plant, which might enjoy different names and, for that matter, have very different medicinal properties. In the text of the *BCGM*, this might even involve the authors creating separate monographs, as in the entry on the "wood of *tong cao*" (*tong cao mu* 通草木). A single numerical identifier is used for each group of related products in this dictionary, that is to say, "wood of *tong cao*" is given the same number as *tong cao* and is identified with the same botanical name. The focus here is on *materia medica* and place, not *materia medica* for its own sake. Readers interested in more precise botanical, mineralogical, and zoological identification may wish to consult the fourth volume of the *Ben cao gang mu Dictionary*.

Most of the *BCGM's materia medica* came from China; however, many areas that were clearly "China" in Li Shizhen's time were not yet China in early times. Yun nan 雲南, for example, only became Chinese in the sixteenth century after it had been part of the earlier Yuan empire. By contrast, many of the places controlled tribally under Ming and considered China by Li Shizhen are part of Vietnam or even Burma today. Nonetheless, many of the mainstream places in China supplying medicinals in Li Shizhen's time continue to produce the same products even today.

Most, but certainly not all, of the foreign *materia medica* seem to have been produced from two main areas. One was Central Asia, here meaning southern Siberia, Inner Mongolia, Mongolia, eastern and western Turkistan and immediately adjacent areas, and a generalized West attached to it, an area much larger in ancient times. The other was Southeast Asia and beyond, the Indian Ocean world that, as time went on, increasingly included Africa.

For China, Central Asia was distant, even mythical terrain until the time of the explorations of Zhang Qian 張騫 (195–114) and the conquests of Han Wu di 漢武

帝, Emperor Wu of Han (r. 140–87 BCE). It did not always remain under direct Chinese control after the time of Emperor Wu but by that time regular commerce along the Silk Road linked points in China to points in Central Asia and beyond.

During Han and thereafter, the Chinese also explored points farther west, their explorers perhaps reaching to the borders of the Roman Empire. In any case, Chinese knowledge of the West grew over time, reaching high points under Tang and then again under Yuan. Nevertheless, many Central Asian and Western products are associated with calcified references in our sources, that is, with a few or even one single source and were hardly common ingredients at the time that the *Ben cao gang mu* was written. The sources and the *Ben cao gang mu* are also full of confusion regarding what was produced where. The tendency was for products from farther afield to be listed in connection with places that were closer, perhaps their shipment points, not the original source of the products in question.

This is the case for asafetida, for example, a plant resin used in cooking and in medicine that is a typical Iranian-area product and is primarily produced in what is now Iran and Afghanistan. Also regularly misassigned is frankincense, one of the key aromatics of the Bible, along with myrrh. The *BCGM* mentions frankincense a number of times and as coming from a number of places, most of them not South Arabia where it was actually produced. But sometimes, when we take into consideration where frankincense was actually marketed in early and more recent times, the *BCGM's* seemingly erroneous assignments are not so strange.

And sometimes the *BCGM* is entirely correct in its seemingly strange assignments. Using very old sources, for example, the *BCGM* authors assign ostriches to a wide range, including Syria and nearby areas, something in fact true about them in early times. Its assignment of hyenas to Central Asia (Western Turkistan) also reflects early reality although they are extinct in Central Asia today. But they were not extinct when first mentioned in Chinese sources. Nonetheless, this tendency on the part of the *BCGM's* authors to mix up periods makes using their information difficult when they are not absolutely clear about their sources and what period they are referring to, which they seldom are. Another problem is that the *BCGM* may, for completeness, list pharmaceutical substances that were certainly not used in its time, a time of known shortage of many of the exotic foreign medicinals.[8]

A major route for imports of medicinals was maritime, from Southeast Asia and later the Indian Ocean, although the Ming trade with the South was heavily focused on interior land routes rather than maritime points. This was largely but not exclusively true of Han times as well. By then sea contacts were assuming enough importance to constitute a second Silk Road, a maritime one. Even more than is

8 The *Hui hui yao fang* 回回藥方, for example shows a progressive modification in its later editions, with one major feature the continuing replacement of more exotic ingredients by those more readily available in late Ming times. See Paul D. Buell, "Eurasia, Medicine and Trade: Arabic Medicine in East Asia: How It Came to Be There, and How It Was Supported, Including Possible Indian Ocean Connections for the Supply of Medicinals," in *Ideology and Knowledge Exchanges across the Indian Ocean*, edited by Angela Schottenhammer (Singapore: University of Singapore Press, forthcoming).

the case with the *BCGM's* Central Asian and West Asian products, a great many of the pharmaceutical substances from these sea routes are misassigned. In fact, there is good reason for this, which becomes apparent when we trace the history of the maritime routes involved and the changing relationships between the various points along them.

The most ancient Chinese maritime trade with points south began with short, coasting trade from point to point, reflecting the limited ancient technology for building ships and also the underdevelopment of the entrepots that were needed for trade to flourish.[9] Some products, for example, cloves, did move a considerable distance from producers in farther Indonesia to Chinese consumers but the trade always seems to have been in stages and was also, in the earliest times, indirect.

This situation began changing with the unification of what was then China, including the Qin conquest of the Canton Delta and associated areas, as well as the first Chinese advances into what is now Vietnam. Under Han, northern Vietnam was (loosely) a Chinese protectorate and, although this situation was not permanent, the Chinese presence in An nan 安南, as it was then termed, "pacifying the South," both reflected a growing trade from points beyond and at the same time stimulated demand. Demand for all exotic products tended to rise once they became available as anything but the greatest of rarities.

In early times, points in what is now Vietnam are listed as producing many products, for example, myrobalans, that were actually produced far afield but were transshipped from points in Vietnam. Ai zhou 愛州, for example, a Chinese administrative center located within what is now Vietnam, is assigned the following local products: *Phyllanthus emblica*, or Indian gooseberry; *Terminalia belerica*, or belleric myrobalan; *Terminalia chebula*, or "black myrobalan"; betel pepper; betel nuts; cloves; and sappan wood. Of them, the Indian gooseberry, the myrobalans, the cloves, and the sappan wood represent transshipping and did not originate in Ai zhou or anywhere else in what is now Vietnam. The myrobalans probably came from India, the nearest major source, and the cloves from Indonesia; the closest source of sappan wood was Thailand. Betel pepper also came from outside Ai zhou, from Malaya or India. Only betel nuts were, strictly speaking, a local product. The *BCGM's* Ai zhou entry is thus strictly historical and refers to a particular period when trade in many of the commodities listed was first developing but when the Chinese still had no good idea of the true origins of many of the products involved.

Indian Ocean trade developed at the ocean's other end similarly to the trade from the south. At first it was strictly a coasting trade but the discovery and use of the monsoon winds soon allowed longer voyages to be made even if these were seasonal and took an entire season. However, largely thanks to these winds, by Roman times the Indian Ocean was dotted with important entrepots, transshipment locations

---

9 See as an introduction Gang Deng, *Maritime Sector, Institutions, and Sea Power of Premodern China*, Contributions in Economics and Economic History (Westport, CT: Greenwood Press , 1999), 212.

that linked Egypt, Iran, and India on the one side with India, Southeast Asia, and ultimately China on the other.[10]

Generally, each stage of a trading journey was served by a different nationality, or at least by people from a different city, but as shipping technology improved, including combinations of eastern and western ship types, longer voyages became possible.[11] In the hands of Persian and Arabic sailors, these became nearly direct by the thirteenth century, although it was, in spite of the Zheng He 鄭和 (1371–1433) voyages, the Portuguese who were to gain full advantage from the new knowledge and approaches involved. The Chinese turned away from maritime exploration after the early fifteenth century. Nevertheless, the older place names and the products associated with them remain in the *BCGM*, even if these products no longer came directly from the places mentioned. The *BCGM*, for example, mentions Aden though in the sixteenth century there were no East Asian contacts in that direction. Frankincense and other local products from Arabia may still have reached China thanks to the Portuguese, whose trade slightly predated the time when the *BCGM* was being compiled.

The Portuguese trade, Chinese maritime exclusion, and even Ming China's great interest penetrating its South, above all the border areas, by land routes was sixteenth-century reality and the present dictionary is a reflection of this sixteenth century reality. It is also a large-scale artifact, a memory of a time or times in the past, of a trade that was largely extinct when the *BCGM* was being written and that was not even fully understood by Li Shizhen himself.

9. The Structure of Entries in the Present Volume

Most entries are structured as in the following example.

Jing zhao 京兆 [3]
Name of a commandery. It was established by Three Kingdoms' Wei 魏. The seat of administration was at a point lying within the ruins

10 Much of what we know about the early trade is from fragmentary textual sources but maritime archaeology is now changing our view of the Indian Ocean past greatly. See for example, this Thailand find with a largely Western cargo: "Arab Dhow Unearthed in Thailand," Archeology, June 3, 2014, www.archaeology.org/news/2160-140603-thailand-dhow-trade.

11 For an introduction see George Hourani and John Carswell, *Arab Seafaring: In the Indian Ocean in Ancient and Early Medieval Times*, expanded (Princeton: Princeton University Press, 1995), and J. Innes Miller, *The Spice Trade of the Roman Empire, 29 B.C.–A.D. 641* (Oxford: Oxford University Press, 1969). See also Paul D. Buell, "The Indian Ocean Trade in Medicinals: Some Indications from Chinese Sources," in *Tribute, Trade and Smuggling*, edited by Angela Schottenhammer (Wiesbaden: Otto Harassowitz Verlag, forthcoming), 133-40. A new survey of all of maritime history that is particularly strong on the Indian Ocean is Lincoln Paine, *The Sea and Civilization: A Maritime History of the World* (New York: Alfred A. Knopf, 2013), see esp. chapters 6, 10, and 13.

of Han 漢 dynasty Chang an 長安, 13 *li* northwest of present-day Xi an 西安 city in Shaan xi 陝西. The administrative territory of the commandery comprised an area extending from the Qin ling 秦嶺 mountain range in present-day Shaan xi toward the North, from Xi an city toward the East, and from Hua 華 county toward the West, and included the counties of San yuan 三原, Jing yang 涇陽, and Gao ling 高陵. Northern Wei 魏 moved the seat of administration to the vicinity of the present-day Xin zhu 新筑 town located northeast of Xi an city. Northern Zhou 周, in 558, again moved the seat of administration to a point 13 *li* northwest of present-day Xi an city in Shaan xi. Sui 隋, in 583, changed the commandery and established Yong zhou 雍州 but, in 607, again established Jing zhao commandery administered in present-day Xi an city. The administrative area was expanded in the north to include Yi jun 宜君 county. In 618, under Tang 唐, the area again became Yong zhou but, in 690, again became Jing zhao commandery, and sequentially again Yong zhou. Mentioned with 204, 631.

First comes the name of the entry, bolded, in pinyin transliteration and Chinese characters, followed, in square brackets, by the number of occurrences of this geographical and administrative designation in the text of the *Ben cao gang mu*. Next, usually, comes the type of administrative unit represented, in this case a commandery or *jun* 郡, and the period of its establishment and administrative headquarters. There follows the scope of administration of the unit in question as it originally existed. Next there usually comes a listing of changes over time, including the type of unit involved, and any moves of the unit's administrative headquarters and any changes in administrative area. Last comes a listing of pharmaceutically relevant items associated with the unit, in this case a type of fish and pears. These items are given as numbers, here 204 and 631 respectively, with their actual Chinese names and a preliminary scientific identification to be recovered from appendix B.

Variations of this basic pattern include compound entries, for occasions when the *BCGM* provides a reference that is ambiguous and there must be a listing of the various possibilities. Subject to similar treatment are places where little more than the same name for multiple places is involved and the *BCGM* does allow readers to distinguish between them. This is illustrated by the following entry.

Nan hai 南海 [1 + 5 + 82 + 5 + 1 + 11 + 10]

□ Regional name. [1] It refers to the areas occupied by various nationalities in the South.

□ Regional name. [5] It refers exclusively to the present-day Ling nan 嶺南 region. Mentioned with 777, 930, 1076, 1335.

□ Regional name. [82] The reference is to the South China Sea. Mentioned with 43, 80, 82, 94, 127, 133, 138, 169, 175, 217, 232, 243, 267, 302, 318, 346, 347, 376, 393, 396, 398, 400, 401, 405, 409, 421, 424, 438, 464, 478, 501, 506, 518, 531, 591, 608, 621, 656, 674, 716, 772, 824, 840, 847, 855, 892, 894, 919, 945, 961, 1012, 1021, 1030, 1044, 1056, 1078, 1084, 1101, 1123, 1170, 1194,

1264, 1273, 1294, 1297, 1341, 1356, 1389, 1421, 1422, 1455, 1463, 1467, 1489, 1508, 1515, 1517, 1576.
□ Regional name. [5] It refers to the area south of the Western Ocean, that is, present-day Qing hai hu 青海湖/Kokonor Lake. Mentioned with 1335.
□ Name of an ocean district. [1] It refers to the ocean east of China. Mentioned with 1030.
□ Name of a commandery. [11] It was established by Qin 秦, in 214 BCE. Its seat of administration was in present-day Guang zhou 廣州 city in Guang dong 廣東 province. Later, during the Qin and during the Han 漢, the area became part of Nan yue 南越. It was reestablished under Western Han in 111 BCE, after it destroyed Nan yue. Its jurisdiction corresponded to the area south of the Weng jiang 滃江 and Da luo 大羅 mountains, the delta of the Pearl River and the area east of the watershed of the Sui jiang 綏江. Later, its territories were reduced. Under Sui 隋, in 589, it was eliminated but, in 607, it was reestablished by renaming Fan zhou 番州. Its seat of administration was in present-day Guang zhou city. Under Tang 唐, in 621, it became Guang zhou but, in 742, it was changed to be Nan hai commandery. It again became Guang zhou in 758. Mentioned with 80, 110, 113, 376, 405, 427, 685, 790, 1335, 1467.
□ Regional name. [10] It refers to a strip of present-day Southeast Asia and its littoral and even as far as the Indian Ocean region. Mentioned with 11, 49, 511, 680, 708, 775, 961, 1030, 1086, 1264.

In this case, the *BCGM* makes it clear specifically which "Southern Ocean" is referred to in each instance. Note that the number of entries is divided by reference although the heading lists all together. Note also that in this and other entries, places mentioned that have entries of their own in the present dictionary are not further explained.

In the following example, however, references are not so certain and the entry indicates this. Pharmaceutically relevant items have, however, been assigned to the county rather than to the commandery as this is more likely.

Xiang yang 襄陽 [9]
Name with several possible applications.
□ Name of a commandery. It was established at the end of Eastern Han 漢. Its seat of administration was in present-day Xiang yang 襄陽 city in Hu bei 湖北. Its territory of administration comprised the present-day cities and counties of Xiang yang, Yi cheng 宜城 and Yuan an 遠安 in Hu bei. At the beginning of Tang 唐, the area was changed to Xiang zhou 襄州.
□ Name of a county. It was established by Western Han. Its seat of administration was in the present-day Xiang zhou 襄州 district in Xiang yang city of Hu bei. In 1951, the seat was moved to Fan cheng 樊城. In 2001, the county was eliminated and became an urban district. Mentioned with 186, 275, 453, 639, 737, 1234, 1285, 1294, 1509.

Another variation of the basic pattern are simple cross-references for instances when the discussion of a place is best placed under a single heading even though the authors of the *BCGM* use one or more abbreviations for the same place in other parts of the *BCGM*. In passing, it should be pointed out that not all places are administrative units or regions. The *BCGM* refers frequently to mountains or mountain ranges, for example, as well as to rivers and other bodies of water. In every case, effort has been made to make references as self-explanatory as possible, while directing readers elsewhere for subentries discussed in more detail in other entries. Also glossed are some plain errors, instances in which the *BCGM* treats a reference as a place name but it is not.

10. Administrative Terminology in Detail

In the identification and translation of administrative terms our authority is generally Charles Hucker, *Dictionary of Official Titles in Imperial China*, which, despite its title, also discusses administrative terminology in some details. Convention has been followed in rendering *xian* 縣 as county and *jun* 郡 as commandery. The authors have supplied their own translations where none exist in Hucker. The following are terms that, where helpful, appear in the dictionary entries in translations together with the original Chinese characters:

an fu si 安撫司	pacification commission
bu zheng shi si 布政使司	provincial administration commission
cheng xuan bu zheng shi si 承宣布政使司	provincial administration commission
ci shi 刺史	regional inspector
ci shi 刺史部	regional inspector division
dao 道	circuit (or simply a route)
du du fu 都督府	area command
du hu fu 都護府	chief protection *fu*
du si 都司	regional military commission
guo 國	country
jie du shi 節度使	military commissioner
jun 軍	army
jun min zong guan fu 軍民總管府	tribal command

jun 郡	commandery
wei 衛	guard
xian 縣	county
xing du si 行都司	regional military commission
xuan wei si 宣慰司	pacification office
zhang guan si 官司	chief's office
zhen 鎮	garrison (except in modern place names where a *zhen* is just a town and is so translated)

Other English translations used in the text of the dictionary for more general terms, sometimes very rarely, include:

ba 壩	dam
chang 場	fair, plantation
he 河	river
hu 湖	lake
jiang 江	river (in general left untranslated to avoid place name ambiguity)
jie 街	market, usually urban as a market street
qu 區	district
shan 山	mountain, mountains
shi 市, *cheng* 城	city
ting 廳	subprefecture

Some terms, for example *fu* 府, *zhou* 州, *xiang* 鄉, and *li* 里, are left untranslated and are explained only here. *Li* was a unit of distance that varied across eras, from an estimated 415 meters during the Han dynasties to 645 during Qing times. A *li* is officially 500 meters today. A *gong li* 公里 is a kilometer. Of course, there were no official *li* or kilometers in early and recent traditional China and kilometers only occur in our locations of traditional names.

The user should note that many Chinese place names have special readings sometimes associated only with a particular place name. Usually these are normal alternative readings that can be found in any dictionary. An example is Zhang zi shan 長子山, "Zhang zi mountain," which could in theory also be read Chang zi shan. In cases where a reading is very specialized or ambiguous, or where a reading is not normal to a character at all, cross-referencing is provided although the main entry for a place is always under the correct reading of the name.

Berlin, 2016

Bibliography

Two kinds of sources were used in preparing this dictionary. First and foremost many primary sources were utilized. These are listed under A below and the catalogue in it is by no means complete. To supplement it the reader is referred to other sources listed and discussed in the published writings of the authors, including many of those listed under C below, which also provides a catalogue of general reference works. In addition, under B are listed the key Chinese-language reference works in the area of historical geography.

The studies in list C are particularly those allowing the identification of problem places and units, usually ones connected with Central Asia, Southeast Asia or points beyond, and contributing to an understanding of the larger issues that are involved with the Indian Ocean trade in particular. There is a considerable literature on the topic and our listings are at best highly selective. Nonetheless, the most important works are listed. In identifying many places a study of the pharmaceutically used items said to have been produced or simply used there is often helpful. Works by Burkill, Laufer, Wang Gungwu, Paul Wheatley and Wolters are thus often of decisive importance. Note author Hua Lin fu's many contributions in this area as well.

A

Primary Sources

Ban Gu 班固, *Han shu* 漢書, "History of the Han," annotated edition, Bei jing 北京: Zhong hua shu ju 中華書局, 1962

Bo Lanxi 孛蘭肸, et al., *Da yuan da yi tong zhi* 大元大一統志, "Great and unified gazeteer of the great Yuan 元," reconstruction by Zhao Wan li 趙萬里, Bei jing 北京: Zhong hua shu ju 中華書局, 1966

Chen Xun 陳循 et al., *Huan yu tong zhi* 寰宇通志, "General record of the world," Zheng Zhen duo 鄭振鐸, ed., Xuan lan tang cong shu xu ji 玄覽堂叢書續集, 1947

Gu Yanwu 顧炎武, *Zhao yu zhi* 肇域志, "Beginning regional record," Annotated by Tan Qixiang 譚其驤 et al., Shang hai 上海: Shang hai gu ji chu ban she 上海古籍出版社, 2004

Gu Zuyu 顧祖禹, *Xu shi fang yu ji yao* 讀史方輿紀要, "A summary after reading the records of regions from the histories," annotated by He Cijun 賀次君 and Shi Hejin 施和金, Bei jing 北京: Zhong hua shu ju 中華書局, 2005

Guo Zizhang 郭子章, *Jun xian shi ming* 郡縣釋名, "Explanations of names for commanderies and counties, 1614 edition

Fang Xuanling 房玄齡, et al., *Jin shu* 晉書, "History of Jin," annotated edition, Bei jing 北京: Zhong hua shu ju 中華書局, 1974

He Shen et al. 和珅, *Da qing yi tong zhi* 大清一統志, "Unified gazeteer of the great Qing 清," revised edition, Si ku quan shu 四庫全書, Shi bu di li lei 史部地理類

Jiang Tingxi 蔣廷錫, et al., *Da qing yi tong zhi* 大清一統志, "Unified gazeteer of the great Qing 清," 1744 first edition, printed by Wu Ying dian 武英殿, and preserved in the library of the National People's University

Li Jifu 李吉甫, *Yuan he jun xian zhi* 元和郡縣志, "Record of the commanderies and counties of the Yuan he period," annotated by He Cijun 賀次君, Bei jing 北京: Zhong hua shu ju 中華書局, 1983

Li Xian 李賢, et al., *Da ming i tong zhi* 大明一統志, "Unified gazeteer of the great Ming 明," reproduction of the 1461 edition by the San qin chu ban she 三秦出版社, 1990

Liu Xu 劉昫, et al., *Jiu tang shu* 舊唐書, "Old Tang history," annotated edition, Bei jing 北京: Zhong hua shu ju 中華書局, 1975

Lü Shibin 呂式斌, *Jin xian shi ming* 今縣釋名, "Explanations of the names of modern counties," Bei jing 北京: Heng he 恒和company, 1931

Mu Zhang'a 穆彰阿, et al., *Da qing yi tong zhi* 大清一統志, "Unified gazetteer of the great Qing," new edition, reproduced from the Si bu cong kan 四部叢刊 supplementary volume, Bei jing 北京: Zhong hua shu ju 中華書局, 1986

Ouyang Min 歐陽忞, *Yu di guang ji* 輿地廣記, "Broad record of the earth," annotated by Li Yongxian 李勇先, Cheng du 成都: Si chuan da xue chu ban she 四川大學出版社, 2003

Ouyang Xiu 歐陽修, et al., *Xin tang shu* 新唐書, "New Tang History," annotated edition, Bei jing 北京: Zhong hua shu ju 中華書局, 1975

Ouyang Xiu, et al., *Xin wu dai shi* 新五代史, "New History of the Five Dynasties," annotated edition, Bei jing 北京: Zhong hua shu ju 中華書局, 1974

Shen Yue 沈約, *Song shu* 宋書, "History of Song," annotated edition, Bei jing 北京: Zhong hua shu ju 中華書局, 1974

Sima Biao 司馬彪, *Xu han shu* 續漢書, "Supplementary Han History," annotated edition, Bei jing 北京: Zhong hua shu ju 中華書局, 1965

Song Lian 宋濂, et al., *Yuan shi* 元史, "History of Yuan," annotated edition, Bei jing 北京: Zhong hua shu ju 中華書局, 1976

Tuo Tuo 脫脫, et al., *Song shi* 宋史, "History of Song," annotated edition, Bei jing 北京: Zhong hua shu ju 中華書局, 1985

Tuo Tuo, et al., *Liao shi* 遼史, "History of Liao," annotated edition, Bei jing 北京: Zhong hua shu ju 中華書局, 1974

Tuo Tuo, et al., *Jin shi* 金史, "History of Jin," annotated edition. Bei jing 北京: Zhong hua shu ju 中華書局, 1975

Wang Cun 王存, *Yuan feng jiu yu zhi* 元豐九域志, "Record of the nine regions from the *yuan feng* period," annotated by Wang Wenchu 王文楚and Wei Songshan 魏嵩山, Bei jing 北京: Zhong hua shu ju 中華書局, 1984

Wang Xiangzhi 王象之, *Yu di ji sheng* 輿地紀勝, "Comprehensive record of the earth," based upon the reproduction of the Zhu ying zhai 懼盈齋 edition of Mr. Cen 岑, Bei jing 北京: Zhong hua shu ju 中華書局, 1992

Wei Shou 魏收, *Wei shu* 魏書, "History of Wei," annotated edition, Bei jing 北京: Zhong hua shu ju 中華書局, 1974

Wei Zheng 魏徵, Yan Shigu 顏師古, et al., *Sui shu* 隋書, "History of Sui," annotated edition, Bei jing 北京: Zhong hua shu ju 中華書局, 1973

Yue Shi 樂史, *Tai ping huan yu ji* 太平寰宇記, "Record of the World from the *tai ping* period," annotated by Wang Wenchu 王文楚 et al., Bei jing 北京: Zhong hua shu ju 中華書局, 2007

Xiao Zixian 蕭子顯, *Nan Qi shu* 南齊書, "History of Southern Qi," annotated edition, Bei jing 北京: Zhong hua shu ju 中華書局, 1972

Xue Juzheng 薛居正, et al., *Jiu wu dai shi* 舊五代史, "Old history of the Five Dynasties," annotated edition, Bei jing 北京: Zhong hua shu ju 中華書局, 1976

You Ji 遊記 et al., *Shui jing zhu* 水經注, "Notes to the water classic," Er shi wu shi bu bian. 二十五史補編

Zhang Yanyu 張廷玉, et al., *Ming shi* 明史, "History of Ming," Bei jing 北京: Zhong hua shu ju 中華書局, 1974

Zhao Erxun 趙爾巽, et al., *Qing shi gao* 清史稿, "Draft History of Qing," Bei jing 北京: Zhong hua shu ju 中華書局, 1977

Zhu Mu 祝穆, revised by Zhu Zhuzeng 祝洙增, *Fang yu sheng lan* 方輿勝覽, "Comprehensive overview of the world regions," annotated by Shi Hejin 施和金, Bei jing 北京: Zhong hua shu ju 中華書局, 2003

B

Chen Chao 陳潮 et al., eds., *Zhong hua ren min gong he guo xing zheng qu hua yan ge di tu ji* 中華人民共和國行政區劃沿革地圖集, "Collection of maps showing the course of changes in the administrative divisions of the People's Republic of China," Bei jing 北京: Zhong guo di tu chu ban she 中國地圖出版社2003

Chen Guirong 陳佳榮, et al., *Gu dai nan hai di ming hui shi* 古代南海地名匯釋, "Collective explanations of early place names from the south seas," Bei jing 北京: Zhong hua shu ju, 1986

Feng Chengjun 馮承鈞, *Xi yu di ming* 西域地名, "Place names of the Western Regions," Bei jing 北京: Zhong hua shu ju, 1980

Li Baoku 李寶庫 and Bu Qingjun 卜慶君, eds., *Zhong hua ren min gong he guo zheng yu biao jun di ming tu ji* 中華人民共和國政區標準地名圖集, "Collection of standard place name maps for the administrative geography of the People's Republic of China," Bei jing 北京: Xing qiu di tu chu ban she 星球地圖出版社, 1999

Li Deqing 李德清, *Zhong guo li dai di ming bi hui kao* 中國歷代地名避諱考, "Investigation of tabu avoidances in historical Chinese place names," Hua dong shi fan da yue chu ban she 華東師範大學出版社, 2002

Li Zhao luo 李兆洛, *Li dai di li zhi yun bian jin shi* 歷代地理志韻編今釋, "Modern explanations of the geography monographs of various periods arranged in rhymes," Guang ling gu ji ke yin she 廣陵古籍刻印社, 1992

Ministry of Civil Affairs, People's Republic of China, *Zhong hua ren min gong he guo xing zheng qu hua jian ce* 中華人民共和國行政區劃簡冊, "Handbook of administrative divisions of the People's Republic of China," issued anually, 1951-

Ministry of Civil Affairs, People's Republic of China, *Zhong hua ren min gong he guo xiang zhen xing zheng qu hua jian ce* 中華人民共和國鄉鎮行政區劃簡冊, "Handbook of administrative divisions for small towns of the People's Republic of China," Bei jing 北京: Zhong guo tong ji chu ban she 中國統計出版社, 2010

Ministry of Civil Affairs, People's Republic of China, *Zhong hua ren min gong he guo di ming ci dian* 中華人民共和國地名詞典, "Place name dictionary for the People's Republic of China," five volumes, Hong Kong: The Commercial Press, 1998-2002

Shi Weile 史為樂, *Zhong guo li shi di ming da ci dian* 中國歷史地名大辭典, "Encyclopedic dictionary of historical Chinese place names," two volumes, Bei jing 北京: Zhong guo she hui ke xue chu ban she 中國社學科學出版社, 2005

Shi Weile 史為樂, chief editor, *Zhong hua ren min gong he guo zheng qu yen ge* 中華人民共和國政區沿革, "The course of changes in administrative units under the People's Republic of China," 2 volumes, Bei jing 北京: Zhong guo she hui ke xue chu ban she 中國社會科學出版社, 2005

Tan Qixiang 譚其驤, chief editor, *Qing ren wen ji di li lei hui bian* 清人文集地理類彙編, "Compilation of collected geographical works of Qing people," 7 volumes, Hang zhou 杭州: Zhe jiang ren min chu ban she 浙江人民出版社, 1986-1990

Tan Qixiang 譚其驤, chief editor, *Zhong guo li shi di tu ji* 中國歷史地圖集, "Collection of Chinese historical maps," 8 volumes, Nan jing 南京: Zhong guo di tu chu ban she 中國地圖出版社, 1982-87

Tan Qixiang 譚其驤, chief editor, *Zhong guo li shi da ci dian* 中國歷史大辭典, "Encyclopedic dictionary of Chinese history," Shang hai 上海: Shang hai ci shu chu ban she 上海辭書出版社, 1996

Tan Qixiang 譚其驤, chief editor, *Ci hai* 辭海, "Sea of phrases," Shang hai 上海: Shang hai ci shu chu ban she, 1979

Wang Mo 王謨, *Han tang di li shu chao* 漢唐地理書鈔, "Selections from geographical books of the Han and Tang," Bei jing 北京: Zhong hua shu ju, 1961

Wei Songshan 魏嵩山 chief editor, *Zhong guo gu dian shi ci di ming ci dian* 中國古典詩詞地名辭典, "Phrase dictionary of place names from Chinese early documents and poetry," volume 1, Nan chang 南昌: Jiang xi jiao yu chu ban she 江西教育出版社, 1989

Wei Songshan 魏嵩山 chief editor, *Zhong guo li shi di ming da ci dian* 中國歷史地名大辭典, "Encyclopedic dictionary of historical Chinese place names," Canton: Guang dong jiao yu chu ban she 廣東教育出版社, 1995

Zang Lihe 臧勵龢, *Zhong guo gu jin di ming da ci dian* 中國古今地名大辭典, "Encyclopedic dictionary of old and modern place names of China," Hong Kong: Hong Kong branch of the Commerical Press, reprinted 1982

Zhong Xingqi 鐘興麒, *Xi yu di ming kao lu* 西域地名考錄, "Investigations of Western Regions' place names," Bei jing 北京: Guo jia tu shu guan chu ban she 國家圖書館出版社, 2008

C

Buell, Paul D. and Eugene N. Anderson, *A Soup for the Qan: Chinese Dietary Medicine of the Mongol Era as Seen in Hu Sihui's Yinshan Zhengyao,* appendix by Charles Perry, second revised and expanded edition, (Sir Henry Wellcome Asian Series 9), Leiden and Boston: E. J. Brill, 2010.

Burkill, J. H., *A Dictionary of the Economic Products of the Malay Peninsula*, London: 1935.

Chen Ming 陳明, "The Transmission of Foreign Medicine via the Silk Roads in Medieval China: A Case Study of the *Haiyao Bencao* 海藥本草," *Asian Medicine, Tradition and Modernity*, 3 (2007), 241-264.

Chaudhuri, K. N., *Asia Before Europe, Economy and Civilization of the Indian Ocean from the Rise of Islam to 1750*, Cambridge: Cambridge University Press, 1990

—, *Trade and Civilization in the Indian Ocean, an Economic History from the Rise of Islam to 1750*, Cambridge: Cambridge University Press, 1985

Chipman, Leigh, *The World of Pharmacy and Pharmacists in Mamlūk Cairo*. (Sir Henry Wellcome Asian Series, 8), Leiden and Boston: E. J. Brill, 2010.

Chu Yaping 褚亞平, *Di ming xue ji chu jiao cheng* 地名學基礎教程, "Basic course of study for place name studies," Bei jing: Zhong guo di tu chu ban she 中國地圖出版社, 1994

Cortesão, Armando, ed. A *Suma Oriental de Tomé Pires e o Livro de Francisco Rodrigues*, Coimbra: University of Coimbra (Acta Universitatis Conimbrigensis), 1978.

Cui Hengsheng 崔恒昇, compiler, *Zhong guo gu jin di li tong ming hui shi* 中國古今地理通名匯釋, "Collection of explanations of ancient and modern Chinese geographical designations," He fei 合肥city: Huang shan shu she 黄山書社, 2003

Deng, Gang, *Maritime Sector: Institutions, and Sea Power of Premodern China*, Westport: Greenwood, 1999

—, *Chinese Maritime Activities and Socioeconomic Development, c. 2100 B.C. – 1900 A.D.*, Westport: Greenwood, 1997

Garcia da Orta, *Colóquios des Simples e Drogas da Índia*, two volumes, edited and annotated by Conde de Ficalho: Lisboa: Imprensa Nacional, 1891.

Hall, Kenneth R., *Maritime Trade and State Development in Early Southeast Asia*, Honolulu: University of Hawaii Press, 1985

Haw, Stephen G., Marco Polo's China, *A Venetian in the Realm of Khubilai Khan*, London and New York: Routledge, Taylor and Francis Group, 2006

Hirth, F., and W. W. Rockill, *Chau Ju-kua: His Work on the Chinese and Arab Trade in the Twelth and Thirteenth Centuries*, Entitled Chu-fan-chi, St. Petersburg, 1911.

Hou Renzhi 侯仁之, chief ed., *Zhong guo gu dai di li ming zhu xuan du* 中國古代地理名著選讀, "Selected readings for ancient Chinese geographical names," first collection. Bei jing 北京: Ge xue chu ban she 科學出版社, 1959

Hourani, George and John Carswell, *Arab Seafaring: In the Indian Ocean in Ancient and Early Medieval Times*, Expanded edition, Princeton: Princeton University Press, 1995.

Hua Linfu 華林甫, Qing qian qi 'shu zhou' kao 清前期屬州考, "Investigation of '*zhou* 州 subordination' during early Qing 清," in *Qing dai zheng zhi yu guo jia ren tong* 清代政治與國家認同, volume 1, Bei jing: She hui ke xue wen xian chu ban she 社會科學文獻出版社, 2012, pp 169-214

——, Qing zhi li sheng di li yang e kao bian shi li 清直隸省地理沿革考辨釋例, "Examples of explanations of geographical changes in the directly administered provinces of Qing times," in *Tan Qixiang xian sheng bai nian yan cheng ji nian wen ji* 譚其驤先生百年誕辰紀念文集, Shang hai 上海: Shang hai ren min chu ban she 上海人民出版社, 2012, pp 506-526

——, Zhong guo zheng qu tong ming gai ge chu yi 中國政區通名改革芻議, "My humble opinion on changes in Chinese administrative terminology," in *Li shi huang jing yu wen ming yan jin—2004 nian li shi di li guo ji xue shu yan tao hui lun wen ji*' 歷史環境與文明演進——2004年歷史地理國際學術研討會論文集, Hong Kong: Commercial Press, December, 2012

——, *Ben cao gang mu* shi di ba shuo 本草綱目釋地八說, "Eight statements on explaining *Ben cao gang mu* place names," Qing hua da xue xue bao 清華大學學報, published by Wu han 武漢: Zhe xue she hui ke xue ban 哲學社會科學版, 2012, 6, 83-91

——, Guan yu bian hui *Qing shi di tu ji* di jian yi 關於編繪清史地圖集的建議, "Regarding the ideas behind the compilation of the Qing history collection of maps," in Qing he Zhu Shiguan jiao shou qi shi hua zhi ji rong xiu lun wen ji 慶賀朱士光教授七十華秩暨榮休論文集, Xi an 西安: San qin chu ban she 三秦出版社, 2008, 515-18

——, Xin xiu *Qing shi di li zhi* di xue shu li lun yu ban zuan shi jian 新修<清史•地理志>的學術理論與編纂實踐, "Scholarly theory for the revised geographical monograph of the Qing history and the process of its compilation," *Qing shi yan jiu* 清史研究, 2008, 3, 117-136

——, Di ming: zheng zhi di qing yu biao 地名: 政治的晴雨錶, "Place names, a governmental barometer," *Zhong guo di ming* 中國地名, 2008, 2, 42-44:

——, Yue Shi *Tai ping huan yu ji* di di ming xue gong xian 樂史太平寰宇記的地名學貢獻, "Contributions to the study of place names in Yue Shi's *Tai ping huan yu ji*," *Dong hua li gong da xue xue bao* 東華理工大學學報, 2008, 1, 1-6

——, Zheng qu yan jiu ying gai da po gu, jin jie xian 政區研究應該打破古,今界限, "Administrative unit research should overthrow old ideas and present-day limitations," *Jiang han lun tan* 江漢論壇, 2005, 1, 101-102

——, Zhong guo zheng qu tong min gai ge cun yi 中國政區通名改革芻議, "My humble opinions on the changes of general designations of Chinese government jurisdictions," in *Li shi huan jing yu wen ming yan jin—2004 nian li shi di li guo zai xue shu yan tao hui lun wen ji* 歷史環境與文明演進--2004 年歷史地理國際學術研討會論文集, Bei jing: Shang wu yin shu guan 北京商務印書館, 2005, 9-33,

——, Chong qing zhi xia shi jian cheng 'yu' di shang que 重慶直轄市簡稱渝的商榷, "Consideration of Yu 渝, the abbreviation for Chong qing directly administered city," *Chong qing shi fan da xue xue bao* 重慶師範大學學報, 2004, 3, 120

——, Zhong guo zhi xia shi tong ming gai ge yan jiu 中國直轄市通名改革研究, "Investigations of the changes in the general designations of Chinese directly-administered cities," *Zhong guo ren min da xue xue bao* 中國人民大學學報, 2003, 5, 148-155

——, Dang dai zhong guo xian cheng tong ming gai ge yan jiu 當代中國縣城通名改革研究, "Investigations of changes in the general designations of present-day Chinese county cities," *Zhong guo li shi di li lun cong* 中國歷史地理論叢, 2003, 4, 57-78

——, Zhong guo xian ji zheng qu tong ming yi hua yi 中國縣級政區通名宜劃一, "General designations of governmental units of China at the country level should be standardized," *Zhong guo fang yu* 中國方域, 2003, 1, 24-26

——, *Zhong guo di ming xue shi kao lun* 中國地名學史考論, "Investigations into the history of Chinese place name studies," Bei jing: She hui ke xue wen xian chu ban she 社會科學文獻出版社, 2002

——, Zhong guo gu dai di ming xue li lun di chu bu tan tao 中國古代地名學理論的初部探討, "Inquiry into the first stages of the methodology of Chinese ancient place name studies," *Shi xue li lun yan jiu* 史学理论研究, 2002, 4, 59-72

——, Qing dai kao ju xue pai di di ming xue gong xian 清代考據學派的地名學貢獻, "The contributions of Qing 清era textual criticism scholars to place name studies," *Zhong hua wen shi lun cong* 中華文史論叢, 2002, 2 (66), 178-241

——, Lun zhong guo di ming wen hua dui chao xian-han guo ban dao di ying xiang 論中國地名文化對朝鮮-韓國半島的影響, "Discussing the influence of the Chinese place name culture on Chao xian and the Korean peninsula," *Zhong guo wen hua yan jiu* 中國文化研究, 2001 issue, 170-177

——, Zhong guo zi zhi qu yi gai ming zi zhi sheng 中國自治區宜改名自治省, "The name 'self-governing region' in China should be changed to be 'self-governing province'." *Zhong guo fang yu* 中國方域, 2001, 3, 13-15

——, Shi xia qu ming cheng cun zai di wen ti 市轄區名稱存在的問題, "The question of the survival of the names of districts under cities," *Shang hai di ming* 上海地名 (internal edition), 2001, 2, 4-6

——, Lue lun zhong guo di ming dui yue nan di ying xiang 略論中國地名文化對越南的影響, "Briefly discussing the influence of Chinese place name culture on Vietnam," *Nan yang wen ti yan jiu* 南洋問題研究, 2001, 2, 49-57

——, Zhong guo li dai geng gai chong fu di ming ji qi xian shi yi yi 中國歷代更改重複地名及其現實意義, "Changes and restorations of place names during Chinese history and its actual meaning," *Li shi yan jiu* 歷史研究, 2000, 4

——, Zhong guo gu dai di ming yuan yuan jie shi fa zhan yuan yin di fen xi 中國古代地名淵源解釋發展原因的分析, "Analysis of the causes of the development of explanations for the origins of Chinese ancient place names," *Zhong guo li shi di li lun cong* 中國歷史地理論叢, 2000, 2, 199-215

——, Lue lun *Jin xian shi ming* di di ming xue jia zhi 略論今縣釋名的地名學價值, "A brief discussion of the value of the place name studies in the *Explanation of the Names of Present-day Counties*" in Fan Yang 潘陽, *Zhong guo di ming* 中國地名, 2000, 18-20

——, Zhong guo di ming xue yuan liu 中國地名學源流, "Origins and course of place name studies in China," Chang sha: Hu nan ren min chu ban she 湖南人民出版社, 1999

——, Lun Li Daoyuan *Shui jing zhu* di di ming xue gong xian 論酈道元水經注的地名學貢獻, "Discussing the contributions of Li Dao yuan's 酈道元 Notes to the *Shui jing* 水經 to place name studies," *Di li yan jiu* 地理研究, 1998, 2, 193-199

——, Lun Tang dai di di ming xue cheng jiu 論唐代的地名學成就, "Discussing achievements in Tang era place name studies," *Zi ran ke xue shi yan jiu* 自然科學史研究, 1997, 1, 35-49

——, Lun xian Qin shi qi wo guo di ming xue de te dian 論先秦時期我國地名學的特點, "Discussing certain special points associated with place name studies for China in pre-Qin times, *Hu bei da xue xue bao* 湖北大學學報, 1996, 4, 104-110

——, Lun liang Han shi qi zhong guo di ming xue di dian ji 論兩漢時期中國地名學的奠基, "Discussing the foundations of studies of Chinese place name during the two Han periods," *Zhong guo shi yan jiu* 中國史研究, 1996, 2, 14-25

——, Ci xi di ming tan wei 慈溪地名探微, "A detailed look at the place name Ci xi 慈溪," *Zhong guo di ming* 中國地名, 1995, 5

——, Lun min guo shi qi zhong guo di xue cong chuan tong xiang xian dai di guo du 論民國時期中國地名-學從傳統向現代的過渡, "Discussing the transition of Chinese place name studies from tradition to modernity during the Republican era," *Li shi di li* 歷史地理, 15 (1995), 348-68

—–, Guo Zizhang ji qi jun xian shi ming shu lun 郭子章及其郡縣釋名述論, "Analysis of Guo Zizhang's 郭子章*Explanation of the names of commanderies and counties*," *Zhong guo li shi di li lun cong* 中國歷史地理論叢, 1995, 3, 235-51

—–, Jian lun wo guo di dan ming xian 簡論我國的單名縣, "Brief discussion of our country's single name counties," *Zhong guo di ming* 中國地名, 1994, 2, 26-29

—–, Wo guo gu dai di shuang fu guo xian 我國古代的雙附郭縣, "Paired suburban counties in ancient times in our country," *Zhong guo fang yu* 中國方域, 1993, 6, 9-11

—–, Wei Jin nan bei chao shi qi di di ming xue cheng jiu 魏晉南北朝時期的地名學成就, "The achievements of studies of place names of the Wei and Jin periods and the Northern and Southern Dynasties era," *Li shi di li* 歷史地理, volume 14, 1994, 216-299

—–, Wo guo li shi shang di ming bi hui 我國歷史上地名避諱, "Place name avoidances of tabus in the history of our country, *Di ming zhi zhi* 地名知识, 1992, 2, 7-9

Hucker, Charles, *A Dictionary of Official Titles in Imperial China*, Stanford, Calif., Stanford University Press, 1985.

Kong, S.Y. 江潤祥et al., *Huihui yaofang* 回回藥, Hong Kong 香港: Xianggang bianyi yinwu youxian gongsi 香港編譯印務有限公司, 1996.

Larner, John, *Marco Polo and the Discovery of the World*, New Haven and London: Yale University Press, 2009

Laufer, Berthold, *Sino-Iranica: Chinese Contributions to the History of Civilization in Ancient Iran, with Special Reference to the History of Cultivated Plants and Products*, Chicago: Field Museum of Natural History, Publication 201, Anthropological Series, Vol. 15, No. 3, 1919

Lev, Efraim and Zohar Amar, *Practical Materia Medica of the Medieval Eastern Mediterranean According to the Carito Genizah*, Leiden and Boston (Sir Henry Wellcome Asian Series, 7), 2008.

Ma Huan, *Ying-yai Sheng-lan, The Overall Survey of the Ocean's Shores* [*1433*], translated and edited by J. V. G. Mills (Hakluyt Society Extra Series XLII), Cambridge: Cambridge University Press, 1970.

Miller, J. Innes, *The Spice Trade of the Roman Empire, 29 B.C. – A.D. 641*, Oxford: Oxford University Press, 1969.

Mills, J.V.G., "Arab and Chinese Navigators in Malaysian Waters in about A.D. 1500," in Wade., ed., 2007: 409-488 (1974).

——"Malaya in the Wu-pei-chih Charts," in Wade, ed., 2007: 367-408 (1937).

——, trans., *Hsing-ch'a Sheng-lan, The Overall Survey of the Start Raft by Fei Hsin*, Wiesbaden: Harrassowitz Verlag, 1996.

Nappi, Carla, "The Monkey and the Inkpot: Natural History and its Transformations in Early Modern China," Harvard University Press, 2006

Paine, Lincoln, *The Sea and Civilization, A Maritime History of the World*, New York: Alfred A. Knopf, 2013

Park, Hyunhee, *Mapping the Chinese and Islamic Worlds, Cross-Cultural Exchange in Pre-modern Asia,* Cambridge: Cambridge University Press, 2012.

Pelliot, Paul, *Notes on Marco Polo*, 3 volumes, ed. L. Hambis, Paris: Imprimerie Nationale, Librairie Adrien-Maisonneuve, 1959-73.

Pulleyblank, Edwin G., *Lexicon of Reconstructed Pronunciation in Early Middle Chinese, Late Middle Chinese, and Early Mandarin*, Vancouver, UBCE Press, 1991.

Sadeh, M. M., *The Arabic Materia Medica of Dioscorides*, Québec: Les Éditions du Sphinx, 1983.

Schafer, Edward, *The Golden Peaches of Samarkand*, Berkeley and Los Angeles: University of California Press, 1963.

Shih Nianhai 史念海, chief editor, *Zhong guo li shi di li lun cong* 中國歷史地理論叢, "Collection of essays on Chinese historical place names," collection 2, Shan xi ren min chu ban she 陝西人民出版社, 1985

Shi Wei le 史為樂, chief editor, Zhong guo di ming kao zheng lun wen ji 中國地名考證論文集, "Collection of essays on the vertification of Chinese place names," Canton: Guang dong sheng di tu chu ban she 廣東省地圖出版社, 1994

Song Xian 宋峴, *Hui hui yao fang kao shi* 回回藥方考釋, two volumes, Beijing 北京: Zhong hua shu ju 中華書局 (Zhong wai jiao tong shi ji cong kan 中外交通史籍叢刊), 2000.

Sun Donghu 孫冬虎, Zhong guo shan ming lun gao 中國山名論稿, "Draft discussion of Chinese names of mountains," Bei jing 北京: Zhong guo di zhi chu ban she 中國地質出版社, 1999.

Tracey, James D., *The Rise of Merchant Empires: Long-Distance Trade in the Early Modern World, 1350-1750*, Cambridge; Cambridge University Press, 1990

Wade, Geoff, "Melaka in Ming Dynasty Texts," in Wade, ed., 2007; 327-366 (1997).

—, ed., *Southeast Asia – China Interactions, Reprint of articles from the Journal of the Malaysian Branch, Royal Asiatic Society*, Singapore: Malaysian Branch of the Royal Asiatic Society, NUS Press, 2007.

— and Sun Laichen, eds., *Southeast Asia in the Fifteenth Century, the China Factor*, Hong Kong: Hong Kong University Press, 2010.

Wang Gungwu, "The Nanhai Trade. A Study of the Early History of Chinese Trade in the South China Sea," in Wade, ed., 2007: 51-166 (1958).

Wang Jitong 王際桐, Wang Ji tong di ming lun gao 王際桐地名論稿, "Draft disscussion of Wang Jitong about place names," Bei jing: She hui ke xue wen xian chu ban she 社會科學文獻出版社, 1999

Wheatley, Paul, *The Golden Khersonese*: Studies in the Historical Geography of the Malay Peninsula before A.D. 1500, Kualalumpur, University of Malaya Press, 1980.

—, "Geographical Notes on Some Commodities Involved in the Sung Maritime Trade," in Wade, ed., 183-295 (1959).

—, "The Malay Peninsula as Known to the Chinese in the Third Century A.D.," in Wade, ed., 2007: 19-37 (1955).

Wolters, O.W., *The Fall of Śrīvijaya in Malay History*, Ithaca, NY: Cornell University Press, 1970.

—, *Early Indonesia Commerce, A Study of the Origins of Śrīvijaya*, Ithaca, NY: Cornell University Press, 1967

Yule, Henry, *Cathay and the Way Thither*, second revision edition, H. Cordier, ed., 3 volumes, London: Hakluyt, 1915 (republished 1967)

—, and Henri Cordier, *The Book of Ser Marco Polo*, 2 volumes third edition, St. Helier: Armorica Book Co. / Amsterdam: Philo Press, 1975 (3 volumes, 1903 (1929)-1920)

Zhou Zhenhe 周振鶴 and You Rujie 遊汝傑, *Fang yan yu zhong guo wen hua* 方言與中國文化, "Dialects and Chinese culture," Shang hai: Shang hai ren min chu ban she 上海人民出版社, 2006

II. GEOGRAPHICAL AND ADMINISTRATIVE DESIGNATIONS

-A-

A dan guo 阿丹國 [1]

Name of a foreign country during Ming 明 times: Aden, located at the northwestern shore of present-day Aden Bay in Yemen. Mentioned with 660, 1196.

A lu zhu guo 阿魯諸國 [1]

Name of a foreign country during Ming 明 times: Aru. It was located on the northwestern coast of Sumatra in the region of Deli and Medan. Its center was the sweet water harbor of present-day Belawan. The Dynastic History of the Ming, *Ming shi* 明史, in its account of foreign countries in *juan* 325, lists aside from Aru the countries of Bo ni 浡泥, Malakka 滿剌加, Su men da la 蘇門答剌, Nan bo li 南渤利 and Rou fo 柔佛. They mostly were situated on Sumatra island, the Malayan peninsula and on Kalimantan island. Mentioned with 344.

A zha li guo 阿吒釐國 [1]

Name of an ancient country, located somewhere at the mid-section of the Ganges river in present-day India. Its exact location is unknown. The *Da tang xi yu ji* 大唐西域記, "Great Tang 唐 Record of the Western Regions," referred to it as A zha li guo. Mentioned with 945.

Ai 愛 → Ai zhou 愛州

Ai lao yi 哀牢夷 [2]

Name of an early country, once located in the western part of present-day Yun nan 雲南 and in northern Myanmar. During the Warring States period and during Qin 秦 and Han 漢, it grew quite large, extending from the Ai lao shan 哀牢山 mountain in the center of present-day Yun nan in the East, and including the entire border region of present-day Myanmar and India in the West, and reaching the border region of present-day Tibet with Myanmar in the North. In the South it reached the territory of present-day Xishuangbanna 西雙版納. The area submitted, in 69, during Eastern Han and became Yong chang 永昌 commandery. Mentioned with 492, 1303.

Ai zhou 愛州 [7]

Name of a *zhou* 州. It was established by Liang 梁 of the Southern Dynasties, in 523. The seat of administration was in a place north of present-day Thanh hóa 清化 city in the Vietnamese province of Thanh hóa, on the southern banks of the Sông Mã river. In 607, the name was changed to Jiu zhen 九真 commandery, but the old name was restored under the Tang 唐, in 621. The administration of the *zhou* was then moved to the present Thanh hóa city. Its territories then comprised present-day Thanh hóa and Nghệ an 義安 provinces in Vietnam. By the Five Dynasties period, the *zhou* had been abolished. Mentioned with 8, 94, 226, 427, 585, 843, 1123.

An 安

→ An zhou 安州.

An cheng 安城 [1]

Place name. Exact location unknown. Mentioned with 1014.

An dong 安東 [2]

Name of a protectorare, *du hu fu*. It was first established during Tang 唐 times, in 668, after the Korean kingdom of Koguryŏ (Gao gou li 高句麗) had been eliminated. The seat of administration was in present-day Pyongyang 平壤 city. The territory administered extended from the present-day Liao 遼 river in the West, reaching the Sea of Japan in the East, and present-day Russia in the North. In the South it reached the Jeolla 全羅 circuit in present-day South Korea. Later the area south of the Taedong 大同 river was gradually taken over by Silla 新羅 and the northern part of the protectorate by the state of Bo hai 渤海, resulting in a downsizing of the territory, and its eventual elimination in 761. Mentioned with 1160, 1351.

An dong dao 安東道 [1]

This is a place name. Its exact location is unknown. Mentioned with 1129.

An feng 安豐 [1]

Name of a region. Towards the end of Western Jin 晉, during the *yuan kang* 元康 reign period (291 – 299), there was an An feng commandery and under it an An feng county. An feng commandery was first established under Wei 魏, in 220, of the Three Kingdoms period. The seat of administration was at a point 20 *li* southwest of present-day Huo qiu 霍邱 county in An hui 安徽. An feng commandery was abolished under Eastern Jin. An Feng county was first established under Qin 秦, and was administered from southeast of present-day Gu shi 固始 county in He nan 河南. During Wei and the Western Jin period, it was subordinated to An feng commandery. It was abolished during Eastern Jin. Mentioned with 1532.

An gu xian 安固縣 [1]
Name of a county. It was established under Western Jin 晉, in 280. It was subordinated to Lin hai 臨海 commandery. The seat of administration was in present-day Rui an 瑞安 city in Zhe jiang 浙江. In 323, it came under Yong jia 永嘉 commandery. It was abolished in 592. In 622, it was reestablished under Dong jia zhou 東嘉州. Later it was subordinated to Wen zhou 溫州. In 903, An gu 安固 became Rui an 瑞安.

An guo xian 安國縣 [1]
This is apparently an error for → An gu xian 安固縣. Mentioned with 968.

An he 闇河 [1]
A place name mentioned in the *Wang Zi nian shi yi ji* 王子年拾遺記, "Wang Zinian's Records of Picked-up Leftovers," as a mythological river associated with supposed events since the time of Fu xi 伏羲. Mentioned with 376.

An li pu 安荔浦 [1]
See → Li pu 荔浦. Mentioned with 682.

An lu 安陸 [2]
Name of an administrative unit, possibly a county or also a commandery. Mentioned with 1266, 1293.
□ There was an An lu county established by Qin 秦. The seat of administration was at a place 53 *li* 里 northwest of present-day An lu city in Hu bei 湖北. At the end of Eastern Jin 晉, the administration was moved to the present An lu city. In 1987, the county was changed to be present-day An lu city.
□ An lu commandery was established under Liu Song 劉宋, in 454. The seat of administration was in present-day An lu city. Its boundaries corresponded to the present-day cities and counties of An lu, Guang shui 廣水, Ying cheng 應城, Xiao Gan 孝感 and Yun meng 雲夢, in Hu bei. It was abolished at the beginning of the *kai huang* 開皇 reign period (581 – 600) in early Sui 隋 times, but reestablished in 607 and in 742. It was abolished in 758.

An lu zhou 安陸州 [1]
Name of a *zhou*. This is an error for → An zhou 安州. Mentioned with 632.

An nan 安南 [15]
During Tang 唐, this was the name of a Chief Protection *fu*, *du hu fu* 都護府. From the Five Dynasties period on, it was the name of a country. During the rule of Tang Emperor Gao zong 高宗, in 679, the Jiao zhou Area Command, Jiao zhou *du du fu* 交州都督府, was changed to An nan Chief Protection *fu*, An nan *du hu fu* 安南都護府. Its seat of administration was in present-day Hanoi. Under Southern Han 漢 of the Five Dynasties, an independent country was established, called by the locals Da qu yue 大瞿越. Under Northern Song 宋, a King of Annan commandery was enfeoffed. During Southern Song a King of An nan country was enfeoffed, and the country became known as An nan in China. An nan was abolished at the beginning of the Ming 明, and a Provincial Administration Commission for Jiao zhi, Jiao zhi *bu zheng shi si* 交阯布政使司, was established instead. In 1427, in connection with the defeat of the Ming

troops attempting to occupy the country, the area became independent again, but the old name An nan was continued. After the establishment of the Nguyen Dynasty (1802 – 1945), the local administration decided to call the country Nan yue 南越, and envisaged it to be a suzerain state. In 1803, the Chinese court entered into negotiations; it considered excessive the territorial claims of the Vietnamese to include Guang dong, Guang xi and An nan. The Nguyen dynasty at first had claimed the former land of the Yue shang 越裳 as their territory. Later, they demanded the entire region of An nan and Jiao zhi south of the Bai yue 百越 region. It was given the name Việt Nam, Chinese: Yue nan, that has persisted ever since. Mentioned with 7, 11, 43, 106, 324, 342, 497, 511, 660, 664, 708, 1074, 1124, 1369, 1403.

An shi guo 安石國 [1]

Name of ancient countries in the western regions, referring to both An guo 安國 and Shi guo 石國. An guo was located in the area of the present-day city of Bukhara in Uzbekistan. Shi guo was located in the area of the present capital Tashkent of Uzbekistan. Mentioned with 10.

An xi 安西 [1]

Name of a Chief Protection *fu,* 都護府 *du hu fu*, established by Tang 唐, in 640. The seat of administration was at a point east of present-day Turfan in Xin jiang 新疆. In its prime time, the area administered covered a huge territory in Central Asia extending from the Yu men Pass (Yu men guan 玉門關) and the Southern Pass (Yang guan 陽關) toward the West, and from the Aral See (Xian hai 鹹海) toward the East. The seat of administration was moved several times. Prior to the life of Chen Cangqi 陳藏器 (713-741), the area was administered from a point in what are today the Eastern suburbs of Kuqa county, Che ku xian 庫車縣, in Xin jiang 新疆. In 790, the administration was abolished since the area it had formerly controlled had been lost to Tibet. Mentioned with 341.

An xi 安息 [1]

See → An xi guo 安息國. Mentioned with 1534.

An xi guo 安息國 [2]

Name of an ancient country in the western regions. Originally, a part of the ancient Persian Empire, it achieved independence between 249 – 247 BCE. The area administered covered the present-day Iranian plateau, Mesopotamia and some surrounding areas. Its capital was moved three times; eventually it was located near present-day Baghdad. In 226 CE, it was eliminated. Mentioned with 11, 1196.

An yi 安邑 [3]

Name of a county. It was established by Qin 秦. The seat of administration was in present-day Yu wang xiang 禹王鄉, located 15 *li* northwest of Xia 夏 county in Shan xi 山西. During the Northern Wei 魏 period, in 487, the county was divided into a northern and a southern part. Sui 隨 changed Southern An yi county to just being An yi county. It was administered at present-day An yi 安邑 town, 10 *li* northeast of present-day Yun cheng 運城 city, in Shan xi. This was continued under later dynasties. In 1915, the county administration was moved to the present-day Yun cheng city and, in 1983, the county became Yun cheng city. The area includes salt lakes and the county was noted for a long time for the production of its famous lake salt. Mentioned with 1057, 1443.

An zhou 安州 [4]

Name of a *zhou* 州. It was established by Western Wei 魏, in 550. The seat of administration was in present-day An lu 安陸 city in Hu bei 湖北. The territory administered comprised the present-day cities and counties of An lu, Guang shui 廣水, Ying cheng 應城, Xiao gan 孝感 and Yun meng 雲夢 in Hu bei 湖北. Its name was changed to De an fu 德安府 in 1119, under the Northern Song 宋. Mentioned with 614, 797, 973, 1034.

-B-

Ba 巴 [1 + 1 +1+ 11]

Refers to various place and regional names, which one not always being clear from context.

□ Name of a *zhou* 州 [1]. It was established by Northern Wei 魏, in 514. The seat of administration was in present-day Ba zhong 巴中 city in Si chuan 四川, controlling the area now administered by the present Ba zhong city and Ping chang 平昌 county. This *zhou* was continued under Sui 隋, Tang 唐, Song 宋 and Yuan 元. Under Ming 明, in 1376, Ba was demoted to become Ba county but, in 1514, its status was raised to Ba zhou 巴州 again, in charge of the two counties of Tong jiang 通江 and Nan jiang 南江. Its administrative area corresponded to the region of present-day Ba zhong 巴中 prefecture-level city. In 1913, the area became Ba zhong county, and it became a city in 1993. Mentioned with 781.

□ Name of an ancient, pre-Qin 秦 country [1]. It was supposedly established as a feudal domain at the beginning of Western Zhou 周. During the Spring and Autumn Period, the ruler was called Ba *zi* 巴子, a minor noble. During the middle Warring States Period, he was called *wang* 王, "king." The capital of Ba was within the area of present-day Chong qing 重慶 municipality. The kingdom ruled the area in present-day Si chuan 四川 extending from the Fu jiang 涪江 and the Jia ling 嘉陵 river in the West, to Feng jie 奉節 county in the East, starting in the North at Da ba 大巴 mountain and in the South reaching the northern portions of present-day Gui zhou 貴州. The kingdom was extinguished in 316 BCE. Mentioned with 1096.

□ Name of a river valley [1]. The Ba river, Ba he 巴河, has it sources at present-day Mi cang 米倉 mountain in Shaan xi 陝西, and in the South flows into Tong jiang 通江 county in Si chuan 四川 and towards the Southwest into Ping chang 平昌 county. The river, eventually being the Qu jiang 渠江 river, finally runs into Jia ling 嘉陵 river.

□ Used as a regional name [11]. The reference is in general to the ancient area of the pre-Qin country of Ba. The BCGM authors refer to the "people of Ba," Ba ren 巴人, five times. These are the inhabitants of the ancient country of Ba. The term Ba jiao ren 巴徼人 refers to the inhabitants of remote regions of Ba. Mentioned with 14, 29, 674, 763, 914, 925, 943, 1158, 1184, 1304, 1475, 1497.

Ba chuan 巴川 [1]

Name of a region based on a reference in the *Cha jing* 茶經, "Tea Classic," of Lu Yu 陸羽 (733-804). There was a commandery and a county. Ba chuan county was established in 734. The seat of administration was in Jiu xian ba 舊縣壩 southeast of Tong liang 銅梁 county within the present-day district of Chong qing 重慶 municipality. At the beginning of the Yuan 元, it became part of Tong liang county. Ba chuan commandery was established, through changing the name of He zhou 合州, in 742. The seat of administration was in present-day He chuan qu 合川區, located in the municipality district Chong qing. In 758, it became He zhou again. Mentioned with 768.

Ba di 巴地 [1]

This is a reference to the general area of the pre-Qin Ba 巴 kingdom (→ Ba). Mentioned with 202.

Ba dong 巴東 [2]

Name of a commandery. Established under Eastern Han 漢, in 201, by renaming Gu ling 固陵 commandery. The seat of administration was in present-day Bai di cheng 白帝城, 10 *li* east of Feng jie 奉節 county of Chong qing 重慶 city. In 216, the name was changed to Gu ling commandery again. During the era of Three Kingdoms' Shu 蜀, in 221, the area was changed to Ba dong commandery. Its administrative territory covered the river valley of the Yang zi 揚子 from Wan zhou qu 萬州區 in Chong qing municipality on down to Wu shan 巫山 county. In 607, during the Sui 隋 dynasty, Xin zhou 信州 had its name changed to again create a Ba dong commandery. Its administration was in the present Feng jie county, and its administrative area in the east reached to the region from Xing shan 興山 and Zi gui 秭歸 in Hu bei 湖北 to the West. Ba dong commandery was abolished at the beginning of Tang 唐. Mentioned with 934, 1335.

Ba dong xian 巴東縣 [1]

Name of a county. It was established under the Sui 隋, in 598. The seat of administration was in present-day Jiu xian ping 舊縣坪 on the northern shore of the Yang zi northwest of Ba dong 巴東 county in Hu bei 湖北. At the beginning of Northern Song 宋, the administrative seat was moved to present-day Xin ling 信陵 town in the present county city. Ming 明 subordinated the area to the Hu guang Provincial Administration Commission, Hu guang *bu zheng shi si* 湖廣布政使司, in Yi ling zhou 夷陵州 of Jing zhou fu 荊州府. Qing 清 put it under Yi chang fu 宜昌府 of Hu bei. Mentioned with 1464.

Ba gong shan 八公山 [1]

Name of a mountain located on the south bank of the Huai 淮 river 5 *li* north of Shou 壽 county in An hui 安徽. Mentioned with 47.

Ba gui 八桂 [1]

Place name. The term is a general reference to present-day Gui lin 桂林 city in Guang xi 廣西. However, there is also a reference in the *Shan hai jing* 山海經, "Classic of Mountains and Seas," to the "eight trees of the cassia forest," which the usage is related to. Guo Pu 郭璞 (276-324) annotated the passage in question to imply that a forest of only eight trees suggests that the trees were very large. Hence the designation Ba gui, "Eight cassia trees." Mentioned with 1535.

Ba jun 巴郡 [8]

This is a commandery established by Qin 秦, in 314 BCE. The seat of administration was at a location in present-day Chong qing 重慶 municipality. During Western Han 漢, the area administered by the commandery corresponded to the entire municipality district of present-day Chong qing and the four cities of Nan chong 南充, Da chuan 達川, Guang an 廣安 and Ba zhong 巴中 in northeastern Si chuan 四川. Under Eastern Han, in 194, Liu Zhang 劉璋 (162-219) divided the commandery into three parts and, in 201, one of the parts, Yong ning 永寧 commandery, became Ba commandery, but administering a much smaller area. Its territory corresponded to a region including Tong liang 銅梁 and Qi jiang 綦江 district in the present Chong qing municipality in the West, Wu sheng 武勝 and Dian jiang 墊江 in the North, Zhong 忠 county and Fu ling 涪陵 in the East, and Tong zi 桐梓 in Gui zhou 貴州 in the South. The commandery was abolished at the beginning of the Sui 隋, but reestablished in 607. In 618, under Tang 唐, the name was changed to Yu zhou 渝州. Mentioned with 19, 66, 202, 462, 781, 1096, 1249.

Ba ling 巴陵 [1]

Name of a county. It was established under Western Jin 晉 in 280. The seat of administration was in present-day's Yue yang 岳陽 city in Hu nan 湖南. It was eliminated, in 1376, but reestablished in 1391. In 1913, Ba ling county became Yue yang county and, in 1961, Yue yang city. Mentioned with 768.

Ba qiong 巴邛 [1]

A general reference to present-day Si chuan 四川, and the area of Chong qing 重慶. → Ba 巴 is an ancient region in Si chuan centered about present Chong qing, but the meaning of qiong 邛 is unclear and could refer to various areas within Si chuan, such as Qiong zhou 邛州, Qiong du 邛都, Qiong hai 邛海 or Qiong lai 邛崍 mountain. Of them, Qiong zhou was located within the present Qiong lai county, while Qiong du and Qiong hai are located southeast of present-day Xi chang 西昌 city. Qiong lai mountain is located between the Min 岷 river and the Da du 大渡 river. Mentioned with 1498.

Ba shu 巴蜀 [5]

Combined regional name referring to the territory comprising present-day Si chuan 四川 and Chong qing 重慶. → Ba 巴 refers to the region of the ancient Ba state with present-day Chong qing in its center. Shu 蜀 refers to the ancient Shu state wth present-day Cheng du 成都 as its center. Mentioned with 19, 585, 675, 793, 1096.

Ba xi 巴西 [7]

Name of a commandery. It was established under the Tang 唐, in 742, by changing the name of Mian zhou 綿州 to Ba xi commandery. The seat of administration was on the east bank of the Fu 涪 river east of present-day Mian yang city in Si chuan 四川. Its administrative area comprised the present-day river valley of the Fu river between the present cities of Jiang you 江油 and Mian yang 綿陽 and the upper reaches of the Luo 羅 river in Si chuan. The commandery became Mian zhou again in 758. Mentioned with 41, 118, 196, 334, 453, 941, 1015.

Ba xia 巴峽 [3]

Abbreviated place name referring to the three gorges (*xia* 峽) of → Ba. These are the Tong luo 銅鑼 gorge, the Ming yue 明月 gorge, and the Huang cao 黃草 gorge, and are located along the Yang zi from the present-day municipality district of Chong qing 重慶 up to Fu ling qu 涪陵區. Mentioned with 674, 789, 1198.

Ba zhong 巴中 [2 + 4]

□ Name of a commandery [2]. It was established under Liang 梁 of the Southern Dynasties. The seat of administration was in present-day Sha ba chang 沙壩場, located northeast of present-day Kai jiang 開江 county in Si chuan 四川. In 555, under the Western Wei 魏, it became Ba qu 巴渠 commandery. Mentioned with 675.

□ General reference to a region [4]. The term refers to the area of the Eastern part of the Si chuan 四川 basin, with the the present-day municipality district of Chong qing 重慶 as its center. Mentioned with 149, 674, 808, 1480.

Ba zhou 霸州 [1]

Name of a *zhou* 州. It was established in Yi jin guan 益津關, in 959, by the Northern Zhou 周 dynasty. The seat of administration was in the present-day Ba zhou 霸州 city in He bei 河北. During Northern Song 宋 times, the area was divided into the three counties of Yong qing 永清, Wen an 文安 and Dai cheng 大城. The territory administered corresponded to much of the present city of Ba zhou and the two counties of Wen an and Dai cheng, as well as towards the southeast the area up to the western river bank of the Zi ya 子牙 river. Under the early Ming 明, the area became a county-level *zhou* and, in 1913, it became Ba 霸 county. In 1990, the county was raised to county city rank. Mentioned with 291.

Bai ji 百濟 [7]

Name of a country located on the Korean Peninsula: Paekche. Its traditional dates are 18 BCE to 660 CE, but the kingdom was probably founded much later, perhaps as late as the fourth century. The Kingdom at first occupied the area around the Han 漢 river with a capital at Hansŏng 漢城 on the Han and, later, at Sabi 泗沘 on the Kŭm 錦 river, but gradually moved south and west due to pressure from Koguryŏ 高句麗, in the north, and Silla 新羅, which conquered Paekche with help from Tang 唐, in 660, in the east. Mentioned with 599, 931.

Bai lang shan 白狼山 [1]
Name of a mountain. It is Da yang 大陽 mountain, located 60 *li* south of the Kharchin Mongolian left wing self-governing banner in Liao ning 遼寧. Mentioned with 1002.

Bai shan 白山 [2]
Name of a mountain. There were many "white mountains" known in China at the time, but this "White Mountain" was roughly east of the present-day city of Nan jing 南京 in Jiang su 江蘇. Mentioned with 978, 1485.

Bai shi 百市 [1]
Minor place name. More research is needed, but it is probably in present-day Lian yun gang 連雲港 city in Jiang su 江蘇. Mentioned with 272.

Bai shui 白水 [7 + 1]
Term used in reference to a number of places.
□ There is a Bai shui that is the river basin of the Bai shui jiang 白水江 in present-day Wen 文 county in Gan su 甘肅. [7] This river has its sources northwest of the Jiu zhai gou 九寨溝 in Si chuan 四川. Towards the southeast, the river flows through Yong le 永樂 town and in the southeast flows into Wen county in Gan su. The river then flows through the Wen county seat, and east of Wen county becomes the Bai long jiang 白龍江. Mentioned with 461, 1096, 1549, 1572.
□ A Bai shui river is found in present-day Bai shui county in Shaan xi 陝西. [1] It has its origins east of Tong chuan 銅川 city. It flows through Bai shui xian 白水縣 city towards the East, and empties into the Luo 洛 river. Mentioned with 461.

Bai yang shan 白羊山 [1]
Name of a mountain located in the general area of present-day Yan zhou 兗州 city in Shan dong 山東, although the exact location is uncertain. Mentioned with 57.

Bai yu he 白玉河 [1]
Name of a river. This is the Yu long 玉龍 or Kash (also: Kax) river, located within the boundaries of Khotan (He tian 和田) county and Khotan city in Xin jiang 新疆. Its source is the Kun lun 昆侖 mountain, located south of Ce le 策勒 county. In the north, it comes together with the Qaraqash river to form the Khotan river. Even further north, it runs through the Taklamakan desert to enter the Tarim river. The river has a seasonal character. Mentioned with 1406.

Ban qiao 板橋 [1]
Minor place name. This is the present town of Ban qiao 板橋, located 15 km southwest of the Zhong hua 中華 gate in Nan jing 南京 city in Jiang su 江蘇. Mentioned with 222, 735.

Ban yang 般陽 [1]
Name of a county. It was established by Western Han 漢. The seat of administration was in present-day Zi chuan 淄川 city southwest of Zi bo 淄博 city in Shan dong 山東. It was abolished under Western Jin 晉. Mentioned with 980.

Bao du 抱犢 [1]
Name of a mountain. The term refers to what is today the Bao du gu 抱犢崮 mountain area, located 33 km northwest of present-day Cang shan 蒼山 county in Shan dong 山東, including the areas bordering on Zao zhuang 棗莊 city and Fei 費 county. Mentioned with 810.

Bao du shan 抱犢山 [1]
Name of a mountain in He bei 河北. It is located 80 km west of present-day Lu quan 鹿泉 city. Mentioned with 1109.

Bao han 抱罕 [1]
This is an error for → Fu han 枹罕. Mentioned with 324.

Bao jing 保靖 [1]
Name of an administrative district. Originally there was a Bao jing zhou 保靖州. The seat of administration was in present-day Bao jing county in Hu nan 湖南. The early Ming 明 changed Bao jing zhou to a Pacification Commission (*an fu si* 安撫司), and, in 1373, established Bao jing zhou as a Pacification Office, *xuan wei si* 宣慰司. In 1729, the *xuan wei si* was changed to Bao jing county. Mentioned with 511.

Bao ling shan 雹零山 [1]
Name of an unidentified mountain. Mentioned with 1521.

Bao qing 寶慶 [1]
Name of a *fu* 府. It was established by Southern Song 宋, in 1225, by promoting Shao zhou 邵州. The seat of administration was in present-day Shao yang 邵陽 city in Hu nan 湖南. Its jurisdiction corresponded to the present-day Shao yang city and the counties and cities of Shao dong 邵東, Xin shao 新邵 and Xin hua 新化. During the Yuan 元, the status of the area was raised to become a *lu* 路, but the *fu* was reestablished at the beginning of the Ming 明. Its administrative area was quite large and extended to the present-day cities and counties of Wu gang 武岡, Xin ning 新寧 and Cheng bu 城步. In 1913, the *fu* was turned into Bao qing county. In 1926, it became Shao yang county. Mentioned with 124.

Bao shan 爆山 [1]
Name of a mountain. It is located more than 20 *li* northwest of present-day Yi shui 沂水 county in Shan dong 山東. Mentioned with 1521.

Bao xie dao 褒斜道 [1]
Name of a route. This was one of the important north-south traffic roads passing through the Qin ling 秦嶺 mountain range. In the north it originated in present-day Mei 眉 county in Shaan xi 陝西 and went south along the Xie gu 斜谷 river, passing through present-day Tai bai 太白 county, moving south along the Bao 褒 river and ending up at Han zhong 漢中. The road was more than 470 *li* long. Mentioned with 781.

Bei 北 [71]
This is a general geographical name for the area located "north" (and west) of China. Mentioned with 80, 96, 101, 102, 103, 137, 142, 145, 170, 176, 180, 288, 321, 329, 371, 422, 445, 447, 450, 470, 477, 550, 565, 614, 626, 631, 637, 660, 667, 673, 685, 712,

782, 787, 801, 804, 810, 817, 861, 861, 893, 1004, 1008, 1026, 1067, 1099, 1219, 1242, 1256, 1270, 1275, 1287, 1296, 1305, 1307, 1336, 1340, 1381, 1398, 1410, 1439, 1447, 1471.

Bei 貝 [1]

Minor place name. This name perhaps lacks an element and is to be understood as Bei qiu 貝丘, a common place name and the *qiu* 丘 often drops off. This Bei or Bei qiu is 5 *li* south of present-day Bo xing 博興 county in Shan dong 山東. Mentioned with 639.

Bei bian 北邊 [2]

General somewhat vague geographical name in LSZ's time for the "northern frontier areas" of Ming China, from adjacent areas of Central Asia into Manchuria. More specifically, the term applies to an area that extends from Jia yu 嘉峪 pass in Gan su 甘肅, then skirts the Great Wall going through the eastern part of Ning xia 寧夏, the northern part of Shaan xi 陝西, the northern part of Shan xi 山西, the northern part of He bei 河北, and goes down to Liao ning 遼寧 in the east. Mentioned with 504, 964.

Bei dai shan 北代山 [1]

Name of a mountain. Its location is uncertain. Mentioned with 595.

Bei dao 北道 [1]

Generalized reference to northern areas. See also → Bei 北, → Bei ren 北人, Bei tu 北土, → Bei fang 北方, → Bei guo 北國, Mentioned with 602.

Bei di 北狄 [1]

This is an ancient term used by the inhabitants of the central regions to refer to northern Asian peoples as a group. During Northern Song 宋, a particular reference was the Khitan Liao 遼 dynasty. Mentioned with 689.

Bei di 北地 [21 + 2]

□ General regional designation for the peoples of the north [21]. Compare ' Bei fang 北方. Mentioned with 126, 182, 195, 213, 223, 417, 656, 738, 871, 873, 901, 924, 1100, 1105, 1241, 1296, 1378, 1381.

□ Name of a commandery [2]. It was established by Qin 秦. In the East, it bordered on Shang 上 commandery. Its seat of administration was at a point southwest of present-day Qing yang 慶陽 county in Gan su 甘肅. The territory administered comprised the eastern part of Gan su, a large part of Ning xia 寧夏 and a section of present-day Inner Mongolia. During Three Kingdoms' Wei 魏, the commandery was moved into the middle sections of Shaan xi 陝西 and, under Western Wei, the name of the commandery was changed to Tong chuan 通川 commandery. Mentioned with 195, 1340.

Bei ding shan 北定山 [1]

Name of a mountain situated at present-day Lin yi 臨沂 city in Shan dong 山東. Further details are unavailable. Mentioned with 1430.

Bei du 北都 [1 + 1]

□ Uncertain regional designation [1]. The name is probably an error for Bei bu 北部, "Northern section," but further information is unavailable. One may hypothesize that the reference is to the northern half of the Yi zhou Regional Inspectorr

Division, Yi zhou *ci shi bu* 益州刺史部, of Eastern Han 漢 times, corresponding to the present-day Si chuan 四川 basin and nearby areas. This was the Xi chuan 西川 region of Tang 唐 times. Thus, the "northern section" of Yi zhou may have corresponded to Xi chuan. Mentioned with 249.

□ Name of a place [1]. The Northern Song 宋 dynasty's Da ming fu 大名府 was made, in 1042, Bei jing 北京. The ruins of this Bei du or Bei jing are 6 km northeast of present-day Da ming 大名 county in He bei 河北 at Da jie xiang 大街鄉. Mentioned with 1105.

Bei fan 北番 [1]

Term used to refer to northern Asian peoples as a group. During Northern Song 宋, a particular reference was the Khitan Liao 遼 dynasty. Mentioned with 1322.

Bei fang 北方 [34]

This is a somewhat vague geographical name for the general "area north" of China but also for northern parts of China itself. See also → Bei 北, → Bei ren 北人, → Bei tu 北土, → Bei dao 北道. Mentioned with 192, 193, 222, 257, 298, 361, 381, 412, 440, 464, 541, 618, 634, 678, 787, 882, 1075, 1100, 1110, 1187, 1238, 1241, 1246, 1283, 1286, 1420, 1532, 1550, 1556.

Bei gan shan 北甘山 [1]

Name of a mountain. It is the Bei gan 北甘 mountain on the eastern bank of the Da ba 大八 river in the northern part of Yang dong 陽東 county, located north of present-day Yang jiang 陽江 city in Guang dong 廣東. Mentioned with 294.

Bei guo 北國 [5]

General designation for north China and points north of that. Compare Bei → 北, → Bei ren 北人, → Bei fang 北方, → Bei tu 北土, → Bei dao 北道. Mentioned with 804, 934, 1313, 1316.

Bei hai 北海 [1 + 8 + 5 + 1]

□ Name of a commandery [1]. In 607, under the Sui 隋, it was established by renaming Qing zhou 青州. In the West it bordered on Zi chuan 淄川 commandery. The seat of administration was in the North of present-day Qing zhou city in Shan dong 山東. The territory administered comprised the cities and counties of present-day Qing zhou, Wei fang 濰坊, Bo xing 博興, Guang rao 廣饒, Lin qu 臨朐 and Chang yi 昌邑, in Shandong. In 621, under the Tang 唐, the commandery was again named Qing zhou, and its administration was moved to the present city of Qing zhou. In 742, Qing zhou was changed to be Bei hai 北海 commandery, but Qing zhou was restored again in 758. Mentioned with 1317.

□ Name of an ocean region [8], in this case the Gulf of Bo hai 渤海. Mentioned with 138, 419, 1057, 1467.

□ Name of an ocean region [5]. The term refers to the ancient Xi hai, 西海, the "Western Sea." This is the present-day Kokonor Lake in Qing hai 青海 province. Mentioned with 1335.

□ Mythological name from the *Shan hai jing* 山海經, "Classic of Mountains and Seas" [1]. No further details available. Mentioned with 1571.

Bei hu 北胡 [2]
This is an ancient pejorative designation for the minority peoples of northern regions. During the Northern Song 宋, the term was specifically applied to the Liao 遼 country. During the Ming 明, it was used to designate Northern Yuan 元 and their successors, the Wala 瓦剌 (known today as Oyrats) and Tartar 韃靼 tribes. Mentioned with 464, 1335.

Bei huang 北荒 [1]
Made-up geographical name generally referring to distant lands in the north. Mentioned with 95.

Bei jian 北間 [3]
General geographical designation to regions "within the North". See also → Bei 北, → Bei ren 北人, → Bei tu 北土, → Bei fang 北方, → Bei dao 北道. Mentioned with 1067.

Bei jie 北界 [1]
Regional name used in Han 漢 times to designate the region of interaction between northern groups such as the Xiong nu 匈奴 and the Han central government. Mentioned with 1382.

Bei lu 北虜 [3]
Ancient pejorative designation as "northern slaves" for the peoples of the north. During the Ming 明, it was used to designate Northern Yuan 元 and their successors, the Wala 瓦剌 (known today as Oyrats) and Tartar 韃靼 tribes. Mentioned with 793, 1115, 1536.

Bei lan ling 北蘭陵 [1]
This is another name for Lan Ling 蘭陵 county. See → Lan ling 蘭陵.

Bei ma dao 北馬道 [1]
In this case, the *bei* 北, "northern," is superfluous and the place name is actually → Ma dao 馬道.

Bei ren 北人 [65]
This is a term generally designating "the people [and area] in the north" of China. → Bei 北, → Bei fang 北人.

Bei shan 北山 [4 + 1 + 1]
□ Name of a mountain [4] but possibly not a reference to a real location. Mentioned with 31, 599, 633, 658, 1505.
□ Name of a mountain [1]. Here referring to an area northeast of present-day Ling bao 靈寶 city in He nan 河南. Mentioned with 658.
□ Name of a mountain [1]. Referred to in the *Ming yi bie lu*, "Further Records of Renowned Physicians.", as Ye bei shan 腋北山, and possibly the same mountain as the → Ye bei shan 液 北山 mentioned elsewhere. In which case this Bei shan was located north of present-day Lai zhou 萊州 city in Shan dong 山東. Mentioned with 463.

Bei tian zhu 北天竺 [1]
General term for "Northern India" and its countries. Compare → Bei tian zhu guo 北天竺國, "Countries of Northern India." Mentioned with 14.

Bei tian zhu guo 北天竺國 [1]
General name for "Northern India." Mentioned with 174.

Bei ting 北庭 [2]
Regional name. Reference is to the greater Beshbaliq area and more specifically to the area administered by the Tang 唐 era Bei ting Chief Protection *fu*, the Bei ting *du hu fu* 北庭都護府. This was established in 702. The seat of administration was at a now defunct city located north of present-day Jimsar, Ji mu sa er 吉木薩爾, county in Xin jiang 新疆. The administration governed huge areas of Central Asia, from the northern part of the Tian shan 天山 to the West towards the Aral Sea. The protectorate was diminished following the An Lushan 安祿山 rebellion (755-763). It was abolished in 790. Mentioned with 811.

Bei ting shan 北庭山 [1]
Name of a mountain. This is Huo yan 火焰 mountain in the northern Turfan basin of present-day Xin jiang 新疆. Mentioned with 811.

Bei tu 北土 [34]
Generalized term for "northern lands" in China and points north (and west). Compare → Bei 北, → Bei ren 北人, → Bei fang 北方, → Bei dao 北道. Mentioned with 43, 56, 159, 176, 314, 440, 495, 507, 614, 631, 651, 743, 769, 823, 886, 1066, 1070, 1090, 1096, 1110, 1117, 1149, 1206, 1221, 1242, 1274, 1316, 1331, 1459, 1499.

Bei yan 北燕 [1]
This is a regional name. It refers to the state of Yan of the Spring and Autumn Period and Warring States time. In the *Shi ji* 史記, "Records of the Historian," this state is referred to as Bei yan 北燕. It is located in the area around present-day Bei jing 北京, the approximate location of its capital. The state controlled what corresponds to the present-day central and northern portion of He bei 河北, and the western part of Liao ning 遼寧. Mentioned with 1480.

Bei yi shan 北邑山 [1]
Name of a mountain. In case this were an error for Ye bei shan 液北山 or Ye bei shan 掖北山, this mountain is located north of present-day Lai zhou 萊州 city in Shan dong 山東. But the exact location of a Bei yi shan remains uncertain. Mentioned with 46.

Bei yuan 北苑 [2]
Minor place name referring to a tea plantation at the Feng 鳳 mountain 15 km northeast of present-day Jian ou 建甌 city in Fu jian 福建. The area was famous for its tea from Northern Song 宋 on. Mentioned with 124.

Bei yue 北岳 [2]
One of the "five mountain ranges," wu yue 五岳, of antiquity. Before late Ming 明, there was the Bei yue heng shan 北岳恒山, "Mount Heng 恒 of the Northern Mountain Range," corresponding to present-day Da mao 大茂 mountain, located northwest of present-day Qu yang 曲陽 county in He bei 河北. In 1661,

a first sacrifice was offered to the Bei yue at present-day Hun yuan 渾源 in Shan xi 山西. Mentioned with 130, 1157.

Bei zhan guo 卑占國 [1]

This is an error for Zhan bei guo 占卑國, the Tang 唐 dynasty name for Jambi, an area associated with the southern Sumatran coast and more specifically with the capital of the Śrīvijayan empire. Mentioned with 842.

Beng cheng 祊城 [1]

Name of an ancient walled city. It was located at present-day Fang cheng 方城 town, east of Fei 費 county in Shan dong 山東. Mentioned with 1171.

Bi 壁 [1]

Name of a *zhou* 州. It was established in 625, and administered from present-day Tong jiang 通江 county in Si chuan 四川. Its territory of administration covered most of present-day Tong jiang county plus the western part of Wan yuan 萬源 city. It was abolished in 1072. Mentioned with 1441.

Bian 汴 [11]

Name of a *zhou* 州, see → Bian zhou 汴州. Mentioned with 169, 283, 338, 530, 639, 665, 729, 768, 861, 896, 1067, 1094.

Bian dong 汴東 [9]

Regional name. During Northern Song, it referred to the area located to the East of the capital of → Bian jing 汴京, generally a strip of land including the eastern part of present-day He nan 河南 and the southwestern part of Shan dong 山東. Mentioned with 99, 202, 272, 623, 687, 748, 1140, 1175, 1215.

Bian du 汴都 [2]

Honorific place name. The Five Dynasties period's Liang 梁, Jin 晉, Han 漢 and Zhou 周 dynasties, as well as Northern Song had their capital in Kai feng fu 開封府. Because the capital city was situated at the Bian he 汴河 river, and because historically this had been Bian zhou 汴州, the capital was called Bian du. This is present-day Kai feng 開封 city in He nan 河南. Mentioned with 509, 550.

Bian jing 汴京 [10]

Place name used in reference to Kai feng fu 開封府, now Kai feng 開封 city. The term was in use during the Five Dynasties period, during Liang 梁, Jin 晉, Han 漢 and Zhou 周, and recalls the connection of the then capital with the Bian 汴 river. The area was also → Bian zhou 汴州. Mentioned with 140, 644, 733, 741, 787, 871, 1017, 1155, 1241, 1294, 1378, 1477, 1573.

Bian liang 汴梁 [1]

This is an old name for present-day Kai feng 開封 city. It harkens back to the old name of the city as Da liang 大梁 when it was the capital of Warring States' Wei 魏. In Sui-Tang 隋唐 times, a → Bian zhou 汴州 was established. Later, it was popularly called Bian liang. During Yuan 元 times, a Bian liang lu 汴梁路 was established there. Mentioned with 1537.

Bian luo 汴洛 [15]

Combined regional designation. Bian 汴 refers to the city on that river, present-day Kai feng 開封 city. Luo 洛 refers to the present-day city of Luo yang 洛陽 in He nan 河南. Mentioned with 100, 158, 167, 171, 196, 423, 440, 1005, 1105, 1122, 1274, 1292, 1301, 1405, 1428.

Bian xi 汴西 [3]

Regional name referring, during Northern Song 宋, to the area "west of (the capital of →) Bian (jing 汴京 or Kai feng 開封 city)." The area corresponded in general to the middle portions of present-day He nan 河南. Mentioned with 130, 202, 1316.

Bian zhong 汴中 [2]

Regional name referring, during Northern Song 宋, to → Bian jing 汴京 and the areas about it, corresponding to a strip around present-day Kai feng 開封 city in He nan 河南. Mentioned with 692, 1140.

Bian zhou 汴州 [2]

Name of a *zhou*. It was established under Northern Zhou 周, in 576. The seat of administration was at a point northwest of present-day Kai feng 開封 city in He nan 河南. It was eliminated in 607, but reestablished in 617. Its administration was moved to present-day Kai feng city. During Tang 唐, its administrative area corresponded to present-day Kai feng city in He nan along with the counties of Kai feng, Feng qiu 封丘, Lan kao 蘭考, Qi xian 杞縣, Tong xu 通許 and Wei shi 尉氏. Under Liang 梁 of the Five Dynasties, Bian zhou was changed, in 907, into Kai feng fu 開封府. Under Later Tang, a Bian zhou was reestablished and, under Later Jin 晉, it was changed to Kai feng fu again. Su Song 蘇頌 (1020 – 1101), who lived during the Song dynasty, did not speak of Kai feng fu; he continued to use the older name and spoke of Bian zhou. Mentioned with 495.

Bin 賓 [2]

Name of a *zhou* 州. → Bin zhou 賓州. Mentioned with 376, 521, 1427.

Bin zhou 賓州 [4]

Name of a *zhou* 州. It was established under Tang 唐, in 631. The seat of administration was in the old city southwest of present-day Bin yang 賓陽 county in Guang xi 廣西. Under Northern Song 宋, in 973, the center of administration was moved to present-day Xin bin 新賓, located north of the present Bin yang county. At the beginning of Yuan 元 a Bin zhou lu 賓州路 was established, but later it was reduced to a Bin zhou. In 1912, the area was renamed Bin yang county. Mentioned with 376, 535, 552, 1047.

Bin zhou 濱州 [1]

Name of a *zhou* 州. Established under Five Dynasties' Zhou 周, in 956. The seat of administration was in present-day Bin zhou city in Shan dong 山東. It governed what is equivalent to Bin zhou city today and the two counties of Li jin 利津 and Zhan hua 沾化 in Shan dong. At the beginning of the *hong wu* 洪武 reign period (1368-1398) of the Ming 明 dynasty, the latter two attached counties were abolished, and became part of Bin zhou. In 1913, the name was changed to Bin 濱 county. In 1982, a Bin zhou city was established. Mentioned with 1057.

Bin zhou 豳州 [1]

Name of a *zhou* 州. It was established by Western Wei 魏. The seat of administration was in present-day Bin 彬 county in Shaan xi 陝西. The area governed comprised present-day Bin 彬 county, along with Yong shou 永壽, Chang wu 長武 and Xun yi 旬邑. In 606, under the Sui 隋, the area became part of Ning zhou 寧州 but, under Tang 唐, it was reestablished in 618. In 725, it became Bin zhou 邠州. Mentioned with 219.

Bin zhou 邠州 [1]

Name of a *zhou*. It was established under the Tang 唐, in 725, by changing the name of Bin zhou 豳州. The seat of administration was in the present Bin 彬 county in Shaan xi 陝西. The area governed comprised the present Bin 彬 county, Yong shou 永壽, Chang wu 長武 and Xun yi 旬邑. Ming 明 established Bin zhou as a Xi an fu 西安府 subordinate *zhou* administrating the counties of Chun hua 淳化, San shui 三水 and Chang wu 長武. In 1725, its status was raised to being a directly administered *zhou*, *zhi li zhou* 直隸州. In 1913, it was demoted again to become Bin 邠 county and, in 1964, it became Bin 彬 county. Mentioned with 219.

Bing 并 [4 + 3]

□ Name of a *zhou* [4]. See → Bing zhou 并州. Mentioned with 188, 239, 494, 1242.
□ Error for *bing* 並 [3] in some editions.

Bing xue 丙穴 [1]

This is a minor place used in reference to the "caves of (Da) bing (大丙 mountain)." This is located southeast of present-day Lue yang 略陽 county in Shaan xi 陝西. Mentioned with 520.

Bing zhou 并州 [10]

Name of a *zhou* 州.
□ The Bing zhou of pre-Qin 秦, an extensive administrative unit, mentioned in *Zhou li* 周禮, Zhi fang 職方, equivalent to present-day Shan xi 山西 and He bei.
□ Name of a *zhou* established by Emperor Wu 武 of Han 漢. It was one of 13 Regional Inspector Divisions, *shi san ci shi bu* 十三刺史部, a "supervised region," *jian cha qu* 監察區. Areas controlled by it administratively included most of Shan xi 山西 and Inner Mongolia, also a corner of He bei. At the end of Eastern Han, this became an administrative region and was governed from the present-day Jin yuan 晉源 town southwest of Tai yuan 太原 city. The *zhou* controlled extensive areas including the northern part of present-day Shaan xi 陝西, and the area around the Great Bend of the Yellow River. After the Three Kingdoms period, the *zhou* was over time greatly reduced in size. During Tang 唐, its administrative area corresponded only to the area of the middle watershed of the Fen 汾 river extending in present-day Shan xi 山西 from Yang qu 陽曲 county in the North to Wen shui 文水 county in the South. In 723, the *zhou* became Tai yuan fu 太原府, and under Northern Song 宋, after it eliminated Northern

Han, it again became Bing zhou and its administration changed to present-day Tai yuan city. In 1059, it became Tai yuan fu again. Mentioned with 556, 702, 816, 931, 934, 941, 1050, 1057, 1538.

Bo 亳 [1]

Name of a *zhou* 州. See → Bo zhou 亳州. Mentioned with 272.

Bo dao 僰道 [1]

Name of a county. It was founded by Warring States Qin 秦, and administered from present-day Yi bin 宜賓 city in Si chuan 四川. According to one tradition, the seat of administration was in An bian chang 安邊場, west of the present-day Yi bin county. Northern Zhou 周 changed the county to be Wai jiang 外江 county. Under Sui 隋, in 607, it again became Bo dao county. Tang 唐, in 842, moved the seat of administration to Jiu zhou ba 舊州垻 located 6 *li* northwest of the present-day Yi bin city. Northern Song 宋, in 1114, changed the county to be Yi bin county. Mentioned with 613.

Bo hai 渤海 [1 + 3]

□ Name of a commandery established in 165 BCE when the feudal country of He jian 河間 was eliminated and Bo hai commandery established in its place. The center of its administration was located southeast of present-day Cang zhou 滄州 city in He bei 河北. The territory administered comprised seven counties including Zhang wu 章武. During Eastern Han 漢, the center of administration was moved to a place northeast of present-day Nan pi 南皮 county in He bei. Under Eastern Wei 魏, the administration was moved to a point east of Dong guang 東光 county in He bei. At the beginning of the *kai huang* 開皇 reign period (581 – 600) of Sui 隋, the commandery was abolished but, at the beginning of the *da ye* 大業 reign period (605 – 618), Cang zhou was changed to be Bo hai commandery. This was abolished at the beginning of Tang 唐. Mentioned with 471.

□ Name of an ocean region [3]. It refers to the Gulf of Bo hai and the areas of present-day Tian jin 天津, He bei 河北, Liao ning 遼寧 and Shan dong 山東 surrounding the gulf, altogether 80,000 square km. Mentioned with 471, 663, 886.

Bo lü guo 波律國 [1]

Name of an ancient country in the Nan yang, "southern oceans" region, including the Malay archipelago and peninsula and Indonesia. This is recent Barus, on the northwest coast of the Indonesian island of Sumatra. Another opinion identifies it as a transcription of Po li 婆利, which may be present-day Brunei, or the Indonesian island of Bali, or Bo ni 渤泥 for Borneo, i.e., present-day Kalimantan island. Mentioned with 680.

Bo ni 渤泥, [3]

Ancient country in the Nan yang, "southern oceans", region, including the Malay archipelago and peninsula and Indonesia. It is generally believed to have been located on the island of Kalimantan/Borneo, but there are divergent references to Brunei in the North and a strip at the Western coast. Mentioned with 144, 511, 1139.

Bo ping jun 博平郡 [1]

Name of a commandery. It was established under Tang 唐, in 742, by changing the name of Bo zhou 博州. The seat of administration was at a place 25 *li* northeast of present-day Liao cheng 聊城 city in Shan dong 山東. The territory controlled comprised the present Liao cheng, Chi ping 茌平, and Gao tang 高唐 cities and counties. The area again became Bo zhou, in 758. Mentioned with 1126, 1539.

Bo si 波斯 [42]

This is the name of an ancient country. In nearly every case the reference is Persia although the name by Song 宋 times had also frequently been applied to a place in southwestern Asia that in part produced substitute products. See also → Bo si guo 波斯國. The list that follows includes products of both Persia and the Malayan Bo si and, in the former case, from adjacent areas of Arabia possibly on into Africa. Mentioned with 103, 106, 122, 157, 202, 285, 332, 357, 367, 368, 427, 449, 535, 592, 698, 720, 777, 779, 861, 866, 885, 890, 945, 1036, 1129, 1140, 1158, 1171, 1239, 1246, 1248, 1252, 1258, 1264, 1375, 1540.

Bo si guo 波斯國 [27]

Name of an ancient foreign country, referring to two places.

First, the Persia of the West, which arose from the western part of the Iranian highland and was founded ca. 550 BCE, with its capital city located in the present-day Iranian province of Chuzestan. During its prime time, the empire extended from the Indus Valley in the East to the Aegean Sea in the West, where at one time it attempted to conquer ancient Greece. In 330 BCE, it was destroyed by Alexander the Great of Macedonia. The Bo si country referred to by Chinese sources in the Middle Ages corresponded to present-day Iran.

Second, the Bo si country of the Southern Ocean region, also called Ba xi, located in the northeastern section of the Indonesian island of Sumatra.

In general, the Bo si country mentioned in Chinese sources until the Five Dynasties period is to be identified as the Bo si in the West, i.e. "Persia." Beginning with the Song dynasty, the name Bo si mostly referred to the region on Sumatra. Mentioned with 11, 14, 15, 85, 89, 110, 478, 585, 680, 700, 720, 770, 772, 779, 851, 890, 961, 1030, 1035, 1196, 1246, 1252, 1299, 1375, 1411, 1497, 1515.

Bo zhou 亳州 [1]

Name of a *zhou* 州. It was established at the end of Northern Zhou 周. The seat of administration was in present-day Bo zhou city in An hui 安徽. During the *da ye* 大業 (605 – 618) reign period of the Sui, and the *tian bao* 天寶 (742 – 756) and *zhi de* 至德 (756 – 758) reign periods of the Tang 唐, the area periodically became Qiao 譙 commandery. During Tang and Song 宋, the territory administered comprised an area equivalent to present-day Bo zhou and the following cities and counties of Guo yang 渦陽 and Meng cheng 蒙城, in An hui, as well as Lu yi 鹿邑 and Yong cheng 永城, in He nan 河南. At the beginning of Ming 明, the *zhou* was reduced to Bo 亳 county. In 1496, it again became Bo zhou, one of the *zhou* subordinate to Feng yang fu 鳳陽府. In 1724, it was elevated to the rank of a directly administered *zhou*, 直隸州 *zhi li zhou*, controlling the two counties of Tai he 太和 and Meng cheng. In 1735, it became one of the "attached" *zhou*, *san zhou* 散州, under Ying zhou fu 穎州府. In 1912, the *zhou* was changed to Bo county. In 1986, Bo zhou city was established. Mentioned with 298.

Bu shan xian 布山縣 [1]

Name of a county. It was established by Western Han 漢 and was a suburbian county under Yu lin 郁林 commandery. The seat of administration was in the former city southeast of present-day Gui ping 桂平 city in Guang xi 廣西. The county was abolished at the beginning of the *da ye* 大業 reign period of Sui 隋, in 605. Mentioned with 474.

-C-

Cai 蔡 [1 + 1]

□ Name of a river, also called Cai he 蔡河. [1] The ancient flow took up the Bian 汴 river east of present-day Kai feng 開封 in He nan 河南, then ran south along a route east of Tong xu 通許 county, and west of Tai kang 太康 county, then to a point directly east of Huai yang 淮陽 county. The river then moved south of Lu yi 鹿邑 county and in the southeast went through Guo yang 渦陽 county in An hui 安徽 and then west of Meng cheng 蒙城 county. It entered the Huai 淮 river southwest of Huai yuan 懷遠 county. Later, the river changed its bed and entered the Ying 潁 through the ancient Lang dang 蒗蕩 channel. During early Northern Song 宋 times, the Min 閔 river was the source of the Cai. Later, following the *kai bao* 開寶 reign period (968 – 976), the name of the Min was changed to Hui min 惠民 river and, subsequently, the Cai was generally called Hui min. From Ming 明 on, the bed of the Cai was frequently taken over by the flow of the Yellow River. Today, only the section below Huai yang that enters the Ying is preserved. According to the BCGM authors, the water of the Cai was suitable for brewing. Mentioned with 1541.

□ Name of a *zhou* 州 [1]. See → Cai zhou 蔡州. Mentioned with 78.

Cai zhou 蔡州 [4]

Name of a *zhou* 州. It was established in 606. Its seat of administration was in present-day Ru nan 汝南 county in He nan 河南. In 621, it was changed to Yu zhou 豫州. In 762, it was changed to Cai zhou again on account of a taboo associated with the name of Tang emperor Dai zong 代宗 (729-779). The territory of the *zhou* corresponded to an area in present-day He nan reaching from the Huai 淮 river in the South to the upper flow of the Hong 洪 river in the North, and to Tong bai 桐柏 mountain in the West. In 1233, the Jin 金 capital was transferred briefly to Cai zhou. In 1293, Cai zhou was changed to Ru ning fu 汝寧府. Mentioned with 275, 535, 823, 1003.

Can ling 蠶陵 [3]

Name of a county. It was established during the *yuan ding* 元鼎 reign period (116 – 111) of Western Han 漢. The seat of administration was in present-day Mao

茂 county in Si chuan 四川. It was abolished during Eastern Jin 晉. Mentioned with 461, 907, 1289.

Cang 滄 [3]
Name of a *zhou* 州. See → Cang zhou 滄州. Mentioned with 338, 1057.

Cang di 傖地 [1]
Name of the region inhabited by the Cang 傖 people. Further details are lacking. Mentioned with 1008.

Cang wu 蒼梧 [4]
Name of a county. It was established in 590. Its seat of administration was in present-day Wu zhou 梧州 city in Guang xi 廣西. In 1897, it was opened to be one of the so-called "treaty ports." In 1952, the seat of administration was moved to Long xu 龍圩 town. Today, this is the administration of Cang wu 蒼梧 county. Mentioned with 141, 520, 624, 1542.

Cang zhou 滄州 [5]
Name of a *zhou* 州. It was established, in 517. Its seat of administration was in present-day Qian tong 千童 town, located southwest of Yan shan 鹽山 county in He bei 河北. It was eliminated at the beginning of the *da ye* 大業 reign period (605 – 618) of Sui 隋. It was reestablished under Tang 唐, in 618. Its seat was moved to present-day Jiu zhou 舊州 town, 40 *li* southwest of Cang 滄 county in He bei 河北. The territory administered comprised an area south of the ocean and river connected with present-day Tian jin 天津 city, and extending from a line formed by Jing hai 靜海, Qing 青 county and Bo tou 泊頭 in the West to a line formed by Dong guang 東光, Ning jin 寧津, Lao ling 樂陵 and Wu di 無棣 in the South. Northern Song 宋 took the *zhou* over and, at the beginning of the *yan you* 延祐 reign period (1314 – 1320) of Yuan 元, the seat of administration was moved to Chang lu 長蘆 town (the present Cang zhou city). Soon the seat was returned to Jiu zhou. In 1369, the seat was again moved to Chang lu town. Under Qing 清, Cang zhou was part of Tian jin fu 天津府. In 1913, it became Cang 滄 county. Mentioned with 471, 675, 1205, 1390.

Cao 曹 [1]
Name of a *zhou* 州. See → Cao zhou 曹州. Mentioned with 687.

Cao zhou 曹州 [2]
Name of a *zhou* 州. It was established under Northern Zhou 周. The seat of administration was at a point 60 *li* northwest of present-day Cao 曹 county in Shan dong 山東. Its administrative area corresponded to present-day He ze 菏澤 city, along with the counties and localities of Ding tao 定陶, Cheng wu 成武, Dong ming 東明 in Shan dong, and Min quan 民權 in He nan 河南. During Northern Song 宋, the *zhou* was promoted to Xing ren fu 興仁府 but, in 1130, it was made Cao zhou again. In 1168, the administrative center was moved to the present He ze city. In 1368, the center was moved to present-day An ling 安陵 village, 26 km southwest of He ze city. In the following year, the administration was transferred to the present Cao county and, in 1372, the area became Cao county. In 1446, Cao

zhou was again established in present-day He ze city. In 1735, the status of the area was promoted to Cao zhou fu 曹州府. Mentioned with 1175.

Cen zhou 岑州 [1]

This place name occurs in the BCGM but appears to be an error since such a place name is otherwise unknown. Mentioned with 1457.

Cha ling 茶陵 [1]

Name of a county. It was established under Western Han 漢. The seat of administration was in present-day Gu cheng ying 古城營, 70 *li* east of Cha ling county in Hu nan 湖南. The county was eliminated under Sui 隋, but again established under Tang 唐 in 698. Its administration was moved to the present Cha ling county. During early Southern Song 宋, the county was promoted into an army (*jun* 軍), but it again became a county under Yuan 元. In 1282, the county was promoted to *zhou* 州 rank, but it became a county again at the beginning of Ming 明, only to be elevated to a *zhou* again in 1482. In 1913, the area became a county again. Mentioned with 768.

Chai sang 柴桑 [1]

Name of a minor region, in this case referring to the area along present-day Jiu jiang 九江 city in Jiang xi 江西. Under Western Han 漢, a Chai sang county was created at present-day Jing lin 荊林 market, located 36 *li* south of Jiu jiang county in Jiang xi. It was abolished during the *kai huang* 開皇 reign period (581 – 600) of Sui 隋. Mentioned with 985.

Chan yu 單于 [1]

One of six Tang 唐 Chief Protection *fu*, *du hu fu* 都護府. It was established in 664. The seat of administration was in Tu cheng zi 土城子, located northwest of present-day He lin ge er xian 和林格爾縣 (Horinger county) in Inner Mongolia. The area administered comprised a strip of territory in Inner Mongolia including the Yin 陰 mountain and the Great Bend of the Yellow River. In 698, the protectorate was combined with the An bei 安北 protectorate. In 720, it was reestablished but, in 845, the name was changed again back to An bei. Mentioned with 945.

Chang an 長安 [18]

Name of an ancient city. The ruins of Chang an of Han 漢 times are found northwest of present-day Xi an 西安. The Chang an of Sui 隋 and Tang 唐 times was located in the area of present-day Xi an. Mentioned with 107, 126, 202, 222, 282, 387, 532, 583, 644, 692, 781, 801, 1204, 1228, 1308, 1406, 1519, 1522.

Chang hua 昌化 [1]

Name of a county. It was established under Northern Song, in 979. The seat of administration was in present-day Chang hua town located 98 *li* west of Lin an 臨安 city in Zhe jiang 浙江. In 1960, it was eliminated and its territory was combined with Lin an county. Mentioned with 1485.

Chang le zhen 長樂鎮 [1]

Name of a garrison or a recent town. Further details are lacking. Mentioned with 793.

Chang li xian 昌黎縣 [1]
Name of a county. It was established, by changing the name of Guang ning 廣寧 county, in 1189. The seat of administration was in present-day Chang li county in He bei 河北. Mentioned with 619.

Chang ming 昌明 [1]
Name of a *xiang* 鄉 or sub-administrative unit. It occupied a strip of present-day Zhang ming 彰明 town southwest of Jiang you 江油 city in Si chuan 四川. Mentioned with 322.

Chang ning 長寧 [1]
Name of a county. It was established, by renaming Chang ning zhou 長寧州, in 1372. The seat of administration was in Shuang he 雙河 town located 70 *li* south of present-day Chang ning county in Si chuan 四川. In 1950, the administration was moved to An ning 安寧 town. This is the present Chang ning county. Mentioned with 1499.

Chang sha 長沙 [1 + 2]
□ Name of a commandery. [1] It was established by Qin 秦 during Warring States times. The seat of administration was in the present-day Chang sha city in Hu nan 湖南. Its administration comprised the eastern and southern part of the present Hu nan, along with the northeastern corner of Guang xi 廣西. During Western Han 漢, the area became a feudal country, but Eastern Han again established the commandery, although its administrative area was gradually reduced. In 758, it was abolished. Mentioned with 869.
□ Name of a *fu* 府. [2] It was established during the Five Dynasties period. The seat of administration was in the present-day Chang sha city in Hu nan. Its administrative area corresponded to the middle of present-day Hu nan, tending towards the eastern areas of Hu nan. It encompassed the area south of Dong ting 洞庭 lake and the Mi luo 汨羅 river, and east of Zi shui 資水 watershed and the region of the line formed by An hua 安化, Xiang xiang 湘鄉 and Cha ling 茶陵 in the South. The *fu* was abolished in 1913. Mentioned with 378, 768.

Chang shan 長山 [1]
Name of a mountain. It is located 25 *li* southwest of the Dan tu 丹徒 region of present-day Zhen jiang 鎮江 city in Jiang su 江蘇. Mentioned with 1238.

Chang shan 常山 [2 + 17]
□ Name of a mountain. It was originally referred to as Bei yue heng shan 北岳恒山, "Mount Heng of the Northern Mountain Range," but the name was later changed due to various taboos associated with the names of Han emperor Wen di 文帝 (202 – 157), Tang emperor Mu zong 穆宗 (795 – 824), and Northern Song emperor Zhen zong 真宗 (968 – 1022). The reference is to Da mao 大茂 mountain located northwest of the present-day Qu yang 曲陽 county in He bei 河北. Mentioned with 130, 1469.
□ Name of a commandery, ' Chang shan jun 常山郡. [17] Mentioned with 192, 299, 359, 361, 431, 579, 599, 631, 652, 816, 997, 1016, 1140, 1324, 1532.

Chang shan jun 常山郡 [2]
Name of a commandery. It was established, by renaming Heng shan 恒山 commandery, in 179 BCE. The seat of administration was at a point northeast of present-day Shi jia zhuang 石家莊 city in He bei 河北. Its administrative territory comprised an area in present-day He bei reaching from the Tang he 唐河 in the North, and the area of Luan cheng 欒城 and Zhao 趙 county in the East, to Nei qiu 內丘 in the South. Northern Wei 魏 moved the administrative center to a point 24 *li* northwest of present-day Gao cheng 藁城 in He bei. In 621, the administrative center was moved to the present Zheng ding 正定 county in He bei. The commandery was abolished in 758. Mentioned with 631, 1396.

Chang yang shan 昌陽山 [1]
Name of a mountain located southwest of present-day Wen deng 文登 city in Shan dong 山東. Mentioned with 233.

Chang yue 常岳 [1]
Name of a mountain range. The reference was later to Bei yue heng shan 北岳恒山, "Heng mountain of the Northern Mountain Range," the name changed due to a taboo associated with the name of Tang 唐 emperor Mu zong 穆宗 (795 – 824). The present-day reference is to Da mao 大茂 mountain located northwest of present-day Qu yang 曲陽 county in He bei 河北. Mentioned with 1469.

Chang zhou 昌州 [1]
Name of a *zhou* 州. It was established in 758. The seat of administration was at a point southwest of present-day Da zu 大足 county in the municipality district of Chong qing 重慶. The territory administered comprised present Da zu, Rong chang 榮昌 and Yong chuan 永川. In 885, the administrative center was moved to Da zu county and, in 1290, the *zhou* was abolished. Mentioned with 558.

Chang zhou 常州 [4]
Name of a *zhou* 州. It was established under the Sui 隋, in 589. The seat of administration was at a point northwest of the present Chang zhou city in Jiang su 江蘇. Its territories embraced the cities and areas of the present-day Chang zhou, Wu xi 無錫, Jiang yin 江陰 and Yi xing 宜興, in Jiang su. In 1277, the status of the *zhou* was raised to Chang zhou lu 常州路. Mentioned with 560, 768, 856, 935, 1055.

Chao 潮 [2]
Name of a *zhou* 州, see → Chao zhou 潮州. Mentioned with 1272, 1297.

Chao ge 朝歌 [1]
Name of an ancient city, located in present-day Qi 淇 county in He nan 河南. Mentioned with 864.

Chao xian 朝鮮 [8 + 2]
□ Name of an ancient country. [8] The name originally referred to the Chao xian region wherein commandaries were established during the Han 漢. These were Le lang 樂浪, Xuan tu 玄菟, Lin tun 臨屯 and Zhen fang 真番. The territories of these four commanderies comprised approximately the northern two-thirds of the Korean peninsula. Mentioned with 501, 1004, 1200, 1205, 1480.

□ In late Chinese usage, this name, the Korean Choson or Joseon, corresponded to the kingdom of the Yi dynasty founded in 1392. [2] It embraced the entire Korean peninsula and ruled until conquered by Japan in 1910. The capital was at Hanseong, the present-day Seoul. Mentioned with 501, 931.

Chao zhou 潮州 [3]

Name of a *zhou* 州. It was established in 591. The seat of administration was in present-day Chao zhou city in Guang dong 廣東. The territory administered comprised the present-day cities and counties of Mei zhou 梅州, Ping yuan 平遠, Feng shun 豐順, Pu ning 普寧 and Hui lai 惠來 in Guang dong. Under Yuan 元, the area became a *lu* 路. Mentioned with 363, 428, 1263.

Che shi guo 車師國[1]

Name of an ancient country in the western regions, It was one of 36 kingdoms said to be existing there in Han 漢 times. Its capital was located at a point 20 *li* northwest of present-day Turfan in Xin jiang 新疆, at the ruined city on the Jiao 交 river. The kingdom later divided into a "former" (*qian* 前) and a "latter" (*hou* 後), and was then, during the Sixteen Dynasties period, destroyed by Ju qu an zhou 沮渠安周 (died 460), the last part around 450. Mentioned with 496.

Chen 郴 [1]

Name of a *zhou* 州. See → Chen zhou 郴州. Mentioned with 217, 1063.

Chen 辰 [1]

Name of a zhou 州. See → Chen zhou 辰州. Mentioned with 202.

Chen 陳 [3]

Name of a region. The reference is to the territories of the pre-Qin 秦 state of Chen. The ruins of the old capital are located in present-day Huai yang 淮陽 county in He nan 河南. Mentioned with 442, 1242.

Chen cang 陳倉 [3 + 1]

□ This is the name of a county. [3] It was established by the Qin 秦. The seat of administration was on the northern bank of the Wei shui 渭水 20 *li* east of present-day Bao ji 寶雞 city in Shaan xi 陝西. Under Tang 唐, the name was changed to Bao ji county. Mentioned with 1155, 1209, 1573.

□ Minor place name. [1] It is present-day Chen cang town east of Bao ji city in Shaan xi 陝西. Mentioned with 495.

Chen liu 陳留 [1]

Name of a region. It is a possible reference to a commandery, but could also be the name of a county. Mentioned with 1346.

□ Chen liu county was established under Qin 秦. The seat of administration was in present-day Chen liu town, 26 *li* southeast of Kai feng 開封 city in He nan 河南. In 1957, it was combined with Kai feng county.

□ The commandery of Chen liu was established under Western Han 漢, in 122 BCE. The seat of administration was in present-day Chen liu county, and its territory comprised an area extending from present-day Kai feng city in the West, to Ning ling 寧陵 county in the East, to Yan jin 延津 in the North, and to the counties of Qi 杞 and Sui 睢 in the South. Under Northern Wei 魏, the administration was moved to the present Kai feng city. In 758, the area was changed to Bian zhou 汴州.

Chen zhou 郴州 [2]

Name of a *zhou* 州. The *zhou* was established under Sui 隋, in 589. The seat of administration was in the present Chen zhou city in Hu nan 湖南. The territory controlled comprised Yong xing county in present-day Hu nan, and south from it the watershed of the Lei shui 耒水 and the areas of Lan shan 藍山, Jia he 嘉禾, Lin wu 臨武 and Yi zhang 宜章. This administrative territory was gradually reduced in size after the Five Dynasties period. Yuan 元 raised the status of the area to become a *lu* 路. Mentioned with 1532.

Chen zhou 辰州 [8]

Name of a *zhou* 州. It was established under Sui 隋, in 589. The seat of administration was in the present Qian cheng 黔城 town northwest of Hong jiang 洪江 City in Hu nan 湖南. Later, the administration was moved to present-day Yuan ling 沅陵 county in Hu nan. Chen zhou's territory comprised the present-day Yuan ling 沅陵 county in Hu nan and the watershed of the Yuan shui 沅水 located south of it. The Yuan 元 raised the area to *lu* 路 rank. Mentioned with 202, 303, 768, 1486, 1518.

Chen zhou 陳州 [3]

Name of a *zhou* 州. It was established by Northern Zhou 周. The seat of administration was in present-day Huai yang 淮陽 county in He nan 河南. The territories governed comprised the present-day cities and counties of Huai yang, Shang shui 商水, Tai kang 太康, Xi hua 西華, Shen qiu 沈丘, Zhou kou 周口 and Xiang cheng 項城 in He nan. Towards the end of Northern Song 宋, its status was raised to Huai ning fu 淮寧府, but Jin 金 again established the *zhou*. Under Ming 明, the area was one of the *zhou* subordinate to Kai feng fu 開封府. In 1734, Chen zhou was raised to the rank of *fu* 府. Mentioned with 857, 1292, 1310.

Cheng 成 [4]

Name of a *zhou*. See → Cheng zhou 成州. Mentioned with 368, 802, 1057, 1523.

Cheng 澄 [1]

Name of a *zhou* 州, see → Cheng zhou 澄州. Mentioned with 521.

Cheng du 成都 [6]

This is the present city of Cheng du in Si chuan 四川. Mentioned with 550, 1096, 1182, 1246, 1279, 1307.

Cheng du fu 成都府 [1]

Name of a *fu* 府. It was formed, in 757, by raising the status of Shu 蜀 commandery. The seat of administration was in the present-day Cheng du 成都 city in Si chuan 四川. Its administrative territory comprised the present-day cities and counties of Cheng du, Shuang liu 雙流 and Pi xian 郫縣 in Si chuan. During Northern Song 宋, it was changed to Yi zhou lu 益州路 and Cheng du fu lu 成都府路. During Ming 明, Cheng du fu was again established with considerably amplified territories. The *fu* was abolished in 1913. Mentioned with 686.

Cheng gao zhu shan 成皋諸山 [1]
Name of a mountain. It is situated at present-day Si shui 汜水 town northwest of Xing yang 滎陽 city in He nan 河南. Mentioned with 908.

Cheng xian 承縣 [1]
Name of a county, a mistake for → **Zheng xian** 氶縣

Cheng zhou 成州 [3]
Name of a zhou 州. It was established at Tang 唐 times in 618. The seat of administration was at a point southwest of present-day Li xian 禮縣 county in Gan su 甘肅. The territory governed comprised the present-day counties of Li xian, Xi he 西和 and Cheng xian 成縣 in Gan su. In 762, it became part of the Tibetan empire, but was again established in 789. At the end of Tang, its administration was moved to the present Cheng xian county. In 1227, its status was raised to Tong qing fu 同慶府. Mentioned with 261, 275, 620.

Cheng zhou 澄州 [3]
Name of a *zhou* 州. It was established in 634. The seat of administration was in present-day Gu cheng 古城 village in Cheng tai xiang 澄泰鄉, located southeast of present-day Shang lin 上林 county in Guang xi. Its administrative area covered the present-day counties of Shang lin and Ma shan 馬山 in Guang xi 廣西. In 972, it was abolished. Mentioned with 535, 552, 816.

Chi 池 [1]
Name of a *zhou* 州. See → Chi zhou. Mentioned with 1302.

Chi mu er cheng 赤木兒城 [1]
Name of a city. This is located west of present-day Huo cheng 霍城 county in Xin jiang 新疆. Mentioned with 1480.

Chi shan 赤山 [1]
Name of a mountain. It is located 30 *li* southeast of present-day Shao xing 紹興 city in Zhe jiang 浙江. Mentioned with 1340.

Chi shui 赤水 [1 +1 +2]
□ This is the name of a river. [1] This is the Chi ting shui 赤亭水, a tributary of the Wei shui 渭水, found east of present-day Long xi 隴西 county in Gan su 甘肅. Mentioned with 461.
□ Name of a *xiang* 鄉, sub-administrative unit, located east of present-day Long xi county in Gan su. Mentioned with 461.
□ Name of a *xiang*. [2] It is a strip of territory along present-day Zhang ming 彰明 town, southwest of Jiang you 江油 city in Si chuan 四川. Mentioned with 322.

Chi shui he 赤水河 [1]
Name of a river. It is the river of the same name in the northwest of present-day Gui zhou 貴州. It is a tributary of the upper river course of the Yang zi. Its headwaters are located east of Zhen xiong 鎮雄 county in Yun nan 雲南. In the east it flows to Xi shui 習水 county in Gui zhou. It passes through the West of Chi shui 赤水 county, and continues in the northeast where it enters the Yang zi at He jiang 合江 county in Si chuan 四川. Mentioned with 569.

Chi zhou 池州 [7]

Name of a *zhou* 州. It was established during the Tang 唐, in 621. The seat of administration was in present-day Chi zhou city in An hui 安徽. Its administrative territory encompassed the present-day cities and counties of Chi zhou, Qing yang 青陽, and Dong zhi 東至. During Northern Song 宋, the jurisdiction of the *zhou* was extended and reached the cities and counties of Shi tai 石台 and Tong ling 銅陵. At the beginning of the Yuan 元, the *zhou* became Chi zhou lu 池州路. Mentioned with 129, 328, 537, 695, 768, 994, 1485.

Chong qing 重慶 [1]

Name of a *fu* 府. It was established under Southern Song 宋, in 1189. The seat of administration was in the present Chong qing 重慶 municipality district. Under Yuan 元, in 1279, it was changed to a *lu* 路. Under Ming 明, in 1371, it again became Chong qing fu 重慶府. Its jurisdiction comprised an area to the east of present-day Xing chang 榮昌 in Si chuan, south of Wu sheng 武勝, west of Fu ling 涪陵 in Chong qing, and the area north of the Qi jiang 綦江. The *fu* was abolished in 1913. Mentioned with 1096.

Chong shan 崇山 [1]

A general reference to high mountains. Further details are unavailable. Mentioned with 345.

Chong wu zhi shan 崇吾之山 [1]

Name of a mountain from the *Shan hai jing* 山海經, "Classic of Mountains and Seas." Further information is unavailable. Mentioned with 577.

Chu 滁 [4]

Name of a *zhou* 州. See → Chu zhou 滁州. Mentioned with 52, 381, 781, 1052.

Chu 楚 [47 + 1]

□ Regional name. [47] Reference is to the Spring and Autumn and Warring States period kingdom in south China. See → Chu guo 楚國. Mentioned with 64, 76, 82, 159, 164, 258, 271, 285, 417, 504, 562, 572, 735, 768, 787, 845, 846, 989, 1051, 1064, 1065, 1083, 1084, 1099, 1105, 1171, 1185, 1210, 1218, 1239, 1242, 1257, 1272, 1283, 1307, 1308, 1310, 1407, 1458, 1471, 1499, 1516.

□ Name of a *zhou* 州. [1] See → Chu zhou 楚州. Mentioned with 1057.

Chu 處 [1]

Name of a *zhou* 州. See → Chu zhou 處州. Mentioned with 981.

Chu di 楚地 [4]

Regional name referring to the ancient territories of the Spring and Autumn and Warring States periods state of Chu. See → Chu 楚, → Chu guo 楚國. Mentioned with 42, 258, 1084, 1509.

Chu guo 楚國 [1]

This is the Spring and Autumn and Warring States period state of Chu. It was enfeoffed during the Western Zhou, with its power increasing steadily during the Spring and Autumn period when it continuously eliminated and took in smaller states. Eventually, it became one of the Five Hegemons of the time. Its capital was Ji nan cheng 紀南城, to the north of present-day Jing zhou 荊州 city in Hu bei 湖北. Its territory reached from the southern part of present-day He nan 河南 and the southeastern part of present-day Shaan xi 陝西 in the West, to present-day Han shan 含山 county in An hui 安徽 in the East, and in the South exceeded Dong ting hu 洞庭湖. During the Warring States periods, it was one of the seven most powerful states. Its territory was extended to the southern part of present-day Shan dong 山東, and the northwestern corner of Guang xi 廣西. After it had abolished the state of Yue 越, it reached the territory of present-day Jiang zhe 江浙. In 223, it was eliminated by Qin 秦.

Chu shan 楚山 [1 + 2]

□ Allusion to mountains. [1] Reference is generally to mountains of present-day Hu bei 湖北 and areas surrounding them. Mentioned with 1214.

□ Allusion to a mountain. [2] This is Shang 商 mountain. It is located west of the present-day Dan feng 丹鳳 county in Shaan xi 陝西, one *li* south of Shang zhen 商鎮. Mentioned with 55, 1214.

Chu zhong 楚中 [1]

General geographical reference used in pointing to Hu bei 湖北. Mentioned with 116.

Chu zhou 滁州 [16]

Name of a zhou 州. It was established in Sui 隋 times at the beginning of the *kai huang* 開皇 reign period (581 – 600). The seat of administration was in present-day Chu zhou 滁州 city in An hui 安徽. Its territories included the present Chu zhou city and the two counties of Lai an 來安 and Quan jiao 全椒 in An hui. In 1912, the area became a county and in 1982 a city was established. Mentioned with 53, 78, 199, 224, 351, 369, 499, 668, 799, 931, 973, 1217, 1478, 1530.

Chu zhou 楚州 [2]

Name of a *zhou* 州. It was established in 581. The seat of administration was at a point southwest of the Huai yin 淮陰 district of present-day Huai an 淮安 city in Jiang su 江蘇. In 592, the administration was moved to the present Huai an city. The territory of the *zhou* embraced the present-day cities and counties of Huai an, Xu yi 盱眙, Bao ying 寶應, Jian hu 建湖, Jin hu 金湖 and Hong ze 洪澤 in Jiang su 江蘇. The *zhou* was changed to Huai an jun 淮安軍 during the Southern Song 宋, in 1228. Mentioned with 700, 1460.

Chu zhou 處州 [8]

Name of a *zhou* 州. It was established, under the Sui 隋, in 589. The seat of administration was in present-day Gu cheng 古城 village, located 7 *li* southeast of Li shui 麗水 city in Zhe jiang 浙江. The area administered comprised the water basins of the Ling jiang 靈江, the Ou jiang 甌江 and the Fei yun jiang 飛雲江, located along a line south of the Tian tai 天台 mountains and the Xian du 仙都 mountains. At the end of Tang 唐, the seat of administration was moved to present-day Li shui city. In 1276, the Mongols changed the name of the *zhou* to Chu zhou lu 處州路. Mentioned with 24, 191, 288, 428, 456, 566, 1017, 1032, 1112.

Chuan 川 [26]
Abbreviation for → Si chuan 四川. During Ming 明, the territories of Si chuan were quite large. In the East, it began from the Three Gorges of the Yang zi and, in the West, it endet at the Da du 大渡 river. In the North, its extension reached Da ba shan 大巴山, mountain of the Qin ling 秦嶺 mountain range and, in the South, it went beyond the Jin sha 金沙 river. Mentioned with 100, 157, 199, 247, 298, 322, 445, 557, 766, 783, 786, 856, 988, 995, 1008, 1036, 1068, 1088, 1096, 1247, 1264, 1408, 1499, 1526.

Chuan dong 川東 [1]
Regional generalization. It refers to the "eastern part of (Si) chuan 四川," more or less the eastern part of present-day Si chuan and the municipality of Chong qing 重慶. Mentioned with 1096.

Chuan guang 川廣 [2]
Combined regional name referring to Si chuan 四川 as well as to Hu guang 湖廣, an area including Hu nan 湖南 and Hu bei 湖北. Mentioned with 550, 1490.

Chuan nan 川南 [1]
General name for the "southern part of Si chuan 四川." Mentioned with 585.

Chuan qian 川黔 [1]
Combined regional name referring to Si chuan 四川 and Gui zhou 貴州, also known as Qian 黔. Mentioned with 875.

Chuan shaan 川陝 [3]
Combined regional name referring to Si chuan 四川 and Shaan xi 陝西. Mentioned with 399, 719, 1119.

Chuan shu 川蜀 [14]
Regional name referring to the plateau centered about present-day Cheng du 成都 city. Mentioned with 100, 199, 323, 330, 462, 491, 524, 698, 752, 905, 949, 1308, 1486.

Chuan xi 川西 [16]
General name for the "western part of Si chuan 四川." Mentioned with 337, 524, 736. 784, 1096.

Chuan xia 川峽 [1]
Regional name apparently in reference to the area of the river gorges, but this is uncertain. Mentioned with 933.

Chuan zhong 川中 [8]
Regional name referring to the "central part of Si chuan 四川." Mentioned with 90, 636, 786, 823, 1308, 1324, 1512.

Chun zhou 春州 [2]
Name of a *zhou* 州. It was established in 621. The seat of administration was in present-day Yang chun 陽春 city in Guang dong 廣東. The territory administered comprised the present area of Yang chun city. It was abolished in 1073. Mentioned with 202, 428.

Chun zhou 淳州 [1]

Name of a *zhou* 州. It was established in 621. The seat of administration was on the eastern bank of the Yu jiang 郁江, north of present-day Luan cheng 欒城 town, located in northwestern part of Heng 横 county in Guang xi 廣西. The area administered was situated within the present-day three counties of Heng xian 横縣, Bin yang 賓陽 and Yong ning 邕寧 in Guang xi. In 805, the area became Luan zhou 巒州, but Luan zhou was abolished under Northern Song 宋, in 972. When Su Song 蘇頌 (1020 – 1101) spoke of Chun zhou, he was borrowing an ancient place name, not a current one. Mentioned with 1430.

Ci shan 慈山 [1]

Name of a mountain but its location is uncertain. Mentioned with 175.

Ci yang 慈陽 [1]

Name of a mountain. No further information is available. Mentioned with 1250.

Ci xi 慈谿 [2]

Name of a county. It was originally Ci xi 慈溪 county but became Ci xi 慈谿 county in 1419. It was administered from present-day Ci cheng 慈城 town, located 32 *li* northwest of Ning bo 寧波 city in Zhe jiang 浙江. The county became Ci xi 慈溪 county in 1949.

Ci zhou 慈州 [3]

Name of a *zhou* 州. It was founded in 634. The seat of administration was in present-day Ji 吉 county in Shan xi 山西. The territory administered comprised present-day Ji county and Xiang ning 鄉寧 county in Shan xi. In 1151, it was changed to be Geng zhou 耿州. In 1190, it became Ji zhou 吉州. Mentioned with 175, 285, 1037, 1250.

Cong long zhi shan 葱聾之山 [1]

This is the name of a mountain from the *Shan hai jing* 山海經, "Classic of Mountains and Seas." It is also called Wu lao 五老 mountain. It is located southeast of present-day Yong ji 永濟 city in Shan xi 山西. Mentioned with 21.

Cong shui 從水 [1]

Mythical place name from the *Shan hai jing* 山海經, "Classic of Mountains and Seas." Further details are unavailable. Mentioned with 805.

-D-

Da bie shan 大別山 [1]

Name of a mountain, also Lu shan 魯山. It is Gui 龜 mountain, located northeast of present-day Han yang 漢陽 in Wu han 武漢 city in Hu bei 湖北. Mentioned with 185.

Da bin xian 大賓縣 [1]
Name of a county. It was established in 595. The seat of administration was at a point 40 *li* northeast of present-day Gui ping 桂平 city in Guang xi 廣西. The county was abolished under Northern Song 宋, in 972. Mentioned with 1138.

Da ci zhi shan 大次之山 [1]
Name of a land from the *Shan hai jing* 山海經, "Classic of Mountains and Seas." Further details are unavailable. Mentioned with 21.

Da da 韃靼 [2]
This name originally referred to the "Tatar" tribal federation of Mongolia, and then to the Mongols themselves. After the end of Yuan 元, the Ming 明 called the eastern part of present-day Inner Mongolia Da da. Mentioned with 215, 1130.

Da heng shan 大横山 [1]
Name of a mountain. It is located south of present-day Ming guang 明光 city in An hui 安徽. Mentioned with 1039.

Da li fu 大理府 [1]
Name of a *fu* 府. It was established in 1382. The seat of administration was in the old city of Da li 大理, located 26 *li* north of present-day Da li city in Yun nan 雲南. The *fu* administered the middle sections of present-day Da li in Yun nan. It was abolished in 1913. Mentioned with 656.

Da niao shan 大鳥山 [1]
Name of a mountain located near present-day Dun huang 敦煌 city in Gan su 甘肅, but additional details are unavailable. Mentioned with 274.

Da qin 大秦 [2]
Name of an ancient country. See → Da qin guo 大秦國. Mentioned with 285, 1406.

Da qin guo 大秦國 [16]
Name of an ancient country. At the time of its earliest mention, the term seems to apply to late Hellenistic Syria and adjacent areas, then to the Seleucid Empire whose capital, Antioch, could be Da'dzin, if this is a transcription, although an older form of the present-day word Tajik (→ Da shi guo 大食國, EMC Da'ẓik country) is possible too and the Da qin here is simply an indication of some country of the extreme west, positioned like Qin 秦 was in China. Following the separation of the ancient Roman Empire into a Western and an Eastern Empire, the term came to mean the Eastern Roman Empire. Mentioned with 104, 229, 245, 511, 542, 670, 772, 799, 935, 945, 1124, 1183, 1237, 1258, 1425, 1427.

Da rou zhi 大月氏 [1]
Name of an ancient country. See → Da rou zhi guo 大月氏國. Mentioned with 1192.

Da rou zhi guo 大月氏國 [1]
Name of an ancient country. During the early years of the rule of Han emperor Wen di 文帝 (202 – 157), it was moved from a region between Dun huang 敦煌 and Qi lian 祁連 river to the West to the region of the Ili (Yi li 伊犁) river in

the western part of present-day Xin jiang 新疆 and regions further to the West. The Rou were forced to migrate even further west to avoid an attack of the Wu sun 烏孫, around 161 BCE. They ended up in Tokharia along the upper ranges of the Amu darya just north of the surviving Greek kingdoms in Bactria where they ultimately founded the Kushan empire in the mid-1st century CE, after the disappearance of the surviving Greek kingdoms in the area. Mentioned with 937.

Da shi 大食 [4]
Name of an ancient country. See → Da shi guo 大食國. Mentioned with 104, 738, 1252, 1272.

Da shi guo 大食國 [9]
Name of an ancient country. This is an ancient form of the present-day Tajik, which now has a very specialized meaning but, from Tang 唐 times on, the term generally referred in Chinese sources to the Arabic world, i.e., the Umayyad and Abbasid caliphates and connected areas. Mentioned with 334, 427, 498, 535, 945, 1124, 1247, 1252, 1544.

Da shi zhu fan 大食諸番 [1]
"The various foreign countries of Da shi." See → Da shi guo 大食國. Mentioned with 209.

Da shi zhu guo 大食諸國 [1]
"The various countries of Da shi." See → Da shi guo 大食國. Mentioned with 887.

Da tong 大同 [1]
Name of a *fu*. See → Da tong fu 大同府. Mentioned with 464.

Da tong fu 大同府 [1]
Name of a *fu* 府. It was established by Liao 遼, in 1044. The seat of administration was in present-day Da tong 大同 city in Shan xi 山西. The territory administered comprised present-day Da tong city in Shan xi and the counties of Zuo yun 左雲, You yu 右玉, Huai ren 懷仁, Da tong, Yang gao 陽高, and Tian zhen 天鎮 , as well as the counties of Feng zhen 丰鎮, Zhuo zi 卓資, and Liang cheng 凉城 in Inner Mongolia, and Yang yuan 陽原 and Huai an 懷安 in He bei 河北. In 1288, the area became Da tong lu 大同路. In 1369, Da tong lu became Da tong fu again. Its administration then corresponded to the northern portions of present-day Shan xi, what was located inside and outside the Great Wall, as well as the counties of present-day Yu xian 蔚縣 and Lai yuan 淶源 in He bei 河北. The area of the Qing 清 period administration was equivalent to the area of present-day Da tong city in Shan xi and surrounding areas. The *fu* was abolished in 1912. Mentioned with 724.

Da wan 大宛 [7]
Name for a kingdom in the Han 漢 era western regions, usually identified with the Ferghana basin in present-day Uzbekistan. Its capital was located in present-day Kasansay in Uzbekistan. Under the Tang 唐, the name of the country was changed to Ning yuan 寧遠. Mentioned with 485, 567, 801, 861.

Da wu 大吳 [1]
Honorific name for the pre-Qin 秦 state of Wu 吳. Wu controlled present-day Jiang su 江蘇, a large part of present-day Shang hai 上海, and parts of An hui 安徽 and Zhe jiang 浙江. Mentioned with 1238.

Da xian 大峴 [1]
Name of a mountain. It is located north of present-day Yi shui 沂水 county in Shan dong 山東. Mentioned with 1521.

Da ya shan 大牙山 [1]
The character *da* 大 is most likely an error for *quan* 犬, and the name of the mountain most likely should be Quan ya shan 犬牙山, but no details are available on the location of a mountain with this name either. Mentioned with 202.

Da yi 大邑 [1]
Name of a county. It was established in 671. The seat of administration was in present-day Da yi county in Si chuan 四川. In 1377, it was eliminated, but was reestablished in 1380. Mentioned with 520.

Da yu ling 大庾嶺 [2]
Name of a mountain range. This is one of China's traditional "five mountain ranges," wu yue 五岳. It is located in the border region of the two present-day counties of Da yu 大余 in Jiang xi 江西 and Nan xiong 南雄 in Guang dong 廣東. Mentioned with 1279, 1307

Da yue shi 大月氏, see → Da rou zhi 大月氏

Da yue shi guo 大月氏國, see → Da rou zhi guo 大月氏國

Dai 代 [4]
Name of a *zhou* 州. See → Dai zhou 代州. Mentioned with 191, 1037, 1137, 1462.

Dai bei 代北 [1]
Regional name. It is a vague reference to Dai 代 commandery of Han 漢 and Jin 晉 times, and to the area north of Dai zhou 代州 from the Tang 唐 period on. Mentioned with 1150.

Dai jun 代郡 [7]
Name of a commandery. It was first established by the state of Zhao 趙 during the Warring States period. During Qin 秦 and Western Han 漢, the administrative center was situated southwest of present-day Yu 蔚 county in He bei 河北. During Western Han, the area administered comprised a territory reaching in present-day He bei from Huai an 懷安 and Yu xian 蔚縣 in the East to Yang gao 陽高 and Hun yuan 渾源 in Shan xi 山西 in the West, an area located inside and outside of the Great Wall, as well as the region passed by the river Dong yang he 東洋河 outside of the Great Wall. During Eastern Han, the center of administration was moved to a point southwest of present-day Yang gao county. The commandery was abolished at the end of Western Jin 晉. Mentioned with 191, 338, 718, 934.

Dai zhou 代州 [5]

Name of a *zhou* 州. It was established in 585. The seat of administration was in present-day Dai 代 county in Shan xi 山西. The area administered comprised the present-day counties of Dai xian 代縣, Fan shi 繁峙, Yuan ping 原平 and Wu tai 五台 in Shan xi. Later, the area became a commandery but, in 758, it again became Dai zhou. In 1369, the *zhou* was demoted to a county, but six years later Dai zhou was reestablished. In 1724, the *zhou* became a directly administered *zhou*, *zhi li zhou* 直隸州. In 1912, it became Dai county. Mentioned with 191, 473, 716, 1449.

Dan 丹 [1]

Name of a *zhou* 州. See → Dan zhou 丹州. Mentioned with 781.

Dan er 儋耳 [1]

Name of a commandery. It was established by Western Han 漢, in 110 BCE. The seat of administration was in present-day Nan tan 南灘, located northwest of Dan zhou 儋州 city in Hai nan 海南 province. The area administered comprised the western portions of the island of Hai nan. In 82 BCE, the area became part of Zhu ya 珠崖 commandery, but Dan er commandery was reestablished under the Sui 隋, in 610. Sui moved the center of administration to Zhong he 中和 town, located northwest of present-day Dan zhou city. In 622, under Tang 唐, the commandery became Dan zhou. Mentioned with 419.

Dan shan zhi nan 丹山之南 [1]

Regional name. Its location is uncertain. Mentioned with 294.

Dan shui 丹水 [2 + 1]

□ River basin. [2] The location is uncertain. Mentioned with 62, 1073.

□ River basin. [1] This is the Dan jiang 丹江, a tributary of the Han jiang 漢江. This Dan shui has its origins from the southern slopes of Feng huang 鳳凰 mountain in the northwestern section of Shang luo 商洛 city in Shaan xi 陝西 province. Leaving Shaan xi, the river goes south through Xi chuan 淅川 county in He nan 河南, and further towards the South where eventually it enters the Han shui 漢水 in Hu bei 湖北 province. Mentioned with 204.

Dan tu 丹徒 [1]

Name of a county. It was established by Qin 秦. The seat of administration was in present-day Dan tu town, located 18 *li* southeast of Dan tu district of Zhen jiang 鎮江 city in Jiang su 江蘇. During the Three Kingdoms period, under Wu 吳, it was changed, in 234, to Wu jin 武進 county. Under Western Jin, in 281, it again became Dan tu county. It was eliminated under the Sui 隋, in 589, but reestablished under Tang 唐, in 620. It was administered in present-day Zhen jiang city. In 1949, it became Dan tu county again. Mentioned with 580.

Dan xi 丹溪 [1]

Not a place name. Dan xi, "cinnabar creek," was an alternative name of the physician and author Zhu Zhen heng 朱震亨 (1281 – 1358).

Dan xue zhi shan 丹穴之山 [1]

Name of a mountain but its location is uncertain. Mentioned with 294.

Dan yang 丹陽 [4 + 7]

□ Name of a county. [4] It was established in 742. The territory administered comprised present-day Dan yang city in Jiang su 江蘇. In 1987, the county became Dan yang city. Mentioned with 376, 928, 1329.

□ Name of a commandery. [7] It was established in 109 BCE. The seat of administration was in present-day Xuan zhou 宣州 city in An hui 安徽. The territory governed ran south of the Yang zi in An hui, to the west of Mao shan 茅 mountain in Jiang su 江蘇 and included a section of the northern portion of Zhe jiang 浙江. During the time of Three Kingdoms' Wu 吳, the administration was moved to the present city of Nan jing 南京. In 589, the commandery was eliminated but later, at the beginning of the reign period *da ye* 大业 (605 – 618) of the Sui 隋, Jiang zhou 蔣州 was renamed Dan yang 丹陽 commandery. In 620, under Tang 唐, the commandery was changed to be Yang zhou 揚州. Mentioned with 87, 135, 157, 429, 572, 1203, 1305, 1375.

Dan yuan 亶爰 [1]

Name of a mountain. Further details are unavailable. Mentioned with 656.

Dan yuan zhi shan 亶爰之山 [1]

Name of a mountain mentioned in the *Shan hai jing* 山海經, "Classic of Mountains and Seas." Further details are unavailable. Mentioned with 656.

Dan zhou 丹州 [2]

Name of a *zhou* 州. Founded by Western Wei 魏, in 554. The seat of administration was in present-day Guo xia 郭下 village northeast of Yi chuan 宜川 county in Shaan xi 陝西. The *zhou* was eliminated under Sui 隋 but reestablished, in 618, and administered from a point northeast of the present Yi chuan county. Later, the *zhou* came under the administration of Yi chuan county. In 1269, it was abolished. Mentioned with 126, 781.

Dang chang 宕昌 [6]

Name of a region. See → Tan chang 宕昌.

Dang shan 碭山 [1]

Name of a mountain. This is Mang dang 芒碭 mountain, located 60 *li* north of present-day Yong cheng 永城 county in He nan 河南. Mentioned with 1509.

Dang yang 當陽 [2]

Name of a county. See → Dang yang xian 當陽縣. Mentioned with 123, 1171.

Dang yang xian 當陽縣 [1]

Name of a county. It was established under Western Han 漢. The seat of administration was at a point southwest of Jing men 荊門 city in present-day Hu bei 湖北. Eastern Han moved the administration to Dang yang 當陽 city in Hu bei. During early Ming 明, the seat of administration was moved to Wan cheng 萬城, northwest of the Jing zhou 荊州 district in what is present-day Jing zhou city. The county was eliminated in 1377, but reestablished in 1380 with the administration moved to present-day Dang yang city. In 1988, the county became Dang yang city. Mentioned with 381.

Dang zhou 當州 [1]

Name of a *zhou* 州. It was established by the Tang 唐, in 647. The seat of administration was at a point on the borders of Hei shui 黑水 county in present-day Si chuan 四川. Its administrative area covered present-day Hei shui county. In 677, the seat of administration was moved to an area east of the present-day Hei shui county. In 742, the *zhou* became Jiang yuan 江源 commandery. In 758, it became Dang zhou again. During Northern Song 宋, the seat of administration was moved to a place northwest of present-day Mao 茂 county in Si chuan. Yuan 元 eliminated Dang zhou. Mentioned with 199.

Dao 道 [1]

Name of a *zhou* 州. See → Dao zhou 道州. Mentioned with 474.

Dao zhou 道州 [3]

Name of a *zhou* 州. It was established in 634. The seat of administration was at a point west of present-day Dao 道 county in Hu nan 湖南. The area administered comprised the present-day Dao county, along with Ning yuan 寧遠, Jiang yong 江永 and Jiang hua 江華 counties in Hu nan. The *zhou* was eliminated in 643, but reestablished in 675. It became Jiang hua 江華 commandery in 742 but, in 758, it was again named Dao zhou. It was administered from present-day Dao county in Hu nan. During early Ming 明, in 1368, Dao zhou was changed to be Dao zhou fu 道州府, but again became Dao zhou in 1377. In 1913, it became a county. Mentioned with 1063, 1091, 1329.

De qing zhou 德慶州 [1]

Name of a *zhou* 州. It was established in 1376. The seat of administration was in present-day De qing 德慶 county in Guang dong 廣東. The area administered comprised the two present-day counties of De qing county and Feng kai 封開, in Hu nan. In 1912, the *zhou* became De qing county. Mentioned with 212.

De shun jun 德順軍 [1]

Name of a regional administration, an army. It was established by Northern Song 宋, in 1043. The seat of administration was in present-day Long de 隆德 county in Ning Xia 寧夏. The area administered comprised the two counties of Long De and Xi ji 西吉 in Ning xia, and Jing ning 靜寧 county in Gan su 甘肅. In 1093, the administrative seat was moved to present-day Jing ning county. In 1142, under Jin 金, the area became De shun zhou 德順州. Mentioned with 816.

Deng 鄧 [3]

Name of a *zhou* 州. See Deng zhou 鄧州. Mentioned with 1005, 1238, 1459.

Deng 登 [1 + 7]

□ Abbreviation for Deng zhou fu 登州府. [1] The *fu* 府 was established in 1376. The seat of administration was in present-day Peng lai 蓬萊 city in Shan dong 山東. The area administered comprised the region extending in present-day Shan dong from the cities and counties of Long kou 龍口, Zhao yuan 招遠, Lai xi 萊西 and Hai yang 海陽 towards the East. It was abolished in 1913. Mentioned with 608.

□ Name of a *zhou* 州. [7] See → Deng zhou 登州. Mentioned with 393, 614, 703, 819, 1027, 1205, 1330.

Deng zhou 登州 [4]

Name of a *zhou* 州. It was established, under the Tang 唐, in 692. The seat of administration was in present-day Ning hai 寧海 town located southeast of Yan tai 煙臺 city in Shan dong 山東. The territory administered comprised the area reaching in present-day Shan dong from Long kou 龍口, Qi xia 栖霞, and Ru shan 乳山 towards the East. In 707, the administration of the *zhou* was moved to Peng lai 蓬萊 city in Shan dong. In 742, the *zhou* was changed to Dong mou 東牟 commandery but, in 758, it again became Deng zhou. Under the Ming 明, in 1376, the status of Deng zhou was raised to Deng zhou fu 登州府. Mentioned with 392, 403, 412, 535.

Deng zhou 鄧州 [7]

Name of a *zhou*. It was founded under Sui 隋, in 587. The seat of administration was in present-day Deng zhou 鄧州 city in He nan 河南. The territory administered comprised the present-day cities of Deng zhou and Nan yang 南陽 in He nan and the counties of Nan yang, Xin ye 新野, Nei xiang 内鄉, Xi xia 西峽, Xi chuan 淅川, Zhen ping 鎮平 and Nan zhao 南召. At the beginning of the *da ye* 大業 reign period (605 – 618) of Sui, it became a commandery but, in 758, the area again became Deng zhou. In 1913, Deng zhou became Deng 鄧 county. Mentioned with 29, 202, 270, 285, 575, 1379.

Deng zhou dao 登州島 [1]

Name of an island. Reference is to an island in the Miao 廟 island group of Shan dong 山東. Mentioned with 632.

Di 氐 [1]

Name of an ancient people. It lived in the border areas of the present provinces of Shaan xi 陝西, Gan su 甘肅 and Si chuan 四川. Mentioned with 298.

Di hu 氐胡 [1]

Name of an ancient people. See → Di 氐. Mentioned with 1433.

Di qiang 氐羌 [1]

Name of a minority people of early times. The name is a combination of that of the → Di 氐 and the Qiang 羌. The groups in question occupied the southern part of present-day Gan su 甘肅. Mentioned with 1307.

Dian 滇 [9]

Name of an ancient country. It was located in the middle part of present-day Yun nan 雲南, in an area near Lake Dian 滇. Its capital was located near present-day Jin cheng 晉城, 32 *li* northeast of Jin ning 晉寧 county in Yun nan. Mentioned with 160, 243, 362, 530, 541, 1339, 1375, 1475.

Dian cang shan 點蒼山 [1]

Name of a mountain. It is located in Yun yang 雲陽 county in Chong qing 重慶. Mentioned with 1069.

Dian guang 滇廣 [1]
Combinded name of a region. Reference is to Yun nan 雲南, Guang xi 廣西 and Guang dong 廣東 as well as the Hai nan 海南 area. Mentioned with 1486.

Dian nan 滇南 [11]
Regional name. It refers to the "southern part of Dian," i.e., Yun nan 雲南. Mentioned with 106, 160, 187, 362, 480, 585, 726, 1102, 1264, 1386.

Ding 鼎 [4]
Name of a *zhou* 州. See → Ding zhou 鼎州. Mentioned with 348, 616, 644, 665.

Ding hai 定海 [1]
Name of a county. It was established under Northern Song 宋. The seat of administration was in the present-day Zhen hai 鎮海 district of Ning bo 寧波 city in Zhe jiang 浙江. In 1687, Ding hai county became Zhen hai county. Mentioned with 319.

Ding ling guo 丁零國 [1]
Name of an ancient country. It was located near present-day Lake Baikal, Russia. Mentioned with 215.

Ding zhou 鼎州 [6]
Name of a *zhou* 州. It was founded under Northern Song 宋, in 1012. The seat of administration was in present-day Chang de 常德 city in Hu nan 湖南, and the area administered comprised the cities and counties of Chang de, Han shou 漢壽, Yuan Jiang 沅江 and Tao yuan 桃源 in Hu nan. In 1165, under Southern Song, its status was raised to Chang de fu 常德府. Mentioned with 188, 768, 783, 1049, 1134, 1448.

Ding zhou 定州 [4]
Name of a *zhou* 州. It was established under Northern Wei 魏, in 400. The seat of administration was in the present-day Ding zhou 定州 city in He bei 河北. Its administrative territory comprised an area extending in present-day He bei from Man cheng 滿城 county in the North, to An guo 安國 city and Rao yang 饒陽 county in the East, and to Jing xing 井陘 county as well as the two cities of Gao cheng 藁城 and Xin ji 辛集 in the South. Afterwards, the area of the *zhou* was gradually reduced and, during the *da ye* 大業 reign period (605 – 618) of Sui 隋 and the *tian bao* 天寶 reign period (742 – 758) of Tang 唐, it periodically became a commandery, but again became Ding zhou after 758. In 1113, the status of the area was promoted to Zhong shan fu 中山府, but became Ding zhou again at the beginning of Ming 明. In 1913, Ding zhou became Ding 定 county. Mentioned with 24, 157.

Dong 東 [9]
Regional name. It refers to the "eastern part" of China. Mentioned with 137, 638, 713, 789, 832, 860, 1122, 1312, 1316.

Dong bei 東北 [1]
Regional name. It refers to the "northeastern part" of China. Mentioned with 1375.

Dong bei hu 東北胡 [1]
Regional indication used to refer to "Hu 胡 minority peoples of the northeast." Mentioned with 1381.

Dong bei yi 東北夷 [1]
Regional indication used to refer to "Yi 夷 minority peoples of the northeast." Mentioned with 1351.

Dong chuan 東川 [1 + 1 +1]
□ Name of a Tang 唐 period regional garrison. [1] It was founded in 757. The seat of administration was the present-day San tai 三台 county in Si chuan 四川. The area administered covered a territory extending from the Fu jiang 涪江 watershed in the central part of the present Si chuan basin in the East, to the lower water basin of the Tuo jiang 沱江 in the West, and the area of Jian ge 劍閣 and Qing chuan 青川. During 763 – 779, the area was briefly combined with Jian nan 劍南 and Xi chuan 西川. At the end of Tang, it was annexed by Wang Jian 王建 (767 – 830). Mentioned with 1091.
□ Name of a *fu* 府. [1] It was established in 1382. The territory of administration comprised the two present-day counties of Hui ze 會澤 and Qiao jia 巧家 in Yun nan 雲南, and the Dong chuan 東川 district in Kun ming 昆明 city. In 1384, the *fu* became a Tribal Office, *jun min fu* 軍民府, and it was administered at the foot of Ma an 馬鞍 mountain, located 10 *li* southwest of Hui ze county. Later, the seat of administration was moved to present-day Hui ze county. The *fu* was abolished in 1913. Mentioned with 768.
□ Name of a region. [1] The location is uncertain.

Dong dao 東道 [1]
Name of region. It refers generally to the east of China. Mentioned with 272.

Dong du 東都 [2]
The term "Eastern capital" was used in reference to Luo yang 洛陽. Mentioned with 268, 634.

Dong e 東阿 [3]
Name of a county. See → Dong e xian 東阿縣. Mentioned with 268, 269.

Dong e xian 東阿縣 [3]
Name of a county. It was established by Qin 秦. The seat of administration was in E cheng 阿城 town located 25 *li* east of present-day Yang gu 陽谷 county in Shan dong 山東. The county was eliminated in 457, under Liu Song 劉宋, but reestablished under Northern Wei 魏. Later, the center of administration was moved several times. In 1373, under the Ming 明, the seat of administration was moved to Dong e 東阿 town, southeast of the present Ping yin 平陰 county. In 1949, the administration was moved to the present-day Tong cheng 銅城 town in Dong e county. Mentioned with 268, 269.

Dong fang 東方 [10]
Regional name. It refers generally to the "eastern section" of China. Mentioned with 93, 113, 634, 702, 867, 948, 1057, 1292, 1538.

Dong guan xian 東莞縣 [1]

Name of a county. It was established under Western Han 漢. The seat of administration was in present-day Yi shui 沂水 county in Shan dong 山東. During Eastern Jin 晉, the administration was moved to present-day Cheng zi 城子, northeast of Yi shui county and, under Liu Song 劉宋, it was moved to Ju 莒 county. At the beginning of Sui 隋, the name of the county was changed to Dong an 東安 county. Mentioned with 1521.

Dong hai 東海 [32 + 4 + 4 + 2 + 1]

□ Name of an ocean. [32]. From Qin 秦 and Han 漢 times on, the term was used to designate a combination of the present-day Huang hai 黃海, "Yellow Sea," and the Dong hai, "East China See." Mentioned with 26, 80, 226, 392, 393, 402, 412, 413, 471, 606, 608, 729, 790, 824, 998, 1024, 1030, 1057, 1134, 1205, 1223, 1261, 1278, 1402, 1414, 1438.

□ Name of an ocean. [4] From Ming 明 times on, the term corresponded to the present-day Dong hai, "East China Sea." Mentioned with 316, 408, 1279, 1525.

□ Legendary place name. [4] Further details are unavailable. Mentioned with 1009, 1141, 1140, 1230.

□ Name of a commandery. [2] See Dong hai jun 東海郡. Mentioned with 790, 975.

□ Name of a county established by Northern Qi 齊. [1] The seat of administration was in present-day Nan cheng 南城 town, located southeast of Lian yun gang 連雲港 city in Jiang su 江蘇. It was eliminated at the beginning of the *kai huang* 開皇 reign period (581 – 600) of Sui 隋, but later reestablished under that dynasty before being finally eliminated in 1283, under the Yuan 元. Mentioned with 693.

Dong hai dao 東海島 [1 + 1]

□ Legendary place name. [1] Further details are unavailable. Mentioned with 1032.

□ Name of an "island in the East China Sea." [1] It is located southeast of Zhan jiang 湛江 city in Guang dong 廣東. Mentioned with 691.

Dong hai jun 東海郡 [1]

Name of a commandery. It was established by Qin 秦. The seat of administration was in present-day Tan cheng 郯城 county in Shan dong 山東. The area administered comprised a region extending in present-day Shan dong from Fei 費 county, Lin yi 臨沂 city, and in Jiang su from Gan yu 贛榆 in the North, to Zao zhuang 棗莊 city in Shan dong, and Pi 邳 county in Jiang su in the West, and, also in Jiang su, to Su qian 宿遷 and Guan nan 灌南 in the South. After Eastern Han 漢, the area came under Xu zhou 徐州 and was reduced in size. During Southern Qi 齊, the seat of administration was moved to present-day Lian shui 漣水 county in Jiang su. Later, the name was changed to Bei dong hai 北東海 commandery. Mentioned with 1030.

Dong hai zhu dao 東海諸島 [1]

Regional place name. The reference is to the islands in the Yellow Sea and East China Sea. Mentioned with 908.

Dong hu 東胡 [1]
Name for an ethnic group. They lived at the Lao ha 老哈 river and the Xi la mu lun 西拉木倫 river (i.e., Xar Moron He), at the upper watershed of present-day Xi liao 西遼 (or: Western Liao) river. Mentioned with 72.

Dong jian 東間 [13]
A vague regional reference to the "eastern part" of China. Mentioned with 64, 129, 317, 616, 639, 740, 781, 823, 867, 879, 1008, 1038, 1241.

Dong jing 東京 [1 + 1]
□ [1] Reference is to the "Eastern Capital," in this case to the Tang 唐 period capital of Luo Yang 洛陽, the city of the same name today in He nan 河南. Mentioned with 341.
□ [1] Reference is to the "Eastern Capital," in this case to the Northern Song 宋 capital of Kai feng 開封, the present city of the same name in He nan 河南. Mentioned with 1083.

Dong jing 東境 [3]
This is a general regional designation used by the BCGM authors in reference to "eastern boundaries", in this case the eastern part of China. Mentioned with 208, 1063, 1485.

Dong jun 東郡 [1]
Name of a commandery. It was established, in Warring States times under Qin 秦, in 242 BCE. The seat of administration was in Gu xian 故縣 village, located 16 *li* southwest of present-day Pu yang 濮陽 county in He nan 河南. During Western Han 漢, its administrative territory comprised an area extending in present-day Shan dong 山東 from Dong e 東阿 and Liang shan 梁山 toward the West, from Yun cheng 鄆城 in Shan dong and Fan xian 范縣 county in He nan toward the North, and from Chi ping 茌平 and Shen 莘 county in Shan dong, and from Nan le 南樂, Qing feng 清豐 and Pu yang 濮陽 in He nan toward the South. After Eastern Han, its jurisdiction was reduced. From the Three Kingdoms on, sometimes the commandery existed, but sometimes it did not. Under Northern Wei 魏, the administration was moved to present-day Cheng guan 城關 town, southeast of Hua 滑 county in He nan. In 589, the commandery was eliminated but shortly thereafter, at the beginning of the *da ye* 大業 reign period (605 – 618), it was reestablished. At the beginning of Tang 唐, the commandery became Hua zhou 滑州. Mentioned with 1227.

Dong lai 東萊 [3]
Name of a commandery. It was established during the reign of Han emperor Gao zu (ruled 202 – 195). The seat of administration was in present-day Dong lai city in Shan dong 山東. The territory administered comprised an area on the east of the Jiao lai 膠萊 river in present-day Shan dong, the area north of Qu yu 嶇嵎 mountain, and the region east of Ru shan 乳山 river. Eastern Han moved the seat of administration to a point southeast of present-day Long kou 龍口 city in Shan dong. Western Jin 晉 turned the commandery into Dong lai country, Dong lai guo 東萊國, and returned the administration to the present-day Lai zhou 萊

州 city. Under Liu Song 劉宋, Dong lai again became a commandery, and the administration was moved to a point 60 *li* northeast of Lai zhou city in Shan dong. Under Northern Wei 魏, it was returned again to Lai zhou city. The commandery was abolished at the beginning of the reign period *kai huang* 開皇 (581 – 600) Sui 隋, but soon revived at the beginning of the reign period *da ye* 大業 (605 – 618). In 621, Tang 唐 turned it into Lai zhou but later, at the beginning of the reign period *tian bao* 天寶 (742 – 756), it became Dong lai commandery and then, at the beginning of the reign period *qian yuan* 乾元 (758 – 760), Lai zhou again. Mentioned with 84, 474.

Dong nan 東南 [11]
Regional name referring to "southeast" China. Mentioned with 298, 305, 362, 503, 518, 723, 724, 861, 986, 1339.

Dong nan hai 東南海 [8]
Regional name. It generally refers to present-day East China Sea and the "Southern Sea" in South-East Asia. Mentioned with 198, 351, 630, 684, 703, 1024, 1046, 1506.

Dong nan hai wai 東南海外 [1]
Possibly mythological place name from the *Shan hai jing* 山海經, "Classic of Mountains and Seas." Further details are unavailable. Mentioned with 293.

Dong nan zhou jun 東南州郡 [1]
Regional name used by the BCGM authors in reference to the "*zhou* 州 and commanderies of the Southeast" of China. Mentioned with 1410.

Dong nan zhu jun 東南諸郡 [1]
Regional name, general referring to the "various commandaries of the southeast" of China. Mentioned with 160.

Dong ping 東平 [1]
Name of a *zhou* 州. It was established by the Ming 明, in 1374. The seat of administration was in Zhou cheng 州城 town located southwest of present-day Dong ping county in Shan dong 山東. Territories administered encompassed the present-day counties of Dong ping, Wen shang 汶上, Dong e 東阿, Ping yin 平陰, Yang gu 陽谷 and Liang shan 梁山 in Shan dong. In 1913, the *zhou* became Dong ping county. Mentioned with 1087.

Dong ping jun 東平郡 [1]
Name of a commandery. It was established at the beginning of the Sui 隋, in the *da ye* 大業 reign period (605 – 618). The seat of administration was at a point 16 *li* east of present-day Yun cheng 鄆城 county in Shan dong 山東. The territory administered comprised the present-day counties of Yun cheng, Jue ye 巨野 and Juan cheng 鄄城 in Shan dong. At the beginning of the *wu de* 武德 reign period (618 – 628) of the Tang 唐, the commandery became Yun zhou 鄆州 and, in 634, the seat of administration was moved to a point northwest of present-day Dong ping 東平 county in Shan dong. In 742, the *zhou* 州 became Dong ping commandery but, in 758, it again became Yun zhou. Mentioned with 268.

Dong shan 東山 [8]
This is a general reference to the "eastern mountains" of China but cannot be determined more closely. Mentioned with 107, 345, 376, 1033, 1105, 1111, 1122, 1509.

Dong ting 洞庭 [2]
Name of a lake. It is located in the northern part of present-day Hu nan 湖南. Mentioned with 67, 573.

Dong ting shan 洞庭山 [1]
Name of a mountain. It is in the middle of Tai hu 太湖 lake west of present-day Su zhou 蘇州 city in Jiang su 江蘇. Actually there are two mountains, an eastern and a western one. Mentioned with 323.

Dong tu 東土 [3]
Name for the central plain of ancient China, identified as "eastern land" from the perspective of the West. Mentioned with 495, 822, 1306.

Dong wu 東吳 [1]
Special regional name. It refers to the entire basin of the present-day Tai hu 太湖 lake. Mentioned with 1036.

Dong wu 東武 [1]
Name of a county. It was established under Western Han 漢. The seat of administration was in present-day Zhu cheng 諸城 city in Shan dong 山東. In 598, Dong wu county became Zhu cheng 諸城 county. Mentioned with 481.

Dong wu cheng 東武城 [1]
Name of a county. It was established under Western Han 漢. The seat of administration was at a point northeast of present-day Qing he 清河 county in He bei 河北. During the reign period *tai kang* 太康 (280 – 289) of Western Jin 晉, it became Wu cheng 武城 county. Mentioned with 111.

Dong xi jing 東西京 [1]
Combined designation of two capital cities, referring to the "eastern and western capitals" of Tang 唐 times, i.e., Chang an 長安 and Luo yang 洛陽. Mentioned with 423.

Dong yang 東陽 [4 + 3 + 2 +3]
□ Name of a county. [4] It was established by Qin 秦. The seat of administration was in present-day Dong yang cheng 東陽城 located 33 km southeast of Xu yi 盱眙 county in Jiang su 江蘇. It was abolished under Southern Dynasties' Chen 陳. Mentioned with 456, 1032, 1311, 1438.
□ Name of a county. [3] It was established under the Tang 唐, in 686. Its seat of administration was in present-day Dong yang city in Zhe jiang 浙江. Its name became Dong chang 東場 county under Liang 梁 of the Five Dynasties. At the beginning of Northern Song 宋, the old name was restored. In 1988, it became a city with county rank. Lu He 盧和, the Ming 明 era author of the *Shi wu ben cao* 食物本草, *Materia medica of Foodstuffs*, came from Dong yang. Mentioned with 1343.
□ Name of a commandery. [2] It was established, under Three Kingdoms' Wu 吳, in 266. The seat of administration was in present-day Jin hua 金華 city in Zhe

jiang 浙江. The territory administered comprised the area along the Jin hua jiang 金華江 and the various present-day counties and cities of the Qu jiang 衢江 basin. In 562, under Southern Dynasties' Chen 陳, the name of the commandery was changed to Jin hua commandery. At the beginning of the reign period *da ye* 大業 (605 – 615) of the Sui 隋, and during the reign periods *tian bao* 天寶 (742 – 756) and *zhi de* 至德 (756 – 758) of Tang 唐, Wu zhou 婺州 periodically was changed to be Dong yang commandery. Its administrative area was reduced. In 758, this Dong yang commandery became Wu zhou again. Mentioned with 292, 298.

□ Designation of a commandery that during Song 宋 times was just a name. [3] During Sui 隋 and Tang 隋, present-day Jin hua 金華 city in Zhe jiang 浙江 was established as Dong yang commandery. During Song, there were no commanderies any more, but the old name was still used to designate the area. Later dynasties continued the practice. Mentioned with 241, 456.

Dong yi 東夷 [3]

General name used in reference to the "Yi 夷 peoples living to the east" of the Chinese central plain, predominately in present-day Shan dong 山東. Mentioned with 404, 535, 817.

Dong yue 東嶽 [1]

Name of a mountain, that is, the Tai shan 泰山, located north of present-day Tai an 泰安 city in Shan dong 山東. Mentioned with 1157.

Dou 竇 [2]

Name of a *zhou* 州. It was established in 634. The seat of administration was in Zhen long 鎮隆 town, located southwest of present-day Xin yi 信宜 county in Guang dong 廣東. The territory administered comprised the present Xin yi county. The *zhou* was abolished under Northern Song 宋, in 1071. Mentioned with 144.

Dou cheng 都城 [1]

Reference to a capital city. In this case, to Bian jing 汴京, the capital of Northern Song 宋. This is present-day Kai feng 開封 city. Mentioned with 1532.

Dou guang 都廣 [1]

Name of an ancient country located in the south. Mentioned with 1469.

Dou kun guo 都昆國 [1]

Name of an ancient country. According to one tradition, it was located in the northeastern part of the Indonesian island Sumatra. Another tradition locates it on the southern part of the Malayan peninsula. Mentioned with 1031.

Dou liang 都梁 [1 + 2]

□ Name of a small place. [1] It was located at the foot of Dou liang mountain, 5 *li* east of present-day Xu yi 盱眙 county in Jiang su 江蘇.

□ Name of a mountain. [2] It is located northeast of present-day Wu gang 武岡 city in Hu nan 湖南. Mentioned with 616.

Dou liang shan 都梁山 [1]
Name of a mountain. It is located south of present-day Xu yi 盱眙縣 county in Jiang su 江蘇. Mentioned with 616.

Dou qu guo 兜渠國 [1]
Legendary country. Details are unavailable. Mentioned with 244.

Dou xia 都下 [4 + 1 + 1 + 1]
□ Reference to the capital. [4] In this case, the Northern Song 宋 capital of Kai feng 開封, the present-day city of that name in He nan 河南. Mentioned with 134, 322, 655.
□ Term for the capital city. [1] In this case, the term refers to the Jin 金 dynasty capital of Zhong du 中都, located near present-day Bei jing 北京 city.
□ Term for the capital city. [1] In this case, the capital was Jian kang 建康, the capital of the Southern Dynasties' Liang 梁 dynasty. This is present-day Nan jing 南京 city in Jiang su 江蘇. Mentioned with 338.
□ Term for the capital city. [1] In this case, the reference is to the Eastern Han 漢 capital of Luo yang 洛陽, the present-day city of that name in He nan 河南. Mentioned with 1340.

Dou xiang 都鄉 [1]
This is the name for a feudal country. It was established under Western Han 漢. The seat of administration was at a point in the West of present-day He bei 河北. Under Eastern Han, it was subordinated to the country of Chang shan 常山, but later it was abolished. Mentioned with 787.

Du shuo shan 度朔山 [1]
Name of a legendary mountain. Its exact location is unknown. Mentioned with 1141.

Duan zhou 端州 [1]
Name of a *zhou* 州. It was established in 589. The seat of administration was in present-day Zhao qing 肇慶 city in Guang dong 廣東. The territory administered comprised the three cities of Zhao qing, Yun fu 雲浮 and Gao yao 高要, the Gao ming 高明 district in Fo shan 佛山 and the two counties of De qing 德慶 and Xin xing 新興, all in Guang dong. It was changed to Xin an 信安 commandery in 607. It became Duan zhou again in 621, but with a reduced administrative area, corresponding to three present-day cities of Zhao qing, Gao yao and Gao ming in Guang dong. In 742, the area became Gao yao commandery. In 758, it became Duan zhou again. Under Northern Song 宋, in 1118, the *zhou* was promoted to Zhao qing fu 肇慶府. Mentioned with 1358.

Dun huang 敦煌 [5 + 1]
□ Name of a commandery. [5] It was established, under Western Han 漢, in 111 BCE. The seat of administration was at a point west of present-day Dun huang city in Gan su 甘肅. The territory administered comprised the area west and south of the Shu le 疏勒 river in Gan su. The commandery was eliminated under Sui 隋, in 583, but reestablished under Tang 唐, in 607. In 619, it became Gua zhou 瓜州 and, in 622, Xi sha zhou 西沙州. In 633, it became Sha zhou 沙州 but,

in 742, it became Dun huang commandery again. In 758, it was again changed to Sha zhou. Mentioned with 1149, 1307, 1335.
□ Dun huang city. [1] Mentioned with 861.

Dun huang shan 敦煌山 [1]
See → Dun huang 敦煌. Mentioned with 1307.

Dun xun guo 頓遜國 [2]
Name of an ancient country, located near Tanintharyi at the southern tip of Myanmar. Mentioned with 489, 1355.

-E-

E 阿 [1]
Name of an early city first mentioned in the *Shi ji* 史記, "Records of the Historian." The site is now E cheng 阿城 town, located 25 km east of Yang gu 陽谷 county in Shan dong 山東.

E 鄂 [1]
Name of a *zhou* 州. See → E zhou 鄂州. Mentioned with 1145.

E jing 阿井 [3]
Name of a well. During Han 漢 and Jin 晉 times, the well was in Dong e xian 東阿縣 city, the ruins of which are found in present-day E cheng 阿城 town, 25 km east of Yang gu 陽谷 county in Shan dong 山東. The waters of the well were known for their clarity and sweetness and they were used to process *E jiao* 阿膠, ass-hide glue. Mentioned with 268.

E mei 峨眉 [2]
Name of a mountain. See → E mei shan 峨眉山. Mentioned with 90, 859.

E mei 峨嵋 [1]
Name of a mountain. See E mei shan → 峨嵋山. Mentioned with 501.

E mei shan 峨眉山 [4]
Name of a mountain. This is written also E mei shan 峨嵋山. The mountain is the E mei shan 峨眉山 located 30 *li* southwest of the present-day E mei shan 峨眉山 city in Si chuan 四川, and is one of the four famous mountains associated with Buddhism. Mentioned with 20, 774, 859, 1018.

E mei shan 峨嵋山 [2]
Name of a mountain. See E mei shan → 峨眉山. Mentioned with 1042, 1325.

E xian cheng 阿縣城 [1]
Name of a city. The county in which this city is found is Dong e xian 東阿縣, "Dong e county," not E xian 阿縣, "E county," as cited incorrectly by Su Song 蘇頌 (1020 – 1101) in whose text the character *dong* 東 has been omitted. A county simply designated as E xian never existed. The E jing well and Dong e xian county were located within the confines of Northern Song Yun zhou 鄆州 in present-day Shan dong 山東, E xian cheng city was administered from pres-

ent-day Da ji cheng 大吉城, located west of Ping yin 平陰 county in Shan dong. Mentioned with 268.

E zhou 鄂州 [1]
Name of a *zhou*. It was established in 589. The seat of administration was in the present-day Wu chang 武昌 district of Wu han 武漢 city in Hu bei 湖北. The territory administered comprised an area extending from present-day Chi bi 赤壁 city in the West, Yang xin 陽新 county in the East, and the Yang zi in the North, to Mu fu 幕阜 mountain in the South. The area became E zhou lu 鄂州路 in 1277. Mentioned with 122.

E zhu 鄂渚 [2]
Name of a sand island. It is situated in the part of the Yang zi west of the Wu chang 武昌 district of Wu han 武漢 city in Hu bei 湖北. Mentioned with 823, 1253.

En zhou 恩州 [4]
Name of a *zhou* 州. It was established in 649. The seat of administration was at a point 20 *li* north of present-day En ping 恩平 city in Guang dong 廣東. The area administered comprised the two present-day cities of En ping and Yang jiang 陽江 in Guang dong. In 891, the seat of administration was moved to the present-day Yang jiang city. In 1048, the *zhou* was changed to Nan en zhou 南恩州. Mentioned with 162, 428, 488, 1437.

Er chuan 二川 [2]
Regional name. See → Liang chuan 兩川. Mentioned with 1274, 1407.

Er guang 二廣 [6]
Regional name. See → Liang guang 兩廣. Mentioned with 9, 330, 362, 367, 674.

Er mao shan 二茅山 [1]
Name of a mountain. This may be a reference to the Mao shan 茅山 mountain located 60 *li* north of present-day Qi chun 蕲春 county in Hu bei 湖北. Mentioned with 1351.

Er zhe 二浙 [4]
Combined regional name. See → Liang zhe 兩浙. Mentioned with 14, 129, 364, 1038.

-F-

Fa xing si 法性寺 [1]
Name of a Zen monastery. It is present-day Guang xiao 光孝 temple located in the northwestern part of Guang zhou 廣州.

Fan 番 [16]
General reference to "foreign regions." Mentioned with 146, 226, 286, 511, 675, 886, 1139, 1140, 1145, 1246, 1252, 1272, 1369.

Fan 梵 [1]
The name refers generally to ancient northern India. It is believed to be a transcription of Sanskrit Brahma. Mentioned with 804.

Fan dong 番峒 [1]
Name of a border region. The term refers to the area occupied by the minority peoples of present-day Nan dan 南丹 county in Guang xi 廣西. Mentioned with 951.

Fan gong quan 范公泉 [1]
Name of a spring. This is now Zhen zhu 珍珠 springs, located east of Bo shan cheng 博山城 in Zi bo 淄博 city in Shan dong 山東. Mentioned with 269.

Fan guo 番國 [2]
General reference to "foreign regions." Mentioned with 585, 1555.

Fan he xian 番禾縣 [1]
Name of a county. It was founded, by renaming Fan he 番和 county, in 619. The seat of administration was in present-day Shui zhai 水寨 city, located two *li* south of Shui mo guan 水磨關, which is 20 *li* west of Yong chang 永昌 county (more popularly known as Bai hu 白虎 city) in Gan su. In 744, Fan he xian was changed to Tian bao 天寶 county. Mentioned with 1037.

Fan shan 樊山 [1]
Name of a mountain. It is located west of present-day E zhou 鄂州 in Hu bei 湖北. Mentioned with 768.

Fan shan 礬山 [1]
Name of a mountain. It is located east of the Wu chang 武昌 district of the present-day Wu han 武漢 city in Hu bei 湖北. Mentioned with 1521.

Fan shui 泛水 [1]
Name of a river. It may be located at Xiang yang 襄陽 city in Hu bei 湖北, but this is uncertain. Mentioned with 666.

Fan yang 范陽 [1]
Name of a commandery. It was established under Three Kingdoms' Wei 魏, by changing the name of Zhuo 涿 commandery, in 226. The seat of administration was in present-day Zhuo zhou 涿州 city in He bei 河北. The territory administered comprised the area in present-day He bei extending from the Tai hang 太行 mountain range in the West, to Yong qing 永清 in the East, and from Ba zhou 霸州, Bao ding 保定, and Zi jing guan 紫荊關 in the South to the Fang shan 房山 district of present-day Bei jing 北京 city in the North. Under Western Jin 晉, the area became Fan yang county. Afterwards, under Later Zhao 趙 of the 16 Dynasties, it again became Fan yang commandery but its administrative domains were reduced. The commandery was abolished, under the Sui 隋, at the beginning of the *kai huang* 開皇 reign period (581 – 600). Mentioned with 635.

Fan zhong 番中 [1]
General reference to foreign areas. Mentioned with 680.

Fang 坊 [1]
Name of a *zhou* 州. It was established in 619. The seat of administration was at a point southeast of present-day Huang ling 黃陵 county in Shaan xi 陝西. The territory administered comprised the two counties of Huang ling and Yi jun 宜君 in Shaan xi. It was abolished in 1269. Mentioned with 1462.

Fang 房 [5]
Name of a *zhou* 州. See → Fang zhou 房州. Mentioned with 107, 503, 654, 1265.

Fang lin yuan 芳林苑 [2]
Name of a park. It was located in an area of the present-day eastern route of Xiao ying 小營, located south of the Tai ping 太平 gate of Nan jing city in Jiang su 江蘇. Originally, it was the old residence of Xiao Daocheng 蕭道成 (427 – 482). After Southern Qi 齊 was established, it became Qing xi 清溪 palace. In 483, the area was rebuilt as a park and the Tai chang ling he 太昌靈和 hall and other buildings were built. This was a favorite place for the emperors to hold ceremonies and to banquet. The Liang 梁 dynasty gave the park to Xiao Wei 蕭偉 (476 – 533), the Minister Prince of Nan ping 南平, Nan ping xiang wang 南平襄王. Under him, the fruits and trees became exceptional and extravagant. Later the park was abolished. Mentioned with 376.

Fang ling 房陵 [4]
Name of a county. See → Fang ling xian 房陵縣. Mentioned with 295, 634, 1147, 1523.

Fang ling xian 房陵縣 [1]
Name of a county. It was established by the Qin 秦. The seat of administration was in present-day Fang 房 county in Hu bei 湖北. At the end of Eastern Han 漢, it was put administratively under Fang ling 房陵 commandery. Under Wei 魏 of the Three Kingdoms, the administration was moved to Xin cheng 新城 commandery. In 563, under Northern Zhou 周, the name of the county was changed to Guang qian 光遷 county. In 636, under Tang 唐, the county again became Fang ling, and was administered from Fang zhou 房州. Under Ming 明, in 1377, it was abolished and combined with Fang zhou. Mentioned with 1147.

Fang shan 方山 [3 + 1]
□ Name of a mountain. [3] There are 33 mountains by this name in the *Da ming yi tong zhi* 大明一統志, "Comprehensive Gazetteer of the Great Ming 明," and 58 in the *Jia qing chong xiu yi tong zhi* 嘉慶重修一統志, "Comprehensive Gazetteer Revised during the Jia qing 嘉慶 era." During the time of Tao Hongjing 陶弘景 (456 – 536), the most famous Fang shan was located near the then capital at Jian kang 建康. This was located southeast of the Jiang ning 江寧 district of present-day Nan jing city in Jiang su 江蘇, near Mao 茅 mountain where Tao Hongjing lived. Maybe this is the Fang shan referred to in the *Ming yi bie lu*, "Further Records of Renowned Physicians." Mentioned with 274, 889.
□ Name of a mountain. [1] It is Wu hu 五虎 mountain, located southeast of Min hou 閩侯 county in present-day Fu jian 福建. Mentioned with 768.

Fang tai shan 方臺山 [1]
Name of a mountain. It is Shi zi 獅子 mountain, located northeast of present-day Hua rong 華容 county in Hu nan 湖南. Mentioned with 1430.

Fang zhou 房州 [4]
Name of a *zhou* 州. It was established under Sui 隋, in 598. The seat of administration was in the present-day Zhu shan 竹山 county in Hu bei 湖北. The territory administered comprised the present-day counties of Fang xian 房縣, Zhu shan, Zhu xi 竹溪, and Bao kang 保康, and the northern areas of Shen nong jia lin 神農架林 district. At the beginning of the *da ye* 大業 reign period (605 – 616) of the Sui, it was eliminated but, in 618, under Tang 唐, it was again reestablished after some restructuring. As before, it was administered from Zhu shan county. In 636, the administrative seat was moved to Fang ling 房陵 county. Under Southern Song 宋, there were many administrative changes, but Yuan 元 changed it back to be Fang ling county. In 1377, the area became Fang 房 county. Mentioned with 130, 290, 629, 1063.

Fei niao shan 飛鳥山 [1]
Name of a mountain. It is located southwest of present-day Wu shan 巫山 county of Chong qing 重慶. Mentioned with 907.

Fen 汾 [4]
Name of a *zhou* 州. See → Fen zhou 汾州. Mentioned with 484, 816, 1017, 1242.

Fen liu shan 分流山 [1]
Name of a mountain. The mountain is located in the Chang cheng ling 長城嶺 mountain range, 38 km south of present-day Hong jia lou 洪家樓 town of the Li cheng 歷城 district of Ji nan 濟南 city in Shan dong 山東. The rivers originating from the mountain flow to Tai an 泰安 in the south and Ji nan 濟南 in the north, thus the name of the mountain ("dividing streams of waters mountain"). Mentioned with 1301.

Fen zhou 汾州 [3]
Name of a *zhou* 州. It was established by Tang 唐, by changing the name of Hao zhou 浩州, in 620. The seat of administration was in the present Fen yang 汾陽 county. In 742, Fen zhou became Xi he 西河 commandery, but again became Fen zhou in 758. In 1595, under the Ming 明, Fen zhou was promoted to Fen zhou fu 汾州府. Mentioned with 499, 693, 1032.

Feng 鳳 [1 + 1]
□ Name of a county. [1] It was established, by demoting Feng zhou 鳳州, in 1374. The seat of administration was in present-day Feng zhou town northeast of Feng xian 鳳縣 in Shaan xi 陝西. In 1950, the administrative seat was moved to Shuang shi pu 雙石鋪, the present county capital. Mentioned with 368.
□ Name of a *zhou* 州. [1] See → Feng zhou 鳳州. Mentioned with 908.

Feng 風 [1]
This is an error for Feng 鳳. See → Feng zhou 鳳州. Mentioned with 1445.

Feng cheng 豐城 [3]

Name of a county. It was founded, by changing the name of Fu cheng 富城 county, in 280. The seat of administration was in present-day Rong tang 榮塘, located west of the Feng shui 豐水, 41 *li* south of Feng cheng 豐城 city in Jiang xi 江西. The county was eliminated under Sui 隋 but then reestablished in 602. It was eliminated again in 617 but reestablished in 622. At the beginning of the *yong hui* 永徽 reign period (650 – 665), the seat of administration was moved to present-day Feng cheng city. Later, during 904 – 907, at the end of Tang 唐, the name was changed to Wu gao 吳皋 county. Under Southern Tang of the Five Dynasties, the county was again named Feng cheng. In 1286, its status was raised to be Fu zhou 富州. In 1369, the area again became Feng cheng county. In 1988, Feng cheng city was established. Mentioned with 578, 856, 1051.

Feng gao 奉高 [4]

Name of a county. It was established under Western Han 漢, and administered by Tai shan 泰山 commandery. Its seat of administration was at Gu xian cun 故縣村, located 38 *li* east of present-day Tai an 泰安 city in Shan dong 山東. Under Northern Qi 齊, the county was abolished and its territory was combined with Dai shan county. In 583, the name of Dai shan county was changed to Feng gao county. The seat of administration was at a point 70 *li* southeast of the present Tai an city. In 586, it became Dai shan county again. Mentioned with 620, 1157.

Feng hua xian 奉化縣 [1]

Name of a county. It was established under Tang 唐, in 738, by splitting Mao 鄮 county. The seat of administration was in present-day Feng hua 奉化 city in Zhe jiang 浙江. In 1295, the county was changed to Feng hua zhou 奉化州. Under the Ming 明, in 1387, it was renamed Feng hua county. In 1988, it was reestablished as Feng hua city. Mentioned with 411.

Feng pei 豐沛 [2]

This is a combination of two place names. One was Feng 豐 county in present-day Jiang su 江蘇 and the other was Pei 沛 county in the same province. Feng county was established by Qin 秦. The seat of administration was in present day Feng county in Jiang su. Pei 沛 county was established by Qin, and administered from present day Pei county in Jiang su. Mentioned with 864, 1405.

Feng shan 豐山 [1]

Name of a mountain. There are many locations of this name in China, and there is no way to determine which one the BCGM authors wished to indicate. Mentioned with 299.

Feng xi xian 封溪縣 [1]

Name of a county. It was founded under Tang 唐, in 621, and was subordinated to Long zhou 隆州, and administered from a point northwest of the present-day Hanoi in Vietnam. Mentioned with 1303.

Feng xiang 鳳翔 [3]

Name of a *fu* 府 It was established under the Tang 唐, in 757, by raising the status of Feng xiang commandery. It was administered from present-day Feng xiang county in Shaan xi 陝西. The territory administered comprised the present-day cities and counties of Feng xiang, Qi shan 岐山, Fu feng 扶風, Lin you 麟遊, Bao ji 寶雞, Mei xian 眉縣 and Zhou zhi 周至 in Shaan xi. The *fu* was abolished in 1913. Mentioned with 1056, 1255, 1532.

Feng zhou 封州 [1]
Name of a *zhou* 州. It was founded under the Sui 隋, by changing the name of Cheng zhou 成州, in 590. The seat of administration was in the old city of Feng chuan 封川, south of present-day Feng kai 封開 county in Guang dong 廣東. The territory administered comprised the area corresponding to present-day Yu nan 郁南 and Feng kai in Guang dong, and the upper watershed of the He jiang 賀江 in Guang xi 廣西. During the *da ye* 大業 (605 – 618) reign period of the Sui, and the *tian bao* 天寶 (742 – 756) and *zhi de* 至德 (756 – 758) reign periods of the Tang 唐, the area periodically became a commandery. In 1277, during Yuan 元, the area became Feng zhou lu 封州路 and, in 1282, it was demoted as Feng zhou 封州. In 1369, the *zhou* was abolished. Mentioned with 141.

Feng zhou 灃州 [1]
This is an error occurring in the BCGM for → Li zhou 澧州.

Feng zhou 鳳州 [2]
Name of a *zhou* 州. It was established, under Western Wei 魏, in 554, by changing the name of Nan qi zhou 南岐州. The seat of administration was in present-day Feng zhou 鳳州 town, located northeast of Feng 鳳 county in Shaan xi 陝西. The territory administered comprised Feng county in present-day Shaan xi, and the two present-day counties of Hui 徽縣 and Liang dang 兩當 in Gan su 甘肅. During the *da ye* 大業 (605 – 618) reign period of the Sui 隋, and the *tian bao* 天寶 (742 – 756) and *zhi de* 至德 (756 – 758) reign periods of the Tang 唐, the area periodically became He chi 河池 commandery. In 1374, it was demoted to Feng county. Mentioned with 797, 1057.

Fo lin 佛林 [1]
Name of an early county. See → Fu lin guo 拂林國. Mentioned with 106.

Fo shi guo 佛誓國 [3]
Name of an ancient country. The name is an abbreviation of Shi li fo shi guo 室利佛逝國, Śrīvijaya. It was located on the island of Sumatra of present-day Indonesia. It had emerged in the 7th century and was conquered by the Majapahit country in the second half of the 14th century. Mentioned with 86, 680, 1035.

Fu 福 [5]
This is an abbreviation for → Fu zhou 福州. Mentioned with 182, 344, 674, 1057.

Fu 撫 [1]
This is an abbreviation for Fu zhou fu 撫州府. Under Yuan 元, in 1362, the Ming 明 rebels led by Zhu Yuanzhang 朱元璋 (1328 – 1399) changed Fu zhou lu 撫州路 to become Lin chuan fu 臨川府, but not long after that changed it again to be Fu zhou fu. The administration of the *fu* 府 was in the Lin chuan 臨川 district of present-day Fu zhou 撫州 city in Jiang xi 江西. At the beginning of Ming, its administrative area corresponded to the present-day districts and counties of Lin

chuan, Dong xiang 東鄉, Jin xi 金溪, Zi xi 資溪, Chong ren 崇仁, Le an 樂安 and Yi huang 宜黃 in Fu zhou city. Later, during the Ming, the administrative area was reduced in size. It was abolished in 1912. Mentioned with 323.

Fu 鄜 [1]

Name of a *zhou* 州. See → Fu zhou 鄜州. Mentioned with 871.

Fu du 涪都 [1]

This is a combined place name. It combines the names of the two counties of Fu ling 涪陵 and Feng du 豐都.

Fu ling county was established under Sui 隋, in 593, and was then administered in the present-day district of Fu ling in Chong qing 重慶. Under Tang 唐, in 618, the administration was moved to Fu zhou 涪州. Under Southern Song 宋, in 1266, Fu ling and Fu zhou 涪州 were both moved to San tai 三台 mountain, northeast of the present-day Fu ling district. Yuan 元 returned the area's administration to the present-day Fu ling district. In 1283, Fu zhou was eliminated as a *zhou* 州 but, in 1913, it was reestablished. In 1983, there was a change and Fu ling city was established. In 1997, the city became a district.

Feng du county was established under the Sui, in 618. It was administered from the present-day Feng du county in Chong qing. Northern Song abolished the county in 1111, but it was reestablished in 1131. In 1377, under Ming 明, the county became part of Fu zhou. In 1380, it was reestablished as an independent entity but changed to be Feng du 酆都 county. In 1958, the name was changed to Feng du 豐都 county. Mentioned with 1126, 1539.

Fu feng 扶風 [1]

Name of a commandery. See → Fu feng jun 扶風郡. Mentioned with 70.

Fu feng jun 扶風郡 [1]

Name of a commandery. It was established by Three Kingdoms' Wei 魏, by changing the name of You fu feng 右扶風. It was subordinated to Yong zhou 雍州. Its seat of administration was at a location 10 *li* southeast of present-day Xing ping 興平 city in Shaan xi 陝西. The territory administered comprised in present-day Shaan xi a region extending from Lin you 麟游 and Qian 乾 county in the East to the Qin ling 秦嶺 mountain range in the South. In 267, the seat of administration was moved to a point northwest of present-day Jing yang 涇陽 county. Later, the extension of the jurisdiction of the commandery underwent many changes. At the beginning of Northern Wei 魏, the seat of administration was moved to a point east of the present Qian county. In 528, the seat of administration was moved to a point 15 *li* southeast of present-day Xing ping city. The administrative area of the commandery corresponded to the three present-day counties and cities of Wu gong 武功, Qian xian 乾縣 and Xing ping in Shaan xi. The commandery was abolished in 583. Mentioned with 1155, 1573.

Fu gao shan gu 傅高山谷 [1]

Unidentified place name. Mentioned with 362.

Fu gou 扶溝 [1]
Name of a county. It was established under Western Han 漢. The seat of administration was in Gu cheng 古城 village, located 44 *li* northeast of present-day Fu gou county in He nan 河南. Western Jin 晉 eliminated the county at first but later reestablished it. Northern Qi 齊 moved the seat of administration to what is present-day Fu gou county.

Fu hai zhou 扶海洲 [1]
This is a legendary land. It was an island, believed to be somewhere deep in the Eastern Ocean. Mentioned with 1438.

Fu han 枹罕
Fu han, given erroneously as Bao han 抱罕 by the BCGM, is the name of several administrative units.
□ Fu han county was established by Qin 秦. The seat of administration was at the northern bank of the Da xia 大夏 river located southeast of present-day Lin xia 臨夏 county in Gan su 甘肅. Western Qin established the seat of administration at that place, but Northern Wei 魏 moved the administration to the present-day Lin xia city.
□ A Fu han commandery was established by Northern Zhou 周. The seat of administration was in present-day Lin xia city.
Fu han commandery was abolished under the early Tang 唐. Fu han county was abolished under the Yuan 元.

Fu jian 福建 [1 + 2]
□ Name of a *lu* 路. [1] It was established under Northern Song 宋, in 985. The seat of administration was in present-day Fu zhou 福州 city in Fu jian 福建. Its administrative area embraced present-day Fu jian province. In 1278, under Yuan 元, a Fu jian Branch Secretariat, Fu jian *xing zhong shu sheng* 福建行中書省, was established. Mentioned with 944.
□ Name of a Provincial Administration Commission, *cheng xuan bu zheng shi si* 承宣布政使司. [2] It was established, by Ming 明, through changing the name of the Fu jian Branch Secretariat, Fu jian *xing zhong shu sheng* 福建行中書省, in 1376. The seat of administration was in present-day Fu zhou city. From the beginning of Qing 清, the area is the present-day Fu jian 福建 province. The administrative area comprised that province. Mentioned with 616, 1036.

Fu jian zhou 福建州 [1]
This is a binome for → Fu zhou 福州 and → Jian zhou 建州.

Fu lang 富浪 [1]
This is a miswriting of Fo lang 佛朗. The name, from the 13th century *Xi shi ji* 西使記, "Record of an Embassy to the West," of Liu Yu 劉郁, is apparently an echo of the Arabic term for the Franks, but in this case probably the crusading states located at the eastern shore of the Mediterranean Sea. Mentioned with 1196.

Fu li zhi shan 鳧麗之山 [1]
Place name, a mountain, from the *Shan hai jing* 山海經, "Classic of Mountains and Seas," which cannot be identified. Mentioned with 83.

Fu liang 浮梁 [1]

Name of a county. It was established, by changing the name of Xin chang 新昌 county, in 742. The seat of administration was in present-day Fu liang 浮梁 county in Jiang xi 江西. In 1295, it was raised to be a *zhou* 州 but, in early Ming 明, it was demoted to a county again. In 1916, its administration was moved to Jing de zhen 景德鎮. In 1960, it was eliminated, but it was reestablished in 1988. This is the Fu liang county of today. Mentioned with 1561.

Fu lin 拂林 [3]

Name of an early country. See → Fu lin guo 拂林國. Mentioned with 1, 1239, 1272.

Fu lin guo 拂林國 [10]

Name of an early county. Also transcribed Fo lin 拂菻/佛林. During Sui 隋 and Tang 唐 times, this name referred to the Eastern Roman Empire, a consequence of the division of the former Roman Empire into a Western and an Eastern empire. Its capital was Constantinople, which is present-day Istanbul in Turkey. It was eliminated by the Osmanic Empire in 1453. Mentioned with 1, 85, 89, 772, 885, 967, 1089, 1091, 1239.

Fu ling 符陵 [3]

This is an error for Fu ling 涪陵. See → Fu ling jun 涪陵郡. Mentioned with 202, 1091.

Fu ling jun 涪陵郡 [1]

Name of a commandery. It was established under Eastern Han 漢 by Liu Bei 劉備, in 216, and administered from present-day Peng shui 彭水 county in Chong qing 重慶. The territory administered comprised the present-day districts and counties of Qian jiang 黔江, Peng shui, Wu long 武隆, Shi zhu 石柱 and You yang 酉陽 in Chong qing. Western Jin 晉 moved the seat of administration to the present-day You yang. The commandery was repeatedly eliminated and reestablished at various times during the *yong jia* 永嘉 reign period (307 – 313) of Western Jin, the *yong he* 永和 reign period (345 – 356) of Eastern Jin and under Qi 齊 of the Southern Dynasties. The commandery was finally eliminated under Sui 隋, in 583. Mentioned with 1297.

Fu lu cheng 福祿城 [1]

Name of a city. This is the same as Fu lu xian cheng 福祿縣城. Fu lu 福祿 county was established under Western Jin 晉 by renaming Lu fu 祿福 county. The seat of administration was in the present-day Jiu quan 酒泉 in Gan su 甘肅. During the time of the Sixteen Kingdoms, it was the capital of the state of Xi liang 西涼. At the end of Sui 隋, Fu lu cheng became Jiu quan county. Mentioned with 1335.

Fu lu xian 福祿縣 [1]

Name of a county. It was established in 619. The seat of administration was at a point southeast of present-day Jiu quan 酒泉 in Gan su 甘肅. In 766, the area came under the Tibetan empire. Mentioned with 934.

Fu nan 扶南 [9]
Name of an early country. See → Fu nan guo 扶南國. Mentioned with 82, 85, 104, 173, 535, 542, 1031.

Fu nan guo 扶南國 [2]
Name of an early country, founded in the 1st century CE. It was located on the lower Mekong in present-day Cambodia and existed until the mid 7th century when it was absorbed by the Khmer Kingdom. Mentioned with 315, 489.

Fu qi 弗其 [1]
Name of an uncertain place. Mentioned with 425.

Fu sang 扶桑 [1]
Name of a mythological country located over the seas. Later, Fu sang was identified with Japan. Mentioned with 1271.

Fu shan 服山 [1]
Name of a mountain. It cannot be identified. Mentioned with 299.

Fu shan 浮山 [1]
Name of a mountain. It is located southeast of present-day Lin fen 臨汾 city in Shan xi 山西. Mentioned with 1329.

Fu tang 福唐 [1]
Name of a county. It was founded under Tang 唐, by changing the name of Wan an 萬安 county, in 742. The seat of administration was in present-day Fu qing 福清 city in Fu jian 福建. During Five Dynasties' Liang 梁, in 908, it was changed to Yong chang 永昌 county. In Later Tang 唐, in 923, the area became Fu tang county again. In 933, the name of the county was changed to Fu qing 福清 county. Mentioned with 674.

Fu xi zhi shan 浮戲之山 [1]
Name of a mountain. It is the origin of the Si shui 汜水 river. It is located southwest of present-day Xing yang 滎陽 city in He nan 河南, that is, a location more than 30 *li* southeast of Si shui town. Mentioned with 1311.

Fu xian 涪縣 [1]
Name of a county. It was established under Western Han 漢, in 201 BCE. The seat of administration was at the eastern bank of the Fu 涪 river of present-day Mian yang 綿陽 city in Si chuan 四川. Western Jin 晉 turned it into Fu cheng 涪城 county, but Liu Song 劉宋 changed it back to Fu 涪 county. Western Wei 魏 changed it to Ba xi 巴西 county. Mentioned with 535.

Fu yan 鄜延 [1]
Name of a *lu* 路. It was established, under Northern Song 宋, in 1041. The seat of administration was in present-day Yan an 延安 city in Shaan xi 陝西. Its administrative area extended from the counties Yi chuan 宜川, Huang long 黃龍, Luo chuan 洛川 and Yi jun 宜君 in the South to Qing jian 清澗 river in the North. It was abolished under the Mongol Empire. Mentioned with 773.

Fu yan zhou 浮炎洲 [1]
Mythological island. No further information is available. Mentioned with 945.

Fu yi xian 扶夷縣 [1]
Name of a county. It was established by Southern Dynasties' Chen 陳 through changing the name of Fu yang 扶陽 county. It was subordinated to Shao ling 邵陵 commandery. The county was administered from the old city of Jin cheng 金城, 2 *li* east of present-day Xin ning 新寧 county, in Hu nan 湖南. The Sui 隋 abolished Fu yi county and made it part of Shao yang 邵陽 county. Mentioned with 1205.

Fu yu 夫餘 [1]
Name of an ancient country, covering the central and lower watershed of the Nen jiang 嫩江 in the two present-day provinces of Ji lin 吉林 and Hei long jiang 黑龍江, the northern watershed of the Song hua jiang 松花江, as well as the watersheds of the La lin he 拉林河 and E shen he 阿什河. Mentioned with 1406.

Fu zhou 涪州 [2]
Name of a *zhou* 州. It was established by Tang 唐, in 618. The seat of administration was in present-day the Fu ling 涪陵 district of Chong qing 重慶. The territory administered comprised the present-day districts of Fu ling 涪陵, Nan chuan 南川, Chang shou 長壽 and Wu long 武隆 in Chong qing. In 1913, the *zhou* was reorganized as Fu ling county. In 1996, the county was replaced by a city. In 1997, the city was turned into a district of Chong qing municipality. Mentioned with 202, 674.

Fu zhou 福州 [16]
Name of a *zhou* 州. It was established, by changing the name of Min zhou 閩州, in 725. The seat of administration was in present-day Fu zhou 福州 city in Fu jian 福建. Its administrative area corresponded to a region extending from the watershed of the Min 閩 river east of present-day You xi 尤溪 to the territory of the cities and counties of Gu tian 古田, Ping nan 屏南, Fu an 福安 and Fu ding 福鼎 in the West, all in present-day Fu jian 福建. After the Five Dynasties period, the area of the *zhou* was reduced in the Southwest. The *zhou* became a commandery later during the Tang 唐. Under Southern Song 宋, in 1276, it was changed to be Fu an fu 福安府. Under Yuan 元, in 1277, the area again became Fu zhou, and next year its status was raised to Fu zhou lu 福州路. Mentioned with 119, 171, 248, 251, 381, 512, 674, 748, 768, 823, 1008, 1011, 1052, 1288, 1513, 1514.

Fu zhou 撫州 [1]
Name of a *zhou* 州. It was founded under Sui 隋, in 589. The seat of administration was at a point west of present-day Lin chuan 臨川 district of Fu zhou 撫州 city. During the *da ye* 大業 reign period (605 – 616) of the Sui, and the *tian bao* 天寶 reign period of the Tang 唐 (742 – 755), the area became Lin chuan commandery. In 762, the seat of administration was moved to the present Lin chuan district. From the time that Sui established Fu zhou its administrative area expanded and contracted. From 624 on, the administrative area corresponded to the Fu he 撫河 watershed south of the present-day Lin chuan district. It was much reduced during Southern Tang of the Five Dynasties period. In 1277, under Yuan 元, the unit became Fu zhou lu 撫州路. Mentioned with 578.

Fu zhou 復州 [1]
Name of a *zhou* 州. It was established by Northern Zhou 周. The seat of administration was in present-day Mian cheng 沔城 town southwest of Xian tao 仙桃 city in Hu bei 湖北. Sui 隋, at the beginning of the *da ye* 大業 reign period (605 – 616), changed the name to Mian zhou 沔州, but the old name was restored under the Tang 唐, in 622. The seat of administration was changed to present-day Tian men 天門 city in Hu bei. In 633, the seat of administration was returned to the old site. The administrative area covered the territories of the three present-day cities of Xian tao 仙桃, Tian men 天門, Hong hu 洪湖, and of Jian li 監利 county in Hu bei 湖北. In 763, the seat of administration was once again moved to the present-day Tian men city and, under Southern Song 宋, during the *duan ping* 端平 reign period (1234 – 1236), the administrative seat was moved to the present Mian cheng town. In 1275, under Yuan 元, the *zhou* became Fu zhou lu 復州路. Mentioned with 75.

Fu zhou 富州 [1]
Name of a *zhou* 州. It was established, by changing the name of Jing zhou 靜州, in 634. The seat of administration was in present-day Zhao ping 昭平 county in Guang xi 廣西. The administrative area of the *zhou* corresponded to the area of present-day Zhao ping county in Guang xi. In 742, the area was changed to Kai jiang 開江 commandery. In 758, the *zhou* was reestablished. In 972, under Northern Song 宋, the *zhou* was abolished. Mentioned with 535.

Fu zhou 鄜州 [3]
Name of a *zhou* 州. It was established under Western Wei 魏, in 554. The seat of administration was at a point 5 *li* southwest of present-day Huang ling 黃陵 county in Shaan xi 陝西. Under Sui 隋, in 607, the seat of administration was moved to present-day Fu xian 富縣 county in Shaan xi, and the *zhou* was changed to be Fu cheng 鄜城 commandery. In 618, under Tang, the commandery became Fu zhou 鄜州 again, but it was still administered from present-day Fu xian 富縣 county. Its administrative area embraced the present-day counties of Fu xian, Gan quan 甘泉 and Luo chuan 洛川 in Shaan xi. Later, during the *tian bao* 天寶 (742 – 756) and *zhi de* 至德 (756 – 758) reign periods of the Tang 唐, the area periodically became a commandery. In 1913, it became Fu xian 鄜縣 county and, in 1964, it became Fu xian 富縣 county. Mentioned with 1040.

-G-

Ga gu luo guo 伽古羅國 [1]
Early country at the Western shore of the Malayan Peninsula. Another tradition locates it at the Kra Isthmus, and still another tradition sees it as situated within the borders of present-day Thailand. Mentioned with 25.

Ga pi guo 伽毘國 [1]
This is an unidentified early country, located somewhere overseas. No further details are available. Mentioned with 1427.

Ga pi ye guo 伽毗耶國 [1]
This is an unidentified early country, located somewhere overseas. No further details are available. Mentioned with 1002.

Ga she na guo 伽闍那國 [1]
Name of an ancient country in western regions, as mentioned in the *You yang za zu* 酉陽雜俎, "Miscellaneous Morsels from Youyang," by Duan Chengshi 段成式 (died 863). In various sources it was referred to as Jia se ni 伽色尼, Ji ci ni 吉慈尼, Ge ji ning 哥疾寧, and He xi na 鶴悉那. It is present-day Ghazni, located 155 km southeast of Kabul, the capital city of Afghanistan. Mentioned with 14.

Gan lu si 甘露寺 [1]
Name of a temple. It was located on Bei gu 北固 mountain, north of present-day Zhen jiang 鎮江 city in Jiang su 江蘇. Mentioned with 1546.

Gan quan dong yuan 甘泉東院 [1]
Minor place name. It is a park at Gan quan 甘泉 mountain, located northwest of present-day Han jiang 邗江 district of Yang zhou 揚州 in Jiang su 江蘇. Mentioned with 1178.

Gan song 甘松 [1]
Name of a mountain. It is also known as Gan song ling 甘松嶺, located southwest of present-day Song pan 松潘 county in Si chuan 四川. Mentioned with 907.

Gan su 甘肅 [4]
Name of a "district under the control of a Ming 明 dynasty inspector-general," a Ming *xun fu xia qu* 明巡撫轄區. It was established, in 1436, and set up in the present-day Zhang ye 張掖 city in Gan su 甘肅 to administer the region of the He xi 河西 corridor of present-day Gan su. The administration was abolished under the Qing 清, in 1754. Mentioned with 746, 1149, 1171, 1364.

Gan zhou 甘州 [1 + 1]
▫ Name of a guard (*wei* 衛). [1] It was established, by changing the name of the Gan su 甘肅 guard, in 1392. It was subordinated to the Shaan xi Regional Military Commission, Shaan xi *xing du si* 陝西行都司, and was administered from present-day Zhang ye 張掖 city in Gan su. The territory administered comprised the present-day cities and counties of Zhang ye, Lin ze 臨澤, Min le 民樂 in Gan su, and Qi lian 祁連 in Qing hai 青海. The next year, the Regional Military Commission, *du si* 都司, was moved there. In 1724, Gan zhou became Gan zhou fu 甘州府. Mentioned with 361.
▫ Name of a *lu* 路. [1] It was established, by changing the name of Gan su lu 甘肅路, in 1271. Later, it was subordinated to the Gan su Branch Secretariat, Gan su *xing zhong shu sheng* 甘肅行中書省. The seat of administration was in present-day Zhang ye 張掖 city in Gan su 甘肅. The territory administered comprised the present-day counties of Zhang ye, Lin ze 臨澤, Gao tai 高臺, Min le

民樂, and Su nan 肅南 in Gan su, and Qi lian 祁連 in Qing hai 青海. In 1281, the Gan su Branch Secretariat was established there. In 1372, the area was changed to Gan su guard. Mentioned with 361.

Gan zhou 贛州 [1]

Name of a *zhou* 州. It was established, by changing the name of Qian zhou 虔州, in 1153. The seat of administration was in present-day Gan zhou city in Jiang xi 江西. Its administrative territory comprised an area extending south from Shi cheng 石城 and Xing guo 興國 counties in present-day Gan zhou city in Jiang xi. In 1277, the *zhou* was promoted to Gan zhou lu 贛州路. Mentioned with 1051.

Gao 高 [4]

Name of a *zhou* 州. It was established under Liang 梁 during the Southern Dynasties period. The seat of administration was at a point west of present-day Yang jiang 陽江 city in Guang dong 廣東. The territory administered comprised an area corresponding to present-day Jian jiang 鑒江 in Guang dong and the watershed of the Mo yang jiang 漠陽江. In 776, the seat of administration was moved to present-day Jiu cheng 舊城 village of Chang po 長坡 town northeast of Gao zhou 高州 city in Guang dong. Its administrative area was reduced and comprised only the section of the present-day city of Gao zhou and Dian bai 電白 county. In 1004, under Northern Song 宋, the *zhou* was eliminated, but it was reestablished again, in 1006. In 1280, the *zhou* was changed to be Gao zhou lu 高州路. Mentioned with 144, 925.

Gao an 高安 [1]

Name of a county. It was established under Tang 唐, in 622, when, as a result of a taboo avoidance, Jian cheng 建城 county was changed to Gao an county. This is the present-day Gao an county in Jiang xi 江西. Mentioned with 926.

Gao chang 高昌 [9]

Name of an ancient city and country. Han 漢 established a Gao chang city and, in 327, Former Liang 涼 established a Gao chang commandery. Under Northern Wei 魏, Juqu Wuhui 沮渠無諱 (died 444) occupied Gao chang and made himself king. His capital was at the old city of Gao chang, located 40 plus *li* east of Turfan city in present-day Xin jiang 新疆. In 460, after the Rou ran 柔然 had destroyed the Juqu 沮渠 clan, another kingdom of Gao chang was established. At the height of its power and extension, in the South it connected with the Tu yu hun 吐谷渾. In the North it neighbored on the Chi le 敕勒. In the East it connected with Dun huang 敦煌, and in the West with Gui ci 龜茲, which is present-day Kuqa/Ku che 庫車 in Xin jiang. In 640, Gao chang was destroyed by Tang 唐. Mentioned with 174, 285, 811, 862, 1030, 1370, 1405.

Gao chang guo 高昌國 [2]

Name of an ancient country. → Gao chang 高昌. Mentioned with 368, 794.

Gao cheng 藁城 [1]

Name of a county. It was established under Western Han 漢. The seat of administration was in present-day Qiu tou 丘頭 town, located 28 *li* southwest of Gao cheng city in He bei 河北. Under Sui 隋, in 606, the administration was moved to Gao cheng. In 1989, the county was converted to a city. Mentioned with 1175.

Gao li 高麗 [15 + 2 + 4]

□ Name of an ancient state, "Koryŏ," in Korea. [15] This is also written Gao gou li 高句麗, "Koguryŏ." The kingdom was established by Zhu Meng (Jumong) 朱蒙 at the end of Western Han 漢, in 37 BCE. The capital was to the east of present-day Ji an 集安 city in Ji lin 吉林 province. It controlled an area extending in present-day Liao ning 遼寧 from the upper watershed of the Hun he 渾河 river toward the East, and from Lang lin 狼林 (Rangrim) mountain in northern Korea toward the West. In the South it reached to the Qing chuan jiang 清川江 (Chongchon river), also in northern Korea. During Eastern Han, in 209, the capital was moved to Shan cheng zi 山城子, located five *li* northwest of Ji an city in Ji lin. In the 4th century, Gao li took over Le lang 樂浪 commandery and, in 427, under Liu Song 劉宋, the capital was moved to present-day Pyongyang. In 668, Gao li was destroyed by Tang 唐 in alliance with Silla. Mentioned with 26, 535, 599, 608, 718, 931, 1254, 1258, 1311, 1375.

□ Name of an early country. [2] This refers to the Korean Koryŏ dynasty (918 – 1392). Mentioned with 1040, 1176.

□ Name of an early country. [4] The term is mistakenly applied to Chosen Korea (1392 – 1910). Mentioned with 215, 493, 535, 670.

Gao li guo 高麗國 [1]

Name of an early country. See the discussion under → Gao li 高麗. Mentioned with 773.

Gao li shan 高麗山 [1]

Name of a mountain. It is located southwest of present-day Lai yang 萊陽 city in Shan dong 山東. Mentioned with 1238.

Gao liang jun 高良郡 [1]

Regional administrative name. A reference to either → Gao liang jun 高涼郡, or → Gao liang 高涼 county. Mentioned with 346.

Gao liang jun 高涼郡 [1]

Name of a commandery. It was established, under Eastern Han 漢, in 220. The seat of administration was at a point west of present-day En ping 恩平 city in Guang dong 廣東. The territory administered comprised the present-day cities and counties of Yang jiang 陽江, Yang dong 陽東, Yang xi 陽西, Yang chun 陽春, En ping, Gao zhou 高州, Mao ming 茂名, and Dian bai 電白 in Guang dong. Under Western Jin 晉, the seat of administration was moved to a point west of Yang jiang city in Guang dong. The seat of administration was restored as before under Liu Song 劉宋. Southern Qi 齊 also moved the administration to a point west of Yang jiang city. Under Sui 隋, in 589, the commandery was eliminated. In 606, Gao zhou was changed to be Gao liang commandery. It was administered from a point west of present-day Yang jiang city. Its administrative area was increased. In 758, Gao zhou was restored again. Mentioned with 533.

Gao liang xian 高涼縣 [1]

Name of a county. It was established under Western Han 漢. The seat of administration was at a point north of present-day Yang dong 陽東 county in Guang dong 廣東. At the end of Eastern Han, the area was subordinated to → Gao liang jun 高涼郡. Under Eastern Jin 晉, the county was abolished.

Gao mi 高密 [1]

Name of a county. It was established under Qin 秦. The seat of administration was in present-day Qian tian 前田 village, located 40 *li* southwest of Gao mi city in Shan dong 山東. The county was eliminated under Northern Qi 齊. It was reestablished during the *kai huang* 開皇 reign period (581 – 600) of Sui 隋, and the administration was moved to Gu xian 故獻 village, located 20 *li* southeast of the present Gao mi city. It was eliminated at the end of Sui. In 620, it was again established at the former Yi cheng bao 義城堡, 1 *li* northwest of the present Gao mi city. In 623, the administration was moved to present-day Gao mi city. In 1994, it was changed to be Gao mi city. Mentioned with 648.

Gao nu xian 高奴縣 [1]

Name of a county. It was established by the Qin 秦. The seat of administration was at the eastern bank of the Yan 延 river east of present-day Yan an 延安 city in Shaan xi 陝西. The county was abolished at the end of Eastern Han 漢. Mentioned with 1040.

Gao ping 高平 [2]

Name of a county. It was established by Northern Wei 魏, under Chang ping 長平 commandery, in 529. The seat of administration was at a point 20 *li* northwest of present-day Gao ping 高平 city in Shan xi 山西. In 550, under Northern Qi 齊, the seat of administration was moved to present-day Gao ping city. In 1993, it was changed to be Gao ping city. Mentioned with 698, 1532.

Gao ping jun 高平郡 [1]

Name of a commandery. It was established, by Northern Wei 魏, and was placed under Yuan zhou 原州, in 524. The seat of administration was in the present Gu yuan 固原 county in Ning xia 寧夏. The territory administered comprised an area corresponding to the two present-day counties of Gu yuan and Peng Yang 彭陽 in Ning Xia. At the end of Western Wei, it was changed to Ping gao 平高 commandery. Mentioned with 595.

Gao shan 高山 [5]

This is a generalized reference to "high mountains", and not a specific place name. Mentioned in connection with this fictive area: 50, 91, 810, 1337, 1428.

Gao shi shan 高石山 [1]

Name of a mountain. It is located in the present-day Long sheng 龍勝 county in Guang xi 廣西. Mentioned with 660.

Gao shi zhi shan 高氏之山 [1]

Name of a mountain. This is Gao shi shan 高氏山, also written Gao shi shan 高是山. It is Cui ping 翠屏 mountain, 7 *li* south of present-day Hun yuan 渾源 county in Shan xi 山西. Mentioned with 83.

Gao tu zhi shan 皋塗之山 [1]
Name of a place from the *Shan hai jing* 山海經, "Classic of Mountains and Seas." Details are lacking. Mentioned with 1435.

Gao xia 高夏 [2]
Name of a mountain. It is probably Gao guan 高冠 mountain in the present-day Wu chang 武昌 district of Wu han 武漢 city in Hu bei 湖北. Mentioned with 661.

Gao you 高郵 [1]
Name of a *zhou* 州. See → Gao you zhou 高郵州.

Gao you zhou 高郵州 [1]
Name of a *zhou* 州. It was established, in 1368, and subordinated to Yang zhou fu 揚州府. It was administered from present-day Gao you 高郵 city in Jiang su 江蘇. The territory administered comprised the two present-day cities of Gao you and Xing hua 興化 in Jiang su and the vicinity of Bao ying 寶應 county. In 1912, the area became Gao you city. Mentioned with 1310.

Gao zhou 高州 [3]
Name of a *zhou* 州. It was established under Southern Dynasties' Liang 梁, in 527 – 528. The seat of administration was at a point west of present-day Yang jiang 陽江 city in Guang dong 廣東. The territory administered comprised the watersheds of the rivers Jian jiang 鑒江 and Mo yang jiang 漠陽江 in Guang dong. Under Sui 隋, in 607, the *zhou* became Gao liang 高涼 commandery but under Tang, in 621, it was reestablished. Later under Tang 唐, in 649, the seat of administration was moved to a point northeast of present-day Gao zhou city in Guang dong. In 776, it was moved to Jiu cheng 舊城 village of Chang bo 長坡 town northeast of the present-day Gao zhou city. The administrative area was reduced being confined only to present-day Gao zhou city and some parts of Dian bai 電白 county. In 1280, Gao zhou became Gao zhou lu 高州路. Mentioned with 346, 428, 1574.

Ge shan 葛山 [1]
Name of a mountain from the *Shan hai jing* 山海經, "Classic of Mountains and Seas." Further details are unavailable. Mentioned with 1574.

Gong shan 宮山 [1]
Name of a mountain. This is the ancient Xin fu 新甫 mountain, located 40 *li* northwest of Xin tai 新泰 city in Shan dong 山東, on the borders to Lai wu 萊蕪 city. This mountain is also called Xiao tai shan 小泰山, "Little Mount Tai," Mentioned with 57.

Gong zhou 龔州 [1]
Name of a *zhou* 州. It was established under Tang 唐, in 633. The seat of administration was in the present-day Ping nan 平南 county in Guang xi 廣西. The territory administered comprised an area corresponding to Ping nan county in present-day Guang xi. In 742, it was changed into Lin jiang 臨江 commandery. In 758, it became Gong zhou again. The *zhou* was abolished under Southern Song 宋, in 1136. Mentioned with 327.

Gu cheng 古城 [1]
Minor place name. Further details are unavailable. Mentioned with 834.

Gu cheng 谷城 [2]
Name of a county. It was established under Qin 秦. The seat of administration was in Dong e 東阿 town, located southwest of present-day Ping yin 平陰 county in Shan dong 山東. The county was eliminated under Western Han 漢, but restored under Eastern Han. It was abolished under Northern Qi 齊. Mentioned with 1443, 1484.

Gu deng zhi shan 鼓鐙之山 [1]
Name of a mountin mentioned in the *Shan hai jing* 山海經, "Classic of Mountains and Seas." It is located east of present-day Yuan qu 垣曲 county in Shan xi 山西. Mentioned with 1185.

Gu du guo 古都國 [1]
This is the name of a region with a "win over", *ji mi* 羈縻, rule whereby the Chinese authorities installed the head of a region inhabited by non-Chinese ethnic groups while respecting their indigenous traditional customs and government structures. The designation "country" (*guo* 國) refers to the territory occupied by the minority people. Tang 唐 established Gu du 古都 county as a "win-over" county subordinate to Liang zhou 諒州 under the Area Command, *du du fu* 都督府, of Yong zhou 邕州. The seat of administration was in the district of Lạng Sơn 諒山 in Tỉnh Lạng Sơn 諒山省 province, in present-day Vietnam. Later it was abolished. Mentioned with 992.

Gu er zhi shui 姑兒之水 [1]
This is a place name from the *Shan hai jing* 山海經, "Classic of Mountains and Seas." Further details are unavailable. Mentioned with 343.

Gu mu 姑幕 [1]
Name of a county. It was established under Western Han 漢, and subordinated to Lang ya 琅琊 commandery. The seat of administration was at a point 40 *li* northwest of present-day Zhu cheng 諸城 city in Shan dong 山東. The county was eliminated under the Liu Song 劉宋, but later reestablished under Later Wei 魏. In 556, it was abolished under Northern Qi 齊. Mentioned with 191.

Gu shu 姑熟 [1]
A wrong writing for → Gu shu 姑孰. Mentioned with 634.

Gu shu 姑孰 [1]
Name of an early city. The walls were built during the time of Three Kingdoms' Wu 吳, between 222 and 229. The city was located in the present-day Dang tu 當塗 county in An hui 安徽. During Southern Tang 唐, in 945, there was an extension of the city walls and additional territory included. In the South, the boundaries went over Gu shu creek to San li dian 三里店, and in the East the city adjoined Ling jia 淩家 mountain. Mentioned with 405.

Gu tao cun 固陶村 [1]
Name of a village. This was located in present-day Li xi xiang 鯉溪鄉 in Wen zhou 溫州 city in Zhe jiang 浙江. Mentioned with 1521.

Gu yao zhi shan 姑媱之山 [1]
Place name from the *Shan hai jing* 山海經, "Classic of Mountains and Seas." Further details are lacking. Mentioned with 1237.

Gu zang 姑臧 [2]
Name of a county. It was established, under Former Han 漢, in 121 BCE, and administered by Wu wei 武威 commandery. Its administrative seat was in the present-day Wu wei city in Gan su 甘肅. Under Three Kingdoms' Wei 魏, during the *huang chu* 黃初 reign period (220 – 226), the administration was moved to Liang zhou 涼州. During the period of the Sixteen Kingdoms, it formed the capital of Former Liang 涼, Later Liang, Southern Liang and Northern Liang. Northern Wei turned this into Lin zhong 林中 county, but Western Wei 魏 restored the name as Gu zang county. After the An lu shan 安祿山 rebellion (755 – 763), the territory became part of the Tibetan empire, and the county was abolished. Mentioned with 721.

Gu zhao 古趙 [1]
Name of an ancient country. This was the Zhao 趙 state of the Warring States period.

Gu zhu 顧渚 [1]
Minor place name. This is present-day Gu zhu village, located 47 *li* northwest of Chang xing 長興 county in Zhe jiang 浙江. The area was noted for its tea, offering a variety from Tang 唐 times on called *zi sun* 紫筍, "purple shoots." Mentioned with 768.

Gua 瓜 [1]
Name of a *zhou*. See → Gua zhou 瓜州.

Gua zhou 瓜州 [3]
Name of a *zhou* 州. It was established under Tang 唐, in 622. The seat of administration was in present-day Suo yang 鎖陽 city, southeast of Gua zhou county in Gan su 甘肅. The territory administered comprised a strip of present-day Gua zhou county. At the end of Xi xia 西夏, the *zhou* was abolished, but it was reestablished under Yuan 元. The seat of administration was moved to Gua zhou kou 瓜州口 located southwest of present-day Gua zhou county. Ming 明 abolished the *zhou*. Mentioned with 449, 695, 738, 1149.

Guan 關 [1 + 5]
□ General name for places. [1] In this case, the reference is to Yu men guan 玉門關 and Yang guan 陽關, both in present-day Gan su 甘肅, northwest of Dun huang 敦煌. Mentioned with 861.
□ General name for places. [5] In this case, the reference is to Han gu guan 函谷關, located 30 *li* northeast of present-day Ling bao 靈寶 city in He nan 河南. Mentioned with 417, 860, 881, 1480, 1547.

Guan 管 [1]
See → Rong guan 容管. Mentioned with 909.

Guan dong 關東 [3]
Regional name. During Han 漢 and Wei 魏 times, the term referred to the area east of the Han gu guan 函谷關 or the Xiao guan 崤關. The area corresponds to the present He nan 河南, Shan dong 山東 and He bei 河北. Mentioned with 20, 1001, 1004.

Guan dong xi 關東西 [1]
Combined designation used to refer to the Guan dong 關東 and Guan xi 關西 areas, and thus a general reference to the Chinese central plain. Mentioned with 442.

Guan fu 關輔 [2]
Combined designation used in reference to the Guan zhong 關中 and San fu 三輔 areas. This corresponded to the present-day Guan zhong region of Shaan xi 陝西 and nearby areas. Mentioned with 663, 1221.

Guan he jian 關河間 [1]
General regional designation. Further details unavailable. Mentioned with 678.

Guan long 關隴 [1]
Regional designation. It was used to designate the Tang 唐 central regions of Guan nei 關內 circuit and Long you 隴右 circuit, corresponding to the present-day Shaan xi 陝西, a large part of Gan su 甘肅, all of Ning xia 寧夏 and a part of Inner Mongolia. Mentioned with 1038.

Guan nei 關內 [1]
Name of a circuit. It was established by Tang 唐, in 627. Its territory corresponded to the whole of Shaan xi 陝西 from the Qin ling 秦嶺 mountain range towards the North, the eastern part of Gan su 甘肅 and a portion of Inner Mongolia. The circuit was later abolished. Mentioned with 132.

Guan shaan 關陝 [8]
Regional name. It is used in reference to the region of Guan zhong 關中 and Shaan zhou 陝州. This is located within the eastern part of the Guan zhong 關中 plateau and the western part of He nan 河南. Mentioned with 126, 300, 579, 1098, 1221, 1308, 1316, 1407.

Guan shan 綸山 [1]
Name of a place from the *Shan hai jing* 山海經, "Classic of Mountains and Seas." No further details are available. Mentioned with 966.

Guan shui 覩水 [1]
Name of a river. Details are lacking. Mentioned with 1230.

Guan shui 灌水 [1]
Name of a river. It is located west of present-day Hua yin 華陰 county in Shaan xi 陝西. Mentioned with 191.

Guan xi 關西 [9 + 6]
□ Regional name. [9]. During Song 宋 times, it referred to the region west of Han gu guan 函谷關 or Yao guan 崤關. This is the territory of present-day

Shaan xi 陝西 and Gan su 甘肅. Mentioned with 117, 158, 504, 583, 628, 804, 1187, 1242, 1428.

□ Regional name. [6] During Ming 明 times, it referred to the region west of the Jia yu guan 嘉峪關, a corner of the western portion of present-day Gan su 甘肅, along with Xin jiang 新疆. Mentioned with 18, 467, 691, 841, 1047, 1367.

Guan you 關右 [1]

Regional name. This is → Guan xi 關西. In early times, the west was considered to be on the "right." Mentioned with 1109.

Guan zhong 關中 [24]

Regional name. This is the Guan zhong 關中 plateau in present-day Shaan xi 陝西. The area is nicknamed the Ba bai li Qin chuan 八百里秦川, "Qin 秦 plain of 800 *li*." Mentioned with 196, 221, 244, 272, 298, 502, 504, 599, 730, 733, 823, 857, 1033, 1038, 1119, 1204, 1221, 1294, 1308, 1392.

Guang 廣 [16 + 4 + 10 + 27 + 3]

□ Abbreviation for ' Guang zhou 廣州. [16] Mentioned with 9, 144, 226, 298, 347, 376, 413, 445, 550, 578, 596, 1028, 1057, 1063, 1463.

□ Territory. [4] Used by the BCGM authors to refer to the territory administered, in Tang 唐 times, by the regional inspector, *ci shi* 刺史, of Guang zhou 廣州 who was jointly military commissioner, *jing lue shi* 經略使, of the five *fu* 府 of Ling nan 嶺南. This territory embraced much of the present province of Guang dong 廣東 and of Guang xi 廣西. Mentioned with 144, 606, 817, 1437.

□ An abbreviation for the Guang nan lu 廣南路 of Song 宋 times. [10] See → Guang nan 廣南. Mentioned with 79, 247, 332, 344, 509, 578, 660, 674, 685, 960, 970, 1008.

□ Abbreviation for → Guang dong 廣東. [27] Mentioned with 133, 157, 212, 243, 323, 347, 362, 367, 603, 746, 766, 777, 783, 915, 1040, 1171, 1272, 1375, 1408, 1475, 1486, 1494, 1499, 1507, 1526.

□ Abbreviation. [3] Used for Guang dong 廣東 and Guang xi 廣西. See → Liang Guang 兩廣. Mentioned with 474, 1247, 1329.

Guang dong 廣東 [4 + 1]

□ Name of a Provincial Administration Commission, *bu zheng shi si* 布政使司. [4] It was established, by Ming 明, in 1376. The seat of administration was in present-day Guang zhou 廣州 city (Canton) in Guang dong province. Its administrative area embraced the two present-day provinces of Guang dong and Hai nan 海南, and the cities of Fang cheng gang 防城港, Qin zhou 欽州 and Bei hai 北海, and their respective administrative areas, in Guang xi 廣西. Qing 清 converted it to Guang dong province. Mentioned with 511, 1139, 1307, 1437.

□ Name of a Pacification Office, *xuan wei si* 宣慰司. [1] It was established, by Yuan 元, in 1278. The seat of administration was in present-day Guang zhou 廣州 city in Guang dong 廣州. The territory administered comprised the portion of Guang dong province east of the geographical strip comprised by the present-day Feng kai 封開, Yu nan 郁南, Luo ding 羅定, Yang chun 陽春 and Yang jiang 陽江. In 1369, this unit was changed to the Branch Secretariat, *xing zhong shu sheng* 行中書省, of Guang dong and other places. Mentioned with 784.

Guang fu 廣府 [1]

This is an abbreviation for the Guang zhou Area Command, Guang zhou *du du fu* 廣州都督府. It was established under Tang 唐, in 624, and administered seven *zhou* 州. The area corresponds to present-day Guang zhou 廣州 city and the nearby region. In 639, its jurisdiction had expanded to cover 14 *zhou*, comprising most of present-day Guang dong 廣東. Between 650 and 655, it was greatly expanded to cover the Ling nan wu guan 嶺南五管, "the five administrations south of the mountain range," i.e., a jurisdiction comprising the so- called Ling nan 嶺南 region, including present-day Guang dong, Guang xi 廣西 and Hai nan 海南 island and the northern portions of Vietnam. Mentioned with 141.

Guang han 廣漢 [4]

Name of a commandery. It was established under Western Han 漢, in 201 BCE. The seat of administration initially was at a point east of present-day Jin tang 金堂 county in Sichuan 四川, but later the administrative seat was moved to present-day Zi tong 梓潼 county in Sichuan. The administration of the commandery embraced an area extending from Wen 文 county in Gan su 甘肅 and Ning qiang 寧強 in Shaan xi 陝西 in the North, Wang cang 旺蒼, Jian ge 劍閣, and Peng xi 蓬溪 in Si chuan in the East, to Tong nan 潼南, Sui ning 遂寧, and Xin du 新都 in Si chuan in the South, and the former Bei chuan 北川 in the West. Eastern Han moved the seat of administration, in 108, to a place east of present-day Mian yang 綿陽 city in Sichuan, and later it was moved to present-day Guang han city in Sichuan. The commandery was abolished under Sui 隋, in 583. Mentioned with 322, 1036, 1096.

Guang ji 廣濟 [1]

Name of a county. It was established under the Tang 唐, in 742. The seat of administration was in present-day Mei chuan 梅川 town, located 62 *li* north of Wu xue 武穴 city in Hu bei 湖北. In 1953, the seat of administration was moved to present-day Wu xue town. In 1987, the county was turned into a city.

Guang jiao guo 廣焦國 [1]

This is the name of an unidentified early foreign country. Further details are unavailable.

Guang ling 廣陵 [2]

Name of a county. It was established by Qin 秦. The seat of administration was at a location on top of Shu gang 蜀岡 hill, northwest of present-day Yang zhou 揚州 city in Jiang su 江蘇. Under Sui 隋, in 598, the county became Han jiang 邗江 county, but at the beginning of the *da ye* 大業 reign period (605 – 616), it became Jiang yang 江陽 county. During the time of Five Dynasties' Tang 唐, the county was changed to Guang ling and the seat of administration was moved to present-day Yang zhou city. In 1072, under Northern Song 宋, the county was combined with Jiang du 江都 county, but it was reestablished again during Southern Song. Yuan 元 eliminated it. Mentioned with 384.

Guang nan 廣南 [26]

Name of a *lu* 路. It was established under Northern Song 宋. The seat of administration was in the present-day city of Guang zhou 廣州. Its area of administration embraced present-day Guang dong 廣東, Guang xi 廣西 and Hai nan 海南 island. Later, there was a division of this territory into two *lu*, eastern and western, but the term Guang nan continued in use. At the beginning of Yuan 元, this practice was gradually abandoned. During Ming 明, the people took up the old designation again. Mentioned with 43, 110, 190, 252, 259, 350, 592, 593, 614, 817, 838, 864, 956, 979, 1020, 1124, 1188, 1340, 1377, 1400, 1425, 1451, 1503.

Guang xi 廣西 [11 + 15]

□ Name of a *lu* 路. [11] This is the Guang nan xi lu 廣南西路. It was established, by Northern Song 宋, in 997. The seat of administration was in present-day Gui lin 桂林 city in Guang xi 廣西. The territory administered comprised present-day Guang xi, Hai nan 海南 and the Lei zhou 雷州 peninsula of Guang dong 廣東. During the *zhi yuan* 至元 reign period (1335 – 1340) of Yuan 元, the *lu* became part of the Branch Secretariat, *xing zhong shu sheng* 行中書省, for Hu guang 湖廣 and other places. Mentioned with 72, 699, 710, 715, 717, 803, 951, 972, 1179, 1239.

□ Name of a Provincial Administration Commission, *bu zheng shi si*. [15] It was established by the Ming 明, in 1376. The seat of administration was in present-day Gui lin 桂林 city in Guang xi 廣西. The territory administered comprised most of present-day Guang xi, Huai ji 懷集 in Guang dong 廣東, and counties in the southwest corner of Gui zhou 貴州. Qing 清 changed this unit to be Guang xi sheng 廣西省, "The Province of Guang xi." Mentioned with 246, 332, 350, 445, 460, 511, 540, 566, 574, 950, 991, 1162, 1279, 1427, 1467.

Guang zhe 廣浙 [1]

Name of a region referring to the two present-day Guang 廣 (Guang dong 廣東 and Guang xi 廣西) provinces and Zhe jiang 浙江. Mentioned with 864.

Guang zhong 廣中 [10]

Regional name. It was used to designate the two present-day Guang 廣 (Guang dong and Guang xi) provinces of the Ling nan region. Mentioned with 127, 578, 635, 685, 930, 939, 954, 967, 1239, 1312.

Guang zhou 廣州 [52 + 2]

□ Name of a *zhou* 州, [52] It was established, under Three Kingdoms' Wu 吳, in 226. The seat of administration was in present-day Wu zhou 梧州 city in Guang xi 廣西. This *zhou* was soon eliminated. In 264, it was reestablished, and the administration was moved to present-day Guang zhou city in Guang dong 廣東. Its administration covered a good part of present-day Guang dong and Guang xi. Its size was slowly reduced after the Southern Dynasties period and, in 592, the seat of administration was moved to the west bank of the Wu shui 武水, 10 *li* south of Shao guan 韶關 city, in Guang dong. At the end of the *kai huang* 開皇 reign period (581 – 600) of the Sui 隋 dynasty, the seat of administration was moved back to present-day Guang zhou city. Under Yuan 元, in 1278, the area became Guang zhou lu 廣州路. Mentioned with 9, 14, 25, 30, 79, 86, 94, 110, 144,

202, 226, 312, 330, 332, 344, 376, 427, 428, 445, 483, 500, 578, 586, 596, 685, 700, 779, 780, 790, 799, 848, 864, 887, 952, 961, 1028, 1057, 1063, 1124, 1246, 1247, 1297, 1324, 1460. Some of the products such as the myrrh, 779, were obviously imports.
□ Name of a *fu* 府. [2] It was established under the Ming 明, in 1368. The seat of administration was in present-day Guang zhou city in Guang dong. The territory administered comprised the central part of present-day Guang dong. It was abolished in 1912. Mentioned with 323, 1375.

Guang zhou 光州 [2]
Name of a *zhou* 州. It was established at the end of Southern Dynasties' Liang 梁. The seat of administration was in present-day Guang shan 光山 county in He nan 河南. Its administrative area included the present-day counties of Huang chuan 潢川, Guang shan, Xin xian 新縣, Gu shi 固始 and Shang cheng 商城 in He nan, and the western part of present-day Jin zhai 金寨 county in An hui 安徽. Under Tang 唐, in 712, the administration was moved to the present Huang chuan county. In 1913, the *zhou* was changed to be Huang chuan county. Mentioned with 986, 1020.

Gui 歸 [1]
Name of a *zhou* 州. See → Gui zhou 歸州.

Gui 貴 [1]
Abbreviation for a Provincial Administration Commission, *bu zheng shi si* 布政使司. See → Gui zhou 貴州.

Gui 桂 [1]
Name of a *zhou* 州. See → Gui zhou 桂州.

Gui ci guo 龜茲國
→ Qiu ci guo 龜茲國.

Gui fang 鬼方 [1]
Ancient designation of a region as "place of demons", located approximately in an area comprising the northern part of present-day Shan xi 山西 and the region in present-day Inner Mongolia north of the Great Bend of the Yellow River. Mentioned with 1532.

Gui fu 桂府 [1]
Name of a village. See → Gui fu cun 桂府村.

Gui fu cun 桂府村 [1]
Name of a village within the borders of present-day Peng lai 蓬萊 city in Shan dong 山東. Mentioned with 474.

Gui guang 桂廣 [1]
Regional name. It is an abbreviation for present-day Guang xi 廣西 and Guang dong 廣東. Mentioned with 925.

Gui hai 桂海 [1]
Regional name. It refers to present-day Guang xi 廣西. Mentioned with 813.

Gui lin 桂林 [7 + 2 + 1 + 2]

□ Name of a *fu* 府. [7] It was founded under the Ming 明, in 1372. The seat of administration was in present-day Gui lin city in Guang xi 廣西. The territory administered comprised the area north from present-day Yong fu 永福 and Yang shuo 陽朔 in the northeastern portion of Guang xi. It was abolished in 1913. Mentioned with 467, 474, 1247, 1283, 1503.

□ Popular local name. [2] During Song 宋 times, the name was used to designate Shi an 始安 commandery and Jing jiang fu 靜江府, that is, present-day Gui lin city of Guang xi. Mentioned with 303, 1063.

□ Name of a commandery. [1] It was established by Qin 秦. The seat of administration was at a point southwest of present-day Gui ping 桂平 city in Guang xi 廣西. Its administrative area included the present-day cities of Liu zhou 柳州, Gui lin and Wu zhou 梧州 in Guang xi, and Zhao qing 肇慶 city and Mao ming 茂名 city in Guang dong 廣東. Under Wu di 武帝 (156 – 87) of Western Han 漢, the name was changed to Yu lin 郁林 commandery. Mentioned with 350.

□ Name of a commandery. [2] It was established, under Three Kingdoms' Wu 吳, in 274. The seat of administration was at a point southeast of present-day Liu zhou 柳州 city in Guang xi 廣西. The territory administered comprised present-day Liu zhou city and other areas. Under Liu Song 劉宋, the seat of administration was moved to a point southwest of present-day Wu xuan 武宣 county. Later the old seat was reestablished. The commandery was abolished at the beginning of the *kai huang* 開皇 reign period (581 – 600) of Sui 隋. Mentioned with 586.

Gui ling 桂嶺 [2]

Name of a county. It was established by Sui 隋, in 598, and administered from Gui ling town northeast of present-day He zhou 賀州 city in Guang xi 廣西. The county was abolished under late Yuan 元. Gui ling became a minor place name only and persists until the present. Mentioned with 376, 1502.

Gui shun 歸順 [1]

Name of a *zhou* 州. It was established at the beginning of Yuan 元. The seat of administration was in present-day Jiu zhou 舊州 village, 10 *li* south of Jing xi 靖西 county, in Guang xi 廣西. At the beginning of Ming 明, it was demoted as Gui shun dong 歸順峒. In 1496, the *zhou* was reestablished and later the seat of administration was moved to the present Jing xi county. In 1886, the *zhou* was promoted to be the Gui shun directly administered *zhou*, *zhi li zhou* 直隸州. In 1912, its status was raised to Gui shun fu 歸順府, but in the next year changed to Jing xi county. Mentioned with 540.

Gui yang 桂陽 [7 + 1]

□ Name of a county [7] See Gui yang xian 桂陽縣.

□ Name of a *zhou* 州. [1] It was established under the Ming 明, in 1376. The seat of administration was in present-day Gui yang county in Hu nan 湖南. The territory administered comprised an area corresponding to the present-day counties of Gui yang, Lan shan 藍山, Jia he 嘉禾 and Lin wu 臨武 in Hu nan. In 1732, its status was raised to a directly administered *zhou*, *zhi li zhou* 直隸州. In 1913, the area was changed into Gui yang county. Mentioned with 1038.

Gui yang xian 桂陽縣 [1]

Name of a county. It was established by Western Han 漢. The seat of administration was in present-day Lian zhou 連州 city in Guang dong 廣東. In 1282, under Yuan 元, the county was promoted to be Gui yang zhou 桂陽州. Mentioned with 217, 376, 635, 818, 1265, 1462.

Gui zhou 桂州 [7]

Name of a *zhou* 州. It was established, under Southern Dynasties' Liang 梁, in 507. The seat of administration was at a point southwest of present-day Liu zhou 柳州 city in Guang xi 廣西. The territory administered extended in present-day Guang xi from Long sheng 龍勝 and Yong fu 永福 in the West to Li pu 荔浦 in the South. Under Southern Song 宋, in 1131, its status was raised to Jing jiang fu 靜江府. Mentioned with 202, 362, 376, 428, 552, 794, 1372.

Gui zhou 貴州 [4]

Name of a Provincial Administration Commission, *bu zheng shi si* 布政使司. It was established in 1413. The seat of administration was in present-day Gui yang 貴陽 city in Gui zhou 貴州. Its administrative area corresponded to most of present-day Gui zhou province. Qing 清 created Gui zhou province, and adjusted its boundaries to slowly form the province as it now is. Mentioned with 157, 569, 1061, 1375, 1427.

Gui zhou 媯州 [1]

Name of a *zhou* 州. It was established under the Tang 唐, in 634. The seat of administration was in Shi hui yao 石灰窯, located southwest of present-day Zhuo lu 涿鹿 county in He bei 河北. The territory administered comprised an area corresponding to present-day Zhang jia kou 張家口 and the counties of Huai lai 懷來, Chi cheng 赤城, Chong li 崇禮, Zhang bei 張北, Huai an 懷安 and Zhuo lu city in He bei. Later under Empress Wu Zetian's (624 – 705) short-lived Zhou 周 dynasty, the seat of administration was moved to old Huai lai, located southeast of present-day Huai lai county. During the Five Dynasties period, the area was conquered by the Khitan. The name was changed to Ke han zhou 可汗州. Mentioned with 931.

Gui zhou 歸州 [1]

Name of a *zhou* 州. It was established under Tang 州, in 619. The seat of administration was in present-day Gui zhou 歸州 town northwest of Zi gui 秭歸 county in Hu bei 湖北. The territory administered comprised the three present-day counties of Zi gui, Ba dong 巴東 and Xing shan 興山 in Hu bei. During Southern Song 宋, the seat of administration was moved to an area southeast of present-day Gui zhou town. The *zhou* was eliminated in 1376, but restored in 1380. In 1561, the seat was returned to present-day Gui zhou town. In 1912, the *zhou* became a county. Mentioned with 1057, 1096.

Guo 虢 [1 + 1]

□ Name of an ancient county. [1] It was located northeast of present-day Ping lu 平陸 county in Shan xi 山西. Mentioned with 261.

□ Name of a *zhou* 州. [1] See → Guo zhou 虢州. Mentioned with 1017.

Guo guo 咼國 [1]

Name of a foreign county. Details are lacking. Mentioned with 1232.

Guo zhou 虢州 [4]

Name of a *zhou* 州. It was established by Sui 隋, in 583. The seat of administration was in present-day Lu shi 盧氏 county in He nan 河南. The territory administered comprised Ling bao 靈寶 and Luan chuan 欒川 to the West in the western part of He nan, and the area of Fu niu 伏牛 mountain to the North. In 607, it was eliminated, but restored under Tang 唐, in 618. In 634, the seat of administration was moved to present-day Ling Bao city in He nan. Under Yuan 元, in 1271, it was abolished. Mentioned with 47, 261, 949, 1017, 1250, 1375.

Guo zhou 果州 [1]

Name of a *zhou* 州. It was established under Tang 唐, in 621. The seat of administration was at a point 5 *li* north of present-day Nan chong 南充 city in Si chuan 四川. The territory administered comprised the present-day cities and counties of Nan chong, Peng an 蓬安, Xi chong 西充, Ying shan 營山 and Yue chi 岳池 in Si chuan. During Southern Song 宋, in 1227, the status of the area as raised to Shun qing fu 順慶府. Mentioned with 956.

-H-

Ha la huo 哈喇火 [1]

See → Huo zhou 火州. Mentioned with 862.

Ha mi 哈密 [1]

See → Ha mi wei 哈密衛. Mentioned with 209.

Ha mi wei 哈密衛 [1]

Name of a guard. It was established under the Ming 明, in 1406. The seat of administration was in present-day Hami City in Xin jiang 新疆. Later, following the *zheng de* 正德 reign period (1506 – 1521), it was subordinated to Turfan and then abolished. Mentioned with 992.

Hai 海 [1 + 1]

□ Name of a *zhou* 州. See → Hai zhou 海州. Mentioned with 1052.

□ General regional name. [1] The precise focus is uncertain. Mentioned with 439.

Hai bei 海北 [3]

Regional name. It is a northern equivalent, "North of the Sea," to the expression Hai nan 海南, "South of the Sea." The term refers to the Lei zhou 雷州 peninsula and the adjacent area north of it, that is the region north of the Qiong zhou 瓊州 strait. Mentioned with 144.

Hai bian guo 海邊國 [1]
General regional name for "Countries at the side of the Sea" without specific application. Mentioned with 489.

Hai bin 海濱 [1]
Regional name. The area designates the region of central China "Along the Sea." Mentioned with 619.

Hai dong 海東 [2]
Regional name. It refers to the areas of the Korean peninsula because they were situated "East of the (Yellow) Sea." Mentioned with 195, 1109.

Hai feng 海豐 [1]
Name of a locality of salt production. It was in the Yang er zhuang Hui nationality town, Yang er zhuang hui zu xiang 羊二莊回族鄉, southeast of the present-day city of Hua shi 驊市. Mentioned with 1057.

Hai guo 海國 [1]
Name of a region. The term refers to the present-day island of Hai nan 海南 and areas in southeast Asia. Mentioned with 86.

Hai kang 海康 [1]
Name of a county. It was established under the Sui 隋, in 590, and administered by He zhou 合州. Its seat of administration was present-day Lei zhou 雷州 city in Guang zhou 廣州. In 1994, it was changed to be Lei zhou city. Mentioned with 1192.

Hai ling 海陵 [1]
Name of a county. It was established by Western Han 漢. The seat of administration was in present-day Tai zhou 泰州 city in Jiang su 江蘇. At the beginning of the *hong wu* 洪武 reign period (1368 – 1398) of Ming 明, it became part of Tai zhou. Mentioned with 760.

Hai nan 海南 [21 + 7]
□ Name of a region. [21] This is the region along the ocean comprising the area south of the Qiong zhou 瓊州 strait, i.e., Hai nan 海南 Island. Mentioned with 144, 175, 330, 480, 509, 523, 585, 587, 680, 777, 838, 855, 1028, 1139, 1230, 1248, 1257, 1369, 1399, 1471.
□ Name of a region. [7] It refers generally to that part of present-day coastal Southeast Asia near China. Mentioned with 86, 483, 493, 511, 779, 1133.

Hai ning 海寧 [1]
Name of a county. It was founded under Western Jin 晉, in 280, by changing the name of Hai yang 海陽 county. Its seat of administration was in present-day Wan an 萬安 town, located 10 *li* east of Xiu ning 休寧 county in An hui 安徽. The county was subordinate to Xin an 新安 commandery. Under Sui 隋, in 589, the county was changed to Xiu ning county.

Hai xi 海西 [1]
Name of a county. It was established under Western 漢 Han. The seat of administration was at a point 20 *li* southeast of present-day Guan yun 灌雲 county in

Jiang su 江蘇. The county was abolished under Western Jin 晉, but reestablished in 549, under Eastern Wei 魏. It was subordinate to Hai xi commandery. Northern Qi 齊 eliminated it. Mentioned with 1210.

Hai xi nan 海西南 [1]

Name of a region. The term applies to the present-day Lei zhou 雷州 peninsula. Mentioned with 1357.

Hai ya guo 海牙國 [1]

Name of a country. It was apparently located around the city Sha ha lu ke ya 沙哈魯克亞, approximately 80 km to the west of the present-day capital Tashkent of Uzbekistan, on the northen bank of the Syr Darya river. The name Hai ya 海牙 is probably the old Turkic tribal name Qay or Qaiya. Mentioned with 14.

Hai yan 海鹽 [3]

Name of a county. It was established by Qin 秦, and subordinated to Kuai ji 會稽 commandery. The seat of administration was at a point south of present-day Zhang yan 張堰 town, 31 *li* southeast of the Jin shan 金山 district in Shang hai 上海. At the end of Western Han 漢, the county sank into Lake Zhe 柘, and the seat of administration was moved to a point east of present-day Ping hu 平湖 city in Zhe jiang 浙江. In 127, under Eastern Han, this site also fell into the same lake. The seat of administration was moved to a point that today lies in the sea southeast of present-day Zha pu 乍浦 town of Ping hu city. In 341, under Eastern Jin 晉, it was moved to the southeastern corner of present-day Hai yan xian cheng 海鹽縣城 in Zhe jiang. In 558, under Southern Dynasties' Chen 陳, the area was separated off and subordinated to Hai ning 海寧 commandery. It was later absorbed by Yan guan 鹽官 county. Under the Tang 唐, in 711, the county was reestablished. It was eliminated again in 712. It was again established in 717 and subordinated to Su zhou 蘇州, and the administration was moved to present-day Hai yan county. Under Yuan 元, in 1295, the status of the county was raised to Hai yan zhou 海鹽州. In 1369, under Ming 明, it became Hai yan county again. Mentioned with 741, 781, 1393.

Hai yang 海陽 [1]

Name of a place. It was established under Ming 明, during the reign period *cheng hua* 成化 (1465 – 1487), and subordinated to the Da song 大嵩 guard. It was located at the garrison at present-day Hai yang suo 海陽所 town of Ru shan 乳山 city of Shan dong 山東. Mentioned with 126.

Hai zhou 海州 [9]

Name of a *zhou* 州. It was established, under Eastern Wei 魏, in 549. The seat of administration was in present-day Long qie 龍且 southwest of Guan yun 灌雲 county in Jiang su 江蘇. Under Northern Qi 齊 it was moved to the present-day Hai zhou 海州 district of Lian yun gang 連雲港 city in Jiang su. The area administered corresponded to present-day Lian yun gang city in Jiang su and the counties of Gan yu 贛榆, Dong hai 東海, Shu yang 沭陽, and Guan yun in Jiang su. Under Southern Song 宋, in 1235, the seat of administration was moved to Nan cheng 南城 town located southeast of the present-day Lian yun gang. In 1252, the administration was returned to the old site. In 1912, the area was changed to be Dong hai 東海 county. Mentioned with 130, 289, 687, 703, 799, 928, 975, 1057.

Han 漢 [2 + 8 + 5]

□ Name of a region. [2] The reference is to the area of the flow of the Han river near Xiang yang 襄陽, including among others the northwestern region of Hu bei 湖北. Mentioned with 793, 848.

□ Name of a *zhou* 州. [8] It was established under Tang 唐, in 686. The seat of administration was in present-day Guang han 廣漢 city in Si chuan 四川. Its administrative area comprised the present-day cities and counties of Guang han, De yang 德陽, Mian yang 綿陽, Shi fang 什邡 and Jin tang 金堂 in Si chuan. Under Southern Song 宋, during the reign period *duan ping* 端平 (1234 – 126), the *zhou* was eliminated. It was reestablished during early Yuan 元, in 1260. In 1913, the *zhou* became Guang han county. Mentioned with 31, 328, 503, 639, 864, 994, 1202, 1396.

□ Name of a river valley. [5] See Han jiang 漢江. Mentioned with 75, 317, 439, 1096.

Han cheng 韓城 [1]

Name of a county. It was established under Sui 隋, in 598. The seat of administration was in Cheng gu 城古 village, located two *li* southeast of Han cheng city in Shaan xi 陜西. Under Tang 唐, in 905, the county became Han yuan 韓原 county. In 926, it again became Han cheng county. Under Jin 金, in 1215, its status was raised to Zhen zhou 禎州. During early Yuan 元, in 1265, it again became Han cheng county. In 1983, it was established as Han cheng city. Mentioned with 816.

Han chuan 漢川 [2]

Name of a commandery. It was established under Sui 隋, in 607. The seat of administration was at a point east of present-day Han zhong 漢中 city in Shaan xi 陜西. The area administered comprised present-day Han zhong city and the present-day counties of Nan zheng 南鄭, Mian 勉, Cheng gu 城固, Yang 洋, Fo ping 佛坪, and Zhen ba 鎮巴 in Shaan xi, and Nan jiang 鎮巴 in Si chuan 四川. Under Tang 唐, in 618, it was renamed Liang zhou 梁州. Mentioned with 1147, 1435.

Han dan 邯鄲 [10]

Name of a county. It was established by Qin 秦, and administered by Han dan commandery. The seat of administration was at the present-day Han dan city of He bei 河北. It was abolished under Eastern Wei 魏, at the beginning of the *tian ping* 天平 reign period (534 – 537), and made part of Zhang 漳 county. In 598, it was reestablished and has continued to exist until the present-day. Mentioned with 21, 272, 816, 931, 1057, 1218, 1412, 1511, 1523.

Han di 漢地 [2]

Regional name. It was situated in the region of the middle and lower watershed of the Yellow River in the Central Plain. Mentioned with 142, 331.

Han gu 函谷 [2]
Name of a pass. It was established during the Warring States period by Qin 秦. It was located 30 *li* northeast of present-day Ling bao 靈寶 city in He nan 河南. Only the old pass gate still exists. Mentioned with 735.

Han guo 韓國 [1]
Name of a country. It was positioned in the South of the present-day Korean peninsula and comprised Ma han 馬韓, Chen han 馬韓, and Bian han 弁韓. Mentioned with 635.

Han jiang 漢江 [1]
Name of a river. This is the Han shui 漢水, the largest tributary of the Yang zi. It has its source in the Bo zhong 嶓冢 mountain located north of present-day Ning qiang 寧強 county in the southwestern part of Shaan xi 陝西. It flows through the southern part of Shaan xi and the northwestern and middle part of Hu bei 湖北, and enters the Yang zi at Wu han 武漢 city. It is 1532 km in length. Mentioned with 535.

Han mian 漢沔 [3]
Regional name. It refers to the middle and lower watershed of the Han shui 漢水 in the northwest section of Hu bei 湖北. Mentioned with 67, 277, 1233.

Han nan 漢南 [1]
Name of a commandery. It was founded under Tang 唐, in 757. The seat of administration was in present-day An kang 安康 city in Shaan xi 陝西. The area administered comprised in present-day Shaan xi an area of the Han shui 漢水 watershed, reaching from Shi quan 石泉 county in the West to Xun yang 旬陽 county in the East. In 758, the commandery was changed to Jin zhou 金州. Mentioned with 931.

Han shang 漢上 [1]
Regional name. Further details are unavailable. Mentioned with 1340.

Han shi shan 寒石山 [1]
Name of a mountain. It is situated northwest of present-day Lin hai 臨海 city in Zhe jiang 浙江. Mentioned with 362.

Han yang 漢陽 [2 + 1]
□ Name of a *fu* 府. [2] Established by Yuan 元, in 1277. The seat of administration was at a location in the Han yang 漢陽 district of present-day Wu han 武漢 city in Hu bei 湖北. The territory administered comprised the Han yang district and the Cai dian 蔡甸 district of present-day Wu han city, and the area of Han chuan 漢川 city. Under the Ming 明, in 1376, the *fu* was demoted to Han yang zhou 漢陽州, but four years later the *fu* was restored. In 1912, it was abolished. Mentioned with 185, 1254.
□ Name of a county. [1] It was established under Sui 隋, in 606. It was administered from a point below Lin zhang 臨嶂 mountain east of the present-day Cai dian 蔡甸 district of Wu han city in Hu bei. Under Tang 唐, in 621, the seat of administration was moved to the present-day Han yang district in Wu han 武

漢 city. In 1949, it was moved to Cai dian town. In 1992, the county became Cai dian district of Wu an City. Mentioned with 75.

Han zhong 漢中 [47 + 2]

□ Name of a commandery. [47] It was established, by Qin 秦, in 312 BCE. The seat of administration was at a point east of present-day Han zhong 漢中 city in Shaan xi 陝西. Its administrative area corresponded to an area in present-day Shaan xi extending from the Qin ling 秦嶺 mountain range in the North, and Liu ba 留壩 and Mian xian 勉縣 in the West, to the watershed of the Qian 乾 river and, in present-day Hu bei, Yun xian 鄖縣 county and Bao kang 保康 in the East, to Mi cang 米倉 mountain and Da ba 大巴 mountain in the South. Under Western Han 漢, the seat of administration was moved to a point north-west of present-day An kang 安康 city in Shaan xi, but Eastern Han restored the old seat of administration. Afterwards, the territories of the commandery were reduced in size. Under Northern Zhou 周, the territories only comprised the cities and counties of Han zhong, Nan zheng 南鄭 and Cheng gu 城固 in Shaan xi. The commandery was eliminated under Sui 隋, at the beginning of the *kai huang* 開皇 reign period (581 – 600), but under Tang 唐, in 742, Liang zhou 梁州 was renamed as Han zhong commandery. It again became Liang zhou in 758. Mentioned with 107, 130, 258, 261, 273, 290, 306, 461, 519, 520, 557, 582, 620, 629, 639, 666, 668, 692, 752, 768, 781, 793, 829, 864, 917, 920, 975, 1020, 1147, 1160, 1178, 1217, 1218, 1241, 1305, 1392, 1449, 1485, 1523.

□ Name of a *fu* 府. [2] It was established under the Ming 明, in 1370. The seat of administration was in present-day Han zhong city in Shaan xi. The territory administered comprised the western half of the area of present-day Shaan xi south of the Qin ling 秦嶺 mountain range. It was abolished in 1913. Mentioned with 511, 520.

Hang 杭 [3]

Name of a *zhou* 州. See → Hang zhou 杭州. Mentioned with 381, 780, 1485.

Hang zhou 杭州 [5 + 3 + 1]

□ Name of a *zhou* 州. [5] It was established under Sui 隋, in 589. The seat of administration was in present-day Yu hang 餘杭 town west of Yu hang district in Hang zhou city in Zhe jiang 浙江. In the following year, the administrative seat was moved to the present-day city of Hang zhou in Zhe jiang. Later, in 591, the seat was moved to a point south of Hang zhou city, at the foot of Feng huang 鳳凰 mountain. During Tang 唐 and Song 宋 times, the administrative area of the *zhou* amounted to what are now the districts and cities of Hang zhou, Hai ning 海寧, Yu hang, Fu yang 富陽 and Lin an 臨安 in Zhe jiang. Under Southern Song 宋, in 1129, the status of the *zhou* was raised to be Lin an fu 臨安府. Mentioned with 345, 365, 456, 1393, 1420.

□ Name of a *fu* 府. [3] It was established under Yuan 元, in 1366. The seat of administration was in present-day Hang zhou city in Zhe jiang. The territory administered comprised the present-day districts and cities of Hang zhou, Hai ning, Yu hang, Fu yang and Lin an in Zhe jiang. It was abolished in 1912. Mentioned with 192, 303, 1563.

□ Name of a *lu* 路. [1] It was established under Yuan 元, in 1278. The seat of administration was in present-day Hang zhou city in Zhe jiang. The territory administered comprised the present-day districts and cities of Hang zhou, Hai ning, Yu hang, Fu yang and Lin an in Zhe jiang. In 1366, it was changed to Hang zhou fu 杭州府. Mentioned with 1106.

Hang yue jian 杭越間 [2]

This is a composite designation. It refers to the Hang zhou 杭州 city, located as today, of Northern Song 宋 times, and to Yue zhou 越州, that is present-day Shao xing 紹興 city. The *jian* 間, "between," refers to the areas in between them. Mentioned with 1254, 1430.

Hao 濠 [1]

Name of a *zhou* 州. See → Hao zhou 濠州. Mentioned with 208.

Hao zhou 濠州 [4]

Name of a *zhou* 州. It was founded under Sui 隋, in 582. The seat of administration was at a point east of present-day Lin huai guan 臨淮關, located northeast of Feng yang 鳳陽 county in An hui 安徽. The territory administered comprised the present-day cities and counties of Bang bu 蚌埠, Ding yuan 定遠, Feng yang 鳳陽 and Ming guang 明光 in An hui. In 1278, the *zhou* became Lin hao fu 臨濠府. In 1291, it became Hao zhou again, but was changed to Lin hao fu in 1367. Mentioned with 64, 474, 556.

He 河 [1 + 4]

□ Regional name. [1] It refers to the He nan 河南 area situated along the middle and lower reaches of the Huang he 黄河 watershed, including the central part and the northern regions of He nan. Mentioned with 99.

□ Name of a river watershed. [4]. This is the Yellow River. It has its sources in Qing hai 青海 at the northern foot of the Ba yan ka la 巴顔喀拉 (Bayan qala) mountains. Its upper reaches pass through Ning xia 寧夏 and ring the Chinese Central Plain in Mongolia. Its middle reaches separate Shan xi 山西 and Shaan xi 陝西. During Tang 唐 and Song 宋, the lower reaches entered the ocean in the present-day Gulf of Bo hai 渤海. Mentioned with 429, 1207, 1335, 1478.

He 合 [1]

Name of a *zhou* 州. See → He zhou 合州. Mentioned with 107.

He 賀 [1]

Name of a *zhou* 州. See → He zhou 賀州. Mentioned with 925.

He bei 河北 [6 + 6 + 20]

□ Name of a region. [6] It refers to the area north of the Yellow River, south of the Yan shan 燕山 mountains, east of the Tai hang 太行 mountains and west of the Gulf of Bo hai 渤海. Mentioned with 599, 665, 856, 861, 1057, 1289.

□ Name of a circuit. [6] It was established by Tang 唐, in 627. Following the *kai yuan* 開元 reign period (713 – 741), the seat of administration was in Da jie xiang 大街鄉, a sub-administrative unit located northeast of present-day Da ming 大名 county in He bei 河北. The territory administered comprised the two present-day cites of Bei jing 北京 and Tian jin 天津, and much of He bei and Liao ning 遼寧, also the region north of the ancient Yellow River watershed in He nan 河南 and Shan dong 山東. The circuit was later abolished. Mentioned with 600, 614, 1033, 1092, 1289, 1473.

□ Name of a *lu* 路. [20] It was established under Northern Song 宋, in 997. The seat of administration was in Da jie xiang 大街鄉, a sub-administrative unit located northeast of present-day Da ming 大名 county in He bei 河北. The administrative area of the *lu* corresponded to present-day Yi 易 county, Xiong 雄 county, and Ba zhou 霸州 city in He bei, the area south of the Hai he 海河 river of Tian jin 天津 city and the largest part of Shan dong 山東 and He nan 河南 north of the Yellow River. Later, during the *xi ning* 熙寧 reign period (1068 – 1077), the *lu* was divided into an eastern and a western part, with the eastern *lu* administered from Da jie xiang, located northeast of present-day Da ming 大名 county, and the western from the present Zheng ding 王定 county. Early Yuan 元 abolished the two *lu*. Mentioned with 158, 196, 202, 542, 572, 612, 648, 667, 730, 768, 931, 1038, 1090, 1160, 1175, 1207, 1215, 1294, 1316, 1467.

He dong 河東 [28 + 5 + 18 + 6]

Ancient regional name. [28] It refers to the southwestern part of the present-day Shan xi 山西. Because the area is intersected by the Yellow River running from north to south forming the western boundary of the area, it is known as "East of the River." Mentioned with 64, 68, 188, 202, 345, 374, 462, 653, 665, 702, 730, 733, 748, 816, 1038, 1057, 1122, 1215, 1254, 1258, 1273, 1340, 1443, 1443, 1562.

□ Regional name. [5] During Ming 明 times, He dong referred to the area of the present-day province of Shan xi 山西. Mentioned with 324, 331, 444, 856, 1057.

□ Name of a *lu* 路. [18] It was established under Northern Song 宋, in 997. The seat of administration was in Tai yuan 太原 city in present-day Shan xi 山西 province. The territory administered comprised in present-day Shan xi an area extending from south of the Great Wall to a line formed by the Long men 龍門 mountains, the Ji 稷 mountains, Jiang 絳 county, and Yuan qu 垣曲 county in the South, and the region of Jia 佳 county in the North, in Shaan xi 陝西, also in the South. In 1128, the *lu* was divided into a southern and a northern *lu*. They were abolished during the period of Mongol rule. Mentioned with 66, 191, 203, 324, 369, 417, 461, 675, 811, 816, 861, 931, 941, 986, 1057, 1242, 1306, 1443.

□ Name of a circuit. [6] It was established under Tang 唐, in 627. Its territory of administration comprised the entire province of Shan xi 山西, and the area within and outside of the Great Wall in the northwestern part of He bei 河北. During Tang, following the *kai yuan* 開元 reign period (713 – 741), it was administered from Pu zhou 蒲州 town, located southwest of present-day Yong ji 永濟 city in Shan xi. Later, the circuit was abolished. Mentioned with 34, 137, 702, 844, 1057, 1340.

He ji 河濟 [1]

This is a regional name. It applied to the region between the Yellow River and the Ji shui 濟水 during Western Han 漢 times, including the southeastern area of present-day He bei 河北 and the northwestern portion of present-day Shan dong 山東. Mentioned with 631.

He jian 河間 [2 + 3 + 2]

□ Name of a commandery. [2] It was established at the beginning of Western Han 漢. The seat of administration was at a point 16 *li* east of present-day Xian 獻 county in He bei 河北. In 178 BCE, the commandery was turned into a feudal country, but under Wei 魏, during the Three Kingdoms period, it was changed back into a commandery. The seat of administration was moved to a point southeast of present-day Xian county. The commandery again became a feudal country under Western Jin 晉. It was made a commandery again under Northern Wei 魏, and the administration was moved to a point south of the present-day He jian city. The commandery was abolished under Sui 隋, at the beginning of the *kai huang* 開皇 reign period (581 – 600), but at the beginning of the reign period *da ye* 大業 (605 – 615) of the Sui 隋, and during the reign periods *tian bao* 天寶 (742 – 756) and *zhi de* 至德 (756 – 758) of Tang 唐, Ying zhou 瀛州 had its name periodically changed to He jian commandery. Under Sui, during the reign period *da ye* 大業, the administration was moved to the present-day He jian city. In 758, the commandery was abolished. Mentioned with 816, 1087.

□ Name of a feudal country. [3] It was established in 178 BCE. The seat of administration was at a point 16 *li* southeast of present-day Xian county in He bei. The territory administered comprised the present Xian county and Bo tou 泊頭 city. It was eliminated at the beginning of Eastern Han, but reestablished in 90 with enlarged jurisdiction. This corresponded to an area extending in present-day He bei from Xiong 雄 county and the Da qing 大清 river in the North, and the Nan yun 南運 river in the East, to Gao yang 高陽 and Su ning 肅寧 in the West, and Fu cheng 阜城 in the South. The area became a commandery under Wei 魏 of the Three Kingdoms. Mentioned with 787, 1321, 1432.

□ Name of a county. [2] It was established under Sui, in 596, and administered from present-day He jian city in He bei. It 1990, this became He jian city. Mentioned with 887, 1308.

He ling guo 訶陵國 [1]

Name of a country. This is She po 闍婆 country. It was located in present Indonesia either on the island of Java, or on the island of Sumatra. Mentioned with 110.

He luo 河洛 [1]

Regional name. It refers to the confluence of the Yellow River and the Luo shui 洛水 and nearby areas including the present-day Luo yang 洛陽 in He nan 河南 and the areas located about it. Mentioned with 72.

He ming 鶴鳴 [1]

Name of a mountain. It is situated on the borders of He ming xiang 鶴鳴鄉, 30 *li* northwest of present-day Da yi 大邑 county in Si chuan 四川. Mentioned with 90.

He nan 河南 [3 + 11 + 5]

□ Name of a *fu* 府. [3] It was established under Tang 唐, in 713. The seat of administration was in the present-day Luo yang 洛陽 city in He nan 河南. The territory administered comprised an area in present-day He nan extending from Ji yuan 濟源 city and the counties of Luo ning 洛寧 and Mian chi 澠池 in the

West, to Xin mi 新密 city and Ba yi 鞏義 city in the East. During the *xing ding* 興定 reign period (1217 – 1222) of the Jin 金 dynasty, it became Jin chang fu 金昌府. Yuan 元 changed it to He nan fu lu 河南府路 and Ming 明 changed this to He nan fu 河南府. It was abolished in 1913. Mentioned with 50, 734, 1057.

□ Regional name. [11] It refers to the region south of the lower watershed of the Yellow River. The reference is primarily to an area in the present-day province of He nan 河南. Mentioned with 339, 428, 443, 648, 934, 1004, 1015, 1126, 1313, 1316, 1335.

□ Name of a Provincial Administration Commission, *bu zheng si* 布政司. [5] It was established under Ming 明, in 1368, as a "Branch of the Central Secretariat," *zhong shu fen sheng* 中書分省, The next year it became He nan Branch Secretariat, He nan *xing sheng* 河南行省, and, in 1377, it became the He nan Provincial Administration Commission, He nan *bu zheng shi si* 河南布政使司. Its seat of administration was located in present-day Kai feng 開封 city in He nan. The territory administered comprised the region of the present-day province of He nan. At the beginning of the Qing 清 dynasty, it became He nan province, He nan sheng 河南省. Mentioned with 270, 905, 927, 976, 1310.

He nan bei 河南北 [2]

Regional name. The reference was to the region of the south and north shores along the lower reaches of the Yellow River. This includes the present He nan 河南, He bei 河北 and Shan dong 山東. Mentioned with 631, 665.

He nei 河內 [2 + 17]

□ Name of a county. [2] It was founded by Sui 隋, in 596. The seat of administration was in present-day Qin yang 沁陽 city in He nan 河南. In 1913, it became Qin yang county. In 1989, the county was changed into a city. Mentioned with 129, 695.

□ Name of a commandery. [17] It was established by Western Han 漢, in 205 BCE. The seat of administration was at a point southwest of present-day Wu zhi 武陟 county in He nan 河南. The territory administered comprised an area in present-day He nan extending from the Yellow River in the South to the Jing guang 京廣 railroad in the East. During Western Jin 晉, the seat of administration was moved to present-day Qin yang 沁陽 city in He nan. During the Sui 隋 period, in 583, the commandery was abolished but reestablished in 607. Under Tang 唐, in 619, the commandery was changed to Huai zhou 懷州 and, in 742, it became He nei commandery again. In 758, it again became Huai zhou. Mentioned with 68, 126, 167, 289, 356, 575, 615, 706, 823, 884, 980, 1092, 1275, 1470, 1478, 1505.

He pu 合浦 [5]

Name of a commandery. It was established under Western Han, in 111 BCE. The seat of administration was at a point south of present-day Xu wen 徐聞 county in Guang dong 廣東. The jurisdiction covered an area reaching from present-day Xin xing 新興 county and Kai ping 開平 city in Guang dong towards the Southwest, and in Guang xi 廣西 from Rong 容 county, Yu lin 玉林 and Heng 橫 county towards the South. During Eastern Han 漢, the seat of administration was moved to present-day Jiu zhou 舊州 village south of Pu bei 浦北 county in Guang xi. The commandery was eliminated, in 589, under Sui 隋 after pacifying Chen 陳, but later reestablished. In 742, under Tang 唐, Lian zhou 連州 was changed to He pu commandery, but in 758 it again became Lian zhou. Mentioned with 319, 376, 514, 533, 1403.

He pu xian 合浦縣 [1]
Name of a county. It was established under Western Han 漢, in 111 BCE. The seat of administration was in present-day Jiu zhou 舊州 village south of Pu bei 浦北 county in Guang xi 廣西. It was eliminated under Ming 明, in 1374, but restored in 1381. Mentioned with 1467.

He shaan 河陜 [8]
Combined regional name. Further details are unavailable. Mentioned with 31, 546, 639, 907, 1067, 1292, 1417, 1449.

He shang 河上 [1]
Minor place name. It is approximately located in the area of Mou 牟 county in He nan 河南. Mentioned with 927.

He shui 涸水 [1]
Name of a river quoted in the BCGM from the *Guan zi* 管子 (7th c. BCE). But no such name is mentioned in the *Guan zi* versions extent today. Mentioned with 87.

He shuo 河朔 [9]
Regional name. It refers generally to the area north of the Yellow River. Mentioned with 364, 614, 633, 667, 1135, 1139, 1242, 1394.

He xi 河西 [27]
Regional name. It refers to present-day Gan su 甘肅 and Qing hai 青海, the area "west of the (Yellow) River," that is, the western corridor of the river and the watershed of the Huang shui 湟水. Mentioned with 140, 188, 239, 285, 324, 361, 504, 934, 1030, 1192, 1242, 1340, 1519, 1258.

He xi shan 河西山 [1]
Name of a mountain. Further details are unavailable. Mentioned with 1030.

He yang 河陽 [6]
Regional name. It refers to a section of He nan with the area from the Tai hang 太行 mountains and the Wang wu 王屋 mountains toward the South, and from the Yellow River toward the North, including the present-day cities and counties of Ji yuan 濟源, Meng zhou 孟州, Jiao zhuo 焦作 and Wen xian 溫縣. Mentioned with 485, 520, 718, 911, 922, 1445.

He yuan 河源 [1]
Regional name. It refers to the "origins of the (Yellow) River." From Han 漢 times on, these origins were assigned to the area of Kun lun 崑崙 mountain in present-day Xin jiang 新疆. Mentioned with 298.

He zhong 河中 [7]
Name of a *fu* 府. See → He zhong fu 河中府. Mentioned with 53, 78, 644, 1324, 1445, 1477, 1519.

He zhong fu 河中府 [10]
Name of a *fu* 府. It was established under Tang 唐, in 720, and administered from present-day Pu zhou 蒲州 town located southwest of Yong ji 永濟 city in Shan xi 山西. In the same year, the *fu* was changed to Pu zhou. In 760, He zhong fu was restored. Its administrative area corresponded to an area in the southern part of present-day Shan xi extending from the Long men 龍門 mountain toward the South, to the Ji shan 稷山, Rui cheng 芮城 county and Yun cheng 運城 city in the East, and the southeastern portion of Da li 大荔 county in Shaan xi 陝西. Under Ming 明, in 1369, the area became Pu zhou. Mentioned with 39, 45, 218, 272, 668, 922, 950, 1062, 1254, 1446.

He zhou 河州 [2]
Name of a *zhou* 州. It was established during the Liang 涼 dynasty of the Sixteen Kingdoms period. The seat of administration was at a point southwest of present-day Lin xia 臨夏 city in Gan su 甘肅. In 445, during Northern Wei 魏, the *zhou* was changed to Fu han 枹罕 town, and the seat of administration was moved to the present Lin xia city. In 492, it was restored as He zhou. In 1269, under the Mongols, it became He zhou lu 河州路. Under Ming 明, in 1451, it was again changed to be He zhou. In 1913, the area became Dao he 導河 county. Mentioned with 447, 1196.

He zhou 河洲 [1]
General place reference to the region of the present-day so-called He xi 河西 corridor. Mentioned with 1282.

He zhou 合州 [6]
Name of a *zhou* 州. It was established, under Western Wei 魏, in 556. The seat of administration was in the present-day He chuan 合川 district in Chong qing 重慶 city. During the early Sui 隋 period, at the end of the *kai huang* 開皇 reign period (581 – 600), it became Fu zhou 涪州 and, in 607, it became Fu ling 涪陵 commandery. In 618, it became He zhou again. Its area of administration embraced the He chuan district, Tong liang 銅梁 county, Wu sheng 武勝 county, and Da zu 大足 county in present-day Chong qing. Under Southern Song 宋, in 1243, the seat of administration was moved to Diao yu cheng 釣魚城, located 10 *li* east of the present-day He chuan district. In 1285, under Yuan 元, the seat of administration was returned to the present-day He chuan district. In 1913, the *zhou* was demoted to be He chuan county. In 1992, the county became a city, and in 2006, it became He chuan district. Mentioned with 58, 110, 328, 781, 1281.

He zhou 和州 [5]
Name of a *zhou* 州. It was established under Northern Qi 齊, in 555. The seat of administration was in the present He 和 county in An hui 安徽. Its administrative area comprised the present-day He county and Han shan 含山 county in An hui. Under Yuan 元, in 1278, its status was raised to He zhou lu 和州路 but,

in 1291, the *lu* 路 was demoted to He zhou. In 1912, it was changed to He county. Mentioned with 653, 738, 781, 1378.

He zhou 賀州 [3]
Name of a *zhou* 州. It was established under Sui 隋, in 589. The seat of administration was in the present-day He jie 賀街 town located southeast of He zhou city in Guang xi 廣西. The *zhou* was eliminated in 606, but reestablished, in 621, under Tang 唐. The territory administered comprised present-day He zhou city, and the counties of Zhong shan 鐘山 and Fu chuan 富川 in Guang xi. The area became He county under Ming 明, in 1377. Mentioned with 428, 1059, 1340.

Hei 黑 [1]
Name of a river. This is the Hei shui 黑水, located northwest of present-day Mao 茂 county in Si chuan 四川. The sources of the river are found in Hei shui county and it is a tributary of the Min jiang 岷江. Mentioned with 1096.

Hei kun lun 黑崑崙 [1]
Name of mountains. These are the Qarakorum mountains located northwest of Tibet on the borders of Pakistan, Afghanistan and India.

Hei qi dan 黑契丹 [1]
Regional and ethnic name of the "Black Khitan". The term refers to the Western Liao 遼 dynasty founded, in 1131, with a capital at Balasaghun (Quz ordo), east of present-day Tokmok in Kirghizia. The territory governed reached from the Amu Darya river in Central Asia east to the present-day western border of Gan su 甘肅 province, in the South to the Kun lun 崑崙 mountains, and in the North to the Altai mountains and Lake Balkhash. The empire was destroyed by the Mongols in 1218. Mentioned with 656.

Hei shui 黑水 [2]
Name of a river. This is the Tao 洮 river, a tributary of the upper reaches of the Yellow River. It has its sources in present-day He nan 河南 county in Qing hai 青海, and towards the northeast flows through the southwestern part of Gan su 甘肅. It flows into the Liu jia xia 劉家峽 reservoir at Yong jing 永靖 county. The river takes its name, "Black Waters," from its comparatively deep color. Mentioned with 199, 461, 1549.

Heng 衡 [2 +1]
□ Name of a *zhou* 州. [2] See → Heng zhou 衡州. Mentioned with 202, 1158.
□ Name of a *fu* 府. [1] See → Heng zhou 衡州. Mentioned with 160.

Heng gao 衡皋 [1]
Place name. It is located north of present-day Fang cheng 方城 county in He nan 河南. Mentioned with 302.

Heng he 恒河 [1]
Name of a river, i.e., the Ganges. It has its origins in Tibet in China, and flows through India and Bangladesh. Mentioned with 542.

Heng jing 横涇 [1]
Name of a town. This is Heng jing town located 30 *li* southwest of the present-day Wu zhong 吳中 district of Su zhou 蘇州 city in Jiang su 江蘇. Mentioned with 1532.

Heng shan 佷山 [1]
This is the name of a county. It was established by Western Han 漢, and subordinated to Wu ling 武陵 commandery. The seat of administration was in Zhou ya ping 州衙坪, 36 *li* west of present-day Chang yang 長陽 county in Hu bei 湖北. Under Eastern Han, it was subordinated to Nan 南 commandery, and, under Three Kingdoms' Wu 吳, to Yi du 宜都 commandery. Under Western Jin 晉, in 280, the area was changed to Xing shan 興山 county. Later it again became Heng shan county. In 588, under Sui 隋, it was changed to Chang yang 長楊 county. Mentioned with 1168.

Heng shan 衡山 [10]
Name of a mountain range in Hu nan 湖南. It is one of the "five mountain ranges," wu yue 五岳. It is located on the borders of present-day Nan yue 南嶽 district of Heng yang 衡陽 city and the counties of Heng shan and Heng yang 衡陽 in Hu nan. The mountains are the dividing ridge for the Xiang shui 湘水 and the Zi shui 資水. Mentioned with 38, 635, 725, 849, 1109, 1155, 1279, 1469, 1491, 1573.

Heng shan 恒山 [2]
Name of a mountain in He bei 河北. It is also called Chang shan 常山, and is the northern one of the "five mountain ranges," wu yue 五岳. It is present-day Da mao 大茂 mountain located northwest of Qu yang 曲陽 county. Mentioned with 816.

Heng shan ceng qing gang 衡山層青岡 [1]
Place name describing mountain terrain, of Heng 衡 mountain. Heng mountain is in present-day Hu nan 湖南, but the exact location remains unidentifiable. Mentioned with 122.

Heng yang 衡陽 [1]
Name of a county. It was established, by Tang, in 732. In 1943, Heng yang 衡陽 city was formed out of it. In 1952, the administration was moved to the present seat of administration, Xi du 西渡 town. Mentioned with 1336.

Heng zhou 衡州 [2 + 1]
□ Name of a *zhou* 州. [2] It was established under Sui 隋, in 589. The seat of administration was in present-day Heng yang 衡 city in Hu nan 湖南. The territory administered comprised the watershed of the Xiang shui 湘水 in present-day Heng yang 衡陽, Chang ning 常寧, and Lei yang 耒陽. Under the Yuan 元, in 1277, it became Heng zhou lu 衡州路. Mentioned with 1257.
□ Name of a *fu* 府. [1] It was established, by Zhu Yuanzhang 朱元璋 (1328 – 1398), in 1364. The seat of administration was in present-day Heng yang 衡陽 city in Hu nan 湖南. The territory administered comprised the three cities of Heng yang, Lei yang 耒陽, and Chang ning 常寧, and the counties of Heng yang, Heng shan 衡山, Heng dong 衡東, An ren 安仁, Yan ling 炎陵, Gui yang

桂陽, Jia he 嘉禾, Lan shan 藍山, and Lin wu 臨武 in present-day Hu nan 湖南. During the Qing 清 period the area of the *fu* was reduced and, in 1913, it was abolished. Mentioned with 1265.

Heng zhou 横州 [6]

Name of a *zhou* 州. It was established, by Tang 唐, in 634. The seat of administration was on the south bank of the Yu jiang 鬱江, seven *li* southwest of present-day Heng 横 county in Guang xi 廣西. The territory administered comprised the present-day Heng county in Guang xi. Under the Yuan 元, in 1279, the status of the county was raised to Heng zhou lu 横州路 but, at the beginning of the *yuan zhen* 元貞 reign period (1295 – 1297), it became Heng zhou again. Under Ming 明, in 1377, it was demoted to Heng county. The seat of administration was moved to the present seat of administration, Heng zhou town. In 1380, its status was raised to Heng zhou. In 1912, it was changed to be Heng county. Mentioned with 113, 350, 460, 574, 710, 925.

Hong 洪 [1]

Name of a *zhou*. See → Hong zhou 洪州. Mentioned with 121.

Hong nong 弘農 [5]

Name of a commandery. See → Hong nong jun 弘農郡. Mentioned with 44, 126, 365, 631, 949.

Hong nong jun 弘農郡 [1]

Name of a commandery. It was established, by Western Han 漢, in 113 BCE. The seat of administration was in the former Han gu guan 函谷關 city located north of present-day Ling bao 靈寶 city in He nan 河南. The territory administered comprised the watersheds of the Luo shui 洛水, Yi shui 伊水, and the Xi chuan 淅川, located south of the Yellow River and west of Yi yang 宜陽 county in present-day He nan 河南, and the upper stretches of the Luo shui 洛水 and She chuan he 社川河, and the watershed of the Dan jiang 丹江 in Shaan xi 陝西. Eastern Han changed the commandery to be Heng nong 恒農 commandery, but Western Jin 晉 reestablished Hong nong commandery. Former Qin 秦 of the era of Sixteen Kingdoms moved the seat of administration to Shaan xian lao cheng 陝縣老城, west of present-day San men xia 三門峽 city of He nan. In 466, under Northern Wei 魏, the area became Heng nong commandery and, in 534, a Western Heng nong commandery was split off and established. It was administered from the former Han gu guan city located north of the present-day Ling bao city. Northern Zhou 周 changed Western Heng nong commandery to be Hong nong commandery. At the beginning of Sui 隋, it was abolished, but the commandery was reestablished in 607. It was administered from the present-day Ling bao city. In 617, it became Feng lin 鳳林 commandery. In 618, under Tang 唐, it was changed to be Ding zhou 鼎州. In 634, it was made part of Guo zhou 虢州 but, in 742, Guo zhou was changed to be Hong nong commandery. In 758, it was again changed to be Guo zhou. Mentioned with 658.

Hong zhou 洪州 [9]
Name of a *zhou* 州. It was founded under Sui 隋, in 589. The seat of administration was at a point west of present-day Nan chang 南昌 city in Jiang xi 江西. During early Tang 唐, the seat of administration was moved to Nan chang city. The territory administered comprised present-day Nan chang city, and the counties of Feng cheng 豐城 city, Yong xiu 永修, Wu ning 武寧 and Xiu shui 修水. During the Five Dynasties period, Southern Tang raised the *zhou* to be Nan chang fu 南昌府, but under Northern Song 宋, in 975, the area again became Hong zhou. In 1165, under Southern Song 宋, the status of the area was raised to Long xing fu 隆興府. Mentioned with 19, 68, 558, 614, 768, 869, 1257, 1370.

Hu 胡 [11]
Regional name. See → Hu di 胡地. Mentioned with 34, 100, 174, 433, 519, 1097, 1193, 1206, 1308, 1337, 1358, 1433.

Hu 湖 [7 + 4]
□ Regional name. [7] It refers to the area located near Dong ting 洞庭 lake. This is principally Hu nan 湖南 province. Mentioned with 22, 100, 439, 537, 789, 958.
□ Name of a *zhou* 州. [4] See → Hu zhou 湖州. Mentioned with 456, 780, 874, 980.

Hu bei 湖北 [1 + 4]
□ Regional name. [1] It refers to the area north of Dong ting 洞庭 lake, that is, primarily present-day Hu bei 湖北 province. Mentioned with 234.
□ Name of a *lu* 路. [4] It is an abbreviation for Jing hu bei lu 荊湖北路. It was established under Northern Song 宋. The seat of administration was in the old Jiang ling 江陵 county city in the present-day Jing zhou 荊州 district in Jing zhou city in Hu bei 湖北. The territory administered comprised an area in present-day Hubei extending from the counties of Xing shan 興山 and Ba dong 巴東 in the West, and from the cities and counties of Da wu 大悟, E zhou 鄂州 and Tong cheng 通城 in the East, to the cities and counties of Yuan an 遠安, Jing men 荊門, Tian men 天門 and Ying cheng 應城 in the North, and including further the watersheds of the Li shui 澧水 and the Yuan jiang 沅江, and the area of Ping jiang 平江 county. It was abolished during the *zhi yuan* 至元 reign period (1264 – 1294) of the Yuan 元 period. Mentioned with 185, 202, 216, 635.

Hu di 胡地 [8]
Name of a region. A general reference to the territories inhabited by minority peoples in the north of China and Central Asia. Mentioned with 441, 476, 484, 485, 1118, 1206, 1532.

Hu guang 湖廣 [3 + 4]
□ Regional name. [3] It refers to present-day Hu bei 湖北 and Hu nan 湖南 provinces. Mentioned with 654, 988, 1329.
□ Name of a Provincial Administration Commission, *bu zheng si* 布政司. [4] It was established under the Ming 明, by changing the name of the Yuan 元 era Hu guang Branch Secretariat, Hu guang *xing sheng* 湖廣行省, in 1376. The seat of administration was in the Wu chang 武昌 district in present-day Wu han 武

漢 city in Hu bei 湖北. The territory administered comprised present-day Hu bei and Hu nan 湖南, as well as parts of Guang dong 廣東 and Gui zhou 貴州. In 1664, under Qing 清, it became the two provinces of Hu bei and Hu nan. Mentioned with 160.

Hu guo 胡國 [5]
This is a regional name. See → Hu di 胡地. Mentioned with 266, 808, 935, 1118, 1335.

Hu ling 湖嶺 [3 + 1]
□ Regional abbreviation. [3] Further details are lacking. Mentioned with 445, 578, 1329.
□ Place name. [1] Located in Wei 威 county in present-day He bei 河北. Mentioned with 628.

Hu mian 湖沔 [1]
Regional abbreviation. Further details are lacking. Mentioned with 67.

Hu nan 湖南 [11 + 10]
□ Regional name. [11] It refers to the area south of Dong ting 洞庭 lake, principally the present Hu nan 湖南 province. Mentioned with 42, 206, 234, 535, 768, 809, 1030, 1171, 1241, 1499.
□ Name of a *lu* 路. [10] This is a designation for Jing hu nan lu 荊湖南路. It was established under Northern Song 宋, in 997. The seat of administration was in Chang sha 長沙 city in Hu nan 湖南. The territory administered comprised an area extending from the cities and counties of Mi luo 汨羅, Yi yang 益陽, An hua 安化, Dong kou 洞口 and Sui ning 綏寧 in present-day Hu nan toward the South, and the northeastern portion of Guang xi 廣西. Yuan 元 abolished the *lu*. Mentioned with 130, 185, 216, 344, 399, 437, 765, 1098, 1155, 1178, 1573.

Hu nan bei 湖南北 [7]
Regional name. It refers to the area on both the northern and southern shores of Dong ting 洞庭 lake in Hu nan 湖南. Mentioned with 535, 566, 576, 583, 786, 848, 1038.

Hu shan 壺山 [1]
Name of a mountain. It is located northeast of the present-day Tang he 唐河 county in He nan 河南. Mentioned with 1485.

Hu shou shan 虎壽山 [1]
This is the name of a mountain. Details are lacking. Mentioned with 1469.

Hu wei zhi shan 虎尾之山 [1]
Name of a mountain from the *Shan hai jing* 山海經, "Classic of Mountains and Seas." Details are lacking. Mentioned with 299.

Hu xian 鄠縣 [1]
Name of a county. It was established under Western Han 漢. The seat of administration was at a point two *li* north of Hu 戶 county in present-day Shaan xi 陝西. Under Sui 隋, in 614, the seat of administration was moved to the present Hu 戶 county. In 1964, it was changed to be Hu 戶 county. Mentioned with 1230.

Hu xiang 湖湘 [4]

Regional name. It refers to the area of Hu nan 湖南 province. Mentioned with 399, 1392, 1507, 1524.

Hu zhong 胡中 [6]

Regional name. See → Hu di 胡地. Mentioned with 92, 368, 485, 770, 1057, 1390.

Hu zhou 湖州 [1 + 1]

□ Name of a *fu* 府. [1] It was established at the end of Yuan 元, by the Ming rebel Zhu Yuanzhang 朱元璋 (1328 – 1398), in 1366. The seat of administration was in present-day Hu zhou 湖州 city in Zhe jiang 浙江. The territory administered comprised present-day Hu zhou city and likewise the three present-day counties of De qing 德清, Chang xing 長興 and An ji 安吉 in Zhe jiang. It was abolished in 1912. Mentioned with 768.

□ Name of a *zhou* 州. [1] It was established under Sui 隋, in 602. The seat of administration was in the present-day Hu zhou 湖州 city in Zhe jiang 浙江. The territory administered comprised present-day Hu zhou city in Zhe jiang, the two present-day counties of Chang xing 長興 and An ji 安吉, and the eastern portion of present-day De qing 德清 county in Zhe jiang. Under Southern Song 宋, in 1225, the *zhou* became An ji zhou 安吉州. Mentioned with 1078.

Hua 滑 [1 + 1]

□ Name of a *zhou* 州. [1] It was established under Sui 隋, in 596. The seat of administration was in present-day Cheng guan 城關 town, located southeast of Hua county in He nan 河南. In 606, the area became Yan zhou 兗州. And in 607, it became Dong 東 commandery. Under Tang 唐, in 618, it was reestablished as Hua zhou. Its administrative area corresponded to the counties of Hua xian 滑縣, Chang yuan 長垣 and Yan jin 延津, all in present-day He nan. It was eliminated under Northern Song 宋, in 1072, but reestablished in 1081. In 1374, under Ming 明, it was demoted to be Hua county. Mentioned with 1122.

□ Name of a county. [1] It was established under Ming, in 1374. The seat of administration was in present-day Cheng guan town southwest of Hua county in He nan. In 1949, the seat of administration was moved to Dao kou 道口 town. Mentioned with 474.

Hua 華 [5 + 1]

□ Name of a *zhou* 州. [5] See → Hua zhou 華州. Mentioned with 126, 473, 802, 1340, 1445.

□ Name of a mountain. [1] See Hua shan 華山. Mentioned with 311.

Hua 化 [3]

Name of a *zhou*. It was established under Northern Song 宋, in 980. The seat of administration was in present-day Hua zhou 化州 city in Guang dong 廣東. The territory administered comprised the two present-day cities of Hua zhou and Lian jiang 廉江 and most of Wu chuan 吳川 city in Guang dong. In 1278, the *zhou* was changed to Hua zhou lu 化州路. Mentioned with 144, 1057.

Hua gai shan 華蓋山 [1]
Name of a mountain located in the Lu cheng 鹿城 district of present-day Wen zhou 溫州 in Zhe jiang 浙江. Mentioned with 1050.

Hua guo 滑國 [2]
Name of a country. It was located within the present-day boundaries of Jimsar (Ji mu sa er 吉木薩兒) county in Xin jiang 新疆. Mentioned with 966, 1192.

Hua rong 華容 [1]
Name of a county. It was established under Western Han 漢. The seat of administration was at a point three *li* west of the Zhou jia zui guan 周家嘴關, located north of Jian li 監利 county in present-day Hu bei 湖北. The county was eliminated, in 280, under Western Jin 晉, but later reestablished until finally dissolved under Northern Zhou 周. Mentioned with 1430.

Hua shan 華山 [15]
Name of a mountain, also called Tai hua shan 太華山. This is one of China's "five mountain ranges", wu yue 五岳. It is located 10 *li* south of the present-day Hua yin 華陰 city in Shaan xi 陜西. Mentioned with 152, 311, 657, 980, 1005, 1134, 1215, 1234, 1311, 1469, 1555.

Hua tai 滑臺 [3]
Name of a place. It is located in present-day Cheng guan 城關 town, 8 *li* southeast of Hua 滑 county in He nan 河南. Mentioned with 322, 1122, 1561.

Hua xia 華夏 [1]
Ancient name used with reference to China by the BCGM authors.

Hua yang 華陽 [2]
Regional name. It is a reference to the area on the "yang side (i.e. the south side) of Hua 華" mountain in Shaan xi 陜西. It corresponds to the area south of the Qin ling 秦嶺 mountain range, along with Si chuan 四川, Gui zhou 貴州 and Yun nan 雲南.

Hua yin 華陰 [12]
Name of a county. It was founded, under Western Han 漢, in 199 BCE. The seat of administration was at a point 5 *li* southeast of present-day Hua yin city in Shaan xi 陜西. During Northern Wei 魏, in 487, the administration was moved to Da li 大荔 county but, in 526, it was moved back to the old location. Under the Sui 隋, in 609, the seat of administration was moved to present-day Hua yin city. Under Tang 唐, the area became Xian zhang 仙掌 county. In 705, it was renamed Hua yin county. In 761, it became Tai yin 太陰 county, but Hua yin county again in 762. The area became a city in 1990. Mentioned with 47, 404, 660, 893, 931, 1038, 1052, 1068, 1311.

Hua yuan 華原 [1]
Name of a county. It was established under Sui 隋, in 586. The seat of administration was in Yao zhou 耀州 district in present-day Tong chuan 銅川 city in Shaan xi 陜西. In 686, it was changed to Yong an 永安 county. In 705, it became Hua yuan again. In 906, next to Hua yuan county, Yao zhou was established.

Under Yuan 元, in 1264, the county was abolished and combined with Yao zhou. Mentioned with 461.

Hua zhou 華州 [9]

Name of a *zhou* 州. It was established under Western Wei 魏, in 554. The seat of administration was at a point west of present-day Hua 華 county in Shaan xi 陝西. At the beginning of the *da ye* 大業 reign period (605 – 618) of Sui 隋, the *zhou* was abolished, but reestablished during the Tang 唐, in 618, and administered from the present Hua county. In 686, the *zhou* was changed to Tai zhou 太州 but, in 705, became Hua zhou again. In 760, it again became Tai zhou and, in 897, its status was raised to be De xing fu 德興府, but became Hua zhou again in 900. The territory administered comprised the three counties of Hua, Hua yin 華陰 and Tong guan 潼關, and the northern part of Wei nan 渭南 city and part of the northeastern part of the Lin tong 臨潼 district in Xi an 西安 city, all in present-day Shaan xi. In 1913, the *zhou* became Hua county. Mentioned with 247, 314, 599, 1005, 1254, 1311, 1393, 1449.

Huai 懷 [4]

Name of a *zhou* 州. See → Huai zhou 懷州. Mentioned with 38, 1289, 1444, 1478.

Huai 淮 [26 + 8]

□ Regional name. [26] It refers to the watershed of the Huai 淮 river including the middle-northern part of present-day An hui 安徽, Jiang su 江蘇, and the southern part of He nan 河南. Mentioned with 22, 75, 130, 271, 389, 444, 572, 730, 857, 877, 958, 980, 1004, 1099, 1171, 1189, 1253, 1302, 1307, 1323, 1380, 1407, 1433, 1441, 1449, 1519.

□ Name of a river. [8] See Huai shui 淮水. Mentioned with 138, 429, 541, 578, 1158, 1400, 1470, 1551.

Huai an 懷安 [1]

Name of a county. It was established during Three Kingdoms times, under Wu 吳. The seat of administration was at a point southeast of present-day Ning guo 寧國 city in An Hui 安徽. It was abolished under Sui 隋, in 589. Mentioned with 298.

Huai bei 淮北 [4]

Regional name. The name refers to the area "north of the Huai" river in present-day An hui 安徽 and Jiang su 江蘇. Mentioned with 631, 719, 776, 794.

Huai dian 淮甸 [4]

General regional reference. It refers to the area on both banks of the Huai 淮 river. Mentioned with 145, 192, 687, 922.

Huai hai 淮海 [2]

Regional name. It refers to the strip of Huai an 淮安 and Lian yun gang 連雲港 in northern Jiang su 江蘇. Mentioned with 760, 1294.

Huai li 槐里 [3]

Name of a county. It was founded by Western Han 漢, in 204 BCE. The seat of administration was at a point near present-day Nan zuo 南佐 village, 10 *li* southeast of Xing ping 興平 city in Shaan xi 陝西. Under Northern Wei 魏, in 446, the administration was moved to a point 25 *li* west of present-day Xing ping city. Under Northern Zhou 周, the county was abolished, in 557. Mentioned with 70.

Huai ling 淮嶺 [1]

Compound place name. Details uncertain. Mentioned with 752.

Huai nan 淮南 [7 + 6 + 1 + 10 + 1]

□ Regional name. [7] It refers the area on the southern bank of the Huai 淮 river. This includes the region in both present-day Jiang su 江蘇 and An hui 安徽 of the Huai river watershed up to its fusion with the Yang zi. Mentioned with 566, 623, 861, 896, 924, 1350.

□ Name of a circuit. [6] It was established under Tang 唐, in 62. The seat of administration was in the area south of the Huai 淮 river and north of the Yang zi, in the east up to the Yellow Sea and in the west to a strip of territory formed by the cities and counties of Ying cheng 應城 and Han chuan 漢川 in Hu bei 湖北. In 733, a Huai nan 淮南 Circuit Investigation and Supervisory Commissioner, Huai nan *dao cai fang chu* 淮南道採訪處, was appointed and his office was in present-day Yang zhou 揚州 city in Jiang su 江蘇. This was later abolished, but the geographical designation was retained until the Five Dynasties period. Mentioned with 224, 328, 797, 1092, 1360.

□ Feudal country/domain. [1] It was established, under Western Han 漢, in 202 BCE. The seat of administration was in Cheng bei xiang 城北鄉, located 10 *li* north of present-day Lu an 六安 city in An hui 安徽. In 196 BCE, the seat of administration was moved to present-day Shou 壽 county in An hui. The domain was eliminated in 173 BCE, but reestablished in 164 BCE. The territory administered comprised the region south of the Huai 淮 river, extending from the counties of Huo shan 霍山 and Qian shan 潛山 (other than Tian chang 天長 city) toward the East, and a portion of the Southeast of He nan 河南 and of the eastern part of Hu bei 湖北, as well as the province of Jiang xi 江西. In 122 BCE, the domain was eliminated and turned into Jiu jiang 九江 commandery. Under Wei 魏 of Three Kingdoms, in 221, Huai nan domain was reestablished and, in 223, it became Huai nan commandery. In 232, it was changed to be the domain of Chu 楚 but, in 249, it became Huai nan commandery again. Mentioned with 242.

□ Name of a 路 *lu*. [10] It was first established under Northern Song 宋. The seat of administration was in present-day Huai an 淮安 city in Jiang su 江蘇. In 976, the *lu* was split up into an eastern and a western *lu*. In 997, the two *lu* were recombined into Huai nan lu 淮南路. The administration was combined and moved to the present city of Yang zhou 揚州. The territory administered comprised an area in the south reaching to the Yang zi, in the north crossing the Huai 淮 river, including the area north of the Huai river in both Jiang su and An hui 安徽, and the cities and counties of Yong cheng 永城 and Lu yi 鹿邑 in He nan 河南. In 1072, Huai nan lu was again divided into an eastern and a western half, two *lu*. Mentioned with 546, 768, 978, 995, 1126, 1167, 1406, 1494, 1516, 1539.

□ Name of a commandery. [1] It was established, under Wei 魏 of the Three Kingdoms, in 223. The seat of administration was in present-day Shou 壽 county in An hui 安徽, and its administrative area corresponded to the area south of the Huai river in present-day An hui, the area north of Chao 巢 lake and east of the Tang 塘 river, and the area reaching from Feng yang 鳳陽 county and Chu zhou 滁州 city toward the West. In 232, the area became the feudal domain of Chu 楚 but, in 249, it again became Huai nan commandery. This was changed to Nan liang 南梁 commandery during the Eastern Jin 晉 period and under Sui 隋, in 607, Shou zhou 壽州 was changed to become Huai nan commandery. Under Tang, in 620, it again became Shou zhou. Mentioned with 1254.

Huai qing 懷慶 [2 + 1 + 2]

□ Name of a *fu* 府. [2] It was established under Ming 明, in 1368. The seat of administration was in present-day Qin yang 沁陽 city in He nan 河南. The territory administered comprised the present-day counties of Xiu wu 脩武 and Wu zhi 武陟 in the West, and the area north of the Yellow River in present-day He nan. It was abolished in 1913. Mentioned with 222.

□ Name of a *lu*. [1] It was established under Yuan 元, in 1319. The seat of administration was in present-day city of Qing yang in He nan. The territory administered comprised an area extending in present-day He nan from the two counties of Xiu wu and Wu zhi toward the West, and from the Yellow River toward the North. Under Ming 明, in 1368, it was changed to Huai qing fu 懷慶府. Mentioned with 99.

□ Name of an army. [2] It was established under Northern Song 宋. The seat of administration was in present-day Qin yang city in He nan. In 1128, it was changed to Nan huai zhou 南懷州. Mentioned with 323, 1306.

Huai shui 淮水 [1]

Name of a river watershed. This is the Huai 淮 river. Its sources arise at Tong bai 桐柏 mountain in He nan 河南 and the river then flows eastward through He nan and An hui 安徽, and enters the ocean in the northern part of Jiang su 江蘇. Mentioned with 203.

Huai xi 淮西 [1]

Name of a *lu* 路. This is Huai nan xi lu 淮南西路, or the "Western Huai nan *lu* 淮南路." See → Huai nan 淮南. The *lu* was founded under Northern Song 宋, in 976. In 997, it was combined with Huai nan dong lu 淮南東路, the Eastern Huai nan *lu* but, in 1072, the combined *lu* was re-divided. The administration of the Huai nan xi lu 淮南西路 was in present-day Feng tai 鳳台 county in An hui 安徽. The Xi lu 西路 administered an area reaching from Feng yang 鳳陽 and He 和 county in present-day An hui toward the West, and in He nan 河南 from Guang shan 光山 county and in Hu bei 湖北 from the Huang pi 黃陂 district of Wu han city toward the East, i.e., areas north of the Yang zi and south of the Huai 淮 river. In 1078, the Xi lu was combined with the Dong lu 東路 as Huai nan lu. In 1085, it was again divided and the Xi lu reestablished. In 1086 there was another recombination. Under Southern Song, a separate Xi lu was again established. Its administration was moved to present-day Shou 壽 county in An hui. Yuan 元 abolished it. Mentioned with 1158.

Huai yang 淮揚 [1]
This is a regional name. The term refers to the middle extent of the Huai 淮 river and the region of the Yang zi. This encompasses the present-day cities and places of Huai an 淮安, Yang zhou 揚州, Yan cheng 鹽城, Nan jing 南京 and Zhen jiang 鎮江 in Jiang su 江蘇. Mentioned with 1378.

Huai yang 淮陽 [1]
Regional name. See → Huai bei 淮北. Mentioned with 1270.

Huai yang jun 淮陽郡 [1]
Name of a commandery. It was established, under Sui 隋, in 607. The seat of administration was in present-day Huai yang 淮陽 county in He nan 河南. The territory administered comprised an area extending in present-day He nan from Xi hua 西華 county toward the East, from Dan cheng 鄲城 county toward the West, from Tai kang 太康 county toward the South, and in An hui 安徽 from the western part of Lin chuan 臨泉 county toward the North. Under Tang 唐, in 618, the area became Chen zhou 陳州. In 742, it again became Huai yang commandery but, in 758, was changed to Chen zhou again. Mentioned with 648.

Huai yi 淮夷 [1]
Name of a tribal group. It refers to an ethnic group located north of the Huai 淮 river. It also generally refers to the entire region between the Yellow River and the Huai river. Mentioned with 1467.

Huai you 淮右 [1]
Regional name. The area "to the right auf the Huai" (as seen from the North) is also called Huai xi 淮西, "West of the Huai." It refers to a region on the northern bank of the Yellow River in the northern part of present-day An hui 安徽 and the western part of He nan 河南. Mentioned with 738.

Huai yuan 淮源 [1]
Place name. It is positioned in present-day Huai yuan 淮源 town in Tong bai 桐柏 county in He nan 河南. Mentioned with 1412.

Huai zhe 淮浙 [1]
Combined regional name. The term refers to An hui 安徽, Jiang su 江蘇 and Zhe jiang 浙江. Mentioned with 272.

Huai zhou 懷州 [2]
Name of a *zhou* 州. It was established, under Northern Wei 魏, in 467. The seat of administration was in present-day Qin yang 沁陽 city in He nan 河南. The *zhou* was eliminated in 494, but reestablished later under Eastern Wei. The territory administered comprised the present-day cities and counties of Jiao zuo 焦作, Qin yang, Wu zhi 武陟, Huo jia 獲嘉, Xiu wu 脩武, and Bo ai 博愛 in He nan. In 1128, under Jin 金, the area was changed to Nan huai zhou 南懷州 but, in 1151, it again became Huai zhou. In 1257, under the Mongols, the area became Huai meng lu 懷孟路. Mentioned with 428, 823.

Huang 黃 [1 + 1]
□ This is the abbreviation for 'Huang zhou fu 黃州府. [1] Mentioned with 1354.
□ Name of a *zhou* 州. [1] See Huang zhou 黃州. Mentioned with 1444.

Huang he 黄河 [2]

This is the Yellow River. It has its sources on the northern slopes of Bayankala (Ba yan ke la 巴顏喀拉) mountain in Qing hai 青. Its upper reaches pass through Ning xia 寧夏 and the Great Bend of the Yellow River in Inner Mongolia. Its middle reaches pass through the two provinces of Shan xi 山西 and Shaan xi 陝西. During the Ming 明 period, the lower reaches of the river overflowed its old channel, took over the channel of the Si shui 泗水 in He nan 河南 and Shan dong 山東 and entered the Huai 淮 river, entering the ocean in the northern portion of present-day Jiang su 江蘇. During the Qing 清, in 1855, the Yellow River broke through its banks at Tong wa xiang 銅瓦廂, and entered the Gulf of Bo hai 渤海 in the northern portion of the Shan dong peninsula. Mentioned with 1330, 1458.

Huang ling 黄陵 [1]

This is an abbreviated name for Huang Di ling 黄帝陵, "tomb of the Yellow Thearch.". It is situated on Qiao 橋 mountain in the northern part of present-day Huang ling county in present-day Shaan xi 陝西. Mentioned with 220.

Huang mei shan 黄梅山 [1]

Name of a mountain. It is situated 40 *li* northwest of present-day Huang mei 黄梅 county in Hu bei 湖北. Mentioned with 1463.

Huang shan 黄山 [3]

Name of a mountain. It is situated in Huang shan 黄山 Scenic Area of present-day Huang shan city in An hui 安徽. Mentioned with 768, 1015, 1228.

Huang shui 黄水 [1]

Name of a river. Another name for it is Huang shi xi 黄石溪. It is located west of present-day Shi men 石門 county in Hu nan 湖南. This is one of the so-called "Nine Li [rivers]," Jiu Li 九澧, including the Li 澧 river and its eight tributaries. Mentioned with 1307.

Huang zhou 黄州 [3 + 1]

□ Name of a *zhou* 州. [3] It was established under the Sui 隋, in 585. The seat of administration was in the Xin zhou 新洲 district of present-day Wu han 武漢 city in Hu bei 湖北. The territory administered comprised the two cities of Huang gang 黄岡 and Ma cheng 麻城 and Hong an 紅安 county and the Huang pi 黄陂 district and Xin zhou 新洲 district of Wu han city in Hu bei. During the Tang 唐, in 885, the administrative seat was moved to Huang zhou district of Huang gang city in Hu bei. Yuan 元 turned the area into Huang zhou lu 黄州路. Mentioned with 641, 1238, 1251.

□ Name of a *fu* 府. [1] See → Huang zhou fu 黄州府. Mentioned with 1412.

Huang zhou 晃州

Name of a *zhou*. It was established, under Tang 唐, in 641, as a minority people's region with a "win over", *ji mi* 羈縻, rule whereby the Chinese authorities installed the head of a region inhabited by non-Chinese ethnic groups while respecting the indigenous traditional customs and government structures. It was administered from Lao Huang cheng 老晃城 located southeast of the Xin

Huang 新晃 self-governing county of the Dong 侗 nationality in present-day Hu nan 湖南. The *zhou* was abolished at the end of Tang. Mentioned with 202.

Huang zhou fu 黄州府 [1]

Name of a *fu*. It was established, during late Yuan 元 times by the Ming 明 rebels under Zhu Yuan zhang 朱元璋 (1328 – 1398), in 1364. The seat of administration was in the Huang zhou 黄州 district in present-day Huang gang 黄岡 city in Hu bei 湖北. The territory administered comprised the Huang zhou district of Huang gang city, the Xin zhou 新洲 district of Wu han 武漢 city, Wu xue 武穴 city and Ma cheng 麻城 city, as well as the counties of Huang pi 黄陂, Hong an 紅安, Da wu 大悟, Luo tian 羅田, Xi shui 浠水, Qi chun 蘄春, and Huang mei 黄梅, all in present-day Hu bei. In 1729, Huang pi county became part of Han yang fu 漢陽府. In 1912, Huang zhou fu was abolished.

Hui 徽 [3]

Name of a *fu* 府. This is Hui zhou fu 徽州府. See → Hui zhou 徽州. Mentioned with 502, 839, 1099.

Hui chang 會昌 [1]

Name of a *xiang* 鄉, sub-administrative unit. It was located near present-day Zhang ming 彰明 town, located south of Jiang you 江油 city in Si chuan 四川. Mentioned with 322.

Hui he 回紇 [3]

This is an alternative transcription of Uighur, → Hui hu 回鶻. Mentioned with 542, 1296.

Hui hu 回鶻 [3]

Ethnic name. Chinese transcription of Ouigour/Uighur. During Tang 唐 times, an Uighur khanate existed covering a territory in present-day Mongolia and north of Tian shan 天山 mountain in Xin jiang 新疆. Its capital, Hui hu ya zhang 回鶻牙帳, i.e. Qara Balgas, was located northwest of Karakorum city at the upper watershed of the Orkhon river in present-day Mongolia. After the khanate was destroyed, at the end of Tang, the Uighurs moved to the West to the Tian shan mountain in Xin jiang and the eastern Tarim basin. During the Yuan 元, they served the Chagatai khanate. During the Ming 明 era, they were conquered by the Ili Baliq. Mentioned with 73, 1206.

Hui hu guo 回鶻國 [1]

Regional name. It refers to the territories of the Uighur (→ Hui hu 回鶻). Mentioned with 1206.

Hui hui 回回 [1 + 13]

This is a word, with various meanings, used by the BCGM authors usually with the meaning Muslim but it can have a geographical connection too. [1] The word is connected with the Chinese term for Uighurs (→ Hui hu 回鶻) and with an even older term, usually pejorative, for another Central Asian people, most commonly written Rou ran 柔然, also Ru ru 茹茹, Ru ru 蠕蠕, etc. The latter form, referring to wriggling worms, has been used to connect with the name of the

Western Avar. Avar is believed to come from a name for serpent, a possible Old Turkic *Apar.

□ As a regional name, the term referred to northwestern China and adjacent areas of Central Asia. [13] When the term Hui hui is applied to medicinals these are mostly of West Asian origin, although some are also Central Asian. Mentioned with 12, 18, 82, 97, 280, 476, 817, 895, 1116, 1139, 1332, 1340, 1396.

□ The term is also used as a synonym for Uighur. [1] Mentioned with 1206.

Hui hui guo 回回國 [1]

Regional name. See under → Hui hui 回回. Mentioned with 284.

Hui shui 徽水 [1]

Name of a river. It is a tributary of the Qing yi jiang 青弋江. It has its sources in the north slopes of the Hui ling 徽嶺 in present-day Ji xi 績溪 county in An hui 安徽. It flows through Jing de 旌德 county and goes north, into Jing 涇 county. Mentioned with 357.

Hui shui wan 會水灣 [1]

Place name. Further details are unavailable. Mentioned with 1085.

Hui zhou 徽州 [1]

Name of a *fu* 府. It was established by Zhu Yuanzhang 朱元璋 (1328 – 1398) and his Ming 明 rebels, in 1367, during late Yuan 元 times. It was administered from Xi xian 歙縣 county in An hui and the area administered comprised Huang shan 黃山 city, and the counties of Xi xian, Xiu ning 休寧, Qi men 祁門, Ji xi 績溪 and Yi xian 黟縣, all in present-day An hui 安徽, as well as Wu yuan 婺源 county in Jiang xi 江西. Hui zhou fu 徽州府 was abolished in 1912. Mentioned with 119.

Hun tong jiang 混同江 [1]

Name of a river. This is present-day Song hua jiang 松花江 and the lower Hei long jiang 黑龍江 after the Song hua jiang has flowed into it. Mentioned with 824.

Hun xi zhi shan 渾夕之山 [1]

Mountain from the *Shan hai jing* 山海經, "Classic of Mountains and Seas." Further information is unavailable. Mentioned with 1497.

Huo shan 霍山 [4]

Name of a mountain. It is Tian zhu 天柱 mountain located southwest of present-day Huo shan county in An hui 安徽. Mentioned with 768, 1216, 1423, 1431, 1469.

Huo shan jun 火山軍 [2]

Name of an administration, an army. It was established under Northern Song 宋, in 982. The seat of administration was at a point southeast of present-day He qu 河曲 county in Shan xi 山西. Under Jin 金, in 1182, it was changed to be Huo shan zhou 火山州. Mentioned with 1341, 1518.

Huo yan shan 火焰山 [1]
Name of a mountain. It is located east of Turfan City in present-day Xin jiang 新疆. Mentioned with 811.

Huo zhou 火州 [2]
Place name. Strictly speaking, this is not a *zhou* 州 since Huo zhou is part of an Uighur name, Qara Qojha. The area was established as an administrative entity under Yuan 元, which controlled the area, and was located south of the present-day Ha la he zhuo 哈拉和卓 (Qara khojha) southeast of Turfan city in Xin jiang 新疆. During early Ming 明, the area was taken over by Ca'adai successor groups and during the middle of the 15th century by Turfan. Mentioned with 174, 811.

Huo zhou 火洲 [1]
Local place name. Details are unavailable, but it was located somewhere in southeast Asia. Mentioned with 14.

-J-

Ji 吉 [2]
Name of a *zhou*. See → Ji zhou 吉州. Mentioned with 344, 981.

Ji 冀 [3]
Name of a *zhou* 州. See → Ji zhou 冀州. Mentioned with 1004, 1057, 1551.

Ji bin guo 罽賓國 [2]
Name of an ancient country. This is essentially present-day Kashmir. Mentioned with 1497.

Ji cui chi 積翠池 [1]
Name of a lake. It was the lake of the Luo yang 洛陽 palaces of Han 漢 and Tang 唐. The lake is now located in the vicinity of Ji cui 積翠 road in present-day Luo yang city. Mentioned with 961.

Ji jun 汲郡 [1]
Name of a commandery. It was established under Western Jin 晉, in 266. The seat of administration was at a point 20 *li* southwest of present-day Wei hui 衛輝 city in He nan 河南. The territory administered comprised the present-day cities and counties of Xin xiang 新鄉, Wei hui, Hui xian 輝縣, Lin zhou 林州 and Qi xian 淇縣 in He nan. At the end of Western Jin 晉, it was eliminated. It was reestablished under Northern Wei 魏, in 488. The seat of administration was at Qi men du 淇門渡 located southwest of present-day Xun xian 浚縣 in He nan 河南. It was eliminated again under Sui 隋, at the beginning of the *kai huang* 開皇 (581 – 600) reign period, but then reestablished at the beginning of the *da ye* 大業 (605 – 618) reign period. It was administered from present-day Wei xian xiang 衛賢鄉, located southwest of present-day Jun county. Under Tang 唐, in 618, it became Wei zhou 衛州. It was again made Ji 汲 commandery in 742, and

administered from present-day Wei hui 衛輝 city. In 758, the commandery became Wei zhou 衛州. Mentioned with 648.

Ji men 薊門 [2]

Variant place name referring to present-day Bei jing 北京 city. Mentioned with 505, 780.

Ji nan 濟南 [1 + 1]

□ Name of a feudal country/domain. [1] It was established by Western Han 漢, in 164 BCE, and had its capital at a point west of present-day Zhang qiu 章丘 city in Shan dong 山東. It controlled the territories of the present-day cities and counties of Ji nan, Tai an 泰安, Chang qing 長清, Fei cheng 肥城, Zhang qiu, Ji yang 濟陽 and Zou ping 鄒平 in Shang dong. In 154 BCE, it became a commandery. Following the time of Emperor Wu 武 (156 – 87), its territories were reduced. In 39, under Eastern Han, it again became a feudal country/domain and, at the beginning of Western Jin 晉, it became a commandery again. Mentioned with 1250.

□ Name of a *fu* 府. [1] It was established under Northern Song 宋, in 1116. The seat of administration was in the present-day Ji nan city in Shan dong 山東. The territory administered included an area in present-day Shan dong extending from the two cities of Xin tai 新泰 and Fei cheng 肥城 toward the North, from De zhou 德州 city and Pin yuan 平原 and the Chang qing 長清 district of Ji nan toward the East, and from the two cities of Zi bo 淄博 and Lai wu 萊蕪 as well as the counties of Huan tai 桓臺, Gao qing 高青 and Li jin 利津 toward the West, as well as from Le ling 樂陵 city and Wu di 無棣 county toward the South. In the Northeast, the *fu* reached to the Ocean. At the beginning of Yuan 元, the *fu* was changed to be Ji nan lu 濟南路. In 1367, it was changed to be Ji nan fu 濟南府. It was abolished in 1913. Mentioned with 545.

Ji nan jun 濟南郡 [1]

Name of a commandery. It was established under Western Han 漢. The seat of administration was at a point west of present-day Zhang qiu 章丘 city in Shan dong 山東. The territory administered comprised the area of the present-day cities and counties of Ji nan 濟南, Tai an 泰安, Chang qing 長清, Fei cheng 肥城, Zhang qiu 章丘, Ji yang 濟陽 and Zou ping 鄒平 in Shan dong 山東. In 164 BCE, under Han Wen di 漢文帝 (202 – 157), the commandery was changed to be Ji nan country/domain. In 154 BCE, it became a commandery again, but became a domain again under Eastern Han, in 39 CE. It again became a commandery under Western Jin 晉. The seat of administration was moved to present-day Ji nan city in Shan dong. Under Sui 隋, the commandery was abolished. Mentioned with 1301.

Ji ning 濟寧 [1]

Name of a *zhou* 州. It was established under Ming 明, in 1385. The seat of administration was in present-day Ji ning city in Shan dong 山東. Its administrative area covered the present-day cities and counties of Ji ning, Jia xiang 嘉祥, Ju ye 巨野 and Yun cheng 鄆城 in Shan dong. Mentioned with 1023.

Ji ning 冀寧 [1]
Name of a *lu* 路. It was established under Yuan 元, in 1305. The seat of administration was in present-day Tai yuan 太原 city in Shan xi 山西. The territory administered comprised an area reaching from Jie xiu 介休 city toward the North, and from the Great Wall toward the South. Under Ming 明, in 1368, Ji ning lu was changed to Tai yuan fu 太原府. Mentioned with 862.

Ji sha shan 積沙山 [1]
This is a sand dune, not a mountain. The reference is to the sand dunes located west of the Yellow River. Mentioned with 324.

Ji shan 箕山 [1 + 1]
□ Name of a mountain. [1] It is also called Fu zhou shan 覆舟山, Wei shan 濰山 and Ji wu shan 箕屋山. It is Wu shan 五山 mountain located 100 *li* northeast of present-day Ju xian 莒縣 county in Shan dong 山東. Mentioned with 1030.
□ Name of a mountain. [1] It is also called Xu you shan 許由山. It is located southeast of present-day Deng feng 登封 city in He nan 河南. Mentioned with 1029.

Ji shan 雞山 [1]
Name of a mountain. Further details are unavailable. Mentioned with 549.

Ji shi shan 積石山 [1]
Name of a mountain. It is also called Da ji shi 大積石 mountain. This is A ni ma qing 阿尼玛卿 (Amye machen) in the southeastern portion of Qing hai 青海. Mentioned with 10.

Ji shui 濟水 [2]
Name of a river. It has its sources at Wang wu 王屋 mountain located west of present-day Ji yuan 濟源 city in He nan 河南, and flows into the Yellow River. A branch forms on the opposite bank of the river where the Ji shui enters the Yellow River, and ancient people considered this to be the lower reaches of the Ji shui. It flows through He nan and enters the sea in Shan dong 山東. At present, the place where the upper flow has its sources still exists but the lower reaches become the Yellow River and are taken over by the great and small Qing 清 river, i.e., the Da qing he 大清河 and the Xiao qing he 小清河. Mentioned with 268, 269.

Ji tou shan 雞頭山 [1]
Name of a mountain. Further details are lacking. This could be Ji gong shan 雞公山 that is located south of present-day Xin yang 信陽 city in He nan 河南. Mentioned with 810.

Ji yang jun 濟陽郡 [1]
Name of a commandery. It was established under Tang 唐, in 742. The seat of administration was at a point southwest of present-day Chi ping 茌平 county in Shan dong 山東. The territory administered comprised Fan xian 范縣 county in He nan 河南, and the counties and cities of Liao cheng 聊城, Dong e 東阿, Fei cheng 肥城, Yang gu 陽谷 and Gao tang 高唐 in present-day Shan dong. In 754, it was abolished. Mentioned with 572.

Ji yin 濟陰 [1]

Name of a commandery. See → Ji yin jun 濟陰郡. Mentioned with 1491.

Ji yin jun 濟陰郡 [1]

Name of a commandery. It was established, by Western Han 漢, in 5 BCE. The seat of administration was at a point 4 *li* northwest of present-day Ding tao 定陶 county in Shan dong 山東. The territory administered comprised present-day He ze 菏澤 city and the counties of Ding tao and Dong ming 東明 in Shan dong. It was abolished under Northern Qi 齊, but reestablished under Sui 隋 at the beginning of the *da ye* 大業 reign period (605 – 618), and administered from a point northwest of present-day Cao xian 曹縣 county in Shan dong. The territory administered comprised present-day He ze city and the areas of Ding tao, Dong ming, Cheng wu 成武, Jin xiang 金鄉 and Shan xian 單縣 county in Shan dong. At the beginning of the *wu de* 武德 reign period (618 – 626) under Tang 唐, it was changed to be Cao zhou 曹州. In 742, it again became Ji yin 濟陰 commandery and, in 758, it was again changed to be Cao zhou. Mentioned with 1417.

Ji yuan 濟源 [2]

Name of a county. It was established under Sui 隋, in 596. The seat of administration was in the present-day Ji yuan 濟源 city in He nan 河南. Mentioned with 1551.

Ji yun guo 吉雲國 [1]

Name of an ancient country. Said to be a Han 漢 period kingdom but information is lacking. Mentioned with 1555.

Ji ze 稷澤 [1]

Place name found in the *Shan hai jing* 山海經, "Classic of Mountains and Seas." Further details are unavailable. Mentioned with 62.

Ji zhou 薊州 [1]

Name of a *zhou* 州. It was established by Tang 唐, in 730, and administered from the present-day Ji xian 薊縣 county of Tian jin 天津 city. The territory administered comprised the area of Ji xian county in Tian jin city and the present-day districts and counties of San he 三河, Yu tian 玉田, Feng run 豐潤 and Zun hua 遵化 in He bei 河北. In 742, the *zhou* was changed to be Yu yang 漁陽 commandery but, in 758, it was again made Ji zhou. In 1913, the *zhou* was changed to be Ji xian county. Mentioned with 566.

Ji zhou 冀州 [6 + 2]

□ Name of a *zhou* 州. [6] It was established under Western Han 漢, during the time of Emperor Wu 武 (reigned 141 – 87). It was one of 13 administrations run by regional inspectors. The territory administered comprised the central and southern sections of He bei 河北, the western tip of Shan dong 山東, and the northern tip of He nan 河南. During Eastern Han, the seat of administration was moved to a point north of Bai xiang 柏鄉 in He bei. Later, the seat of administration was moved to a point southwest of the present Lin zhang 臨漳 county. During Three Kingdoms' Wei 魏, it was moved to the present-day Ji zhou city. Under Jin 晉, the administration was moved to a point southwest of the present Gao yi 高邑 county. Its administrative area was then reduced somewhat. Northern Wei 魏 returned the administration to the present Ji zhou city. During Tang 唐, in 623, the administration was moved to a point southeast of the present-day Shen zhou 深州 city. In 627, it was returned to Ji zhou city. During Qing 清 times, in 1724, the status of the *zhou* was raised to be a directly administered *zhou*, *zhi li zhou* 直隸州. In 1913, the *zhou* was changed to be Ji xian 冀縣 county. In 1993, there was a change and Ji zhou city established. Mentioned with 639, 931, 1160, 1254, 1389, 1448.

□ One of the nine ancient *zhou*. [2] The term referred to the area east from the main trunk of the Yellow River, the area north of the Yellow River between He nan and Shan xi 山西, the western sections of Shan dong, and the southeastern portions of He bei. Mentioned with 504, 1538.

Ji zhou 吉州 [3]

Name of a *zhou* 州. It was established during the *kai huang* 開皇 reign period (581 – 600) of Sui 隋. The seat of administration was at a point north of present-day Ji shui 吉水 county in Jiang xi 江西. The territory administered comprised the watershed of the Gan jiang 贛江 between Xin gan 新淦 and Tai he 泰和 and the areas of the present-day counties of An fu 安福 and Yong xin 永新 in Jiang xi. Later, during the reign period *da ye* 大業 (605 – 618) of the Sui 隋 and during the mid-8th century under Tang 唐, at the beginning of the reign period *tian bao* 天寶 (742 – 756), it was periodically changed to be a commandery. In 1277, under Yuan 元, its status was raised to be Ji zhou lu 吉州路. Mentioned with 348, 389, 535.

Ji zhou 箕州 [1]

Name of a *zhou* 州. It was established under Tang 唐, in 625. The seat of administration was in present-day Zuo quan 左權 county in Shan xi 山西. The territory administered comprised an area corresponding to the present-day counties of He shun 和順, Zuo chuan 左權, and Yu she 榆社 in Shan xi 山西, and the northern portion of She xian 涉縣 county in He bei 河北. In 712, it was changed to be Yi zhou 儀州 Mentioned with 931.

Jia 嘉 [1]

Name of a *zhou* 州. See → Jia zhou 嘉州. Mentioned with 674.

Jia ding 嘉定 [1]

Name of a *zhou* 州, established under the Ming 明, in 1376. The seat of administration was in present-day Le shan 樂山 city in Si chuan 四川. The territory administered comprised the present-day cities, counties and regions of Le shan 樂山, E mei shan 峨眉山, Jia jiang 夾江, Hong ya 洪雅, E bian 峨邊, Qian wei 犍為, Rong xian 榮縣, and Wei yuan 威遠 in Sichuan. Under Qing 清, in 1734, the area became Jia ding fu 嘉定府. Mentioned with 768.

Jia qing fang 嘉慶坊 [1]

Name of a mill. This was a mill in the Tang 唐 eastern capital of Luo yang 洛陽, the city of that name still existing in He nan 河南. Mentioned with 634.

Jia xing 嘉興 [1]
Name of a county. See → Jia xing xian 嘉興縣. Mentioned with 249.

Jia xing xian 嘉興縣 [1]
Name of a county. It was established, under Three Kingdom's Wu 吳, in 242. The seat of administration was at a point south of present-day Jia xing 嘉興 city in Zhe jiang 浙江. The county was eliminated under the Sui 隋 but restored again in 624 under Tang 唐, although eliminated again the next year only to be restored in 634. In 896, the seat of administration was moved to Jia xing city. In 938, under Later Jin 晉, Wu yue 吳越 established Xiu zhou 秀州 there. In 1912, this was combined with Xiu shui 秀水 county to establish Jia he 嘉禾 county. Mentioned with 631.

Jia zhou 嘉州 [7]
Name of a *zhou* 州. It was established under Northern Zhou 周, in 579. The seat of administration was in present-day Le shan 樂山 city in Si chuan 四川. The territory administered comprised the cities and counties of Le shan, E mei shan 峨眉山 and E bian 峨邊 in present-day Si chuan 四川. Under Sui 隋, the area became a commandery but, under Tang 唐, the area again became Jia zhou. The administrative area was greatly expanded and included the territories of present-day Jia jiang 夾江, Qian wei 犍為 and Ma bian 馬邊 counties. Under Southern Song 宋, in 1196, the status of the area was promoted to Jia ding fu 嘉定府. Mentioned with 19, 395, 520, 778, 859, 866, 1040.

Jian 建 [1]
Name of a *zhou*. It was established under Tang 唐, and administered from the present-day Fu zhou 福州 city in Fu jian 福建. The territory administered comprised the present Fu jian province. In 623, it was changed to be Quan zhou 泉州. Mentioned with 124.

Jian an jun 建安郡 [1]
Name of a commandery. It was established in 742. The seat of administration was in present-day Jian ou 建甌 city in Fu jian 福建. The territory administered comprised present-day Nan ping 南平 city in Fu jian and the area of the watershed of the Min jiang 閩江 above it. In 758, the commandery became Jian zhou 建州. Mentioned with 575.

Jian chang 建昌 [1]
Name of an army. It was established, under Northern Song 宋, in 979. The seat of administration was in present-day Nan cheng 南城 county in Jiang xi 江西. The territory administered comprised the present-day counties of Nan cheng, Nan feng 南豐, Guang chang 廣昌, Li chuan 黎川 and Zi xi 資溪 in Jiang xi. Its status was raised during the Yuan 元 to be Jian chang lu 建昌路. Mentioned with 67.

Jian jin shan 揀金山 [1]
Name of a mountain. It is located on the outskirts of present-day Ji nan 濟南 city in Shan dong 山東. Mentioned with 1344.

Jian kang 建康 [2 + 1]

□ Name of a county. [2] It was established under Western Jin 晉, in 313, when Jian ye 建鄴 was changed to be Jian kang. It was administered from the present-day Nan jing 南京 city in Jiang su 江蘇. Eastern Jin and all the Southern Dynasties made this their capital. After Sui 隋 destroyed Chen 陳, Jian kang county became a part of Jiang ning 江寧 county. Mentioned with 623, 718.

□ Name of a *fu* 府. [1] It was established under Southern Song 宋, in 1129. The seat of administration was in the present-day Nan jing 南京 city in Jiang su 江蘇. The territory administered comprised the present Nan jing city and the counties of Jiang ning 江寧, Ju rong 句容, Li yang 溧陽 and Li shui 溧水, in Jiang su. Under Yuan 元, in 1277, the status of the area was promoted to be a *fu*. Mentioned with 579.

Jian nan 劍南 [9 + 5]

□ Regional name. [9] The reference is to the area south of present-day Jian ge 劍閣 to the Yun nan 雲南 and Gui zhou 貴州 plateau. Mentioned with 123, 453, 558, 596, 748, 781, 956, 1480.

□ Name of a circuit. [5] It was founded under Tang 唐, in 627. Its administrative territory covered an area extending in present-day Si chuan 四川 from the watershed of the Fu jiang 涪江 toward the West, from the watershed of the Da du 大渡 river and the lower watershed of the Ya long jiang 雅礱江 toward the East, and in present-day Yun nan 雲南 from the Lan cang jiang 瀾滄江 river and Ai lao 哀牢 mountain toward the East, as well as from the Qu jiang 曲江 river and the Nan pan jiang 南盤江 river toward the North. Furthermore, in Gui zhou 貴州, an area extending from Shui cheng 水城 and Pu an 普安 toward the West, and also Wen xian 文縣 in Gan su 甘肅. Later, during the *kai yuan* 開元 reign period (713 – 741) of the Tang, the seat of administration was moved to present-day Cheng du 成都 city in Si chuan. Later there was a division into an east Chuan (Dong chuan 東川) and a west Chuan (Xi chuan 西川). After the Five Dynasties period the name of the circuit gradually disappeared. Mentioned with 615, 642, 658, 1092, 1282.

Jian ning 建寧 [2 + 1]

□ Name of a *fu* 府. [2] It was established under Southern Song 宋, in 1162. The seat of administration was in present-day Jian ou 建甌 city in Fu jian 福建. The territory administered comprised the Jian xi 建溪 watershed north from Jian ou city, and the counties of Shou ning 壽寧 and Zhou ning 周寧 in Fu jian. In 1279, the *fu* was promoted to Jian ning lu 建寧路. Under the Ming 明, in 1368, it again became a *fu*. Its administrative area corresponded to the Jian xi watershed north from Jian ou city and the counties of Shou ning and Zhou ning in Fu jian, as before. It was abolished in 1913. Mentioned with 243, 634, 768.

□ Name of a *lu* 路. [1] It was established under Yuan 元, in 1279. The seat of administration was in present-day Jian ou 建甌 city in Fu jian 福建. The territory administered comprised the Jian xi 建溪 watershed north from Jian ou city and the counties of Shou ning 壽寧 and Zhou ning 周寧 in Fu jian. It became a *fu* again under Ming 明, in 1368. Mentioned with 634.

Jian ning jun 建寧郡 [1]

Name of a commandery. It was established, under Three Kingdoms Shu 蜀, in 225. The seat of administration was in present-day San cha 三岔, located 15 *li* northwest of Qu jing 曲靖 city in Yun nan 雲南. Its administrative area comprised present-day Dian dong 滇東 (Eastern Yun nan) and Dian zhong 滇中 (Central Yun nan), and it reached in the southwest to Shuang bo 雙柏 and Xin ping 新平 east of Ai lao 哀牢 mountain. During Eastern Jin 晉, the administrative territory only corresponded to the area east of the present-day Yun nan counties of Xun dian 尋甸, Yi liang 宜良, and Mi le 彌勒. During Southern Qi 齊, the administrative seat was moved to an old site 3 *li* south of present-day Lu liang 陸良 county in Yun nan. At the end of the Liang 梁 period of the Southern Dynasties the commandery was abolished. Mentioned with 1253.

Jian ping 建平 [21 + 1]

▫ Name of a commandery. [21] See Jian ping jun 建平郡. Mentioned with 66, 130, 216, 261, 273, 275, 437, 456, 535, 577, 620, 629, 660, 934, 995, 1052, 1096, 1168, 1250, 1254.

▫ Name of a postal station, *yi zhan* 驛站. [1] It was established by Ming 明 and located east of Gui zhou 歸州 town northwest of Zi gui 秭歸 county in present-day Hu bei 湖北. Mentioned with 841.

Jian ping jun 建平郡 [1]

Name of a commandery. It was established, under Three Kingdoms' Wu 吳, in 260. The seat of administration was at a point south of present-day Zi gui 秭歸 county in Hu bei 湖北. After Wei 魏 destroyed Shu 蜀, it was established again and administered from present-day Wu shan 巫山 county in Chong qing 重慶 municipality. In 280, the two Jian ping 建平 counties were combined and administered from Wu shan count

y in Chong qing. The administrative area corresponded to the present-day Wu shan and Wu xi 巫溪 in Chong qing, the two counties of Xing shan 興山 and Zi gui in Hu bei, and the middle and upper watershed of the Qing jiang 清江. The commandery was abolished under Sui 隋. Mentioned with 462.

Jian wei 犍為

See → Qian wei 犍為

Jian yang 建陽 [1]

Name of a county. It was established, under Western Jin 晉, during the *tai kang* 太康 reign period (280 – 289). The seat of administration was at a point northeast of present-day Jian yang 建陽 city in Fu jian 福建. Under the Sui 隋, in 590, it was eliminated but restored, in 621, under the Tang 唐. It was abolished again in 625. In 688, it was reestablished, but the seat of administration was moved to the present-day Jian yang city. Under Southern Song 宋, in 1260, the county was changed to be Jia he 嘉禾 county. Mentioned with 415.

Jian zhou 劍州 [5]

Name of a *zhou* 州. It was established by Tang 唐, in 713. The seat of administration was in Jian ge 劍閣 in present-day Si chuan 四川. Its administrative area corresponded to the areas of the counties of Jiang ge and Zi tong 梓潼 in Si chuan. In 742 it was changed to be Pu an 普安 commandery. In 758 the area again became Jian zhou. Under Southern Song 宋, in 1164, the status of the area was promoted to Pu an Army. Mentioned with 45, 669, 866, 1324.

Jian zhou 建州 [3]

Name of a *zhou* 州. It was founded, under Tang 唐, in 621. The seat of administration was in present-day Jian ou 建甌 city in Fu jian 福建. Its administrative area corresponded to the Min jiang 閩江 watershed north of present-day Nan ping 南平 in Fu jian. During Northern Song 宋, its administrative area in the northwest and in the south was reduced. It only included the watershed of the Jian xi 建溪 north of present-day Jian ou city, and Shou ning 壽寧 and Zhou ning 周寧 counties. Under Southern Song, in 1162, its status was raised to Jian ning fu 建寧府. Mentioned with 214, 768, 1348.

Jian zhou 簡州 [3]

Name of a *zhou* 州. It was established under Sui 隋, in 603. The seat of administration was in the northern bank of the Jiang xi he 綘溪河 located northwest of present-day Jian yang 簡陽 city in Si chuan 四川. The territory administered comprised present-day Jian yang city and a portion of Jin tang 金堂 county in Si chuan. In 1373, under Ming 明, it was changed to be Jian xian 簡縣. In 1513, the county was promoted to be Jian zhou 簡州, and the administrative seat was moved to present-day Jian yang city. The *zhou* was abolished in 1913, and changed to be Jian yang county. Mentioned with 44, 82, 1054.

Jiang 江 [2 + 2 + 1 + 2]

□ Abbreviation referring to the Jiang xi 江西 area. [2] See → Jiang xi. Mentioned with 472, 766.

□ Name of a *zhou* 州. [2] See Jiang zhou 江州. Mentioned with 22, 456.

□ Name of a river, i.e., the Yang zi. [1] Mentioned with 439.

□ Regional name. [2] This is Jiang nan lu 江南路. It was established under Northern Song 宋, in 997. The seat of administration was in present-day Nan jing 南京 city in Jiang su 江蘇. Its administrative area corresponded to the whole province of present-day Jiang xi, and, in present-day Jiang su 江蘇, a line extending from the area south of the Yang zi, Zhen jiang 鎮江 city, and Da mao 大茅 mountain as well as Chang dang 長蕩 lake toward the West. Furthermore, in present-day An hui 安徽 the area south of the Yang zi, and the counties of Yang xin 陽新 and Tong shan 通山 in Hu bei 湖北. In 1018, the area was divided into an eastern and a western *lu* 路. Mentioned with 509. 1105.

Jiang 絳 [2]

Name of a *zhou* 州. See → Jiang zhou 絳州. Mentioned with 1052, 1324.

Jiang bei 江北 [9]

This is a regional name. It is a general allusion to the area "north of the Yang zi river." Mentioned with 614, 757, 794, 1067, 1087, 1253, 1287, 1470, 1553.

Jiang biao 江表 [3]
Regional name. It refers to the area south of the Yang zi. Mentioned with 264, 495, 1242.

Jiang dong 江東 [104]
Regional name. Traditional designation of the territory on the southern bank of the Yang zi down the river from its South-South-West and North-North-East passage between the two present cities of Wu hu 蕪湖 and Nan jing 南京. Mentioned with 33, 40, 48, 60, 145, 152, 159, 163, 170, 189, 191, 203, 206, 208, 221, 222, 231, 240, 263, 272, 314, 319, 321, 330, 338, 344, 364, 371, 421, 440, 456, 508, 530, 572, 600, 614, 623, 637, 639, 641, 649, 651, 665, 667, 668, 687, 688, 745, 810, 861, 871, 881, 893, 896, 905, 910, 982, 989, 1026, 1032, 1060, 1064, 1067, 1119, 1137, 1158, 1161, 1178, 1184, 1188, 1226, 1231, 1232, 1244, 1251, 1302, 1308, 1360, 1387, 1392, 1404, 1405, 1420, 1430, 1443, 1453, 1463, 1477, 1480, 1486, 1490, 1505, 1512, 1522, 1554.

Jiang guang 江廣 [2]
This term refers to an area of a broad river basis without being specific. Mentioned with 410, 719.

Jiang han 江漢 [7]
This is a regional name. It refers to the alluviation area where the Yang zi and the Han jiang 漢江 flow into each other. It corresponds to the present Jiang han plain. Mentioned with 67, 729, 1008.

Jiang he 江河 [1]
Regional name. With the two words for river, it is a general reference to the river basins of the southern rivers. Mentioned with 761, 1486.

Jiang hu 江湖 [19 + 5]
□ This is a regional name. [19] It refers to the region in south China thickly covered by rivers. Mentioned with 126, 145, 171, 364, 678, 752, 768, 924, 1038, 1088, 1105, 1152, 1158, 1194, 1215, 1279, 1470, 1573.
□ Regional name generally referring to an area of rivers and lakes. [5] Mentioned with 128, 258, 635, 729, 1448.

Jiang hu nan bei 江湖南北 [1]
Term for all of China. Mentioned with 385.

Jiang hua xian 江華縣 [1]
Name of a county. It was established in 621. The seat of administration was at a point southwest of present-day Jiang hua 江華 county in Hu nan 湖南. In 684, it became Yun xi 雲溪 county but, in 705, the old name was restored. The seat of administration was moved to a point 10 *li* southeast of the present-day Jiang hua county. In 1462, it was moved to present-day Tuo jiang 沱江 town in Jiang hua county. Mentioned with 1063.

Jiang huai 江淮 [5 + 50]
□ Combined designation for a region. [5] It refers to the Yang zi and the Huai he 淮河, Huai river. Mentioned with 79, 1314, 1330, 1458.
□ Regional name. [50] It refers to the area north of the Yang zi, and south of the Huai he 淮河 corresponding to the present-day Jiang su 江蘇 and the middle

part of An hui 安徽, along with the eastern part of Hu bei 湖北. Mentioned with 6, 31, 38, 42, 66, 119, 158, 188, 234, 247, 249, 263, 272, 429, 437, 442, 445, 562, 572, 725, 730, 799, 823, 871, 900, 931, 950, 958, 980, 985, 1033, 1096, 1135, 1139, 1158, 1167, 1178, 1216, 1219, 1241, 1287, 1311, 1329, 1445, 1449, 1458, 1472, 1495, 1516.

Jiang lai zhi xu 姜賴之墟 (虛) [2]
Name of place in the western regions. Jiang lai 姜賴 was located in present-day southeastern Xin jiang near the old ruins of Lop-nor. Mentioned with 1335.

Jiang lin shan 江林山 [2]
This is the name of a mountain. It might be Qing cheng shan 青城山 mountain of present-day Du jiang yan 都江堰 city in Si chuan 四川. Mentioned with 130.

Jiang ling 江陵 [4]
Name of a county. It was established by Qin 秦. The seat of administration was in the former Jiang ling 江陵 county located in the present-day Jing zhou 荊州 district of Jing zhou city in Hu bei 湖北. In 1994, the county was eliminated and, in 1998, a Jiang ling county was separately established at Hao xue 郝穴 town. Mentioned with 616, 1063, 1242.

Jiang ling 江嶺 [2]
Regional name. This is the region south of the Yang zi and north of the Five Ranges, Wu ling 五嶺. Mentioned with 793, 1463.

Jiang ling fu 江陵府 [2]
Name of a *fu* 府. It was established under Tang 唐, in 761. The seat of administration was in the old Jiang ling 江陵 county in the present-day Jing zhou 荊州 district of Jing zhou city in Hu bei 湖北. Its administrative territory corresponded to an area extending in present-day Hu bei toward the East from Zhi jiang 枝江 city, toward the West from Qian jiang 潛江 city, and toward the South from Jing men 荊門 city. Under Southern Song 宋, it was changed to be Jing nan fu 荊南府. Mentioned with 78, 1310.

Jiang nan 江南 [143 + 2 + 4]
□ Regional name. [143] It refers in general to the area south of the Yang zi and north of the Five Ranges, Wu ling 五嶺. This is the area "South of the Yang zi" of present-day Hu bei 湖北, and Hu nan 湖南 and Jiang xi 江西. Mentioned with 13, 54, 63, 70, 78, 100, 105, 113, 135, 150, 163, 164, 166, 178, 179, 192, 205, 211, 227, 247, 261, 298, 320, 322, 323, 330, 340, 345, 360, 362, 364, 377, 381, 383, 389, 395, 428, 440, 451, 455, 475, 501, 509, 539, 541, 558, 578, 588, 590, 597, 601, 614, 616, 631, 632, 634, 644, 649, 662, 663, 668, 680, 735, 751, 792, 794, 797, 801, 804, 806, 831, 839, 872, 886, 899, 949, 953, 958, 969, 988, 1004, 1067, 1078, 1087, 1113, 1117, 1136, 1154, 1165, 1171, 1177, 1181, 1221, 1229, 1238, 1257, 1273, 1279, 1287, 1292, 1293, 1298, 1301, 1302, 1308, 1316, 1336, 1340, 1342, 1378, 1391, 1400, 1416, 1430, 1442, 1443, 1447, 1460, 1465, 1470, 1475, 1477, 1490, 1498, 1504, 1516, 1526, 1553.
□ Name of a *lu* 路. [2] This was one of 15 *lu* established by the Song, during the *zhi dao* 至道 reign period (995 – 997). The seat of administration was in the present-day Nan jing 南京 city in Jiang su 江蘇. The territory administered comprised an area including the entire province of Jiang xi 江西, and the area south

of the Yang zi in Jiang su 江蘇, the area toward the West from the line formed by Zhen jiang 鎮江, Da mao 大茅 mountain, and the Chang dang 長蕩 lake, along with the portion of An hui 安徽 south of the Yang zi, and the counties of Yang xin 陽新 and Tong shan 通山 in Hu bei 湖北. In 1030, the area was divided into an eastern and a western *lu*. Mentioned with 216, 1098.

□ Name of a Branch Secretariat, *xing sheng* 行省. [4] It was established in 1356 by the Ming 明 rebel and founder of the Ming dynasty Zhu Yuanzhang (1328 – 1398). The seat of administration was in the present-day city of Nan jing 南京 in Jiang su 江蘇. The territory administered comprised an area corresponding to the two present-day provinces of Jiang su and An hui 安徽 along with Shang hai 上海 up to present-day Wu yuan 婺源 county in Jiang xi 江西 province. Under the Ming, in 1368, the area became a Province under the Central Secretariat, *zhong shu sheng* 中書省. Mentioned with 29, 809, 969, 1499.

Jiang nan bei 江南北 [1]

Regional name. It refers to the area located north and south of the Yang zi. Mentioned with 1098.

Jiang nan zhu dao 江南諸道 [1]

Collective designation for several circuits in the Jiang nan 江南 area. The reference is to the various Tang 唐 era circuits located south of the Yang zi, namely Jiang nan dong 江南東, Jiang nan xi 江南西, Fu jian 福建 and Ling nan 嶺南. Territorially this corresponds to the present-day provinces, municipalities and autonomous regions of Zhe jiang 浙江, Shang hai 上海, Jiang xi 江西, Hu nan 湖南, Fu jian 福建, Guang dong 廣東, Guang xi 廣西 and Hai nan 海南, and the sections of the three provinces Jiang su 江蘇, An hui 安徽 and Hu bei 湖北 south of the Yang zi. Mentioned with 428.

Jiang ning 江寧 [4 + 2]

□ Name of a *fu* 府. [4] See → Jiang ning fu 江寧府. Mentioned with 615, 644, 687, 1052.

□ Name of a county. [2] It was established under Western Jin 晉, in 281. The seat of administration was in Jiang ning 江寧 town located southwest of the present-day Jiang ning district in Nan jing 南京 city in Jiang su 江蘇. In 590, the seat of administration was moved to the Chao tian 朝天 palace compound in Nan jing city. In 620, Jiang ning county became Gui hua 歸化 county. In 761, it was changed to be Shang yuan 上元 county. In 917, under Wu 吳 of the Five Dynasties, it was reestablished as Jiang ning county. In 1934, the seat of administration was moved to present-day Dong shan 東山 town of the Jiang ning district. Mentioned with 222, 735.

Jiang ning fu 江寧府 [8]

Name of a *fu*. It was established under Southern Tang 唐 of the Five Dynasties period, in 937. The seat of administration was in the present-day Nan jing 南京 city in Jiang su 江蘇. Its administrative area corresponded to the present-day Nan jing city, and the areas of the cities and counties of Jiang ning 江寧, Liu he 六合, Jiang pu 江浦, Gao chun 高淳, and Ju rong 句容. Under the Northern Song 宋, in 975, the *fu* became Sheng zhou 昇州 and, in 1018, its status was raised to be Jiang ning fu. Under Southern Song, in 1129, it was changed to Jian kang fu 建康府. Mentioned with 53, 199, 381, 441, 706, 875, 1378, 1510.

Jiang pu 江浦 [1]

Area along the Yang zi. The reference is to both banks of the Yang zi. Mentioned with 1400.

Jiang shan 江山 [1]

Name of a mountain. Reference is to Jiang lang 江郎 mountain located south of present-day Jiang shan 江山 county in Zhe jiang 浙江. Mentioned with 1038.

Jiang shan 蔣山 [2]

Name of a mountain. This is Zhong 鐘 mountain. It is located outside the Zhong shan men 中山門 gate of present-day Nan jing 南京 city in Jiang Su 江蘇. Mentioned with 978, 1485.

Jiang wai 江外 [1]

Regional name. It refers to the Jiang nan 江南 area. This name is from the perspective of inhabitants of the Chinese central plain. The Jiang nan area is "beyond the Yang zi," thus the name. Mentioned with 1459.

Jiang xi 江西 [14 + 6+ 9 + 2]

□ Abbreviated name of a *lu*. [14] In 1018, Northern Song 宋 established a Jiang nan xi lu 江南西路. The seat of administration was in present-day Nan chang 南昌 city in Jiang xi 江西. The territory administered comprised most of present-day Jiang xi and the counties of Da ye 大冶, Tong shang 通山 and Yang xin 陽新 in Hu bei 湖北. It was abolished under Yuan 元. Mentioned with 58, 75, 216, 550, 558, 848, 886, 1038, 1051, 1407, 1425, 1460, 1485, 1499, 1530.

□ Abbreviated name of a circuit. [6] Under Tang 唐, in 733, a Jiang nan xi 江南西 circuit was established. The seat of administration was in present-day Nan chang 南昌 city in Jiang xi 江西. The territory administered comprised the region "south of the river (Yang zi)", including present-day Jiang xi and Hu nan 湖南 (other than the watershed of the Yuan shui 沅水 south of Yuan ling 沅陵), the southern part of An hui 安徽, and eastern part of Hu bei 湖北, as well as, in Guang dong 廣東, the cities and counties of Lian zhou 連州, Yang shan 陽山 and Lian nan 連南. The circuit was abolished during the Five Dynasties period. Mentioned with 389, 739, 873, 1013, 1113, 1178.

□ Name of an administrative area. [9] This is an abbreviation for the Jiang xi Provincial Administration Commission, Jiang xi *bu zheng shi si* 江西布政使司. It was established in 1376. The seat of administration was in the present Nan chang 南昌 city in Jiang xi 江西. Its administrative area in the North went as far as the present-day Jiu jiang 九江 city of Jiang xi, in the east it went as far as Yu shan 玉山 county in present-day Jiang xi, in the South it went as far as present-day An yuan 安遠 county in Jiang xi, and in the West it went to present-day Yong ning 永寧 county in Jiang xi. Its extent more or less corresponded to the present-day province of Jiang xi. The Qing 清 turned the area into Jiang xi province. Mentioned with 100, 328, 476, 566, 578, 928, 1208, 1243.

□ Regional name. [2] Before the Sui-Tang 隋唐 period, people customarily called the area on the northern banks of the lower Yang zi and south of the Huai shui 淮水 Jiang xi. Mentioned with 1099, 1486.

Jiang xia 江夏 [5 + 6]

□ Name of a county. [5] It was established under Sui 隋, in 589. The seat of administration was in present-day Wu chang 武昌 district in Wu han 武漢 city in Hu bei 湖北. In 1912, Jiang xi was changed to be Wu chang county. Mentioned with 780, 833, 1222, 1233, 1521.

□ Name of a commandery. [6] It was established under Western Han 漢, in 201 BCE. The seat of administration was at a point 2 *li* west of present-day Xin zhou 新洲 district in Wu han 武漢 city in Hu bei 湖北. The territory administered comprised an area in present-day Hu bei extending from Zhong xiang 鐘祥 city, Qian jiang 潛江 city, Jia yu 嘉魚 county and Chi bi 赤壁 city toward the East, from the counties of Hong an 紅安, Xin zhou, Qi chun 蘄春 and Yang xin 陽新 toward the West, from the counties of Chong yang 崇陽 and Tong shan 通山 toward the North, and from An lu 安陸 city, as well as in He nan 河南 the counties of Xin yang 信陽, Luo shan 羅山, and Guang shan 光山 toward the south. At the beginning of the *jian an* 建安 reign period (196 – 220) of Eastern Han, the seat of administration was moved to present-day Han kou 漢口 in Wu han city. In 208, the seat of administration was moved to the present-day Han yang 漢陽 district in Wu han city. Later that year, General Wen Pin 文聘 moved the seat of administration to a point west of the present-day Huang pi 黃陂 district in Wu han city. Under Three Kingdoms' Wei 魏, in 251, the seat of administration was moved to a point southwest of the present-day Yun meng 雲夢 county. Under Western Jin 晉, it was moved to a point north of the present An lu 安陸 city. In 454, under Liu Song 劉宋, the seat of administration was moved to the present-day Wu chang 武昌 district in Wu han city. The commandery was abolished in 589, under the Sui 隋. Mentioned with 33, 291, 533, 1233, 1443, 1532.

Jiang yang 江陽 [1]

Name of a commandery. It was established under Eastern Jin 晉. The seat of administration was at a point northeast of present-day Peng shan 彭山 county in Si chuan 四川. The area administered comprised the connected territories of the counties of Peng shan, Shuang liu 雙流 and Ren shou 仁壽. Northern Zhou 周 abolished the commandery. Mentioned with 1096.

Jiang yang shan 江陽山 [1]

Name of a mountain. This is Qing cheng 青城 mountain of present-day Du jiang yan 都江堰 city in Si chuan 四川. Mentioned with 130.

Jiang yin 江陰 [3]

Name of a county. It was founded, under Southern Dynasties' Liang 梁, in 558. The seat of administration was in present-day Jiang yin city in Jiang su 江蘇. Mentioned with 429, 519.

Jiang yuan 江源 [1]

Name of a county. It was established under Western Han 漢. The seat of administration was at a point east of present-day Jiang yuan chang 江源場, located 30 *li* southeast of Chong zhou 崇州 city in Si chuan 四川. It was eliminated at the end of Western Jin 晉, but reestablished under Eastern Jin during the *yong he* 永和 reign period (354 – 356). The seat of administration was moved to present-day Huai yuan 懷遠 town, located 60 *li* northwest of Chong zhou city in Si chuan. Under Northern Zhou 周, Jiang yuan county became Duo rong 多融 county. Mentioned with 550.

Jiang zhe 江浙 [18 + 8]

□ Combined regional name. [18] During the Song 宋 period, it referred to the Eastern *lu* of Jiang nan 江南, the Western *lu* of Jiang nan, and the Liang zhe lu 兩浙路. This corresponded to present-day Jiang xi 江西 province, Zhe jiang 浙江 province and the Su nan 蘇南 region from Da mao 大茅 mountain east. Mentioned with 76, 100, 185, 344, 348, 358, 566, 589, 838, 858, 905, 1207, 1262, 1407, 1486, 1493, 1499.

□ Name of a Branch Secretariat, *xing sheng* 行省. [8] It was established during the Yuan 元, in 1284. The seat of administration was in present-day Hang zhou 杭州 city in Zhe jiang. The territory administered reached from the present-day Zhe jiang province, Shang hai 上海 city, and, in Jiang xi, the area east of Po yang 鄱陽 lake toward the East, and, in the two provinces of Jiang su 江蘇 and An hui 安徽, the area south of the Yang zi. In 1299, the administrative area was expanded to include the whole province of Fu jian 福建. In 1366, the Ming 明 rebels changed Jiang zhe to be the Zhe jiang Branch Secretariat, Zhe jiang *xing sheng* 浙江行省. Mentioned with 76, 222, 399, 550, 572, 1486, 1340, 1379.

Jiang zhou 江州 [7]

Name of a *zhou* 州. It was established under Western Jin 晉, in 291. The seat of administration was at a point east of present-day Nan chang 南昌 city in Jiang xi 江西. Its administrative area comprised both the two present-day provinces of Jiang xi and Fu jian 福建, and, in Hu bei 湖北, the area east of the Lu shui 陸水 and south of the Yang zi, as well as, in Hu nan 湖南, the region east of the middle and upper flow of the Chong ling shui 舂陵水. Later, its jurisdiction was reduced. In 477, the seat of jurisdiction was moved to a point southwest of present-day Jiu jiang 九江 city in Jiang xi. In 557, under Southern Dynasties' Liang 梁, the seat of administration was moved to a point east of present-day Nan chang city. Under the Chen 陳 dynasty, at the beginning of the *tian jia* 天嘉 reign period (560 – 566), it was again moved to present-day Jiu jiang city. During the reign period *da ye* 大業 (605 – 615) of the Sui 隋, and during the reign periods *tian bao* 天寶 (742 – 756) and *zhi de* 至德 (756 – 758) of the Tang 唐, the *zhou* was periodically changed to a commandery. During the Tang, the jurisdiction of the commandery comprised the present-day cities and counties of Jiu jiang, De an 德安, Peng ze 彭澤, Hu kou 湖口 and Du chang 都昌 in Jiang xi. In 1277, during Yuan 元, the status of the area was promoted to Jiang zhou lu 江州路. Mentioned with 81, 555, 1020, 1078, 1160, 1430.

Jiang zhou 絳州 [6]
Name of a *zhou* 州. It was established under Northern Zhou 周, in 560. The seat of administration was at a point 28 *li* northeast of present-day Wen xi 聞喜 county in Shan xi 山西. Later, Zhou Emperor Wu 武 (543 – 578) moved the seat of administration to Bai bi 柏壁 village, located 20 *li* southwest of present-day Xin jiang 新絳 county. In 577, the seat of administration was moved to the southern bank of the Fen he 汾河, 12 *li* southwest of the present-day Ji shan 稷山 county. The administrative area of the *zhou* comprised the counties of He jin 河津, Ji shan, Xin jiang, Qu wo 曲沃, Jiang xian 絳縣 and Yi cheng 翼城 in Shan xi. During Sui 隋, in 607, the area became Jiang 絳 commandery. Under Tang 唐, in 618, its status was raised to become the Jiang zhou 絳州 area command, Jiang zhou *zong guan fu* 絳州總管府. In 620, the area again became Jiang zhou. The seat of administration was moved to the present Xin jiang county in Shan xi. In 1912, the area became Xin jiang county. Mentioned with 617, 927, 1318, 1393, 1412, 1443.

Jiang zuo 江左 [23]
Regional name. This is Jiang dong 江東, referring to the area east of the flow of the Yang zi between present-day Wu hu 蕪湖 city and Nan jing 南京 city. Mentioned with 78, 123, 178, 254, 322, 346, 359, 456, 502, 519, 691, 810, 863, 906, 1008, 1020, 1036, 1087, 1407, 1460.

Jiao 交 [12]
Name of a *zhou* 州. See → Jiao zhou 交州. Mentioned with 9, 144, 202, 226, 347, 367, 376, 445, 746, 772, 843, 1028, 1272.

Jiao dong 膠東 [1]
Regional name. The reference is to the area of the Jiao dong peninsula east from present-day Wei fang 濰坊 city in Shan dong 山東. Mentioned with 556.

Jiao guang 交廣 [24]
Combined regional name. It is a combination of the names of Jiao zhou 交州 and Guang zhou 廣州. The area corresponded to the region of present-day Ling nan 嶺南 and the northern part of Vietnam. Mentioned with 51, 94, 135, 164, 187, 287, 288, 336, 373, 453, 533, 535, 596, 794, 1080, 1307, 1371, 1386, 1457, 1463, 1499, 1557.

Jiao he 交河 [5]
Name of an ancient city. The ruins of the old city of Jiao he are found at a site 13 km west of present-day Turfan city in Xin jiang 新疆. Mentioned with 174, 484, 584, 1370.

Jiao ling 交嶺 [1]
Regional name. It refers to the Ling nan 嶺南 area. Mentioned with 886.

Jiao zhi 交趾 [21+ 5 + 8]
Name of a commandery. [21] It was established by Zhao Tuo 趙佗 (230 – 137) of Nan Yue 南越 at the beginning of the Western Han 漢. It came under the jurisdiction of Han, in 111 BCE. The seat of administration was at a point northwest of present-day Hanoi. It controlled present-day northern Vietnam. Eastern Han moved the seat of administration to a point east of the present-day Tiên Du 仙

游 in Bắc Ninh province of Vietnam. The jurisdiction of the commandery was reduced and limited to a strip of the Red River delta. In 590, under Sui 隋, it was eliminated but later, at the beginning of the *da ye* 大業 reign period (605 – 615), reestablished. The administration was moved to present-day Hanoi city in Vietnam. Tang reestablished a Jiao zhou 交州. Mentioned with 61, 136, 144, 252, 307, 376, 437, 489, 514, 534, 586, 596, 680, 759, 878, 1128, 1264, 1396, 1506.

□ Regional name. [5] During Tang 唐 and Song 宋 times, it referred to the northern part of present-day Vietnam. Mentioned with 243, 963, 1086, 1272, 1399.

□ Name of a province-level administrative unit. [8] Ming 明 established the Jiao zhi Provincial Administration Commission, Jiao zhi *bu zheng shi si* 交趾布政使司, in 1407. The seat of administration was in present-day Hanoi city. Its administrative territory comprised 17 *fu* 府, 47 *zhou* 州 and 157 counties. Simultaneously, Ming established a Regional Military Commission (*du zhi hui shi si* 都指揮使司), and under it were 11 guards and 3 bases. The jurisdiction of the province-level unit comprised the region north of the middle section of present-day Vietnam. In 1427, the area was abandoned by the Chinese, and Annam restored itself as a country. Mentioned with 106, 144, 197, 480, 758, 834, 1028, 1303.

Jiao zhou 膠州 [1]

Name of a *zhou* 州. It was established by Northern Wei 魏, in 529. The seat of administration was in present-day Zhu cheng 諸城 city in Shan dong 山東. The territory administered comprised the present-day cities of Zhu cheng, Gao mi 高密, An qiu 安丘, Jiao zhou 膠州 and Jiao nan 膠南 in Shan dong. Under the Sui 隋, in 585, it became Mi zhou 密州. Mentioned with 111.

Jiao zhou 交州 [23]

Name of a *zhou* 州. It was established under Eastern Han 漢, in 203. The seat of administration was in present-day Wu zhou 梧州 city in Guang xi 廣西. In 210, the seat of administration was moved to present-day Guang zhou 廣州 city in Guang dong 廣東. The administrative area of the *zhou* comprised most of present-day Guang dong and Guang xi, and all provinces north of present-day Tỉnh Thừa in central Vietnam. In 226, under Three Kingdoms' Wu 吳, the *zhou* was divided into the two *zhou* of Jiao 交 and Guang 廣. Jiao zhou was subsequently administered from a point east of the present-day Tiên Du in Bắc Ninh province of Vietnam. Its administrative area comprised present-day Qin zhou 欽州 city in Guang xi, the Lei zhou 雷州 peninsula in present-day Guang dong and the region of northern and central Vietnam. Sui 隋 eliminated the *zhou* but it was reestablished under the Tang 唐, in 622, and administered from a location northwest of present-day Hanoi city in Vietnam. In 825, the seat of administration was moved to present-day Hanoi city. During the Five Dynasties period, the *zhou* was eliminated but the area was still called Jiao zhou in Song times. Mentioned with 30, 51, 94, 144, 226, 376, 388, 427, 432, 585, 586, 772, 794, 1078, 1123, 1264, 1406, 1515.

Jie 階 [3]

Name of a *zhou* 州. See → Jie zhou. 階州. Mentioned with 368, 1057, 1063.

Jie di 階地 [1]
Term referring in general to places above and below, high and low in topography. Mentioned with 1382.

Jie gu guo 結骨國 [1]
This is the name of an ancient country located apparently in Central Asia. Further details are unavailable. Mentioned with 1205.

Jie qiao 界橋 [1]
Minor place name. It is located on the borders of present-day Yi chun 宜春 city in Jiang xi 江西, but further details are lacking. Mentioned with 768.

Jie zhou 階州 [11]
Name of a *zhou* 州. It was established by Tang 唐, in 892. The seat of administration was at a point west of present-day Kang xian 康縣 county in Gan su 甘肅. The territory administered comprised present-day Long nan 隴南 city and the area of Kang xian county in Gan su. In 932, during the Five Dynasties period, the seat of administration was moved to Long nan city. Yuan 元 moved the seat of administration to Liu shu cheng 柳樹城 in Jiao gong xiang 角弓鄉, located 70 *li* northwest of the present Wu du 武都 county. Under Ming 明, in 1371, the *zhou* was reduced to a county and, along with this, the seat of administration was moved to the present Long nan city. In 1377, the county became a *zhou* again. In 1729, the status of the area was raised to be a directly administered *zhou*, *zhi li zhou* 直隸州. In 1913, the area was changed to a new Wu du county. Mentioned with 27, 202, 368, 1307, 1378, 1406, 1435.

Jin 金 [6]
Name of a *zhou* 州. See → Jin zhou 金州. Mentioned with 202, 654, 660, 864, 908, 1265.

Jin 錦 [2]
Name of a *zhou* 州. See → Jin zhou 錦州. Mentioned with 202.

Jin 晉 [14 + 3]
□ Name of a Spring and Autumn period country. [14] Most of it was in the southern portion of present-day Shan xi 山西. The capital was at Qu wo 曲沃 in present-day Shan xi. Later, its territory was much extended and came to include much of Shan xi, the southwest portion of He bei 河北, the northern part of He nan 河南 and a corner of Shaan xi 陝西. During the middle of the 4th century BCE, Jin became divided into the three states of Han 韓, Zhao 趙 and Wei 魏. Mentioned with 64, 285, 444, 614, 620, 856, 1065, 1171, 1258, 1301, 1410, 1443, 1551.
□ Name of a *zhou* 州. [3] See → Jin zhou 晉州. Mentioned with 1052, 1324, 1519.

Jin an 晉安 [10]
Name of a county. It was established under Western Jin 晉, at the beginning of the *tai kang* 太康 reign period (280 – 289). The seat of administration was in Feng zhou 豐州 town located east of present-day Nan an 南安 city in Fu jian 福建. Under the Sui 隋, in 589, the area became Nan an county. Mentioned with 298, 535, 790, 925, 1238, 1457, 1460.

Jin bian bei di 近汴北地 [1]
Regional name. It refers to region north of the Bian he 汴河 river, in the northern part of present-day Kai feng 開封 city in He nan 河南. Mentioned with 145.

Jin cheng 金城 [1]
Minor place name. It was located on the southern shore of the Yang zi northeast of present-day Nan jing 南京 city in Jiang su 江蘇. Mentioned with 1443.

Jin chi 金齒 [2]
Name of a base (*suo* 所). It was established during early Ming 明, and administered from present-day Bao shan 保山 city in Yun nan 雲南. Later, in 1585, the *suo* was changed to be the Zhen an Independent Battalion, Zhen an *shou yu qian hu suo* 鎮安守禦千戶所, and was moved to Meng lin 猛淋. Mentioned with 493, 726.

Jin di 晉地 [10]
Name of a feudal domain. See → Jin 晉. Mentioned with 78, 102, 285, 604, 675, 695, 733, 819, 1443.

Jin hua 金華 [5]
Name of a *fu* 府. It was established, by the Ming 明 rebels, under Zhu Yuanzhang 朱元璋 (1328 – 1398), in 1360. The seat of administration was in present-day Jin hua 金華 city in Zhe jiang 浙江. The territory administered comprised the Jin hua jiang 金華江 watershed and the cities and counties of Lan xi 蘭溪 and Pu jiang 浦江 in the present province of Zhe jiang. The *fu* was abolished in 1912. Mentioned with 4, 566, 768.

Jin kang 晉康 [1]
Name of a commandery. It was established under Eastern Jin 晉, in 351. The seat of administration was at a point east of present-day De qing 德慶 county in Guang dong 廣東. During the era of Liu Song 劉宋 of the Southern Dynasties, the seat of administration was moved to a point south of present-day Luo ding 羅定 city in Guang dong. Thereafter, during the *yuan jia* 元嘉 reign period (424 – 453), it was moved to present-day De qing county. Under Southern Qi 齊, it was moved to a point south of present-day Yu nan 郁南 county in Guang dong but, under Liang 梁, it went back again to De qing county. The commandery was eliminated under Sui 隋, during the *kai huang* 開皇 reign period (582 – 600). It was reestablished, in 742, under Tang 唐 and administered the cities and counties of present-day De qing, Yu nan and Yun fou 雲浮 in Guang dong. In 758, the area became Kang zhou 康州. Mentioned with 1096.

Jin ling 金陵 [7]
Alternative place name. It refers to the city of Nan jing 南京 in Jiang su 江蘇. Mentioned with 303, 566, 738, 928, 1222, 1391, 1435.

Jin ling 晉陵 [1]
Name of a commandery. See → Jin ling jun 晉陵郡. Mentioned with 768.

Jin ling jun 晉陵郡 [1]
Name of a commandery. It was established under Western Jin 晉, in 311. The seat of administration was in present-day Dan tu 丹徒 town of Zhen jiang 鎮江 city

in Jiang su 江蘇. The territory administered comprised the present-day cities and counties of Zhen jiang, Chang zhou 常州, Wu xi 無錫, Jiang yin 江陰, Wu jin 武進, Dan yang 丹陽 and Jin tan 金壇 in Jiang su. In 318, under Eastern Jin, the seat of administration was moved to present-day Zhen jiang city in Jiang su and, in 413, it was moved to present-day Chang zhou city in Jiang su. In 589, under Sui 隋, the commandery became Chang zhou. Under Tang 唐, at the beginning of the *tian bao* 天寶 reign period (742 – 756), it again became Jin ling 晉陵 commandery. In 758, it was again changed to Chang zhou. Mentioned with 768.

Jin ning xian 晉寧縣 [1]

Name of a county. It was established under Western Jin 晉, in 280, and administered from present-day Jiu shi 舊市 city southeast of Zi xing 資興 city in Hu nan 湖南. The county was abolished at the beginning of Sui 隋. Mentioned with 1390.

Jin xi zhu man 晉溪諸蠻

Jin xi 晉溪 is probably an error for Jin xi 晉熙. This is the name of a commandery. It was established by Eastern Jin 晉, during the *yi xi* 義熙 reign period (405 – 419). The seat of administration was in present-day Qian shan 潛山 county in An hui 安徽. The territory administered comprised the present-day cities and counties of An qing 安慶, Qian shan, Huai ning 懷寧, Yue xi 岳西, Tong cheng 桐城, Zong yang 樅陽, Wang jiang 望江, Tai hu 太湖 and Su song 宿松. The commandery was abolished at the beginning of the *kai huang* 開皇 reign period (581 – 600) of the Sui 隋. Mentioned with 986.

Jin xing xian 晉興縣 [1]

Name of a county. It was established under Tang 唐, in 622. The seat of administration was at a point 30 *li* south of present-day Wu ming 武鳴 county in Guang xi 廣西. In 972, under Northern Song 宋, it became Le chang 樂昌 county. Mentioned with 428.

Jin ya tuan 金牙湍 [1]

Name used for a section of the upper flow of the Han shui 漢水. The area is located on the outskirts of present-day Han zhong 漢中 city in Shaan xi 陝西. Details are lacking. Mentioned with 557.

Jin yang 晉陽 [1 + 2]

□ Ancient place name. [1] It was a city in the state of Jin 晉 in the Spring and Autumn period. It was located southwest of present-day Tai yuan 太原 city in Shan xi 山西. Mentioned with 966.

□ Name of a county. [2] It was established under Qin 秦, in 248 BCE. The seat of administration was in Gu cheng ying 古城營 village southwest of present-day Tai yuan 太原 city in Shan xi 山西. Under Northern Qi 齊, in 565, the seat of administration was moved to a point east of the Fen shui 汾水. Under Sui 隋, in 590, the seat of administration was returned to Gu cheng ying. Under Northern Song 宋, in 979, the county was abolished. Mentioned with 290, 444.

Jin yang xiang 晉陽鄉 [1]
Minor place name. It was located on the borders of present-day Lian zhou 連州 city in Guang dong 廣東. Mentioned with 21.

Jin yun 縉雲 [3]
Name of a county. It was founded under Tang 唐, in 696. The seat of administration was in present-day Jin yun county in Zhe jiang 浙江. Mentioned with 456, 1032, 1279.

Jin zhou 金州 [8]
Name of a *zhou* 州. It was founded under Western Wei 魏, in 554. The seat of administration was in present-day An kang 安康 city in Shaan xi 陝西. Its jurisdiction comprised an area of the Han shui 漢水 watershed in present-day Shaan xi extending from Shi quan 石泉 county toward the East and Xun yang 旬陽 county toward the West. Under Ming 明, in 1583, the area became Xing an fu 興安府. Mentioned with 130, 202, 291, 629, 864, 1096, 1485.

Jin zhou 錦州 [2]
Name of a *zhou* 州. It was founded under Tang 唐, in 687. The seat of administration was at Lu shui kou 盧水口 on the border of present-day Ma yang 麻陽 county in Hu nan 湖南. Later the seat of administration was moved to Du rang 杜壤, located 75 *li* southwest of Ma yang 麻陽 county. The jurisdiction of the *zhou* comprised present-day Feng huang 鳳凰 county and Ma yang county in present-day Hu nan, and Tong ren 同仁 county in Gui zhou 貴州. During the Five Kingdoms period, it was abolished. Mentioned with 202.

Jin zhou 晉州 [3]
Name of a *zhou* 州. It was established under Northern Wei 魏, in 528. The seat of administration was in present-day Lin fen 臨汾 city in Shan xi 山西. Its administrative area included in present-day Shan xi the two cities of Lin fen and Huo zhou 霍州, and the counties of Hong tong 洪洞, Fu shan 浮山, An ze 安澤, and Fen xi 汾西. Under Tang 唐, in 618, the seat of administration was moved to present-day Lin fen city and, later again, it was moved to present-day Jin dian 金殿 town, located 18 *li* southwest of Lin fen city. During the Five Dynasties period, it was again moved to Lin fen city. Under Northern Song 宋, in 1116, its status was raised to Ping yang fu 平陽府. Mentioned with 285, 1443.

Jin zhou 靳州 [1]
This is an error for → Qin zhou 勤州. Mentioned with 635.

Jing 荊 [10 + 3]
□ Name of a *zhou* 州. [10] See → Jing zhou 荊州. Mentioned with 38, 79, 99, 369, 456, 980, 1067, 1184, 1446, 1493.
□ Name of a *fu* 府. [3] See under → Jīng zhou 荊州. Mentioned with 637, 958, 1375.

Jing 京 [1]
This is a term meaning capital. The reference in this case is to the Tang 唐 capital of Chang an 長安, now Xi an 西安, in Shaan xi 陝西.

Jing chu 荊楚 [18]
Regional name. The reference is to a strip of Hu bei 湖北 province or the surrounding areas. Mentioned with 178, 180, 378, 546, 572, 787, 893, 901, 1119, 1312, 1498.

Jing de zhen 景德鎮 [1]
Originally this was the name of a garrison (*zhen* 鎮). It was established during Northern Song 宋 and is now Jing de town in Jiang xi 江西, the garrison connotation in the name having long been lost. Mentioned with 24.

Jing dong 京東 [1]
Name of a *lu* 路. It was founded under Northern Song 宋, in 997. The seat of administration was at a point south of present-day Shang qiu 商丘 in He nan 河南. The territory administered comprised the area southeast of the Tu hai he 徒駭河 in present-day Shan dong 山東, Dong ming 東明 in Shan dong, as well as the area of Ning ling 寧陵 and Zhe cheng 柘城 county toward the East in He nan 河南, and the northwestern corner of Jiang su 江蘇. In 1074, the area was divided into an eastern and a western *lu*. Mentioned with 191.

Jing du 京都 [1]
This is a term for "capital city." It refers to the Northern Song 宋 capital of Bian jing 汴京, this is the present-day Kai feng 開封 city in He nan 河南. Mentioned with 692.

Jing fu 荊府 [1]
Term used as reference to the Jing zhou 荊州 Princely Establishment, Jing zhou *wang fu* 荊州王府, conferred during the Ming 明. This was in present-day Jing zhou city in Hu bei 湖北. Mentioned with 322.

Jing hu 荊湖 [5]
Name of a *lu* 路. It was established at the beginning of Northern Song 宋, during the *yong xi* 雍熙 reign period (984 – 987). The seat of administration was in former Jiang ling 江陵 county city in the present-day Jing zhou 荊州 district of Jing zhou city in Hu bei 湖北. The territory administered comprised the whole province of present-day Hu nan 湖南, Hu bei south of Jing 荊 mountain and Da hong 大洪 mountain, the area from E zhou 鄂州 and Chong yang 崇陽 county toward the West, the area of Ba dong 巴東 county and Wu feng 五峰 county toward the East, and the watersheds of the Xiang shui 湘水 and Guan jiang 灌江 east of the Yue cheng ling 越城嶺 mountain range in Guang xi 廣西. In 997, the area was divided into a southern and a northern *lu*. Later on, people used the term Jing hu for the region of Hu bei and Hu nan. Mentioned with 535, 1274, 1446.

Jing kou 京口 [6]
Place name. At the end of Eastern Han 漢 and during Three Kingdoms' Wu 吳, this area was called Jing cheng 京城, but afterwards it became known as Jing kou. This is the present-day Zhen jiang 鎮江 city in Jiang su 江蘇. Mentioned with 338, 634, 969, 1238, 1546.

Jing le xian 靜樂縣 [1]

Name of a county. It was established by Sui 隋, in 608, and administered from present-day Jing le 靜樂 county in Shan xi 山西. Mentioned with 1532.

Jing lu 京陸 [1]

Minor place name. Details are lacking. Mentioned with 1157.

Jing luo 京洛 [1 + 6]

□ This was the collective designation for the Tang capital of Chang an 長安 and the city of Luo yang. [1] This is now Xi an 西安 in Shaan xi 陝西, and Luo yang 洛陽 in He nan 河南. Mentioned with 189.

□ This is the term used for Kai feng 開封 and Luo yang 洛陽 of the Song 宋 period. [6] It refers to the whole regional strip from present-day Kai feng in He nan 河南 to present-day Luo yang. Mentioned with 927, 1038, 1110, 1275, 1287, 1407.

Jing man 荊蠻 [1]

This is the ancient country of Chu 楚. The term refers in general to the region of the country of Chu, now a strip of territory in Hu bei 湖北 province. Mentioned with 1272.

Jing men jun 荊門軍 [1]

Name of a region. Five Dynasties' Liang 梁 established a Jing men 荊門 army. The seat of administration was in present-day Dang yang 當陽 city in Hu bei 湖北. It was soon eliminated. Northern Song 宋 reestablished the army, in 972, and moved the seat of administration to present-day Jing men city in Hu bei. It was eliminated in 1073, but reestablished in 1088. In 1236, the seat of administration was moved to the present-day Dang yang city. Under the Yuan 元, in 1277, the army was changed to a new Jing men fu 荊門府. Mentioned with 381.

Jing nan 荊南 [4]

Name of a regional garrison. It was established under the Tang 唐, in 757. The seat of administration was in the old Jiang ling xian 江陵縣 city in the present-day Jing zhou 荊州 district of Jing zhou city in Hu bei 湖北. The territory administered comprised, in present-day Hu bei, an area of the Yang zi watershed extending from Shi shou 石首 and Jing zhou city toward the West, and from Dian jiang 墊江 of Chong qing 重慶 municipality and Feng du 豐都 toward the East, as well as a strip formed by the lower watersheds of the two rivers of the Li shui 澧水 and the Yuan shui 沅水 rivers in Hu nan reaching from Dong ting 洞庭 lake in Hu nan 湖南 toward the West. Under Five Dynasties' Later Tang, in 925, the area became independent as Nan ping guo 南平國. Mentioned with 208, 1152, 1486.

Jing shan 荊山 [4]

Name of a mountain. It is located west of present-day Nan zhang 南漳 county in Hu bei 湖北. Mentioned with 636, 746, 839, 966.

Jing shan 景山 [1]

Place name from the *Shan hai jing* 山海經, "Classic of Mountains and Seas." Details are lacking. Mentioned with 1105.

Jing shan xian 荊山縣 [1]
Name of a county. It was established in 619. The seat of administration was at a point west of present-day Nan zhang 南漳 county in Hu bei 湖北. In 730, this was changed to the new Nan zhang county. Mentioned with 381.

Jing shi 京師 [1 + 4 + 2 + 3 + 1]
□ Designation for the capital. [1] It refers to the Eastern Han 漢 capital city of Luo yang 洛陽. This is the old city of Han and Wei 魏 times located northeast of present-day Luo yang city in He nan 河南. Mentioned with 1558.
□ Another designation for the capital. [4] In this case, it refers to the Northern Song capital of Bian jing 汴京, the present-day Kai feng 開封 in He nan 河南. Mentioned with 21, 185, 243, 660.
□ Another designation for the capital. [2] In this case, it refers to the Tang 唐 capital of Chang an 長安, present-day Xi an 西安 in Shaan xi 陝西.
□ Another designation for the capital. [3] In this case, the term refers to the Ming 明 capital of Bei jing 北京. Mentioned with 2, 913, 1316.
□ Another designation for the capital. [1] In this case, the term refers to the Yuan 元 capital of Da du 大都, present-day Bei jing 北京. Mentioned with 1532.

Jing xi 京西 [1]
General regional name. It refers to approximately the area of He nan 河南 west of present-day Kai feng 開封 city. Mentioned with 768.

Jing xia 京下 [2 + 1]
□ Another designation for the capital. [2] In this case, the reference is to the Northern Song capital of Bian jing 汴京, the present-day Kai feng 開封 city in He nan 河南. Mentioned with 226, 249.
□ Another designation for the capital. [1] In this case, the reference is to Tang 唐 Chang an 長安, the present-day Xi an 西安 city in Shaan xi 陝西. Mentioned with 1446.

Jing xiang 荊湘 [1]
Combined regional name. The term refers to the region formed by the present Hu bei 湖北 and Hu nan 湖南. Mentioned with 119.

Jing xiang 荊襄 [10]
Regional name. It refers to the region between Jing zhou 荊州 and Xiang yang 襄陽. This area more or less corresponds to the northern part of present-day Hu bei 湖北. Mentioned with 51, 298, 538, 578, 830, 871, 900, 924, 950, 1020.

Jing yang 荊揚 [4]
Combined name for the two ancient *zhou* 州 of Jing zhou 荊州 and Yang zhou 揚州 in what is today a region in the South. Mentioned with 164, 1093, 1538.

Jing yang 涇陽 [1]
Name of a county. It was established by Former Qin 秦 of the Sixteen Kingdoms. The seat of administration was in Gu xian 故縣 village, located 30 *li* southeast of present-day Jing yang 涇陽 county in Shaan xi 陝西. It was eliminated, in 446, but shortly thereafter, at the beginning of the *jing ming* 景明 reign period (500

– 504), reestablished. Under the Sui 隋, in 583, the seat of administration was moved to the present-day Jing yang county. Mentioned with 441.

Jing ying 荊郢 [1]
Regional name. It refers to the area between present-day Jing zhou 荊州 and Zhong xiang 鍾祥. This area more or less corresponds to the middle portion of Hu bei 湖北. Mentioned with 1320.

Jing yuan 涇原 [1]
Name of a *lu* 路. It was founded under Northern Song 宋, in 1041. The seat of administration was in present-day Ping liang 平涼 city in Gan su 甘肅. Its administrative area corresponded in present-day Gan su to an area extending from the Pu he 蒲河 river to the west, from the Hu lu 葫蘆 river to the East, from Zhang jia chuan 張家川 county toward the North, and included in Ning xia 寧夏 the areas of Gu yuan 固原, Long de 隆德, Jing yuan 涇源 and Xi ji 西吉. The *lu* was abolished by Jin 金, in 1142. Mentioned with 188.

Jing zhao 京兆 [3]
Name of a commandery. It was established by Three Kingdoms' Wei 魏. The seat of administration was at a point lying within the ruins of Han 漢 dynasty Chang an 長安, 13 *li* northwest of present-day Xi an 西安 city in Shaan xi 陝西. The administrative territory of the commandery comprised an area extending from the Qin ling 秦嶺 mountain range in present-day Shaan xi toward the North, from Xi an city toward the East, and from Hua 華 county toward the West, and included the counties of San yuan 三原, Jing yang 涇陽, and Gao ling 高陵. Northern Wei 魏 moved the seat of administration to the vicinity of the present-day Xin zhu 新筑 town located northeast of Xi an city. Northern Zhou 周, in 558, again moved the seat of administration to a point 13 *li* northwest of present-day Xi an city in Shaan xi. Sui 隋, in 583, changed the commandery and established Yong zhou 雍州 but, in 607, again established Jing zhao commandery administered in present-day Xi an city. The administrative area was expanded in the north to include Yi jun 宜君 county. In 618, under Tang 唐, the area again became Yong zhou but, in 690, again became Jing zhao commandery, and sequently again Yong zhou. Mentioned with 204, 631.

Jing zhou 景州 [1]
Name of a *zhou* 州. It was established under Tang 唐, in 786. The seat of administration was at a point northeast of present-day Fu cheng 阜城 county in He bei 河北. The territory administered comprised an area corresponding to present-day Fu cheng and Dong guang 東光 county in He bei. In 821, it was eliminated, but reestablished the next year. In 830, it was eliminated again, but reestablished in 892. During Five Dynasties' Liang 梁, it was administered from present-day Jing xian 景縣 in He bei. In 955, during Later Zhou 周, it was eliminated but reestablished, at the beginning of the Jin 金 dynasty, and administered, as before, from Fu cheng county. Its administrative area comprised the counties of Dong guang, Fu cheng, Jing xian and Wu qiao 吳橋 in He bei, and De zhou 德州 city and Ning jin 寧津 county in Shan dong 山東. Later, during the *da an* 大安 reign period (1209 – 1211), the area was changed to Guan zhou 觀州. Under

the Yuan 元, in 1265, the *zhou* again became Jing zhou, and the seat of administration was moved to present-day Jing xian county in He bei. In 1913, the *zhou* became Jing xian county. Mentioned with 1224.

Jing zhou 涇州 [3]

Name of a *zhou* 州. It was established under Northern Wei 魏, in 430. The seat of administration was at a point southeast of present-day Zhen yuan 鎮原 county in Gan su 甘肅. The seat of administration was later moved to a point 5 *li* north of Jing chuan 涇川 county in Gan su. The territory administered comprised the counties of Jing chuan, Chong xin 崇信, Ping liang 平涼, Hua ting 華亭 and Ling tai 靈臺 in Gan su, and the cities and counties of Bin xian 彬縣, Xun yi 旬邑 and Yong shou 永壽 in Shaan xi 陝西, and Jing yuan 涇源 in Ning xia 寧夏. The *zhou* was abolished at the beginning of the *kai huang* 開皇 reign period (581 – 600) of Sui 隋, but it was periodically reestablished during the reign period *da ye* 大業 (605 – 615), and, under Tang 唐, during the reign periods *tian bao* 天寶 (742 – 756) and *zhi de* 至德 (756 – 758). Under the Ming 明, in 1370, the administration was moved to present-day Jing chuan county. In 1913, the area was demoted to Jing xian 涇縣 county. Mentioned with 462, 907, 1449.

Jing zhou 荊州 [23 + 4 + 2]

□ Name of a *zhou* 州. [23] It was established under Western Han 漢, in 106 BCE, and was one of the 13 Regional Inspector Divisions, *shi san ci shi bu* 十三刺史部. Its administrative area was the equivalent of the two provinces of present-day Hu bei 湖北 and Hu nan 湖南, and portions of He nan 河南, Gui zhou 貴州, Guang xi 廣西 and Guang dong 廣東. Under Eastern Han, it was administered from a point northeast of present-day Chang de 常德 city in Hu nan. In 190, the seat of administration was moved to the Xiang zhou 襄州 district on the southern bank of the Han shui 漢水 at present-day Xiang yang 襄陽 city in Hu bei. During Eastern Jin 晉, the seat of administration was in the present-day Jing zhou district at Jing zhou city in Hu bei. At the beginning of Sui 隋, the *zhou* was eliminated but reestablished, in 621, under Tang 唐. In 742, the *zhou* was changed to Jiang ling 江陵 commandery. In 758, it again became Jing zhou, but its territories were reduced. They corresponded to the northern part of the Yang zi watershed from Song zi 松滋 to Shi shou 石首. They also included present-day Jing zhou and Dang yang 當陽. In 760, the area became Jiang ling fu 江陵府. Mentioned with 28, 78, 148, 221, 328, 375, 381, 562, 572, 578, 828, 994, 1000, 1020, 1034, 1051, 1147, 1176, 1435, 1545, 1561.

□ One of the ancient nine *zhou* of China. [4] Reference is to the region of Hu bei and Hu nan south of Jing shan 荊山 mountain, this is in present-day Nan zhang 南漳 county in Hu bei. Mentioned with 42, 462, 1041, 1418.

□ Name of a *fu* 府. [2] It was established under the Yuan 元, in 1364. The seat of administration was in the former Jiang ling xian 江陵縣 city in the present-day Jing zhou district of Jing zhou city in Hu bei. During the Ming 明, in 1376, its administrative territory more or less comprised an area extending from the present-day Ba dong 巴東 and Chang yang 長陽 county toward the East, and from Jian li 監利 county toward the West, as well as from the counties and cities of

Yuan an 遠安, Zhi jiang 枝江 and Jing zhou toward the South in Hu bei. It was abolished in 1912. Mentioned with 323, 768.

Jiu he 九河 [1]

Common popular designation for China's river system in ancient times. The term refers to the water flow system of the Yellow River through the He bei 河北 plain with most of the rivers involved flowing into the sea. The reference is not specific to any given "nine rivers."

Jiu hua 九華 [1]

Name of a mountain. This is the Jiu hua mountain located 40 *li* southwest of present-day Qing yang 青陽 county in An hui 安徽. Mentioned with 768.

Jiu jiang 九江 [1 + 3]

□ Name of a *fu* 府. [1] It was established, by the Ming 明 rebels under Zhu Yuan-zhang 朱元璋 (1328 – 1398), in 1361. The seat of administration was in present-day Jiu jiang 九江 city in Jiang xi 江西. The territory administered comprised the area of the present-day cities and counties of Jiu jiang, De an 德安, Hu kou 湖口, Rui chang 瑞昌 and Peng ze 彭澤, in Jiang xi 江西. It was abolished in 1912. □ Name of commandery. [3] It was established by Qin 秦. The seat of administration was in present-day Shou xian 壽縣 county in An hui 安徽. The territory administered comprised an area from the Huai he 淮河 river in present-day An hui and He nan 河南 toward the south, from Huang gang 黃岡 in Hu bei 湖北 toward the East, and the whole province of Jiang xi 江西. During Western Han 漢, in 203 BCE, the area became the Huai nan 淮南 kingdom, but was later restored as Jiu jiang commandery. Its jurisdiction comprised the area in present-day An hui south of the Huai he 淮河 river, and from Wa bu 瓦埠 lake toward the East, as well as from Chao hu 巢湖 lake to the North. At the beginning of Three Kingdoms' Wei 魏, in 221, the area was changed to be Huai nan country again. Mentioned with 672, 673, 823.

Jiu keng 鳩坑 [1]

Name of a mountain. It is located on the boundary of present-day Chun an 淳安 county in Zhe jiang 浙江. Mentioned with 768.

Jiu ling 鷲嶺 [1]

Name of a range of mountains. They are located in the central part of India and are a land of Buddhist legend. Mentioned with 1420.

Jiu quan 酒泉 [1]

Name of a commandery. It was established under Western Han 漢, in 121 BCE. The seat of administration was in present-day Jiu quan 酒泉 city in Gan su 甘肅. The territory administered comprised the area from the Shu le 疏勒 river toward the East, and from Gao tai 高台 county to the West, in present-day Gan su. The commandery was eliminated under Northern Wei 魏 during the reign of Emperor Tai wu 太武 (408 – 452), but reestablished later, during the *xiao chang* 孝昌 reign period (525 – 528). It was eliminated under Sui 隋, in 583, but reestablished under Tang 唐, in 742. In 758, it became Su zhou 肅州. Mentioned with 1335.

Jiu xian shan 九仙山 [1]

Name of a mountain, located 30 *li* southeast of present-day Wu lian 五蓮 county in Shan dong 山東. Mentioned with 1424.

Jiu yi shan 九疑山 [1]

Name of a mountain located 60 *li* south of present-day Ning yuan 寧遠 county in Hu nan 湖南. Mentioned with 1414.

Jiu yuan 九原 [1]

Name of a commandery. It was established by Qin 秦, in 214 BCE. The seat of administration was in the ancient city at present-day San ding zhang fang 三頂帳房 village of Hei liu zi xiang 黑柳子鄉 located southeast of the Urad Front Banner, Wu la te qian qi 烏拉特前旗, in the Inner Mongolian Autonomous Region. One tradition places it west of Bao tou 包頭 city, with the territory administered having comprised the area reaching from the lower section of the Great Bend of the Yellow River, Hou tao 後套, toward the East up to Bao tou 包頭 city, and the northern part of Yi ke zhao meng qi 伊克昭盟 Banner, in Inner Mongolia, on the southern banks of the Yellow River. Here the old place names are used. Mentioned with 361.

Jiu zhen 九真 [16 + 1]

□ Name of a commandery. [16] It was established at the beginning of Western Han 漢 and in 111 BCE it was taken over fully by the Han. The seat of administration was in present-day Thanh Hóa 清化 province in Vietnam, in 楊舍 Dương xá Village in Đông Sơn 東山 county. The territory administered comprised the area of Thanh Hóa province, Nghe an 義安 province, and the eastern portion of Thành phố 河靜 province. During the Three Kingdoms period and thereafter the administrative area of the commandery was gradually reduced. Under Liu Song 劉宋 of the Southern Dynasties, the seat of administration was moved to a place on the southern bank of the Sông Mã river (Ma jiang 馬江) north of Thanh Hóa. Sui 隋 moved the seat to Thanh Hóa city. The commandery was eliminated at the beginning of the Tang 唐 dynasty but, in 742, it was reestablished. In 758, the commandery was changed to Ai zhou 愛州. Mentioned with 22, 136, 252, 300, 381, 405, 489, 534, 759, 963, 1087, 1123, 1506, 1515.

□ Name of a *zhou* 州. [1] It was established under Ming 明, in 1407. The seat of administration was in present-day Tĩnh Gia 靖嘉 county in the southeast portion of Vietnam's Thanh Hóa province. The territory administered comprised the southern portion of Thanh Hóa province in central Vietnam. In 1427, the *zhou* was abolished and abandoned and the territory went over to Annam. Mentioned with 1264.

Jiu zhou 九州 [6 + 1 + 1]

□ General regional name. [6] This is a traditional way of referring to all of China. Mentioned with 10, 1551, 1538, 1559.

□ Term used by the BCGM authors in reference to the Nine *Zhou* 州 of the "Tribute of Yu 貢" section of the Book of History, *Shang shu* 尚書. [1] The nine *zhou* are Ji 冀, Yan 兖, Qing 青, Xu 徐, Yang 揚, Yu 豫, Jing 荊, Liang 梁 and Yong 雍.

□ These are Nine *Zhou* of the *Zhi fang* 職方 section of the *Zhou li* 周禮. [1] They are You 幽, Ji, Yan, Qing, Bing 并, Yang, Yu, Jing and Yong.

Ju jia cun 劇家村 [1]
Minor place name. It is located within the borders of present-day Shen zhou 深州 city in He bei 河北. Mentioned with 544.

Ju ku zhou 聚窟州 [1]
Legendary place name. Details are lacking. Mentioned with 282.

Ju lu 鉅鹿 [1]
Name of a commandery. It was founded by Qin 秦, in 222 BCE. The seat of administration was in present-day Ping xiang 平鄉 town in Ping xiang county in He bei 河北. The territory administered comprised an area extending in present-day He bei from Bai yang dian 白洋淀 and Wen an wa 文安洼 toward the South, from the Nan yun he 南運河 toward the West, from Gao yang 高陽, Bai xiang 柏鄉, Ning jin 寧晉 and Ren xian 任縣 county toward the East, and from Ping xiang and, in Shan dong 山東, Lin qing 臨清 to the North. Eastern Han 漢 moved the seat of administration to a place southeast of the present Ning jin county. Jin 晉 changed the commandery to Ju lu 巨鹿 country. Mentioned with 631.

Ju luo shan 拘羅山 [1]
Name of a mountain. It is located in present-day Qi ting 岐亭 town in Ma cheng 麻城 city in Hu bei 湖北. Mentioned with 210.

Ju qing shan 句青山 [1]
This is the name of a mountain. Further details are unavailable. Mentioned with 1014.

Ju qu shan 句曲山 [1]
Name of a mountain. This is Mao shan 茅山 mountain located in the southwestern portion of Jiang su 江蘇.

Ju yan 舉巖 [1]
Name of a mountain. It is located on the borders of present-day Jin hua 金華 city in Zhe jiang 浙江. Mentioned with 768.

Ju ye 鉅野 [1]
Name of a county. It was established by Western Han 漢. The seat of administration was at a point northeast of present-day Ju ye 巨野 county in Shan dong 山東. Liu Song 劉宋 of the Southern Dynasties moved the seat of administration to a point one *li* south of present-day Ju ye county. Northern Qi 齊 eliminated the county. It was reestablished, in 596, under Sui 隋 but eliminated under the Jin 金, in 1150. It was reestablished under Yuan 元, in 1269, and the seat of administration moved to the present Ju ye county. Mentioned with 631.

Juan shan 卷山 [2]
Name of a mountain. Details are lacking. Mentioned with 35, 474.

Juan xian 卷縣 [1]
Name of a county. It was established under Western Han 漢. The seat of administration was in present-day Juan cheng 圈城 to the west of Yuan yang 原陽 county in He nan 河南. The county was eliminated under Northern Wei 魏, in 447, but revived later, in 487. Northern Qi 齊 eliminated it. Mentioned with 474.

Jue shui 決水 [2]
Place name from the *Shan hai jing* 山海經, "Classic of Mountains and Seas." Details are unavailable. Mentioned with 825, 932.

Jun 均 [3]
Name of a *zhou* 州. See → Jun zhou 均州. Mentioned with 328, 503, 654.

Jun shan 君山 [1]
Name of a mountain. This is Tong guan 銅官 mountain, located 20 *li* southwest of present-day Yi xing 宜興 city in Jiang su 江蘇. 805.

Jun shui 均水 [1]
Name of a river. The upper reaches are called the Xi shui 淅水. It emerges in He nan 河南, in Lu shi 盧氏 county, from where the river flows south through the West of Xi xia 西峽 county. When the river reaches a point south of Xi chuan 淅川 county, it combines with the Dan shui 丹水 to become the Jun shui 均水. At Dan jiang kou 丹江口 city in Hu bei 湖北, it enters the Han shui 漢水. Mentioned with 204.

Jun zhou 筠州 [9]
Name of a *zhou* 州. It was established under Tang 唐, in 624. The seat of administration was in present-day Gao an 高安 county in Jiang xi 江西. It was eliminated the following year but reestablished, in 952, under Southern Tang. The territory administered comprised the cities and counties of Gao an, Yi feng 宜豐, Shang gao 上高, Wan zai 萬載, and Zhang shu 樟樹 in Jiang xi. During Northern Song 宋, it was reduced in size and only corresponded to the lands of the present-day counties of Gao an, Shang gao and Yi feng. In 1225, under Southern Song, it became Rui zhou 瑞州. Mentioned with 304, 405, 513, 568, 874, 1053, 1077, 1279, 1281.

Jun zhou 均州 [7]
Name of a *zhou* 州. It was established under Sui 隋, in 585. The seat of administration was in the North of Bei guan yan 北關岩, located northwest of present-day Dan jiang kou 丹江口 city in Hu bei 湖北. At the beginning of the *da ye* 大業 reign period (605 – 618), the *zhou* was abolished. It was reestablished under Tang 唐. In 659, the seat of administration was moved to the old Jun xian 均縣 city east of present-day Guan men yan 關門岩, located northwest of Dan jiang kou city in Hu bei. Its administrative area corresponded to the two present-day cities of Dan jiang kou and Shih yan 十堰, as well as Yun xian 鄖縣 county, all in Hu bei. In 1912, the *zhou* became Jun county. Mentioned with 131, 570, 622, 653, 921, 1147, 1217.

-K-

Kai ming shan 開明山 [1]

This is a mountain name from the *Shan hai jing* 山海經, "Classic of Mountains and Seas." Details are lacking. Mentioned with 895.

Kai yuan si 開元寺 [1]

Name of a temple. It is located in present-day Zhen jiang 鎮江 city in Jiang su 江蘇. Mentioned with 361.

Kai zhou 開州 [3]

Name of a *zhou* 州. It was founded under 唐, in 618, by changing Wan zhou 萬州 to Kai zhou. Its seat of administration was in Kai xian 開縣 county in present-day Chong qing 重慶 municipality. In 742, it was changed to be Sheng shan 盛山 commandery but, in 758, again become Kai zhou. The territory administered comprised the area of the present-day Kai xian county. In 1373, the area was reduced to be Kai xian county. Mentioned with 145, 524.

Kang qian he 康乾河 [1]

Name of a river in the western regions. The location is uncertain. Mentioned with 493.

Kang guo 康國 [2]

Name of ancient country in the western regions of Han 漢 and Tang 唐 times with a capital at A lu di 阿祿迪 city, located 7 *li* north of present-day Samarkand in Uzbekistan. The then royal family was called Wen 溫, and was of Rou zhi 月氏 (Tokharian Indo-European) extraction. They formerly resided in Zhao wu cheng 昭武城, north of Qi lian shan 祁連山 mountain in northeast Qing hai 青海 province. The Rou zhi were forced to move by the Xiong nu 匈奴, and thus came to settle further west in the Pamir high plateau. Later, an original Kang kingdom broke up into a number of smaller kingdoms, all of them retaining Zhao wu as family name. Mentioned with 310, 1196.

Kang zhou 康州 [4]

Name of a *zhou* 州. It was founded under Tang 唐, in 621. Its seat of administration was in the present-day De qing 德慶 county in Guang dong 廣東. The territory administered encompassed the present-day cities and counties of De qing, Yu nan 郁南 and Yun fu 雲浮 in Guang dong. The *zhou* was eliminated in 626, but again established in 638. Under Southern Song 宋, in 1131, the *zhou* was changed to De qing fu 德慶府. Mentioned with 26, 141, 428, 1051.

Ke shan 騍山 [1]

Name of a mountain from the *Shan hai jing* 山海經, "Classic of Mountains and Seas." Further details are lacking. Mentioned with 73.

Kuang lu 匡廬 [2]

This is Lu shan 廬山 mountain. It is located in the northern portion of present-day Jiang xi 江西. It towers over Po yang 鄱陽 lake on the bank of the Yang zi. The name is connected with a story supposedly going back to Yin 殷 and

Zhou 周 times, when Kuang Su 匡俗 and his brothers, altogether seven persons, retired there to cultivate the DAO and built a cottage on the mountain. Mentioned with 859, 1499.

Kuang shui 狂水 [1]
Name of a river from the *Shan hai jing* 山海經, "Classic of Mountains and Seas." It was located somewhere in the southern part of He nan 河南. Mentioned with 81.

Kuai ji 會稽 [13 + 2 + 1]
□ Name of a commandery. [13] It was established in 222 BCE. Its seat of administration was in the present-day Su zhou 蘇州 city in the province of Jiang su 江蘇. The territory administered comprised the area south of the Yang zi in present-day Jiang su, and an area extending from present-day Shang hai 上海 city, Tian tai 天台 mountain in Zhe jiang 浙江, Da pan 大盤 mountain and the Xian xia ling 仙霞嶺 mountain range toward the North, as well as a portion of present-day southern An hui 安徽 province. During Western Han 漢, the commandery was extended toward the South into the two provinces of Zhe jiang and Fu jian 福建. In 129, under Eastern Han, the seat of administration was moved to present-day Shao xing 紹興 city in Zhe jiang. In 589, under Sui 隋, the commandery was eliminated. It was reestablished in 607. Under Tang 唐, in 621, it became Yue zhou 越州. In 742, the *zhou* 州 was changed to be Kuai ji commandery again. Its jurisdiction was reduced and comprised the basins of the Pu yang jiang 浦陽江 (other than Pu yang 浦陽 county), the Yong jiang 甬江 and the Cao e jiang 曹娥江 in Zhe jiang. In 758, it was changed again to be Yue zhou. Mentioned with 80, 261, 344, 362, 381, 394, 635, 641, 768, 1134, 1521.
□ Name of a county. [2] It was established by Chen 陳 of the Southern Dynasties. The seat of administration was in present-day Shao xing 紹興 city in Zhe jiang 浙江 and abolished in 1913. Mentioned with 1324, 1342.
□ Name of a mountain. [1] It is located south of present-day Shao xing 紹興 city in Zhe jiang 浙江. Mentioned with 1438.

Kui 夔
See → 夔州. Mentioned with 58, 456, 468, 730.

Kui chuan 夔川 [1]
This is an alternative name for Kui zhou 夔州. See → Kui zhou. Mentioned with 585.

Kui lu 夔路 [1]
This is an abbreviation for Kui zhou lu 夔州路. It was established under Northern Song 宋, in 1001. The seat of administration was in present-day Feng jie 奉節 county in the Chong qing 重慶 municipality. The territory administered reached, in present-day Si chuan 四川, from Wan yuan 萬源, Da chuan 達川 and He jiang 合江, and from Dian jiang 墊江 and Bi shan 璧山 county in Chong qing toward the West, and in Hu bei 湖北 from Jian shi 建始 and He feng 鶴峰 toward the West, and also included parts of Gui zhou 貴州. The *lu* 路 was abolished at the beginning of Yuan 元. Mentioned with 389.

Kui zhou 夔州 [6 + 2]

□ Name of a *zhou* 州. [6] Kui zhou was founded under Tang 唐, in 619. Its seat of administration was in Bai di 白帝 city, located 10 *li* east of present-day Feng jie 奉節 county in the Chong qing 重慶 municipality. The territory administered comprised the counties of Feng jie, Wu xi 巫溪, Wu shan 巫山 and Yun yang 雲陽, in the present-day Chong qing municipality. In 742, the area became Yun an 雲安 commandery but, in 758, again Kui zhou. Under Northern Song 宋, the administrative area of the *zhou* was reduced. In 1006, the seat of administration was moved to the present-day Feng jie county. In 1278, under Yuan 元, the area became Kui zhou lu 夔州路. Mentioned with 58, 468, 730.

□ Kui zhou is the name of a *fu* 府. [2] It was established, in 1371, by changing the name of Kui zhou lu 夔州路. Its seat of administration was in present-day Feng jie 奉節 county in the Chong qing 奉節 municipality. The administrative area comprised the northeastern section of the present-day Chong qing municipality and a corner of Hu bei 湖北. In 1376, Kui zhou was reduced to being a subordinate *fu* to Chong qing. In 1380, the area was raised again to being Kui zhou fu 夔州府. In 1913, the *fu* was abolished. Mentioned with 768, 1096.

Kun lun 昆崙 [17]

Name of an ancient country. During Tang 唐 and Song 宋 times, the name referred to the Indo-China peninsula and Southern Asia. There are, in fact, a number of Kun lun countries located in that region and referred to in classic Chinese sources. The name is a stand-in for southeast Asia and nearby areas. Mentioned with 14, 94, 98, 226, 288, 333, 799, 845, 886, 935, 1123, 1124, 1205, 1272, 1399, 1406, 1515, 1532.

Kun lun guo 崑崙國 [4]

Name of an ancient country. See → Kun lun 昆崙. Mentioned with 14, 226, 386, 1030.

Kun lun pan pan guo 崑崙盤盤國 [1]

Name of an old country, It was located on the east coast of Bandon Bay in South Thailand and was powerful enough to long carry on independent and harmonious relations with China from Liu Song 劉宋 times (420 – 479) on to the beginning of the Tang 唐 dynasty. Mentioned with 1139.

Kun lun shan 崑崙山 [2]

Name of a mountain from the *Shan hai jing* 山海經, "Classic of Mountains and Seas." Further details are lacking. Mentioned with 895.

Kun lun xu 崑崙墟 [1]

Name of mountains. This refers to the Kun lun 崑崙 range in present-day Xin jiang 新疆 and the Qaraqorum range. Mentioned with 895.

Kun ming chi 昆明池 [1]

Name of a lake and marsh land located between the Feng shui 豐水 and Jue shui 潏水, west of the present-day Chang an 長安 district of Xi an 西安 city in Shaan xi 陝西. This is the low-lying land southeast of Dou men 斗門 town. Mentioned with 562.

Kun shan 崑山 [3]
Name of mountains. This refers to the Kun lun 崑崙 range in Xin jiang 新疆.

Kun wu shan 昆吾山 [1]
Name of a mountain. Details are lacking. Mentioned with 517.

Kuo 括 [2]
Name of a *zhou* 州. It was established under Sui 隋, in 592, by changing the name of Chu zhou 處州. Its seat of administration was in Gu cheng 古城 village, located 7 *li* southeast of present-day Li shui 麗水 city in Zhe jiang 浙江. The territory administered comprised the watersheds of the Ling jiang 靈江, Ou jiang 甌江 and Fei yun jiang 飛雲江, south of the line formed by the Tian tai 天台 and Xian du 仙都 mountains. Under Tang 唐, in 779, the area became Chu zhou again. Mentioned with 278, 1248.

Kuo cang 括蒼 [3]
Alternative name of a place. Reference is to Chu zhou 處州 because it has a Kuo cang mountain on its borders. This is the present Li shui 麗水 city in Zhe jiang 浙江. Mentioned with 1277, 1535, 1560.

Kuo zhou 廓州 [1]
Name of a *zhou* 州. It was established under Northern Zhou 周, in 576. Its seat of administration was at a location south of present-day Gui de 貴德 county in Qing hai 青海. Under Tang 唐, in 619, the seat of administration was moved to a point on the northern bank of the Yellow River, located 60 *li* west of present-day Hua long 化隆 county in Qing hai. The territory administered comprised the present-day counties of Hua long and Jian zha 尖扎 in Qing hai. The *zhou* was abolished under Northern Song 宋, during the *da guan* 大觀 reign period (1107 – 1110). Mentioned with 1335.

-L-

Lai 萊 [7 + 1]
□ Name of a *zhou* 州. [7] See → Lai zhou 萊州. Mentioned with 393, 474, 608, 614, 703, 1027.
□ Name of a city. [1] This is located southeast of present-day Chang yi 昌邑 city in Shan dong 山東. Mentioned with 1330.

Lai zhou 萊州 [8]
Name of a *zhou* 州. The *zhou* was founded under the Sui 隋, in 585. Its seat of administration was in the present-day Lai zhou city in Shan dong 山東. The territory administered comprised the present-day cities and counties of Lai zhou, Lai yang 萊陽, Ji mo 即墨, Ping du 平度, Lai xi 萊西 and Hai yang 海陽 in Shan dong. At the beginning of the reign period *da ye* 大業 (605 – 615) of the Sui 隋, and during the reign periods *tian bao* 天寶 (742 – 756) and *zhi de* 至德 (756 – 758) of Tang 唐, it periodically became Dong lai 東萊 commandery. Under the Ming

明, in 1376, its status was raised to Lai zhou fu 萊州府. Mentioned with 412, 606, 819, 1027, 1205, 1223.

Lan cang 瀾滄 [1]

Name of a region. It was located in the western part of what is now Yun nan 雲南. Today, this is the watershed of the Lan cang jiang 瀾滄江 river. Mentioned with 896.

Lan ling 蘭陵 [2 + 2]

□ Name of a county. [2] It was established during Warring States times by Chu 楚. Its seat of administration was in Lan ling 蘭陵 town, located 45 *li* southwest of the present-day Cang shan 蒼山 county. The county was eliminated under Northern Qi 齊, but again established under Sui 隋, in 596. In 606, it was again eliminated, but Cheng 丞 county was renamed Lan ling county. Its seat of administration was in present-day Yi cheng 嶧城 town, located southeast of Zao zhuang 棗莊 city in Shan dong 山東. In 621, Lan ling county administered from Yi cheng town was eliminated, and the Lan ling county administered at present-day Lan ling town was established in its place. In 627, it was eliminated again. In 1195, under the Jin 金, Cheng county was changed to become Lan ling county again, administered in the present Yi cheng town. In 1336, it was eliminated. Mentioned with 566.

□ Name of a commandery. [2] It was established, in 291, under Western Jin 晉. Its seat of administration was at a location 1 *li* northwest of present-day Yi cheng 嶧城 town of Zao zhuang 棗莊 city in Shan dong 山東. The territory administered comprised the present Zao zhuang city, the eastern and southeastern part of Teng zhou 滕州 city, and the southwestern part of Cang shan 蒼山 county in Shan dong. During Liu Song 劉宋, the seat of administration was moved to a point 60 *li* southeast of Teng zhou city in Shan dong. During Eastern Wei 魏, in 547, the seat of administration was again moved to a point 1 *li* northwest of Yi cheng town of Zao zhuang city in Shan dong. It was abolished under Sui 隋, in 583. Mentioned with 272, 1417.

Lan tian 藍田 [13]

Name of a county. It was established, in 379 BCE, under the Warring States kingdom of Qin 秦. Its seat of administration was at a location 30 *li* west of present-day Lan tian county in Shaan xi 陕西. It was eliminated under Northern Wei 魏, in 446, but reestablished in 487. In 573, under Northern Zhou 周, the seat of administration was moved to the present Lan tian county. Mentioned with 62, 88, 902, 908, 1254, 1406, 1486.

Lan ting 蘭亭 [1]

Minor place name. This is located below Lan zhu 蘭渚 mountain, 27 *li* southwest of Shao xing 紹興 county in Zhe jiang 浙江. Mentioned with 785.

Lan xian 蘭縣 [1]

Name of a county. It was established under Ming 明, in 1369, by changing the name of Lan zhou 蘭州. Its seat of administration was in the present-day Lan zhou city in Gan su 甘肅. In 1477, the status of the area was promoted to Lan zhou. Mentioned with 811.

Lan zhou 蘭州 [2]

Name of a *zhou* 州. It was established under Sui 隋, in 581. Its seat of administration was in the present Lan zhou 蘭州 city in Gan su 甘肅. The territory administered comprised the city of Lan zhou and the county of Lin tao 臨洮. Later it was changed to be Jin cheng 金城 commandery, but under Tang 唐, in 619, it again became Lan zhou. Its administration was reduced to the areas near present-day Lan zhou city. In 763, the area was lost to the Tibetans. In 1081, under Northern Song 宋, it was reconquered. In 1104, Lan quan 蘭泉 county was established to be the seat of administration of the *zhou*. In 1369, the area was demoted to become Lan xian 蘭縣 county. In 1477, it again became Lan zhou. In 1666, it was administered by the Gan su Provincial Administration Commission, Gan su *bu zheng shi si* 甘肅布政使司. In 1738, it became Lan zhou fu 蘭州府. Mentioned with 361, 595.

Lang 朗 [1]

Name of a *zhou* 州. See Lang zhou 朗州. Mentioned with 1063.

Lang ling 朗陵 [3]

Name of a county. It was established under Western Han 漢. Its seat of administration was in Ren dian 任店, located 35 *li* southwest of Que shan 確山 county in present-day He nan 河南. At the end of Liu Song 劉宋, the county was abolished. Mentioned with 322, 1253.

Lang ya 琅邪 [1]

This is the same as Lang ya 琅琊. See → Lang ya 琅琊. Mentioned with 667.

Lang ya 琅琊 [9]

Name of a commandery. It was established by Qin 秦. Its seat of administration was in Lang ya town located southwest of present-day Jiao nan 膠南 city in Shan dong 山東. Western Han 漢 moved the seat of administration to Zhu cheng 諸城 city in Shan dong. The territory administered comprised the cities of Qing dao 青島, Jiao zhou 膠州, Jiao nan 膠南, Ji mo 即墨, Zhu cheng and Ri zhao 日照, as well as the counties of Yi shui 沂水, Wu lian 五蓮, Hai yang 海陽, Ju nan 莒南 also in Shang dong, and Gan yu 贛榆 county in Jiang su 江蘇. During Eastern Han, in 80, the area became Lang ya country/domain, and the seat of administration was moved to a point north of present-day Lin yi 臨沂 city in Shan dong. The southwestern part of its administration was expanded, but during the Three Kingdoms period it was reduced. After Eastern Jin 晉, the area became a commandery. Under Northern Wei 魏, the seat of administration was moved to a point 20 *li* west of Lin yi city in Shan dong. The area was eliminated under Sui 隋, during the *kai huang* 開皇 reign period (581 – 600), but later, at the beginning of the *da ye* 大業 reign period (605 – 618), it was reestablished as Lang ya commandery. Its seat of administration was in Lin yi city in Shang dong. At the beginning of Tang 唐, the area became Yi zhou 沂州 and, in 742, it was changed to Lang ya commandery. It was abolished in 758. Mentioned with 272, 356, 538, 908, 975, 1344, 1430.

Lang zhong 閬中 [2]

Name of a county. It was established by Warring States Qin 秦. Its seat of administration was in present-day Lang zhong city in Si chuan 四川. During the Sui 隋, at the beginning of the *kai huang* 開皇 reign period (581 – 600), the area became Lang nei 閬內 county. In 618, under Tang, it became Lang zhong county again. In 1991, it became Lang zhong city. Mentioned with 1096.

Lang zhou 閬州 [1]

Name of a *zhou* 州. It was created in 713 in response to a taboo avoidance of the name of Tang 唐 emperor Xuan zong 玄宗, Li Longji 李隆基, when the Long 隆 of Long zhou 隆州 was changed to Lang zhou. Its seat of administration was at Lang zhong 閬中 city in Si chuan 四川. The territory administered comprised the cities and counties of Lang zhou, Nan bu 南部 and Cang xi 蒼溪 in Si chuan. In 742, the area became Lang zhong commandery but, in 758, again became Lang zhou. Under Southern Song 宋, in 1243, the seat of administration was moved to Wang du xiang 王渡鄉, located southeast of Cang xi 蒼溪 county in Si chuan. Under Yuan 元, in 1276, it became Bao ning fu 保寧府. Mentioned with 869.

Lang zhou 朗州 [1]

Name of a *zhou* 州. It was founded under Sui 隋, in 596. Its seat of administration was in present-day Chang de 常德 city in Hu nan 湖南. The territory administered comprised Chang de city and the two present-day counties of Han shou 漢壽 and Tao yuan 桃源 in Hu nan. At the beginning of the reign period *da ye* 大業 (605 – 615) of the Sui 隋, and during the reign periods *tian bao* 天寶 (742 – 756) and *zhi de* 至德 (756 – 758) of Tang 唐, the area several times became Wu ling 武陵 commandery. Under Northern Song 宋, in 1012, the area became Ding zhou 鼎州. Mentioned with 780.

Lao 佬 [1]

This term refers to the area in which the Lao ethnic group lives. In general, this is a region of Hu nan 湖南 and Gui zhou 貴州. Mentioned with 1242.

Lao shan 牢山 [2]

Name of a mountain. This is Lao shan 勞山 mountain or Lao shan 嶗山 mountain. It is located northeast of the present-day Lao shan 嶗山 district of Qing dao 青島 city in Shan dong 山東. Mentioned with 880, 1523.

Lao shan 勞山 [2]

Name of a mountain. The name is also written Lao shan 牢山 and Lao shan 嶗山. It is located northeast of the present-day Lao shan 嶗山 district of Qing dao 青島 city in Shan dong 山東. Mentioned with 425, 1155, 1573.

Lao shui 澇水 [1]

Name of a river. This is the ancient Liao shui 潦水. It emerges from Lao gu 澇谷 of Niu shou 牛首 mountain, located south of present-day Hu xian 戶縣 county in Shaan xi 陕西, and flows north to a point southwest of Xian yang 咸陽 city where the river enters of the Wei he 渭河 river. Mentioned with 1230.

Lao wo 老撾 [1]
Name of a regional administration. In 1404, the Ming 明 established a Lao wo 老撾 Tribal (i.e., Laos) Pacification Commissioner's Office, Lao wo *jun min xuan wei shi si* 老撾軍民宣慰使司, to be administered from what is today the Lang bo la 琅勃拉 domain in Laos. Its administrative area corresponded to the northern part of present-day Laos. Toward the end of Ming this was abolished. Mentioned with 1236.

Le bi guo 勒畢國 [1]
Legendary Han 漢 era kingdom. Details of its location are lacking. Mentioned with 753.

Le lang 樂浪 [3]
Name of a commandery. It was established under Western Han 漢, in 108 BCE. Its seat of administration was at Tu cheng dong 土城洞 on the south bank of present-day Pyongyang city in Korea or, according to one tradition, in present-day Pyongyang city. The territory administrated corresponded to the area of the present-day provinces of South Pyŏngan, South Hwanghae, North Hwanghae, Kangwon and Hamgyong. Under Western Jin 晉, in 313, the seat of administration was moved to a point southwest of Yi 義 county in present-day Liao ning 遼寧. In 432, under Northern Wei 魏, it was eliminated but reestablished again later, around 525. Its seat of administration was moved to the present Yi county, and the name was changed to Le liang 樂良 commandery. Mentioned with 207, 501, 1330.

Le ping 樂平 [3]
Name of a county. It was established under Tang 唐, in 621. Its seat of administration was in Luo kou 洛口, located east of present-day Le ping city in Jiang xi 江西. In 626, it was eliminated, but reestablished later during the *kai yuan* 開元 reign period (713 – 741). The seat of administration was moved to present-day Le ping city. Under Yuan 元, in 1295, its status was raised to be Le ping zhou 樂平州. Under Ming 明, in 1371, it was again demoted to a county. In 1992, Le ping city was established. Mentioned with 866, 1375.

Le ping jun 樂平郡 [1]
Name of a commandery. It was established at the end of Eastern Han 東. Its seat of administration was at a location southwest of present-day Xi yang 昔陽 county in Shan xi 山西. The territory administered corresponded to the present-day counties of Xi yang, Zuo quan 左權, He shun 和順 and Ping ding 平定 in Shan xi. Under Northern Wei 魏, in 448, it was eliminated, but reestablished in 526, with the seat of administration located in Le ping county. It was abolished under Sui 隋, in 583. Mentioned with 1375.

Le you yuan 樂游苑 [1]
Name of a park in Chang an 長安 established during Western Han 漢 in the spring of 59 BCE. It was located in the area of present-day Tie lu miao 鐵爐廟 village, southeast of Xi an 西安 city in Shaan xi 陝西. Mentioned with 801.

Le zhou 勒州 [1]
This is an error for Qin zhou 勤州. See → Qin zhou.

Lei 雷 [3]
Name of a *zhou*. See → Lei zhou. Mentioned with 144, 596, 1357.

Lei chi 雷池 [1]
Name of a lake. The ancient Lei shui 雷水 flowed from the eastern boundary of present-day Huang mei 黃梅 county in Hu bei 湖北, and passed through present-day Su song 宿松 county in An hui 安徽 to enter the Wang jiang 望江 river at a point southeast of the county. The waters accumulated into a lake and this was known as Lei chi. After Tang 唐, Song 宋 and Yuan 元, the lake diminished in size and broke up into parts, and the name Lei chi was subsequently replaced by different local lake names. Mentioned with 877.

Lei yang 耒陽 [1]
Name of a county. It was established by Qin 秦. Its seat of administration was in present-day Lei yang 耒陽 city in Hu nan 湖南. Sui 隋 changed it to be Lei yin 洡陰 county. In 621, Tang 唐 restored the former name Lei yang county. Under the Yuan 元, in 1282, its status was raised to be Lei yang zhou 耒陽州. Under Ming 明, in 1370, it was again changed to be Lei yang county. In 1986, the county became a county rank city. Mentioned with 1471.

Lei zhou 雷州 [9 + 1]
□ Name of a *zhou* 州. [9] It was founded under Tang 唐, in 634. Its seat of administration was in present-day Lei zhou 雷州 city in Guang dong 廣東. The territory administered comprised the Lei zhou peninsula south of Sui xi 遂溪 and Zhan jiang 湛江. In 742, the area became Hai kang 海康 commandery but, in 758, became Lei zhou again. Under the Yuan 元, in 1278, the status of the *zhou* was raised to be the Lei zhou Pacification Commission, Lei zhou *an fu si* 雷州安撫司. In 1280, Lei zhou lu 雷州路 was established. Mentioned with 405, 627, 844, 925, 995, 1257, 1399, 1425.
□ Name of a *fu* 府. [1] It was established under the Ming 明, in 1368. Its seat of administration was in Lei zhou city in present-day Guang dong. The territory administered corresponded to the present-day cities and counties of Lei zhou, Zhan jiang, Sui xi and Xu wen 徐聞 in Guang dong. The *fu* was abolished in 1912. Mentioned with 627.

Lei ze 雷澤 [3]
Name of an ancient wet land, also called the Lei xia ze 雷夏澤. It was located northeast of present-day He ze 菏澤 in Shan dong 山東. After Song 宋 times, the wet lands dried up. Mentioned with 645, 1083, 1094.

Li 澧 [2]
Name of a *zhou* 州. See → Li zhou 澧州. Mentioned with 348, 1063.

Li 漓 [1]

Name of a river, also written Li shui 離水 and also named Gui jiang 桂江. The river is located in the eastern part of Guang xi 廣西, and is a tributary of the Xi jiang 西江. It has its sources on Mao er 貓兒 mountain in present-day Xing an 興安 county, and flows through the cities and counties of Xing an, Ling chuan 靈川, Gui lin 桂林, Yang shuo 陽朔, Ping le 平樂, Zhao ping 昭平 and Cang wu 蒼梧. The river enters the Xi jiang at Wu zhou 梧州 city. Mentioned with 1503.

Li 利 [1]

Name of a *zhou*. See → Li zhou 利州. Mentioned with 644.

Li cheng 歷城 [1]

Name of a county. It was established by Qin 秦. Its seat of administration was in present-day Ji nan 濟南 city in Shang dong 山東. Western Han 漢 placed the area under Ji nan commandery, and Eastern Han placed it under Ji nan country. Western Jin 晉 put it under Ji nan commandery and later, following the *yong jia* 永嘉 reign period (307-313), it was administered from Ji nan commandery. Under Tang 唐, it was administered from Qi zhou 齊州 and, under Song 宋, it was administered from Ji nan fu 濟南府. Yuan 元 placed it under Ji nan lu 濟南路. Under Ming 明 and Qing 清, it was administered by Ji nan fu. In 1987, this was canceled and the area became Li cheng district under Ji nan city. Mentioned with 510.

Li dong 黎峒 [2]

Name of a mountain occupied by the Li 黎 people. The reference is to the area surrounding Wu zhi 五指 mountain in the middle part of Hai nan 海南 province. Mentioned with 144.

Li guo zhi shui 歷虢之水 [1]

River name mentioned in the *Shan hai jing* 山海經, "Classic of Mountains and Seas." Details are lacking. Mentioned with 1434.

Li jiang 麗江 [1]

Name of a *fu* 府. It was established under Ming 明, in 1382. In 1397, it was changed to a Tribal Office, *jun min fu* 軍民府. Its seat of administration was in present-day Yu long 玉龍 county in Yun nan 雲南. The territory administered comprised an area in the Northwest of present-day Yun nan, extending from the counties of Li jiang, Lan ping 蘭坪 and Fu gong 福貢 toward the North. Under Qing 清, the administrative area was made to comprise in addition the present-day counties of Jian chuan 劍川 and Hao qing 鶴慶. The *fu* was abolished in 1913. Mentioned with 493.

Li mu shan 黎母山 [1]

Name of a mountain range. This is Li mu ling 黎母嶺, north of present-day Qiong zhong 瓊中 county in Hai nan 海南. Mentioned with 144.

Li pu 荔浦 [1]

Name of a county, established under Western Han 漢, and subordinated to Cang wu 蒼梧 commandery. Its seat of administration was at what is now Qing shan xiang 青山鄉, located 40 *li* southwest of Li pu county in Guang xi 廣西. Under

Three Kingdoms' Wu 吳, it was subordinated to Shi an 始安 county. Southern Dynasties Song subordinated it to Shi jian 始建 country. Qi 齊 subordinated it to Shi an 始安 commandery again. During the reign period *da ye* 大業 (605 – 615) of the Sui 隋, and during the reign periods *tian bao* 天寶 (742 – 756) and *zhi de* 至德 (756 – 758) of Tang 唐, it was again part of Shi an commandery. During Northern Song 宋, it was subordinated to Gui zhou 桂州, and under Southern Song to Jing jiang fu 靜江府. Yuan 元 made it part of Jing jiang lu 靜江路, and the administration of the county was moved to a point south of the present-day county. Under Ming 明, it was subordinated to Gui lin fu 桂林府 and, in 1456, administration was transferred to its present-day seat.

Li shan 歷山 [1]
Name of a mountain. This is Lei shou shan 雷首山, located south of present-day Pu zhou 蒲州 town of Yong ji 永濟 city in Shan xi 山西. Mentioned with 391.

Li shan 黎山 [1]
Name of a mountain. It is also called Li yang 山 黎陽 and Da pi 大伾山. It is located two *li* southeast of present-day Xun xian 浚縣 county in He nan 河南. Mentioned with 300.

Li shan 驪山 [2]
Name of a mountain. It is also called Li shan 麗山 or Li rong zhi shan 麗戎之山. It is situated at a point southeast of the Lin tong 臨潼 region of present-day Xi an 西安 in Shaan xi 陝西. Mentioned with 1176, 1228.

Li shui 澧水 [2]
Name of a river. It is located in the northwestern corner of the present Hu nan 湖南 province. Its source comes from a point north of Sang zhi 桑植 county, and the river then flows east to cross the boundaries of the cities and counties of Zhang jia jie 張家界, Ci li 慈利, and Li xian 澧縣. At Xin zhou 新洲 in Li xian it enters Dong ting 洞庭 lake. Mentioned with 1574.

Li xia 歷下 [1]
Name of a city. This is a Qi 齊 city of the Spring and Autumn period. It was located west of present-day Ji nan 濟南 city in Shan dong 山東. Mentioned with 269.

Li xian 酈縣 [1]
Name of a county. It was established by Qin 秦. Its seat of administration was at a location northwest of present-day Nan yang 南陽 city in He nan 河南. During Eastern Han 漢, the seat of administration was moved to Li cheng 酈城 village, located 10 *li* north of present-day Nei xiang 內鄉 county in He nan. Northern Wei 魏 changed Li xian to be Nan li 南酈 county. Northern Zhou 周 restored the name Li county. At the beginning of the *kai huang* 開皇 reign period (581 – 600) of Sui 隋, the area became Ju tan 菊潭 county. Mentioned with 575.

Li yang 歷陽 [7]
Name of a commandery. It was established under Western Jin 晉, in 304. Its seat of administration was in present-day He 和 county in An hui 安徽. The territory administered comprised the area of He county, and Han shan 含山 county

in An hui. Under Liu Song 劉宋, in 421, a Nan yu zhou 南豫州 was established in the commandery. Qi 齊 subordinated it to Yu zhou and, in 484, it was subordinated to Nan yu zhou 南豫州. Northern Qi 齊 established He zhou 和州 at the same time. In 589, the commandery was abolished. During the reign period *da ye* 大業 (605 – 615) of the Sui 隋, and during the reign periods *tian bao* 天寶 (742 – 756) and *zhi de* 至德 (756 – 758) of Tang 唐, He zhou was periodically changed to be Li yang 歷陽 commandery. This was abolished in 758. Mentioned with 199, 222, 771, 1308.

Li zhou 利州 [4]

Name of a *zhou* 州. It was established under Western Wei 魏, in 554. Its seat of administration was in Guang yuan 廣元 city in Si chuan 四川. The territory administered comprised territories of the present-day cities and counties of Guang yuan, Wang cang 旺蒼, and Qing chuan 青川 in Si chuan 四川, and of Ning qiang 寧強 in Shaan xi 陝西. During the reign period *da ye* 大業 (605 – 615) of the Sui 隋, and during the reign periods *tian bao* 天寶 (742 – 756) and *zhi de* 至德 (756 – 758) of Tang 唐, it periodically became a commandery. Under Northern Song 宋, in 1001, the area came under Li zhou lu 利州路. Its territory was reduced. Under Yuan 元, in 1277, the area was changed to Guang yuan lu 廣元路. Mentioned with 547, 767, 866, 1155.

Li zhou 黎州 [1]

Name of a *zhou* 州. The *zhou* was established under Northern Zhou 周, in 568. Its seat of administration was at a location northeast of present-day Han yuan 漢源 county in Si chuan 四川. It was eliminated under Sui 隋 but reestablished under Tang 唐, in 701. Its seat of administration was in present-day Jiu xiang 九襄 town, located north of Han yuan county in Si chuan. It was abolished in 707, but restored in 716. In 742, it was changed to be Hong yuan 洪源 commandery. In 758, it again became Li zhou. Its administration included the counties of Han yuan, Shi jin 石棉, and Gan luo 甘洛, and portions of the counties Lu ding 瀘定, Yue xi 越西, and E bian 峨邊 in present-day Si chuan 四川. During the *zhen yuan* 貞元 reign period (785 – 805), the Han yuan county of the Sui 隋 had its seat of administration moved to Qing xi xiang 清溪鄉 north of the present county. In 1375, under the Ming 明, the area was changed to become the Li zhou Chief's Office, Li zhou *zhang guan si* 黎州長官司." Mentioned with 111.

Li zhou 澧州 [5]

□ Name of a *zhou* 州. [5] It was established in 589. Its seat of administration was at a location southeast of present-day Li xian 澧縣 county in Hu nan 湖南. Tang moved the seat of administration to the present Li xian county. During the reign period *da ye* 大業 (605 – 615) of the Sui 隋, and during the reign periods *tian bao* 天寶 (742 – 756) and *zhi de* 至德 (756 – 758) of Tang 唐, the *zhou* several times became Li yang 澧陽 commandery, and under Yuan 元, in 1277, its status was raised to be Li zhou lu 澧州路. In 1364, Zhu Yuanzhang 朱元璋 (1328 – 1398) changed the area to be Li zhou fu 澧州府. In 1376, it was demoted to be Li zhou. In 1729, its status was raised to be a directly administered *zhou*, *zhi li zhou* 直隸州. In 1913, it was changed to be Li county. Mentioned with 456, 616, 665, 694.

Lian 連 [2]

Name of a *zhou* 州. It was established under Sui 隋, in 590. Its seat of administration was in present-day Lian zhou 連州 city in Guang dong 廣東. The territory administered comprised the present-day cities and counties of Lian zhou, Yang shan 陽山, Lian shan 連山 and Lian nan 連南, in Guang dong. During the *da ye* 大業 (605 – 618) reign period of the Sui, and the *zhi de* 至德 (756 – 758) and *qian yuan* 乾元 (758 – 760) reign periods of the Tang 唐, the area several times was made a commandery. Under Yuan 元, in 1280, the status of the area was raised to be Lian zhou lu 連州路. In 1282, it was again changed to be Lian zhou. Under Ming 明, in 1369, Gui yang zhou 桂陽州 was combined with Lian zhou, but it was later abolished. In 1381, it was reestablished. In 1912, the area was changed to Lian county. Mentioned with 1063.

Lian 廉 [1]

Name of a *zhou* 州. See under Lian zhou 廉州. Mentioned with 909.

Lian shui 廉水 [1]

Minor place name. Located north of present-day Zhang ming 彰明 town and south of Jiang you 江油 city in Si chuan 四川. Mentioned with 322.

Lian zhou 廉州 [1 + 2]

□ Name of a *fu* 府. [1] It was founded under Ming 明, in 1368. Its seat of administration was in present-day He pu 合浦 county in Guang xi 廣西. The territory administered comprised the present-day counties of He pu, Pu bei 浦北 and Ling shan 靈山, and the three cities of Fang cheng gang 防城港, Qin zhou 欽州 and Bei hai 北 in Guang xi 廣西. In 1374, the area was demoted to be Lian zhou but, in 1381, was reestablished as Liang zhou fu 廉州府. It was abolished in 1912.
□ Name of a *zhou* 州. [2] Established under Tang 唐, in 634. Its seat of administration was in Jiu zhou 舊州 village south of present-day Pu bei 浦北 county in Guang xi 廣西. The territory administered comprised the two present-day counties of He pu 合浦 and Pu bei, and the territory of Bei hai 北海 city, in Guang xi. Under Northern Song 宋, in 983, the *zhou* was eliminated but, in 998, it was reestablished, and the seat of administration was moved to the present-day He pu county. Under Yuan 元, in 1280, the area became Lian zhou lu 廉州路. Under the Ming 明, in 1368, this was changed to Lian zhou fu 廉州府. In 1374, the area was demoted to be Lian zhou but again became Lian zhou fu, in 1381. Mentioned with 1467.

Liang 梁 [6 + 1]

□ This is the name of a *zhou* 州. [6] See under → Liang zhou 梁州. Mentioned with 535, 675, 1004, 1202, 1396.
□ One of the feudal domains of Western Zhou 周 times and the Spring and Autumn period. [1] This is present-day Xi shao liang 西少梁, 20 *li* southwest of Han cheng 韓城 city in Shaan xi 陝西. Mentioned with 1174.

Liang 涼 [1]

Name of a *zhou*. See under → Liang zhou 涼州. Mentioned with 239.

Liang chuan 兩川 [1]
Regional name. The name refers to the territories of both the Xi chuan Military Commissioner, Xi chuan *jie du shi* 西川節度使, and the Dong chuan Military Commissioner, Dong chuan *jie du shi* 東川節度使. The area more or less corresponds to present-day Si chuan 四川. Mentioned with 1499.

Liang guang 兩廣 [1]
This is a combined designation for Guang dong 廣東 and Guang xi 廣西, corresponding to the territory of the present-day provinces of Guang dong, Guang xi and Hai nan 海南. Mentioned with 585.

Liang guo 梁國 [1]
Feudal domain. It was established under Western Han 漢, in 202 BCE, with a capital city located northwest of present-day Ding tao 定陶 county in Shan dong 山東. Later, during the reign of Han emperor Wen di 文帝 (202 – 157), the capital was moved to a point south of present-day Shang qiu 商丘 city in He nan. The administrative area of the domain corresponded to the present-day Shang qiu city, with the counties of Yu cheng 虞城, and Min quan 民權 in He nan 河南, as well as Dang shan 碭山 county in An hui 安徽. During early Three Kingdoms Wei 魏, the area became Liang 梁 commandery. During Western Jin 晉, it was made Liang 梁 domain. Liu Song 劉宋 changed this to Liang commandery. Mentioned with 631.

Liang han 梁漢 [3]
Regional name. This is a combined designation for Liang zhou 梁州 and Han zhong 漢中. The area corresponds to the present-day cities and counties of Han zhong, Cheng gu 城固, Nan zheng 南鄭 and Mian xian 勉縣, as well as the northern portion of Ning qiang 寧強 county in Shaan xi. Mentioned with 434, 871, 1461.

Liang huai 兩淮 [1]
Regional designation. At the beginning of Yuan 元, a Salt Distribution Administration of the Liang huai, Liang huai *yan yun si* 兩淮鹽運司, was established in present-day Yang zhou 揚州 city in Jiang su 江蘇. Its production area included all the salt fields of present-day Huai nan 淮南 and Huai bei 淮北 north of the Yang zi in Jiang su. Mentioned with 1057.

Liang jiang 兩江 [1]
Regional name. During Yuan 元 and Ming 明, the watershed of the rivers to the left and to the right of Guang xi 廣西, namely the Yu jiang 郁江 and Qian jiang 黔江 rivers, was called Liang jiang 兩江, "Two Rivers". Since the two rivers had a great deal of precious jade and because they passed the settlements of the Zhuang 僮 nationality, the area was called the "the caves along the streams of two rivers", *liang jiang xi dong* 兩江溪峒. Mentioned with 332.

Liang jing 兩京 [1]
The name, as used by the BCGM authors, refers to the "two (Tang 唐) capitals" of Chang an 長安 and Luo yang 洛陽. That is, the reference is to the Xi an 西安 of today in Shaan xi 陝西 and present-day Luo yang 洛陽 city in He nan 河南.

Liang shan 梁山 [3 + 1 +1]

□ Name of a mountain. [3] It is located west of Han cheng 韓城 city in Shaan xi 陝西, connecting with He yang 合陽 county. Mentioned with 594, 1389.

□ Name of a county. [1] It was established by Northern Zhou 周, in 567. Its seat of administration was in present-day Ju kui 聚奎 town, located west of Liang ping 梁平 county in Chong qing 重慶 municipality. Under Northern Song 宋, in 965, the seat of administration was moved to present-day Liang ping county. Because this duplicated names with Liang shan county in Shan dong 山東, the county was renamed Liang ping county in 1952. Mentioned with 520.

□ Name of a mountain. [1] It is also called Liang zhou 梁州 mountain. It is located southeast of present-day Nan zheng 南鄭 county in Shaan xi 陝西. Mentioned with 1272.

Liang yi 梁益 [3]

Name of a region. The name is a combination of Liang zhou 梁州 and Yi zhou 益州 and refers to the southern part of present-day Shaan xi 陝西, a large section of Si chuan 四川, as well as Yun nan 雲南 and Gui zhou 貴州. Mentioned with 1057, 1371.

Liang zhe 兩浙 [1]

This is a combined designation for "the two Zhe", i.e., Zhe dong 浙東 and Zhe xi 浙西. This corresponds to the entire province of present-day Zhe jiang 浙江, Shang hai 上海 city, as well as the section of Jiang su 江蘇 south of the Yang zi. Mentioned with 1279.

Liang zhou 涼州 [12 + 2]

□ Name of a *zhou* 州. [12] It was established by Western Han 漢, in 106 BCE, and was one of the 13 Regional Inspector Divisions, *shi san ci shi bu* 十三刺史部. Eastern Han placed the administration in present-day Zhang jia chuan 張家川 county in Gan su 甘肅. The administrative area of the *zhou* corresponded to the present day Gan su, Ning xia 寧夏, and the watershed of the Huang shui 湟水 in Qing hai 青海, to Ding bian 定邊, Wu qi 吳起, Feng xian 鳳縣, Lue yang 略陽, in Shaan xi 陝西, and to a strip of the Ejina banner, E ji na qi 額濟納旗, in the Inner Mongolian Autonomous Region. During the *huang chu* 黃初 reign period (220 – 226) of Three Kingdoms' Wei 魏, the seat of administration was moved to present-day Wu wei 武威 city in Gan su. After Wei 魏 and Jin 晉, the administrative area of the *zhou* was reduced in size, and the *zhou* was confined solely to the region west of the Yellow River in Gan su. During the reign period *da ye* 大業 (605 – 615) of the Sui 隋, and during the reign periods *tian bao* 天寶 (742 – 756) and *zhi de* 至德 (756 – 758) of Tang 唐, the area several times was made Wu wei 武威 commandery. At the beginning of Tang, its administrative territory only comprised a strip in present-day Gan su extending from Yong chang 永昌 county toward the East and from Tian zhu 天祝 county toward the West. In 764, the area was lost to Tibet. During the Five Dynasties period and under Xi xia 西夏, the area was renamed Xi liang fu 西涼府. Mentioned with 26, 140, 188, 196, 301, 337, 496, 595, 804, 1307, 1335.

□ Name of a guard. [2] It was established under Ming 明, in 1376. Its seat of administration was in Wu wei 武威 city in Gan su 甘肅. The territory administered comprised the area of present-day Wu wei city. In 1724 the area became Liang zhou fu 涼州府. Mentioned with 804, 1335.

Liang zhou 梁州 [3+ 19]

□ One of the nine *zhou* 州 found in the *Book of History's* "Yu gong 禹貢," "Tribute of Yu 禹." [3] This is the approximate area south of present-day Xi yue hua shan 西岳華山 mountain. Mentioned with 1041,1538, 1551.

□ Name of a *zhou* 州. [19] It was established under Three Kingdoms' Wei 魏, in 263. Its seat of administration was in present-day Jiu zhou pu 舊州鋪 located east of Mian 勉 county in Shaan xi 陝西. In 282, under Western Jin 晉, the seat of administration was transferred to a point east of present-day Han zhong 漢中 city. The administrative area corresponded to the area in present-day Shaan xi, from the Qin ling 秦嶺 mountain range to the South, and from Da ba 大巴 mountain and Wu shan 巫山 mountain toward the West. Further, in present-day Si chuan 四川, from the counties and cities of Qing chuan 青川, Jiang you 江油, Zhong jiang 中江 and Sui ning 遂寧, as well as Bi shan 璧山 and Qi jiang 綦江 of Chong qing 重慶 muncipality, to the East, and also, in Gui zhou 貴州, the counties of Tong zi 桐梓 and Zheng an 正安. After that, the administrative area was gradually shifted, and over time the *zhou* ruled the area northwest of present-day An kang 安康 city, Da zhong si 大鐘寺 northwest of present-day Han zhong city, and the area east of present-day Cheng gu 城固 county. Under Liu Song 劉宋, in 434, the administration was moved to Nan zheng 南鄭 county. In 607, under Sui 隋, the *zhou* was eliminated but it was restored under Tang 唐, in 618. The territory administered comprised the present-day cities and counties of Hang zhong, Cheng gu, Nan zheng and Mian xian 勉縣, as well as the area north of Ning qiang 寧強 county, in Shaan xi 陝西. In 784, the status of the area was raised to be Xing yuan fu 興元府. Mentioned with 129, 130, 167, 216, 219, 441, 576, 639, 660, 666, 819, 864, 1004, 1014, 1032, 1147, 1305, 1324.

Liao 僚 [1]

Term used in reference to the region in the South where minority peoples live, partly spread in present-day Guang dong 廣東, Guang xi 廣西, Hu nan 湖南, Si chuan 四川, Yun nan 雲南 and Gui zhou 貴州. It also vaguely refers to the minority peoples of the south in general. Mentioned with 1242.

Liao 獠 [1]

This is a variant of Liao 僚. See → Liao 僚. Mentioned with 1532, 1535.

Liao 遼 [2 +4]

□ [2]. See under 'Liao dong 遼東. Mentioned with 931, 1057, 1538.

□ Name of a *zhou* 州. [4] See → Liao zhou 遼州. Mentioned with 620, 748, 931, 1462.

Liao 蓼 [1]

Name of a mountain. It is located somewhere in the central part of present-day Xian ju 仙居 county in Zhe jiang 浙江. Mentioned with 1134.

Liao ban shan 遼坂山 [1]

Name of a mountain. It is located in present-day Dan jiang kou 丹江口 city in Hu bei 湖北. Mentioned with 131.

Liao cheng xian 膋城縣 [1]

Name of a county. Its history and location are unknown. Mentioned with 474.

Liao dong 遼東 [1 + 13 + 8 + 2]

□ Name of a *lu* 路. [1]. It was established under Yuan 元, in 1267. Its seat of administration was in the present-day Nong an 農安 county in Ji lin 吉林 province. The *lu* administration extended, in the west, from present-day Kai yuan 開原 in Liao ning 遼寧, Si ping 四平 in Ji lin 吉林, and the Song hua jiang 松花江 watershed. In the North, it reached the mouth of the Amur/Hei long jiang 黑龍江 river northeast of the Khabarovsk border region in Russia. Toward the South it reached to the northeast parts of the Korean peninsula, and in the East to the sea. In 1286, Liao dong lu 遼東路 was changed to Kai yuan lu 開元路. Mentioned with 1458, 1551.

□ Name of a Regional Military Commission, *du zhi hui shi si* 都指揮使司, abbreviated as *du si* 都司. [13] The Ming 明 established a Liao dong guard in 1371 but, in 1375, this was changed to Liao dong Regional Military Commission, Liao dong *du si* 遼東都司. Its seat of administration was in the old city of present-day Liao yang 遼陽 city in Liao ning 遼寧, and had an administrative area corresponding to much of present-day Liao ning, and parts of Inner Mongolia and Ji lin 吉林. The *du si* was abolished at the end of Ming. Mentioned with 72, 73, 213, 215, 356, 404, 439, 447, 448, 464, 691, 931, 1004, 1364.

□ Name of a commandery. [8] It was established by Yan 燕 during the Warring States period. Its seat of administration was in the old city in present-day Liao yang 遼陽 city in Liao ning 遼寧. The territory administered included the area, in present-day Liao ning, from the Da ling 大凌 river toward the East, from Kai yuan 開原 city toward the South, and, in Korea, the area north of the lower water course of the Qing chuan 清川 river. Western Jin 晉 changed the commandery to be Liao dong country/domain, but later restored the commandery. During the era of Later Yan of Sixteen Kingdoms, the area became part of the Korean state of Koguryŏ, Gao gou li 高句麗. During the era of Northern Yan 燕, a new Liao dong commandery was established in the western part of present-day Liao ning. Northern Wei 魏 abolished this. Mentioned with 430, 639, 690, 931, 1149, 1253, 1330.

□ Name of a region. [2] The general reference is to the area east of the Liao he 遼河 river in Liao ning. Mentioned with 26, 1462.

Liao hai 遼海 [2 + 5]

□ Name of a guard. [2] It was established under the Ming 明, in 1390. Its seat of administration was at a location west of Chang tu 昌圖 county in Liao ning 遼寧. In 1393, the seat of the administration was moved to the old city located northeast of present-day Kai yuan 開原 city in Liao ning. The guard was abolished at the beginning of Qing 清. Mentioned with 1109, 1381.

□ Regional name. [5] Reference is to the area east of the Liao he 遼河 watershed up to the ocean region. Mentioned with 407, 896, 1330, 1458.

Liao she 聊攝 [1]
Name of an ancient city. It was a city in Qi 齊 during the Spring and Autumn period, and was located at the site of the Liao gu miao 聊古廟 near today's Yan jue si 閻覺寺 temple, 22 *li* northwest of Liao cheng 聊城 city in Shan dong 山東. Mentioned with 70.

Liao xi 遼西 [1]
Regional name. [1] The reference is to the area "west of the Liao 遼 (he 河)" in Liao ning 遼寧. Mentioned with 1205.

Liao yang 遼陽 [2]
Name of a *lu* 路. It was established under Yuan 元, in 1288. Its seat of administration was in the old city of present-day Liao yang 遼陽 city in Liao ning 遼寧. The territory administered comprised a region south from Liao yang city including the Liao dong 遼東 peninsula in Liao ning 遼寧. It was eliminated in 1371 but restored in 1373. It was finally eliminated in 1377. Mentioned with 501, 1110.

Liao zhou 遼州 [4]
Name of a *zhou* 州. It was founded under Sui 隋, in 596. Its seat of administration was at a location near Xi zhai 西寨 village, more than 40 *li* southwest of present-day Xi yang 昔陽 county in Shan xi 山西. The administrative area comprised present-day Zuo quan 左權, Yu she 榆社 and He shun 和順 in Shan xi. It was eliminated at the beginning of the *da ye* 大業 reign period (605 – 618) of the Sui 隨, but revived under the Tang 唐, in 620. In 623, the seat of administration was moved to present-day Zuo quan county in Shan xi. In 625, the area became Ji zhou 箕州. Liao zhou was reestablished in 883. Under Northern Song 宋, in 1074, it was eliminated but revived again in 1085. Under Southern Song, in 1128, the area became Nan liao zhou 南遼州, but again Liao zhou in 1151. In 1912, the area became Liao xian 遼縣 county. Mentioned with 52, 337, 653, 931.

Lin an 臨安 [3 + 2]
□ Name of a county. [3] It was founded under Western Jin 晉, in 280. Its seat of administration was in present-day Gao hong xiang 高虹鄉, located 18 *li* north of Lin an city in Zhe jiang 浙江. The county was eliminated under Sui 隋 but restored by Tang 唐, in 688. In 908, during the time of Five Dynasties' Liang 梁, Wu yue 吳越 changed it to be An guo 安國 county. Under Northern Song 宋, in 978, the area was again named Lin an county. Under Southern Song, during the *jing ding* 景定 reign period (1260 – 1264), the seat of administration was moved to present-day Xi shu jie 西墅街 located northwest of Lin an county city in Zhe jiang. At the beginning of Ming 明, the seat of administration was moved to the present Lin an city. Mentioned with 312, 712, 1182.
□ Name of a *fu* 府. [2] It was established, in 1382, under Ming 明. Its seat of administration was in present-day Jian shui 建水 county in Yun nan 雲南. The territory administered was most of the Hong he Hani Yi Autonomous Prefecture 紅河哈尼族彝族自治州, the Wen shan Zhuang Miao 文山壯苗 autonomous

zhou, Wen shan Zhuang Miao Autonomous Prefecture 文山壯苗族自治州, the counties of present-day Tong hai 通海, Hua ning 華寧, E shan 峨山 and Xin ping 新平, in Yun nan, and a part of Vietnam. During the Qing 清, the administrative area corresponded more or less to the present-day Hong he Hani Yi Autonomous Prefecture, the counties of Tong hai, Hua ning and E shan and a part of Vietnam. In 1913, the *fu* was abolished. Mentioned with 664, 1120.

Lin chuan 臨川 [8]

Name of a commandery. It was established by Three Kingdoms' Wu 吳, in 257. Its seat of administration was at a location 5 *li* west of the present-day Lin chuan 臨川 district of Fu zhou 撫州 city in Jiang xi 江西. The territory administered comprised the watersheds of the 盱江 and the Yi huang shui 宜黃水 from the present-day Lin chuan district of Fu zhou city in Jiang xi toward the South, and toward the West to the borders of Le an 樂安 county. Southern Qi 齊 moved the seat of administration to a point southeast of present-day Nan cheng 南城 county in Jiang xi. Southern Dynasties' Chen 陳 again moved the seat of administration to a point 5 *li* west of the present-day Lin chuan district. Under Sui, in 589, the area was changed to be Fu zhou. Later under Sui 隋, at the beginning of the *da ye* 大業 reign period (605 – 618), it was made Lin chuan commandery again. Under Tang 唐, in 622, it was changed again to be Fu zhou and, in 742, was again made Lin chuan commandery. In 758, it was changed again to be Fu zhou. Mentioned with 64, 202, 357, 455, 1524, 1561.

Lin feng zhou 麟鳳洲 [1]

Legendary place name. Details are lacking. Mentioned with 294.

Lin hai 臨海 [4 + 2]

▫ Name of a commandery. [4] It was established, in 257, under Three Kingdoms' Wu 吳. Its seat of administration was in present-day Lin hai city in Zhe jiang 浙江. Subsequently the seat of administration was moved to present-day Zhang an 章安 town in the Shu jiang 椒江 district of Tai zhou 台州 city in Zhe jiang. The territory administered comprised all the cities and counties of the Ling jiang 靈江, the Ou jiang 甌江, and the Fei yun jiang 飛雲江 watersheds in Zhe jiang. The administrative area was reduced under Eastern Jin 晉, in 323. The area was changed to Chi cheng 赤城 commandery under Southern Dynasties' Liang 梁, but subsequently Lin hai commandery was restored. Chen 陳, in turn, changed it to Zhang an 章安 commandery, but later changed the area again to Lin hai commandery. In 589, under Sui 隋, the commandery was eliminated. Under Tang 唐, in 742, Tai zhou was changed to be Lin hai commandery. Its seat of administration was in present-day Lin hai city in Zhe jiang. The commandery was abolished in 758. Mentioned with 298, 328, 1311.

▫ Name of a county. [2] It was established under Three Kingdoms Wu 吳, in 257. Its seat of administration was in present-day Lin hai city in Zhe jiang. Mentioned with 456, 1050.

Lin he 臨賀 [3]

Name of a commandery. It was established under Three Kingdom's Wu 吳, in 226. Its seat of administration was in present-day He jie 賀街 town, located southeast of He zhou 賀州 city in Guang xi 廣西. The territory administered comprised the three counties of He zhou, Zhong shan 鐘山 and Fu chuan 富川 in present-day Guang xi, and the counties of Jiang yong 江永 and Jian hua 江華 in present-day Hu nan 湖南. The area became He zhou during the *kai huang* 開皇 reign period (581 – 600) of the Sui 隋. It again became Lin he commandery under Tang 唐, in 742. In 758, this was changed to He zhou. Mentioned with 1265.

Lin huai 臨淮 [1]

What the BCGM authors are referring to is an old commandery name. It was established by Western Han 漢. Its seat of administration was at a location south of present-day Si hong 泗洪 county in Jiang su 江蘇. The territory administered comprised the central part of present-day Jiang su from Tai zhou 泰州, Jiang yan 姜堰 and Liu he 六合 toward the North, and toward the South from Sui ning 睢寧, Su qian 宿遷 and Lian shui 漣水, and in addition, in present-day An hui 安徽, Tian chang 天長 and Ming guang 明光. Western Jin moved the administrative seat to a point northeast of Xu yi 盱眙 county in Jiang su. Eastern Jin 晉 abolished the commandery. Mentioned with 616.

Lin jiang jun 臨江軍 [1]

Name of an administrative unit, an army. In 992, Northern Song 宋 established a Lin jiang 臨江 army. Its seat of administration was in present-day Lin jiang town southwest of Zhang shu 樟樹 city in Jiang xi 江西. The territory administered comprised the two cities of present-day Xin yu 新余 and Zhang shu, and the counties of Xin gan 新淦 and Xia jiang 峽江 in Jiang xi. Under the Yuan 元, the status of the area was raised to Lin jiang lu 臨江路. Mentioned with 1159.

Lin ju 臨沮 [1]

Name of a county. It was founded by Western Han 漢. Its seat of administration was at a location northwest of present-day Yuan an 遠安 county in Hu bei 湖北. Eastern Han changed the county to be Lin ju hou guo 臨沮侯國. Later, the county was restored. Under Western Jin 晉, following the *yong ning* 永寧 reign period (301 – 302), the seat of administration was moved to a point northwest of present-day Dang yang 當陽 city in Hu bei. Eastern Jin, during the *xian he* 咸和 reign period (326 – 334), put the county under Ju yang 沮陽 commandery. Sui 隋 abolished it. Mentioned with 932.

Lin lü shan 林慮山 [1]

Name of a mountain. The original name was Long lü shan 隆慮山. Under Eastern Han 漢, the name was changed because of a taoo on the short-lived Han ruler Liu Long's 劉隆 (105 – 106) name. The mountain is located 20 *li* northwest of present-day Lin zhou 林州 city in He nan 河南. Mentioned with 1043.

Lin ping 臨平 [1]

Name of a town. This is present-day Lin ping 臨平 town of the Yu hang 余杭 district of Hang zhou 杭州 city in Zhe jiang 浙江. Mentioned with 1418.

Lin qiong 臨邛 [1]

Name of a county. It was established by Qin 秦 during the Warring States period. Its seat of administration was in present-day Qiong lai 邛崍 city in Si chuan

四川. After the end of the period of Cheng Han 成漢 (306 – 347), the county was abolished. It was reestablished under Western Wei 魏, in 553. Under Yuan 元, in 1284, it was abolished. Its territory became part of Qiong zhou 邛州. Mentioned with 550.

Lin qu 臨朐 [3]

Name of a county. It was established by Western Han 漢. Its seat of administration was in present-day Lin qu county in Shan dong 山東. It was eliminated under Liu Song 劉宋, but reestablished under Sui 隋, in 606. Under Yuan 元, in 1266, it was combined with Yi du 益都 county. In 1278, it was reestablished. Mentioned with 823, 1037, 1105.

Lin ren xian 林任縣 [1]

Name of a county. There is no information available about its administrative changes, and exact location. Mentioned with 952.

Lin ru 臨汝 [1]

Name of a commandery. It was established by Tang 唐, in 742. Its seat of administration was in present-day Ru zhou 汝州 city in He nan 河南. The territory administered comprised the two present-day cities of Ru zhou and Ping ding shan 平頂山, and the counties of Ru yang 汝陽, Bao feng 寶豐, Lu shan 魯山, Ye xian 葉縣 and Xiang cheng 襄城 in He nan. Under Tang, in 758, the commandery was changed to Ru zhou 汝州. Mentioned with 1092.

Lin tao 臨洮 [5]

Name of a *fu* 府. It was established under Jin 金, in 1142. Its seat of administration was in present-day Lin tao 臨洮 county in Gan su 甘肅. The territory administered comprised the three present-day counties of Lin tao, Kang le 康樂 and Wei yuan 渭源 in Gan su. The territory administered was expanded under the Ming 明, and corresponded to the present-day cities and counties of Lan zhou 蘭州, Yu zhong 榆中, Wei yuan 渭源 and Lin tao, and the Lin xia Hui Autonomous Prefecture 臨夏回族自治 in Gan su, and the counties of Xun hua 循化, Jian zha 尖扎, Gui de 貴德, Gui nan 貴南 and Tong ren 同仁 in Qing hai 青海. In 1738, the seat of administration was moved to Lan zhou city in Gan su, and the name of the *fu* was changed to Lan zhou fu 蘭州府. Mentioned with 447, 467, 747, 811, 1143.

Lin ting 臨汀 [3]

Name of a Song 宋 times military establishment. This is present-day Ting zhou 汀州 in Chang ting 長汀 county in Fu jian 福建. Mentioned with 823, 1014, 1546.

Lin tong 臨潼 [1]

Name of a county. It was established under Northern Song 宋, in 1015. Its seat of administration was in present-day Lin tong 臨潼 district in Xi an 西安 city in Shaan xi 陝西. Mentioned with 1122.

Lin wu 臨武 [1]

Name of a county. It was established under Western Han 漢. Its seat of administration was in present-day Gu cheng du 古城渡, located 15 *li* east of Lin wu 臨武 county in Hu nan 湖南. Under Tang 唐, in 692, the area became Long wu 隆

武 county. In 705, the area again became Lin wu county. Under Five Dynasties' Jin 晉, in 936, it was eliminated and its territory became part of the Gui yang jian 桂陽監. Under Southern Song 宋, in 1146, Lin wu county was reestablished. The seat of administration was moved to the present Lin wu county. Mentioned with 685.

Lin yi 林邑 [11]

Name of an ancient country. At the end of Eastern Han 漢, it was established in Xiang lin 象林 county of the Western Han Ri nan 日南 commandery. Its center comprised present-day Vietnam's Tỉnh Quảng Nam province and Đà Nẵng municipality. Its original territory of administration extended from Hải vâ (Cape Varella) in the southern part of Khánh hòa province or the Phiền lãng area of Ninh thuận province. Later it gradually expanded toward the North and went up to the vicinity of Hoành 横 mountain in the northern part of Quảng bình province. Later on, Lin yi was gradually absorbed by Annam/An nan 安南. Mentioned with 82, 173, 406, 493, 535, 787, 1030, 1369, 1375, 1521.

Lin yi 臨沂 [1]

Name of a county. It was established, by retaining the name of a place formerly occupied elsewhere, under Eastern Jin 晉, in 341, west of Qi xia 栖霞 mountain, located 38 *li* northeast of present-day Nan jing 南京 city in Jiang su 江蘇. It was administered by Lang ya 琅琊 commandery. In the North, it came up to the Yang zi. Under Southern Qi 齊, the seat of administration was moved to a point outside the Jin chuan 金川 gate of present-day Nan Jing city. Sui eliminated the county. Mentioned with 1443.

Lin yi zhu guo 林邑諸國 [1]

Term used by the BCGM authors in reference to "various countries of Lin yi 林邑," i.e., central Vietnam and surrounding areas. Mentioned with 794.

Lin yuan xian 臨沅縣 [1]

Name of a county. It was established by Qin 秦. Its seat of administration was in present-day Chang de 常德 city in Hu nan 湖南. Sui 隋 changed this to be Wu ling 武陵 county. Mentioned with 202.

Lin zhang 臨漳 [1]

Name of a commandery, also written as Lin zhang jun 臨瘴郡 and Lin zhang jun 臨障郡. Its seat of administration was at a location east of present-day Jiu zhou 舊州 village, in the south of Pu bei 浦北 county in Guang xi 廣西. Southern Qi 齊 established a Zhang ping 漳平 county, and this was administered from Lin zhang 臨漳 commandery. The territory administered corresponded to the connected territories of the three present-day counties of He pu 合浦, Pu bei and Ling shan 靈山 in Guang xi. The commandery was abolished during Liang 梁 and Chen 陳. Mentioned with 202.

Lin zi 臨淄 [4]

Name of a commandery. See → Lin zi jun 臨淄郡. Mentioned with 131, 275, 631, 987.

Lin zi jun 臨淄郡 [1]
Name of a commandery. It was established under Qin 秦, in 221 BCE. Its seat of administration was in present-day Qi du 齊都 town of the Lin zi 臨淄 district of Zi bo 淄博 city in Shan dong 山東. The territory administered included the cities and counties of Zi bo, Bo xing 博興, Gao qing 高青, Li jin 利津, Shou guang 壽光, Guang rao 廣饒, Chang le 昌樂, Bin zhou 濱州, Qing zhou 青州 and Lin Qu 臨朐 in Shan dong. Western Han changed it to Qi 齊 commandery. Mentioned with 572.

Lin zi xian 臨淄縣 [1]
Name of a county. It was established by Qin 秦. The seat of administration was in present-day Qi du 齊都 town of Lin zi 臨淄 located northeast of Zi bo 淄博 city in Shan dong 山東. Under Western Han 漢, it came under the administration of Qi 齊 commandery. Eastern Han made this Lin zi 臨菑. Northern Qi 齊 moved the administration of Qi commandery to present-day Qing zhou 青州 city in Shan dong, and it was eliminated and its territory became part of Yi du 益都. In 596, under Sui 隋, it was reestablished. Tang 唐 made it part of Qing zhou, and the administration was moved to present-day Lin zi town located northeast of Zi bo city. In 1969, the county was revoked and the territory was made part of Zi bo city. Mentioned with 131.

Ling 陵 [2]
Name of a *zhou* 州. It was established under Northern Zhou 周, in 557. The seat of administration was at a location two *li* east of present-day Ren shou 仁壽 county in Si chuan 四川. The territory administered corresponded to the two present-day counties of Ren shou and Jing yan 井研 and part of Jian yang 簡陽 city and Shuang liu 雙流 county in Si chuan. During the reign period *da ye* 大業 (605 – 615) of the Sui 隋, and during the reign periods *tian bao* 天寶 (742 – 756) and *zhi de* 至德 (756 – 758) of Tang 唐, the area temporarily became a commandery. In 627, the seat of administration was moved to the present Ren shou county. Under Northern Song 宋, in 1072, the area became Ling jing jian 陵井監. Mentioned with 368, 1054.

Ling 嶺 [5]
Regional name. See → Ling nan 嶺南. Mentioned with 376, 541, 674, 789, 848.

Ling bei 嶺北 [2]
Regional name. The reference is to the area "north of the (Five) Ranges," (Wu) ling (五)嶺. Mentioned with 376, 1557.

Ling biao 嶺表 [9]
Regional name. This is the same as Ling nan 嶺南, and refers to present-day Guang dong 廣東, Guang xi 廣西 and Hai nan 海南, and the north of Vietnam. Mentioned with 94, 187, 376, 500, 535, 753, 1185, 1497.

Ling chuan xian 陵川縣 [1]
Name of a county. It was established under Sui 隋, in 596. The seat of administration was in present-day Ling chuan 陵川 county in Shan xi 山西. It was eliminated under the Yuan 元, in 1266, but restored in 1294. Mentioned with 1250.

Ling ling 零陵 [6 + 2]

□ Name of a commandery. [6] It was established under Western Han 漢, in 111 BCE. Its seat of administration was at a location southwest of present-day Quan zhou 全州 in Guang xi 廣西. The territory administered comprised in present-day Hu nan 湖南 an area reaching from Shao yang 邵陽 city and Heng yan 衡陽 county toward the South, from Yong zhou 永州 city and Ning yuan 寧遠 county toward the West, from Wu gang 武岡 city and, in present-day Guang xi, Gui lin 桂林 city toward the East, and from Yang shuo 陽朔 county in Guang xi and, in Hu nan, Dao xian 道縣 county toward the North. Eastern Han moved the center of administration to a point located 2 *li* north of the present-day Ling ling district in Yong zhou city in Hu nan. After the Three Kingdoms period, the area of the commandary was reduced. Under Sui 隋, in 589, Yong zhou was established in its place. At the beginning of the reign period *da ye* 大業 (605 – 615) of the Sui 隋, Ling ling commandery was reestablished, and the seat of administration was transferred to present-day Ling ling district of Yong zhou city in Hu nan. Under Tang 唐, in 621, it was once more changed to be Yong zhou. In 742, the area again became Ling ling commandery, but in 758 Yong zhou again. Mentioned with 789, 1329, 1384, 1435.

□ Name of a county. [2] It was established, in 589, under Sui 隋. Its seat of administration was in the Ling ling district of Yong zhou city in Hu nan. In 1982, it became Yong zhou city. Mentioned with 171, 1058.

Ling ling xian 零陵縣 [1]

Name of a county. It was established by Qin 秦. Its seat of administration was at a location southwest of present-day Quan zhou 全州 county in Guang xi 廣西. It was abolished under Sui 隋, in 589. Mentioned with 1307.

Ling nan 嶺南 [162]

Regional name. Also called Ling wai 嶺外 and Ling biao 嶺表. The term designates the area "south of the (Five) Ranges," (see → Wu ling 五嶺), the so-called Ling nan. This includes Guang dong 廣東, Guang xi 廣西, Hai nan 海南 and the northern part of Vietnam. Mentioned with 4, 9, 15, 30, 58, 60, 85, 94, 106, 110, 121, 127, 130, 143, 144, 149, 162, 189, 190, 214, 236, 243, 250, 255, 258, 296, 300, 322, 323, 324, 327, 330, 332, 335, 344, 346, 350, 362, 367, 376, 389, 405, 419, 427, 428, 465, 468, 474, 479, 483, 486, 489, 521, 522, 529, 534, 535, 547, 552, 564, 585, 590, 602, 611, 615, 624, 628, 642, 654, 674, 679, 724, 730, 736, 762, 770, 780, 791, 793, 798, 821, 832, 834, 836, 843, 857, 860, 873, 899, 909, 925, 929, 935, 956, 979, 981, 991, 1004, 1027, 1028, 1035, 1068, 1092, 1127, 1139, 1151, 1157, 1177, 1190, 1192, 1212, 1222, 1226, 1231, 1237, 1238, 1245, 1257, 1267, 1276, 1309, 1329, 1335, 1339, 1342, 1350, 1367, 1369, 1371, 1399, 1425, 1446, 1460, 1467, 1497, 1499, 1526.

Ling nan xi dong 嶺南溪峒 [1]

Regional name. It refers to the region of Ling nan 嶺南 inhabited by minority nationalities. Mentioned with 1532.

Ling qiao 嶺嶠 [1]

This is another name for the "Five Ranges" (see → Wu ling 五嶺). Mentioned with 519.

Ling qiu 靈丘 [1]

Name of a county. It was established by Western Han 漢. Its seat of administration was in present-day Gu cheng 固城 village, located 10 *li* east of Ling qiu county in Shan xi 山西. It was eliminated at the beginning of Eastern Han, but restored during the last years of Eastern Han. Western Jin 晉 eliminated it, but Northern Wei 魏 reestablished it. It was once more eliminated at the end of Sui 隋, but restored under Tang 唐, in 623. Its administration was assigned to present-day Yang qu 陽曲 town, located 15 *li* northeast of Tai yuan 太原 city in Shan xi. In 624, the administration was entrusted to a point west of the present Fan shi 繁峙 county. In 625, the administration was returned to the present Ling qiu county. Mentioned with 698.

Ling shan xiang 靈山鄉 [1]

Name of a sub-administrative unit. This is today's Ling shan xiang 靈山鄉鄉 of Shang rao 上饒 city in Jiang xi 江西. Mentioned with 552.

Ling wai 嶺外 [10]

Regional name. This is also given as Ling nan 嶺南. From the standpoint of an inhabitant of the Chinese central plain, the area of Ling nan was "beyond the (Five) Ranges" (see → Wu ling 五嶺), thus the name. Mentioned with 110, 378, 400, 428, 483, 558, 641, 983, 1030, 1400.

Ling wai zhou jun 嶺外州郡 [1]

Regional name. It refers to the "*zhou* and commanderies beyond the (Five) Ranges" (see → Wu ling 五嶺), i.e., the region of the three provinces of Guang dong 廣東, Guang xi 廣西 and Hai nan 海南 and northern Vietnam. Mentioned with 94.

Ling yin 陵陰 [1]

Not a real place name but just designates a frozen underground, a cold place. Mentioned with 1483.

Ling yin si 靈隱寺 [2]

Name of a temple. This is today's Ling yin 靈隱 temple on the northwestern side of the West Lake in Hang zhou 杭州 city in Zhe jiang 浙江. Mentioned with 1420.

Ling zhou 靈州 [4]

Name of a *zhou* 州. It was established under Northern Wei 魏, during the *xiao chang* 孝昌 reign period (525 – 528). Its seat of administration was at a location north of present-day Wu zhong 吳忠 city in Ning xia 寧夏. During the reign period *da ye* 大業 (605 – 615) of the Sui 隋, and during the reign periods *tian bao* 天寶 (742 – 756) and *zhi de* 至德 (756 – 758) of Tang 唐, the area temporarily became Ling wu 靈武 commandery. Its jurisdiction included the area extending in present-day Ning xia from Zhong wei 中衛 city and Zhong ning 中寧 county toward the North. It was abolished at the beginning of the *hong wu* 洪武 reign period (1368 – 1398) of the Ming 明 but, under Qing 清, in 1725, a Ling zhou was again established. In 1913, the area became Ling wu 靈武 county. Mentioned with 191, 361, 650, 1057.

Liu 柳 [1 + 1]

□ Name of a *fu* 府. [1] The name is an abbreviation of Liu zhou fu 柳州府. See → Liu zhou 柳州. Mentioned with 1427.

□ Name of a *zhou* 州. [1] See → Liu zhou. Mentioned with 376.

Liu cheng jun 柳城郡 [1]

Name of a commandery. It was established under Sui 隋, at the beginning of the *da ye* 大業 reign period (605 – 618). Its seat of administration was in present-day Chao yang 朝陽 city in Liao ning 遼寧. The territory administered comprised an area extending from the Shan hai guan 山海關 toward the East, and, in Liao ning, from the flood plains of Da ling he 大凌河 and Xiao ling he 小凌河, as well as from the area of Jin zhou 錦州 and Chao yang 朝陽 toward the West. Under Tang 唐, in 618, it became Ying zhou 營州. In 742, it became Liu cheng 柳城 commandery. In 758, it was changed back to Ying zhou. Mentioned with 572.

Liu qiu 琉球 [5]

Name of an early country, that is, the Ryukyu Islands. See → Liu qiu guo 琉球國. Mentioned with 511, 566, 1535.

Liu qiu guo 琉球國 [2]

Name of an early country. Originally this was a common designation from the outside of the three separate kingdoms Shan nan 山南, Zhong shan 中山 and Bei shan 北山. Later, the name referred to the kingdom resulting from their unification. In 1879, this united kingdom was conquered by Japan and organized into a Japanese *ken* 縣. Much of it became Okinawa 沖繩 *ken*. The northern part was divided to establish Kagoshima 鹿兒島 *ken*. Mentioned with 1030, 1041, 1535.

Liu sha 流沙 [2]

Regional name. [2] It refers to the "flowing sands" deserts to the northwest of China. Mentioned with 294, 1230.

Liu zhou 柳州 [4 + 1]

□ Name of a *fu* 府. [4] It was established under Ming 明, in 1368. Its seat of administration was in present-day Liu zhou city in Guang xi 廣西. Its administrative territory comprised an area in present-day Guang xi extending from the Luo qing he 洛清河 and Da yao 大瑤 mountain toward the West, from Da ming 大明 mountain toward the North, and from Luo cheng 羅城 and Bin yang 賓陽 toward the East. It was abolished in 1913. Mentioned with 202, 540, 1427, 1500.

□ Name of a *zhou* 州. [1] It was established by Tang 唐, in 634. Its seat of administration was in present-day Liu zhou city in Guang xi. The territory administered comprised Liu zhou city and the counties of Liu jiang 柳江, Liu cheng 柳城 and Lu zhai 鹿寨 in Guang xi. In 1265, under Southern Song 宋, the seat of administration was moved to a point southwest of present-day Liu cheng county. Under Yuan 元, in 1279, the status of the area was promoted to be Liu zhou lu 柳州路. Mentioned with 456.

Long 龍 [1]

Name of a *zhou* 州. See → Long zhou 龍州. Mentioned with 660.

Long 隴 [7]
Name of a *zhou* 州. See → Long zhou 隴州. Mentioned with 468, 478, 660, 741, 801, 802, 1008.

Long an 龍安 [1]
Name of a county. It was established under Tang 唐, in 620. Its seat of administration was at a location northeast of present-day An chang 安昌 town of An xian 安縣 county in Si chuan 四川. Under Northern Song 宋, in 1119, the area became An chang county. Under Southern Song, in 1131, it once again became Long an 龍安 county. Under Yuan 元, in 1264, it was abolished. Its territory became part of An zhou 安州. Mentioned with 322.

Long cheng 龍城 [1]
Name of a county. It was established under Northern Wei 魏, in 487. Its seat of administration was at a location northeast of present-day Min xian 岷縣 county in Gan su 甘肅, on the eastern bank of the Tao he 洮河 river. It was abolished under Northern Zhou 周. Mentioned with 1335.

Long chuan xian 龍川縣 [1]
Name of a county. It was established by Qin 秦. Its seat of administration was in Tuo cheng 佗城 town, located 20 *li* southwest of present-day Long chuan 龍川 county in Guang dong 廣東. It was eliminated by Sui 隋, in 591, but early Tang 唐 reestablished it. Later, at the beginning of the *zhen guan* 貞觀 reign period (627 – 649), it was again eliminated. In 917, under Southern Han 漢 of the Five Dynasties, it was reestablished. The seat of administration was moved to a point northwest of present-day Long chuan county. Northern Song 宋, in 1121, changed the county to be Lei jiang 雷江 county, and Southern Song, in 1131, renamed the county as Long chuan county. In 1145, the seat of administration was moved to present-day Tuo cheng town. In 1912, it was moved to the present-day Lao long 老隆 town. Mentioned with 347.

Long dong 龍洞 [1]
Name of a mountain grotto. It is located in the northwest of present-day Ning qiang 寧強 county in Shaan xi 陕西. Mentioned with 907.

Long ji shan 龍濟山 [1]
Name of a mountain. It is located south of present-day Yi zhou 宜州 city in Guang xi 廣西. Mentioned with 1247.

Long men 龍門 [1 + 4]
□ Name of a mountain. This refers to Yi que 伊闕. [1] It is located 25 *li* south of present-day Luo yang 洛陽 city in He nan 河南, at the Long men mountain and Xiang shan 香山 mountain gorge passed by the Yi he 伊河 river, like a gate, thus the name. Mentioned with 341.
□ Name of a mountain. [4] This is Yu men kou 禹門口 located northwest of present-day He jin 河津 city in Shan xi 山西, and northeast of present-day Han cheng 韓城 city in Shaan xi 陕西. Mentioned with 583, 675, 1458.

Long men shan 龍門山 [1]
Name of a mountain. It is located in the northwest of present-day He jin 河津 city in Shan xi 山西. On the west it is bordered by present-day Han cheng 韓城 city in Shaan xi 陝西 and the Yellow River. Mentioned with 381.

Long nao gang 龍腦岡 [1]
Name of a mountain ridge. It is located in present-day Dong ping 東平 county in Shan dong 山東. Mentioned with 1087.

Long shan 蠪山 [1]
Name of a mountain. It is located north of present-day Hu zhou 湖州 city in Zhe jiang 浙江. Mentioned with 1521.

Long shan 龍山 [1]
Name of a mountain. It is located west of present-day Zhang qiu 章丘 city in Shan dong 山東. Mentioned with 272.

Long shang 隴上 [1]
Regional name. The reference is to the present-day Shaan bei 陝北 (northern Shaan xi 陝西) area, Gan su 甘肅 and the area further in the West. Mentioned with 361.

Long shu 隴蜀 [1]
Regional name. Reference is to the two present-day provinces of Gan su 甘肅 and Si chuan 四川. Mentioned with 1386.

Long xi 隴西 [20 + 2 + 5]
□ Name of a commandery. [20] It was established by Warring States Qin 秦, in 279 BCE. Its seat of administration was at a location south of present-day Lin tao 臨洮 county in Gan su 甘肅. The territory administered comprised an area in present-day Gan su extending from Long shan 隴山 mountain toward the West, from the Yellow River toward the East, from the Western Han shui 漢水 and the upper watershed of the Bai long jiang 白龍江 toward the North, and from the Zu li 祖厲 river and Liu pan 六盤 mountain toward the South. After Eastern Han 漢, the commandery was gradually reduced in size. Three Kingdoms' Wei 魏 moved the seat of administration to a point southeast of present-day Long xi county in Gan su. At the end of Northern Wei, the administrative area of the commandery only included the area about Long xi county in Gan su. Later, at the beginning of the *kai huang* 開皇 reign period (581 – 600), the commandery was abolished, but it was reestablished in 607. During early Tang 唐, the area became Wei zhou 渭州 and, in 742, the area was changed to Long xi commandery. It again became Wei zhou in 758. Mentioned with 188, 199, 249, 285, 454, 461, 819, 861, 908, 934, 1199, 1289, 1323.
□ Name of a county. [2] It was established under Northern Song 宋, in 109. Its seat of administration was in present-day Long xi county in Gan su. Mentioned with 461, 1428.
□ Regional name. [5] It refers to the area west of Long shan 隴山 mountain. Mentioned with 249, 275, 331, 620, 1126.

Long zhou 隴州 [1]
Name of a *zhou* 州. It was founded by Western Wei 魏, in 554. Its seat of administration was at a location 16 *li* southeast of Long xian 隴縣 county in present-day Shaan xi 陝西. The territory administered corresponded to the Qian shui 千水 watershed in Shaan xi, and Hua ting 華亭 county in Gan su 甘肅. It was eliminated under Northern Zhou 周, in 569, but shortly thereafter revived, in 580. The seat of administration was moved to the present-day Long xian county. It was eliminated again under Sui 隋, in 607, but reestablished under Tang 唐, in 618. Subsequently, the territory administered was gradually reduced in size. Jin 金 moved the seat of administration to a point northwest of present-day Qian yang 千陽 county in Shaan xi. At the beginning of Yuan 元, it was moved again to Qian yang county. In 1913, the area became Long county. Mentioned with 914.

Long zhou 龍州 [5]
Name of a *zhou* 州. It was established under Western Wei 魏, in 553. Its seat of administration was in the present-day Jiu zhou 舊州 of Nan ba 南壩 town, located southeast of Ping wu 平武 county in Si chuan 四川. During the reign period *da ye* 大業 (605 – 615) of the Sui 隋, and during the reign periods *tian bao* 天寶 (742 – 756) and *zhi de* 至德 (756 – 758) of Tang 唐, the area temporarily became a commandery. Under Tang 唐, in 627, the area was changed to be the Long men win-over *zhou*, Long men *ji mi zhou* 龍門羈縻州, whereby the Chinese authorities installed the head of a region inhabited by non-Chinese ethnic groups while respecting the indigenous traditional customs and government structures. Later, during the *chui gong* 垂拱 reign period (685 – 688), the area became Long men zhou 龍門州. The territory administered included present-day Ping wu county along with a section of Qing chuan 青川 county and Jiang you 江油 city, in Si chuan. Under Northern Song 宋, in 1115, the area was named Zheng zhou 政州. Later, in 1131, the area became Long zhou. In 1258, during Southern Song, the seat of administration was moved to present-day Jiu xian ba 舊縣壩 of Da kang 大康 town, located north of Jiang you city. Under the Ming 明, in 1373, it was moved to present-day Qing xi 青溪 town, southwest of Qing chuan 青川 county in Si chuan and, in 1389, it was moved to present-day Ping wu county in Si chuan. In 1566, Long an fu 龍安府 was established. Mentioned with 322, 437, 1168.

Lu 廬 [1]
Name of a *zhou* 州. See under → Lu zhou 廬州. Mentioned with 873.

Lu 瀘 [1 + 1]
□ Name of a guard unit. [1] See Lu zhou 瀘州. Mentioned with 585.
□ Name of a *zhou* 州. [1] It was established under Southern Dynasties' Liang 梁. Its seat of administration was at present-day Lu zhou 瀘州 city in Si chuan 四川. During the reign period *da ye* 大業 (605 – 615) of the Sui 隋, and during the reign periods *tian bao* 天寶 (742 – 756) and *zhi de* 至德 (756 – 758) of Tang 唐, the area temporarily became Lu chuan 瀘川 commandery. Its jurisdiction included the lower watershed of the Tuo jiang 沱江 in Si chuan 四川 and the watersheds of the Chang ning he 長寧河, Yong ning he 永寧河, and Chi shui he 赤水河.

Under Southern Song 宋, in 1243, the seat of administration was moved to present-day Nan lao lu 南老瀘 in Jiao tan xiang 焦灘鄉, located northwest of He jiang 合江 county in Si chuan. In 1261, the area became Jiang an zhou 江安州. Under Yuan 元, in 1275, the area became Lu zhou again. The seat of administration was moved to a place on the eastern bank of the Yang zi, east of present-day Lu zhou city. Under Ming 明, in 1373, the status of the area was promoted to be a directly administered *zhou*, *zhi li zhou* 直隸州, and the seat of administration was moved to present-day Lu zhou city. Mentioned with 9.

Lu 魯 [8]

Regional name. It refers to the watersheds of the Wen 汶, Si 泗, Yi 沂 and Shu 沭 south of Tai shan 泰山 mountain in Shan dong 山東. Mentioned with 22, 485, 614, 832, 1105, 1197, 1242, 1444.

Lu 潞 [4]

Name of a *zhou* 州. See → Lu zhou 潞州. Mentioned with 111, 178, 980, 1178.

Lu an 六安 [2 + 1]

□ Name of a feudal lord's country/domain. [2] It was established under Eastern Han 漢. Its seat of administration was in present-day Cheng bei xiang 城北鄉, 10 *li* north of Lu an city in An hui 安徽. Three Kingdoms Wei 魏 changed the country to Lu an county. Mentioned with 1020, 1266.

□ Name of a *zhou* 州. [1] It was established by the Yuan 元. Its seat of administration was in today's Lu an city in An hui. The territory administered comprised the counties of Lu an and Huo shan 霍山 in present-day An hui, and Ying shan 英山 county in Hu bei 湖北. At the beginning of Ming 明, Lu an county was abolished and made part of the *zhou*. In 1912, the *zhou* was abolished and became a county. Mentioned with 768.

Lu di 魯地 [2]

Regional name. It refers to the watersheds of the Wen 汶, Si 泗, Yi 沂 and Shu 沭 south of Tai shan 泰山 mountain in Shan dong 山東. Mentioned with 667, 1208.

Lu guo 魯國 [2]

Feudal country of the Zhou 周 era. Its capital was at present-day Gu cheng 古城 village, 2 *li* northeast of Qu fu 曲阜 city in Shan dong 山東. Its boundaries, at their greatest extent, extended from Teng zhou 滕州 and Shan xian 單縣 county toward the South, and included the counties of Yun cheng 鄆城 and Ju ye 巨野 in the West. In the Northwest, it reached to the boundary of Fan 范 county in He nan 河南, in the East it reached the region of Lin yi 臨沂 and the Yi shui 沂水. In the Northeast, it reached the region of Tai an 泰安 and Xin tai 新泰 and bordered on Qi 齊. In 256 BCE, Lu 魯 was destroyed by Chu 楚. Mentioned with 706, 830.

Lu jiang 廬江 [3 + 1]

□ Name of a commandery. [3] A Lu jiang commandery was established both by Three Kingdoms Wei 魏 and by Wu 吳. The Lu jiang commandery of Wei was administered at Cheng bei xiang 城北鄉, 10 *li* north of present-day Lu an 六安

city in An hui 安徽. The territory administered comprised the cities and counties of Lu an, Shu cheng 舒城, Huo shan 霍山 and Lu jiang and part of Shou xian 壽縣 county in An hui. The Lu jiang commandery of Wu was administered at Qian shan 潛山 county in An hui. The territory administered comprised the southwestern part of present-day An hui. Western Jin 晉 combined the two commanderies into one, and moved the seat of administration to Shu cheng county. The administrative area was expanded toward the South to the northern bank of the Yang zi. Liu Song 劉宋 moved the seat of administration to a point northeast of present-day Huo shan county. Under Southern Qi 齊, in 480, it was moved to Shu xian 舒縣 county. Liang 梁 moved the seat of administration to present-day Lu jiang county. The commandery was abolished under Sui 隋, in 589. Mentioned with 562, 768, 1149.

□ Name of a commandery. [1] It was established during the era of the states of Chu 楚 and Han 漢. The territory administered comprised an area extending in present-day An hui 安徽 from the Yang zi toward the South, and from Jing xian 涇縣 county and Xuan zhou 宣州 toward the West, as well as in present-day Jiang xi 江西 the Xin jiang 信江 watershed and the area in the North of it. After the era of Emperor Wu 武 of Han (156 – 87), the seat of administration was moved to present-day Cheng chi xiang 城池鄉, located 30 *li* southwest of Lu jiang county in An hui. The administrative area of the commandery extended in present-day An hui from Chao hu 巢湖 city, Shu cheng 舒城 and Huo shan 霍山 county toward the South, and from the Yang zi toward the North; it comprised in Hu bei 湖北 the counties of Ying shan 英山, Guang ji 廣濟, and Huang mei 黃梅, as well as in He nan 河南 the county of Shang cheng 商城. The commandery was abolished at the end of Eastern Han. Mentioned with 911.

Lu ling 廬陵 [3]

Name of a commandery. See → Lu ling jun 廬陵郡. Mentioned with 344, 348, 890.

Lu ling jun 廬陵郡 [1]

Name of a commandery. It was founded, in 195, under Eastern Han 漢. Its seat of administration was at a location northeast of present-day Ji an 吉安 city in Jiang xi 江西. The territory administered comprised in present-day Jiang xi an area extending toward the South from Yong xin 永新, Xia jiang 峽江, Le an 樂安 and Shi cheng 石城. Three Kingdoms' Wu 吳 moved the seat of administration to a point 3 *li* northwest of Tai he 泰和 county in Jiang xi. Under Western Jin 晉, during the *tai kang* 太康 reign period (280 – 289), the seat of administration was moved back to a point northeast of present-day Ji an city, but the administrative area was reduced. The present-day Wan an 萬安, and the area south of Guang chang 廣昌, in Jiang xi, were detached and made part of Nan kang 南康 commandery. Under Sui 隋, during the *kai huang* 開皇 reign period (581 – 600), the area was reestablished as Ji zhou 吉州 but, in 607, Lu ling commandery was reestablished. During Tang 唐, in 622, it was changed to be Ji zhou but, in 742, became Lu ling commandery again. In 758, the area became Ji zhou again. Mentioned with 788.

Lu meng shan 魯蒙山 [1]
Referenced by the BCGM authors, possibly in error. Should perhaps be 魯地的蒙山, "Meng shan 蒙山 of Lu di 魯地," rather than Lu meng shan 魯蒙山. Mentioned with 1017.

Lu rong 盧容 [1]
Name of a county. It was established by Western Han 漢. Its seat of administration was at the place where the Dông hương giang 東香江 and the Bồ giang 蒲江 rivers come together in the eastern part of present-day Tỉnh Thừa Thiên - Huế province in Vietnam. After Southern Qi 齊, the county was abolished. Mentioned with 1406.

Lu shan 盧山 [6 + 1]
□ Name of a mountain. [6] It is located 30 *li* southeast of present-day Zhu cheng 諸城 city in Shan dong 山東. Mentioned with 666, 1017, 1344.
□ Name of a mountain. [1] It is located north of present-day Long ting 龍廷 town of Xin tai 新泰 City in Shan dong 山東. Mentioned with 1017.

Lu shan 廬山 [10]
Name of a mountain. This is anciently called Nan zhang shan 南障山. It is also called Kuang shan 匡山 and Kuang lu 匡廬. This is Lu shan 廬山 mountain at present-day Jiu jiang 九江 city in Jiang xi 江西. Mentioned with 132, 559, 725, 768, 810, 942, 1015, 1051, 1228, 1430.

Lu shan 魯山 [3]
Name of a mountain, also called Lu shan 露山. It is located 18 *li* east of present-day Lu shan 魯山 county in He nan 河南. Mentioned with 270, 1293.

Lu shi 盧氏 [1]
Name of a county. See → Lu shi xian 盧氏縣. Mentioned with 866.

Lu shi xian 盧氏縣 [1]
Name of a county. It was established under Western Han 漢. Its seat of administration was in the present-day Lu shi 盧氏 county in He nan 河南. Mentioned with 1250.

Lu tai 鹿臺 [1]
Place name. Another name is Nan dan tai 南單台. This is in present-day Qi 淇 county in He nan 河南. Mentioned with 733.

Lu zhong 虜中 [1]
Regional name. It refers to areas occupied by minority groups in the North. Mentioned with 1340.

Lu zhou 潞州 [10]
Name of a *zhou* 州. It was established under Northern Zhou 周, in 578. Its seat of administration was at a location north of present-day Xiang yuan 襄垣 county in Shan xi 山西. Sui 隋, during the *kai huang* 開皇 reign period (581 – 680), moved the seat of administration to a point southeast of present-day Hu guan 壺關 county in Shan xi. In 618, under Tang 唐, the area was changed to Lu zhou 潞州, and the seat of administration was moved to the present-day Zhang zhi

長治 city in Shan xi. The administrative area of the *zhou* corresponded to Zhang zhi city and the present-day counties of Wu xiang 武鄉, Qin xian 沁縣, Xiang yuan, Li cheng 黎城, Tun liu 屯留, Lu cheng 潞城, Ping shun 平順, Zhang zi 長子 and Hu guan, in Shan xi, and She xian 涉縣 county in He bei 河北. Under Northern Song 宋, in 1104, its status was raised to Long de fu 隆德府. Jin 金 again made it Lu zhou. Under early Yuan 元, it was changed to Long de fu 隆德府 but, in 1231, it became Lu zhou. Under Ming 明, in 1529, its status was raised to Lu an fu 潞安府. Mentioned with 131, 426, 818, 931, 1134, 1186, 1250, 1435, 1438.

Lu zhou 瀘州 [1]
Name of a guard. It was established under the Ming 明, in 1392. Its seat of administration was in Lu zhou city in Si chuan 四川. In 1468, the seat of administration was moved to Xing wen 興文 county in Si chuan. Under the Qing 清, in 1685, the guard was abolished and made part of Lu zhou. Mentioned with 768.

Lu zhou 廬州 [3 + 3]
□ Name of a *fu* 府. [3] It was established under Yuan 元, in 1364. Its seat of administration was in present-day He fei 合肥 city in An hui 安徽. The territory administered comprised the present-day counties and cities of He fei, Lu jiang 廬江, Wu wei 無為, Chao hu 巢湖 in An hui, and Ying shan 英山 in Hu bei 湖北. It was abolished in 1912. Mentioned with 64, 712, 768.
□ Name of a *zhou* 州. [3] It was founded under Sui 隋, in 581. Its seat of administration was in present-day He fei 合肥 city in An hui 安徽. The territory administered corresponded to the cities and counties of He fei, Chao hu 巢湖, Lu jiang 廬江, Wu wei 無為, Shu cheng 舒城, Lu an 六安, Huo shan 霍 mountain and Jin zhai 金寨 in An hui. During the Five Dynasties, the area first belonged to Wu 吳 and then to Southern Tang 唐. Under Southern Song 宋, during the *shao xing* 紹興 reign period (1131 – 1162), the administrative seat was moved to present-day Chao hu city. Under Yuan 元, in 1277, the area became Lu zhou lu 廬州路. Mentioned with 186, 293, 1020.

Lü yu he 緑玉河 [1]
Name of a river. It is also called the Hei yu 黑玉 river. It is the Karakash 喀拉喀什河 river in present-day Khotan (He tian 和田) city in Xin jiang 新疆 that is a Western affluent of the Khotan/Hotan river. Mentioned with 1406.

Lü xiang xian 呂鄉縣 [1]
The *xiang* 鄉 is an error for *xiang* 香. See → Lü xiang xian 呂香縣.

Lü xiang xian 呂香縣 [1]
Name of a county. It was founded under Tang 唐, in 627. Its seat of administration was near present-day Xi po 西坡 town, located 52 *li* southwest of Xiang ning 鄉寧 county in Shan xi 山西. In 634, the county was put under Ci zhou 慈州, and it was abolished under Five Dynasties' Zhou 周, in 956. Mentioned with 1250.

Luo 羅 [2]
Zhou 州 name. See → Luo zhou 羅州. Mentioned with 596, 1357.

Luo 洛 [1 + 10 + 1]
□ [1] See Shang luo shan 商洛山. Mentioned with 660.

□ Name of an ancient capital. [10] See Luo yang 洛陽. Mentioned with 298, 421, 440, 495, 639, 1005, 1025, 1067, 1306, 1367, 1535.
□ Name of a river. [1] See Luo shui 洛水. Mentioned with 1176.

Luo cha guo 羅刹國 [1]
Name of an ancient country. This is certainly Lochac on Borneo, known in Marco Polo's time, but this Luo cha 羅刹 is only defined in terms of other locations of uncertain identification themselves, despite the phonological connection. It was said to have been located near the Kelantan in Malaysia, or on the islands of Luzon or Sulu in the Philippines, or has been identified with Maluku in Malaysia. Mentioned with 492.

Luo cheng xian 羅城縣 [1]
Name of a county. It was established, in 972, under Northern Song 宋. Its seat of administration was at a location near present-day Wu yang 武陽 of Huang jin 黃金 town north of Luo cheng 羅城 county in Guang xi 廣西. Under Northern Song, in 1074, the county was eliminated. It was reestablished under Ming 明, in 1369, when the seat of administration was moved to the present-day Luo cheng county. Mentioned with 1427.

Luo fu shan 羅浮山 [4]
Name of a mountain. It is located northwest of present-day Bo luo 博羅 county in Guang dong 廣東. Mentioned with 547, 828, 983.

Luo gu 駱谷 [1]
Minor place name. It was located southwest of present-day Zhou zhi 周至 county in Shaan xi 陝西. It was an important thoroughfare between the Guan zhong 關中 area and Han zhong 漢中. Mentioned with 443.

Luo jiang 羅江 [1]
Name of a river. It is the Fei yun jiang 飛雲江, located in present-day Zhe jiang 浙江 province. Mentioned with 138.

Luo shui 洛水 [3]
Name of a river. It is the Luo he 洛河, located in present-day He nan 河南 province. Mentioned with 599, 1144, 1435.

Luo xi 洛西 [2]
Regional designation. The reference is to the area "west of Luo (yang 洛陽)." Mentioned with 1417, 1470.

Luo yang 洛陽 [16]
Name of an old capital. It is so-called because it is located on the north side of the Luo shui 洛水. The original name of the city was Cheng zhou 成周, but it was renamed during the Warring States period. Eastern Han 漢 established its capital at Luo yang in 25 and the foundations of the old city of Han and Wei 魏 are located northeast of present-day Luo yang city in He nan 河南. Luo yang was again the capital under Three Kingdoms Wei 魏, Western Jin 晉 and Northern Wei 魏. Sui 隋 established its eastern capital 18 *li* west of the old city of Han and Wei. A capital continued thereafter to be at Luo yang into the Five Dynasties period. The old city is along the southern and northern banks of the Luo shui

of present-day Luo yang city in He nan. Mentioned with 50, 77, 170, 339, 437, 572, 631, 922, 978, 1095, 1435.

Luo zhong 洛中 [4]

Another name for Luo yang 洛陽. See → Luo yang. Mentioned with 1140, 1157, 1266, 1385.

Luo zhou 洛州 [2]

Name of a *zhou* 州. It was established under Northern Wei 魏, in 423. Its seat of administration was in the northwest corner of the old city of Han 漢 and Wei 魏, northeast of present-day Luo yang 洛陽 city in He nan 河南. In 493, the seat of administration was moved to the old city of Han and Wei, located northeast of Luo yang city in He nan, and the *zhou* became a Metropolitan Area, *si zhou* 司州. Under Eastern Wei, during the *tian ping* 天平 reign period (534 - 537), it again became Luo zhou. At the beginning of the *da ye* 大業 reign period (605 – 618) of the Sui 隋, it was moved to the present-day Luo yang city, and the *zhou* was changed to be He nan 河南 commandery. In 621, under Tang 唐, it was again named Luo zhou. Later, at the beginning of the *yong chun* 永淳 reign period (682 – 683) of the Tang, the territory administered included Ji yuan 濟源 city and the area of Wen xian 溫縣 county in the South, Song xian 嵩縣 county and the two cities of Deng feng 登封 and Yu zhou 禹州 in the North, the counties of Luo ning 洛寧 and Mian chi 澠池 in the East, and the Si shui 汜水 town of Xing yang 滎陽 city as well as Xin mi 新密 city in the West in present-day He nan. In 713, the status of the status of the area was raised to be He nan fu 河南府. Mentioned with 47, 693.

Luo zhou 羅州 [1]

Name of a *zhou* 州. It was established under Southern Dynasties' Liang 梁. Its seat of administration was in present-day Hua zhou 化州 city in Guang dong 廣東. The territory administered comprised the area of Hua zhou city and the two cities of Zhan jiang 湛江 and Wu chuan 吳川 in Guang dong. The *zhou* was abolished under Sui 隋, at the beginning of the *da ye* reign period (605 – 618), but reestablished under Tang 唐, in 622. The next year, the seat of administration was moved to a point northeast of present-day Lian jiang 廉江 city in Guang dong. Under Northern Song 宋, in 972, the *zhou* was abolished. Mentioned with 144.

-M-

Ma cheng 麻城 [1]

Name of a county. It was established under Sui 隋, in 598, by changing the name of Xin an 信安 county. It was under Huang zhou 黄州. It was located 15 *li* east of present-day Ma cheng city in Hu bei 湖北. At the beginning of the *da ye* 大業 reign period (605 – 618) of the Sui, it became subordinate to Yong an 永安 commandery, but Tang 唐 put it under Huang zhou. In 808, it was eliminated but re-established in 849. During Southern Song 宋, in 1236, the seat of administration was moved to Shi zi 什子 mountain, located 80 *li* east of the present-day county. Yuan 元 put it under Huang zhou lu 黃州路 but, during the *zhi yuan* 至元 reign period (1264 – 1294), the seat of administration was moved from Shi zi mountain to the old seat. At the end of Yuan, the seat of administration was moved to the present seat of administration. In 1986, the county became a city.

Ma dao 馬道 [1]

Minor place name. This is now Ma dao postal station of Ma dao town, located 22 km south of present-day Liu ba 留壩 county in Shaan xi 陝西. Mentioned with 1147.

Ma gu 麻姑 [1]

Name of a mountain. It is located southwest of present-day Nan cheng 南城 county in Jiang xi 江西. The mountain has a "spring offering divine service," Shen gong quan 神功泉, and the water of the spring is said to be good for brewing. Mentioned with 732.

Ma hu 馬湖 [2]

Name of a lake. It was in present-day Bo bai 博白 county in Guang xi 廣西, but has now dried up. Mentioned with 474.

Ma ling shan 馬嶺山 [1]

Name of a mountain. It is on the boundary of present-day Bo bai 博白 county in Guang Xi 廣西. Mentioned with 474.

Ma yang 麻陽 [3]

Name of a county. It was established under Tang 唐, in 620. It was placed under Chen zhou 辰州. Its seat of administration was in the old county of Huang sang xiang 黃桑鄉, located east of present-day Gao cun 高村 town of Ma yang county in Hu nan 湖南. Under Northern Song 宋, during the *xi ning* 熙寧 reign period (1068 – 1077), the seat of administration was moved to present-day Jin he 錦和 town, located southwest of Gao cun town. It was subordinated to Yuan zhou 沅州. Yuan 元 put it under Yuan zhou lu 沅州路. Ming 明 put it under Yuan zhou, and Qing 清 put it under a Yuan zhou fu 沅州府. In 1953, the county had its administration moved to present-day Gao cun. Mentioned with 202.

Man gu 滿谷 [1]

Name of a mountain valley. It was located 500 *li* east of Heng 衡 mountain in Hu nan 湖南 but further details are unavailable. Mentioned with 1109.

Man jie 蠻界 [1]

Large regional designation. It refers to the present-day Liang guang 兩廣, and the western and southern part of Si chuan 四川, once occupied by minority tribes, the "region of the Man 蠻." Mentioned with 9.

Man la jia guo 滿剌加國 [1]

Early country. This is Malacca, a kingdom based on an island off the southwestern coast of the Malayan peninsula. As an independent kingdom it flourished between the 14th and 16th centuries including as a Chinese ally during the reign of King Paramesvara (1402 - 1414) after the Zheng he 鄭和 (1371 – 1433) voyages.

Malacca was conquered by the Portuguese, in 1511, and ceased to be an independent kingdom. Mentioned with 1265.

Man yi 蠻夷 [1]

Large regional name. It refers in general to the area in early times occupied by minority peoples in the south of China. Mentioned with 164.

Mang bu 芒部 [1]

Name of a *lu* 路. Early Yuan 元, during the *zhi yuan* reign period (1264 – 1294), established Mang bu lu 芒部路, a *lu* 路 subordinate to the Wu sa wu meng Pacification Office, Wu sa wu meng *xuan wei si* 烏撒烏蒙宣慰司. Its seat of administration was at a location north of present-day Zhen xiong 鎮雄 county in Yun nan 雲南. The territory administered comprised the area of present-day Zhen xiong, Wei xin 威信, and Yi liang 彝良 in Yun nan. Under Ming 明, in 1382, the area was changed to Mang bu fu 芒部府, and was made subordinate to the Yun nan Provincial Administration Commission, Yun nan *bu zheng si* 雲南布政司. The seat of administration was moved to a point 7 *li* northwest of the present-day Zhen xiong county. The following year, the area was changed to be subordinate to the Si chuan Administration Commission, Si chuan *bu zheng si* 四川布政司. In 1526, the area was changed to be the Zhen xiong Tribal Office, Zhen xiong *jun min fu* 鎮雄軍民府. Mang bu was subordinate to it. Under Qing 清, in 1727, the area was detached and made part of Yun nan. Mentioned with 1018.

Mao 茂 [1]

Name of a *zhou* 州. See → Mao zhou 茂州. Mentioned with 585.

Mao ling 茂陵 [1]

Name of a county. It was established under Western Han 漢 by changing the name of Mao ling yi 茂陵邑. It was subordinated to You fu feng 右扶風. Its seat of administration was in present-day Mao ling village of Nan wei xiang 南位鄉, located 19 *li* northeast of Xing ping 興平 city in Shaan xi 陝西. Western Jin 晉 eliminated it, and made it part of Shi ping 始平 county. Mentioned with 801.

Mao luo dao 毛羅島 [1]

Name of an island. This was originally Tun luo dao 屯羅島. In the *Ben cao yan yi* 本草演義, "Elucidations of *materia medica*," it was incorrectly named Mao luo dao 毛羅島. The island is the same as the Dan luo 耽羅 of the *Yuan shi* 元史, "Dynastic History of Yuan," that is Jeju-do 濟州島 island located south of present-day Korea. Mentioned with 195.

Mao shan 茅山 [21]

Name of a mountain. This is Da mao shan 大茅山 in the southwestern portion of Jiang su 江蘇. Its expanse covers the present-day counties and cities of Ju rong 句容, Jin tan 金壇, Li shui 溧水 and Li yang 溧陽. Under Qi 齊 of the Southern Dynasties, Tao Hong jing 陶弘景 (456-536) of Liang 梁 lived there as a recluse. Mentioned with 428, 455, 631, 894, 978, 1039, 1063, 1238, 1438.

Mao zhou 茂州 [5]

Name of a *zhou* 州. It was founded by Tang 唐, in 634, by changing the name of Nan hui zhou 南會州. Its seat of administration was in present-day Mao xian

茂縣 county in Si chuan 四川. In 742, it became Tong hua 通化 commandery. In 758, it again became Mao zhou. The territory administered corresponded to Mao county and Bei chuan 北川 county in present-day Si chuan. Yuan 元 subordinated it to the Tu bo Pacification Office, Tu bo *xuan wei si* 吐蕃宣慰司. Ming 明 subordinated it to Cheng du fu 成都府. It abolished Wen shan 汶山 county and made it part of Mao zhou. Qing 清 raised it to the status of a directly administered *zhou*, *zhi li zhou* 直隸州. In 1913, it was demoted to be Mao county. Mentioned with 111, 557, 1289, 1481.

Mei 眉 [1]
Name of a *zhou* 州. See → Mei zhou 眉州. Mentioned with 208.

Mei ling 梅嶺 [1]
Name of a mountain range. It was one of China's "five mountain ranges," (see → Wu ling 五嶺). This is the Da yu 大庾 range, located on the border of Jiang xi 江西 and Guang dong 廣東. Mentioned with 1279.

Mei shan 禖山 [1]
Name of a mountain. Details are lacking. Mentioned with 757.

Mei shan 眉山 [1]
Name of a county. It was established under Northern Song 宋, in 976, by renaming Tong yi 通義 county. Its seat of administration was in present-day Mei shan 眉山 county in Si chuan 四川. Under Yuan 元, in 1283, it became part of Mei zhou 眉州. In 1913, Mei zhou was reduced to being Mei shan county. Mentioned with 1475.

Mei xian 郿縣 [1]
Name of a county. It was established by Warring States Qin 秦. Its seat of administration was at a location on the northern bank of the Wei he 渭河 river, 15 *li* east of present-day Mei xian 郿縣 county in Shaan xi 陝西. Northern Wei 魏 changed the county to be Ping yang 平陽 county but Western Wei changed it to be Mei cheng 郿城 county. Northern Zhou 周 changed it to be Zhou cheng 周城 county, and Sui 隋, during the *kai huang* 開皇 reign period (581 - 600), changed the county to be Wei bin 渭濱 county, but later, during the *da ye* 大業 reign period (605 – 618), changed it to be Mei xian county. In 620, under Tang 唐, the seat of administration was moved to present-day Mei xian county. In 1964, the county became Mei xian county. Mentioned with 1532.

Mei zhou 眉州 [7]
Name of a *zhou* 州. It was founded under Western Wei 魏, in 554. Its seat of administration was in present-day Mei shan 眉山 county in Si chuan 四川. Under Northern Zhou 周, its administrative territory corresponded to the counties of present-day Mei shan, Dan ling 丹棱 and Qing shen 青神 in Si chuan. Sui 隋 eliminated it but it was reestablished under Tang 唐, in 619. Later in Tang, during the *tian bao* 天寶 reign period (742 – 756), it became Tong yi 通義 commandery but, in 758, again became Mei zhou. Its jurisdiction was expanded to include Peng shan 彭山 and Hong ya 洪雅. Its size was reduced from Song 宋 on. Yuan 元 put it under Jia ding lu 嘉定路, and Mei shan county was eliminated

as it became part of a *zhou*. At the beginning of Ming 明, it was reduced to Mei county but later, in 1380, its status was raised to be Mei zhou. In 1913, a Mei shan county was established. Mentioned with 19, 184, 359, 456, 787, 1028, 1491.

Meng 蒙 [1]

Name of a mountain. See→ Meng shan 蒙山. Mentioned with 768.

Meng 孟 [3]

Name of a *zhou* 州. See → Meng zhou 孟州. Mentioned with 38, 1017, 1523.

Meng shan 蒙山 [5 + 1]

□ Name of a mountain. [5] It is the Meng shan 蒙山 mountain connecting the west part of present-day Ming shan 名山 county in Si chuan 四川 with Ya an 雅安 city. It lies across the northwestern side of the county city of Ming shan county. The northern part is higher than the south. In a northeast-southwest zonal distribution, the mountain extends to the city of Ya an. It is about 10 km long and 4 km wide. The top is divided into 5 peaks, arranged like a lotus blossom. The highest peak is called Shang qing feng 上清峰, 1456 m above sea level. Mentioned with 768.

□ Name of a mountain. [1] It is also called Dong meng shan 東蒙山. It is located southwest of present-day Meng yin 蒙陰 county in Shan dong 山東, on the border of Ping yi 平邑 county. Mentioned with 1017.

Meng xi 孟溪 [1]

Name of a town. It is located 100 *li* northwest of present-day Tong ren 銅仁 city in Gui zhou 貴州 on the northern bank of the Meng xi 孟溪 river. The town is located at the eastern foot of Fan jing 梵淨 mountain in the hinterland, in the middle part of Song tao 松桃 county. The town was once one of the five major market towns in the eastern part of ancient Gui zhou. Mentioned with 1277.

Meng xi 夢溪 [1]

Name of a park located at the southeastern corner of present-day Zhen jiang 鎮江 city district in Jiang su 江蘇 province. During Northern Song 宋 times, this park was said to have been designed by the famous government official and scientist Shen Kuo 沈括 (1031 – 1095). The name comes from a small stream in the park.

Meng xian 鄳縣 [1]

Name of a county. This is Meng 鄳 county. It was established by Western Han 漢. Its seat of administration was at a location west of present-day Luo shan 羅山 county in He nan 河南. Northern Qi 齊 changed it into Gao an 高安 county. This was abolished under Sui 隋, in 583. Mentioned with 1250.

Meng yang 孟養 [1]

Name of a Ming 明 area Tribal Administration, *tu si* 土司. It began during the *zhi yuan* 至元 reign period (1264 – 1294) of Yuan 元 times, when a Tribal Command was established for Yun yuan lu 雲遠路 at Meng yang 孟養, the Yun yuan lu *jun min zong guan fu* 雲遠路軍民總管府. Later, during the *hong wu* 洪武 reign period (1368 – 1398) of the Ming 明, it was changed to be Yun yuan fu 雲遠府, but shortly thereafter a Meng yang Tribal Pacification Office, Meng yang *jun min xuan wei si* 孟養軍民宣慰司, was established. It was focused on the Burmese Kachin Kingdom, and staffing of the administration were local Thai people. The territory administered comprised much of the Kachin Kingdom, from the Irrawaddy River toward the West, up to a strip of land including Jie sha 傑沙, located northeast of Shi jie 實階 district, and Shang qin dun 上欽墩 county in the Northwest. After the *wan li* 萬曆 reign period (1573 – 1620), the area was gradually absorbed by a local Toungoo (Chinese: Dong wu 洞吾) kingdom (1531 - 1752) and disappeared. The territory ceased to be Chinese. Mentioned with 664.

Meng zhou 孟州 [4]
Name of a *zhou* 州. It was established under Tang 唐, in 843. Its seat of administration was at a location 15 *li* south of present-day Meng 孟 county in He nan 河南. The territory administered comprised the counties and cities of Ji yuan 濟源, Meng xian 孟縣, and Wen xian 溫縣, as well as the strip of the two towns of Si shui 汜水 and Guang wu 廣武 on the southern bank of the Yellow River. Under Yuan 元, the size of the *zhou* was somewhat reduced. Under Ming 明, in 1377, it was demoted to a county. Mentioned with 668, 871, 1444, 1459.

Mi 密 [2]
Name of a *zhou* 州. See → Mi zhou 密州. Mentioned with 703, 1057.

Mi shan 密山 [1]
Name of an ancient mountain. It could have been located in the southwestern suburb of present-day Luo yang 洛陽 or possibly in Xin jiang 新疆, but additional details are lacking. Mentioned with 62.

Mi yun 密雲 [1]
Name of a mountain. It is located on the borders to present-day Feng ning 豐寧 county in He bei 河北. Northern Wei 魏 established a Mi yun county using the name of the mountain. Mentioned with 1443.

Mi zhou 密州 [5]
Name of a *zhou* 州. It was established by Sui 隋, in 585, by changing the name of Jiao zhou 膠州. Its seat of administration was in present-day Zhu cheng 諸城 city in Shan dong 山東. During Tang 唐, the territory administered comprised an area in Shan dong extending from Yi shan 沂山 and Ju nan 莒南 toward the East, and from Jiao zhou and An qiu 安丘 toward the South. After the Jin 金 period, the southern part was reduced in size. The *zhou* was abolished under Ming 明, in 1368. Mentioned with 20, 221, 481, 819, 1424.

Mian dian 緬甸 [2]
Name of a Pacification Office, *xuan wei si* 宣慰司. It was founded under Ming 明, in 1394, as the Mian zhong *xuan wei si* 緬中宣慰司. Later, a Mian dian 緬甸 Tribal Pacification Commission, *jun min xuan wei shi si* 軍民宣慰使司, was established. In 1427, the Mian zhong Tribal Pacification Commission was combined with it and became part of a Mian dian 緬甸 Pacification Commission. It was subordinate to the Yun nan Provincial Administration Commission. Its seat of administration was in present-day Ava in Myanmar, Mian dian a wa 緬甸阿瓦. Its jurisdiction corresponded to the region of the middle watershed of the

Ayeyarwady River south of Katha in Myanmar. In 1527, the area was occupied by the kingdom of Meng yang 孟養. Mentioned with 1040, 1102.

Mian shang 綿上 [3]

This is an early place name from Spring and Autumn times, located in the old state of Jin 晉, southeast of present-day Jie xiu 介休 city in Shan xi 山西. Jie Zhitui 介之推, a government official noted for his loyalty to Duke Wen 文 of Jin, lived as an hermit there. He died there in 636 BCE. In the same year, Duke Wen turned an area of Mian shang into a sacrificial field for Jie Zhitui. Mentioned with 461.

Mian shui 沔[水] [5]

Name of a river. In ancient times, the Han shui 漢水 was generally called Mian shui. According to the *Shui jing zhu* 水經注, "Classic of Waters, Notes," a river in the North called Ju shui 沮水, originating from a point west of present-day Liu ba 留壩 in Shaan xi 陝西, is the Mian 沔 river, while a second river originating in the West from a point north of present-day Ning qiang 寧強 is the Han 漢 river. After the two sources come together they are called the Mian shui or Han shui. The northern source is long and the western one is short. Thus the northern source, i.e., the Mian river, is considered the real source of the river. The western Han shui is also called the Han. Mentioned with 75, 317, 1079, 1088.

Mian xian 沔縣 [1]

Name of a county. It was founded under the Ming 明, in 1374, by changing Mian zhou 沔州. It was subordinated to Han zhong fu 漢中府. Its seat of administration was in Wu hou 武侯 town west of the present-day Mian county in Shaan xi 陝西. In 1935, the seat of administration was moved to the present-day Mian xian county and, in 1964, it was changed to be Mian county. Mentioned with 520.

Mian zhou 沔州 [1]

Name of a *zhou* 州. It was established by Western Wei 魏, in 554, by changing Jiang zhou 江州 to Mian zhou. Its seat of administration was at a location southeast of present-day Han chuan 漢川 city in Hu bei 湖北. The *zhou* was eliminated under Northern Zhou 周, but reestablished under Tang 唐. The seat of administration was moved to present-day Han yang 漢陽 district of Wu han city in Hu bei. In 826, it became a part of E zhou 鄂州. Mentioned with 75.

Mian zhou 綿州 [4]

Name of a *zhou* 州. It was founded by Sui 隋, in 585. Its seat of administration was at a location east of the present Mian yang 綿陽 city. During the Tang 唐, the administrative area of the *zhou* corresponded to the watershed of the Fu jiang 涪江 between the Jiang you 江油 and Mian yang, west of the Tong he 潼河 river and east of the upper watershed of the Luo jiang 羅江 in Si chuan 四川. Later there were changes. Under the Qing 清, in 1728, the status of the *zhou* was raised to be a directly administered *zhou*, *zhi li zhou* 直隸州. In 1913, it became Mian yang county. Mentioned with 322, 548, 1168.

Miao 苗 [1]

Allusion to a place name. It refers to the areas in Hu nan 湖南 and Gui zhou 貴州 occupied by the Miao nationality. Mentioned with 1242.

Min 岷 [1]

Name of a river. This is the Min jiang 岷江. From the time of the *Book of History's* "Yu gong 禹貢," "Tribute of Yu 禹," on down, the Min was universally regarded as the source of the Yang zi. Only later was this corrected by Xu Xia ke 徐霞客 (1587-1641). To be sure, the Min is an affluent of the Yang zi providing much of its water. Its sources are from the southern slopes of Min shan 岷山 mountain north of Song pan 松潘 county in Si chuan 四川. The river then flows south through the present-day cities and counties of Song pan, Mao xian 茂縣, Wen chuan 汶川 and Du jiang yan 都江堰 and runs into the Yang zi on the east of Yi bin 宜賓 city. The entire length is 793 km. Mentioned with 1096.

Min 閩 [48 + 5]

□ Abbreviation for Fu jian 福建. [48] The area was originally occupied by Min yue 閩越 peoples, but Qin 秦 established Min zhong 閩中 commandery and, at the beginning of Han 漢, there was a Min yue 閩越 country. The area was in the Asian subtropical zone and from antiquity there were many snakes. The snake was worshipped as a totem by the ancient Yue tribes that lived in the area. The name Min comes from this. Mentioned with 71, 79, 139, 182, 247, 298, 322, 323,332, 351, 456, 472, 537, 572, 578, 603, 608, 616, 660, 685, 748, 768, 807, 848, 915, 960, 963, 1028, 1057, 1170, 1171, 1204, 1239, 1269, 1407, 1455, 1493, 1494, 1508.

□ Name of a *zhou* 州. [5] It was established under Southern Dynasties' Chen 陳. Its seat of administration was in present-day Fu zhou 福州 city. In 564, it was eliminated but under Sui 隋, during the *da ye* 大業 reign period (605 – 618), it was reestablished by changing the name of Quan zhou 泉州 to Min zhou 閩州. Under Tang 唐, in 725, it was renamed Fu zhou. Mentioned with 71, 79, 139, 182, 247, 298, 322, 323, 332, 351, 456, 472, 537, 572, 578, 603, 608, 616, 660, 685, 748, 768, 807, 848, 915, 960, 963, 1028, 1057, 1170, 1171, 1204, 1239, 1269, 1407, 1455, 1493, 1494, 1508.

Min guang 閩廣 [8]

Regional name. It is primarily Fu jian 福建 province as well as Guang dong 廣東 and Guang xi 廣西. Because this area is located in China's South, the climate is favorable to humans, and the area has abundant production. Mentioned with 94, 262, 330, 344, 590, 1198, 1460

Min ling 閩嶺 [1]

General regional name. It refers to the mountainous areas in the North of Fu jian 福建. Mentioned with 160.

Min shan 岷山 [1]

Name of a mountain. It is also called Wen shan 汶山 and Wen jiao 汶焦. The mountain is located in the northwestern part of present-day Si chuan 四川 on the borders of Si chuan and Gan su 甘肅. This is the area where the water of the Min jiang 岷江 system and the Jia ling jiang 嘉陵江 system originate, with the white snow of tall mountains shining white. The highest peak in the range, the Xue bao ding 雪寶鼎, is 5588 m above sea-level. Mentioned with 1407.

Min yue 閩越 [3]
Name of an ancient country, also called Min yue guo 閩越國. It was located in the northern part of what is now Fu jian 福建. This was jointly founded by Yue people who had fled there, after their state had been destroyed during the Warring States times by Chu 楚, and local Bai yue 百越 people. When it existed, it was large, reaching a high point between 334 and 110 BCE. The royal city built by the Min yue king Wu Zhu 無諸 (died 192 BCE) at present-day Xing tian 興田 town on the south side of Wu yi shan 武夷山 city in Fu jian was the largest city of the whole area of the Southeast of that period. Mentioned with 914, 962, 1349.

Min yue 閩粵 [1]
Name of an ancient country. See → Min yue 閩越. Mentioned with 823.

Min zhong 閩中 [18]
Name of a commandery. It was established by Qin 秦. Its seat of administration was in present-day Fu zhou 福州 city. The territory administered corresponded to the entire province of present-day Fu jian 福建 and Ning hai 寧海, and the watersheds of the Ling jiang 靈江, the Ou jiang 甌江 and the Fei yun jiang 飛雲江 south of Ning hai in Zhe jiang. The commandery disappeared at the end of Qin. In olden times the name became an alternative designation for Fu zhou fu 福州府. For example, everything mentioned in the *Min zhong kao* 閩中考 of Ming 明 writer Chen Mingshu 陳鳴樹 took place within Fu zhou. Mentioned with 94, 288, 330, 400, 407, 588, 674, 687, 790, 931, 1064, 1105, 1245, 1400, 1407, 1486.

Min zhou 岷州 [1]
Name of a *zhou* 州. It was established under Western Wei 魏, in the 6th century, and was named after Min shan 岷山 mountain. Its seat of administration was in present-day Min xian 岷縣 county. The territory administered corresponded to an area of present-day Min xian county. In the middle of the 8th century, the area was conquered by the Tibetans. Following the *xi ning* 熙寧 reign period (1068 – 1077) of Northern Song 宋, the jurisdiction of the *zhou* comprised the counties of Xi he 西和, Li xian 禮縣 and Min xian in Gan su 甘肅, and the southeastern part of the Gan nan Zang Autonomous Prefecture, Gan nan Zang zu *zi zhi zhou* 甘南藏族自治州. During the *shao xing* 紹興 reign period (1131 – 1162), the area became Xi he zhou 西和州 and the administration was moved to present-day Xi he. Yuan 元 reestablished Min zhou at the present Min county. Ming 明 changed the *xian* 縣 to Min zhou guard but Qing 清, during the *yong zheng* 雍正 reign period (1722 – 1735), restored Min zhou. In 1913, the *zhou* was demoted to Min county. Mentioned with 799.

Ming 明 [4]
Name of a *zhou* 州. It was established under Tang 唐, in 738, and the *zhou* was named because of the presence of Si ming 四明 mountain within its boundaries. Its seat of administration was at a location south of present-day Ning bo 寧波 city. The territory administered comprised the Yong jiang 甬江 watershed, and

present-day Ci xi 慈溪 and Zhou shan 舟山 archipelago in Zhe jiang 浙江. Under Southern Song 宋, in 1194, the status of the area was promoted to be Qing yuan fu 慶元府. Mentioned with 468, 741, 908, 1057.

Ming sha xian 鳴沙縣 [1]
Name of a county. It was founded under Sui 隋, in 599. Its seat of administration was in present-day Ming sha 鳴沙 town, located northeast of Zhong ning 中寧 county in Ning xia 寧夏. Under Tang 唐, in 706, the area was taken by the Turks (Tu jue 突厥). The county city was laid to waste and abandoned. It was recovered in 849. During the Ming 明, the county was abolished and became the territory of Guang wu ying bao 廣武營堡. Mentioned with 191.

Ming shan 明山 [1]
Name of a mountain in the southern part of present-day Hu nan 湖南 but details of its exact location are lacking. Mentioned with 141.

Ming shan xian 茗山縣 [1]
Name of a county. The text is perhaps corrupt and this may be an error. Mentioned with 1017.

Mo bei 漠北 [2]
General regional term. It refers to the great deserts of Mongolia and the term was in use from Han 漢 times on with the variant Mu bei 幕北. During the Qing 清 period, all of Mongolia was called Mo bei. Mentioned with 229, 1332.

Mo luo duan cha guo 抹羅短叱國 [1]
Name of an ancient Indian kingdom. The Sanskrit name was also transliterated Mo luo ju zha guo 秣羅矩吒國. It was located in the extreme southern part of the Indian peninsula, covering the watersheds of the Kaveri river and the Vaigai river of Tamil Nadu. Mentioned with 680.

Mo qie tuo guo 摩伽陀國 [3]
Ancient Indian country. This is the Magadha of the Buddhist sources, a name transliterated in various forms in Chinese. Magadha is associated with considerable Buddhist legend and was the center of several Indian empires. It was located in the region of present-day Bihar.

Mu 睦 [3]
Name of a *zhou* 州. See → Mu zhou 睦州. Mentioned with 121, 278, 871.

Mu fu shan 幕阜山 [1]
Name of mountains. They are also called Tian yue 天嶽 mountains. They are on the border area of the three provinces of Hu nan 湖南, Hu bei 湖北 and Jiang xi 江西, running in a northeast-southwest direction. The highest peak in the range is 1596 m above sea level and is located on the northeastern boundary of present-day Ping jiang 平江 county in Hu nan. Mentioned with 1485.

Mu lan zhou 木蘭洲 [1]
Local place name. This is a small island in the Xun yang jiang 潯陽江 river, located in a section of the river north of present-day Jiu jiang 九江 city flowed

through by the Yang zi. It gets its name, "Magnolia Island", because of the many magnolias growing there. Mentioned with 789.

Mu men 木門 [1]
Name of a town. This is Mu men town located southeast of present-day Wang cang 旺蒼 county in Si chuan 四川. Later, during the *wu de* 武德 reign period (618 – 628) of Tang 唐, Jing zhou 靜州 was established there. Mentioned with 322.

Mu yang 牧羊 [1]
Name of an early city. It is also called Mu yang cheng 木羊城. It was located at present-day Jin zhou 金州 town northeast of Da lian 大連 city in Liao ning 遼寧, about 500 m from the ocean. From Qin 秦 and Han 漢 times on, this city was associated with important maritime transport routes and a strategic coastal defense area in north China. Mentioned with 1030, 1171.

Mu yang shan 牧羊山 [1]
Name of a mountain. It was located southwest of present-day Xu yi 盱眙 county in Jiang su 江蘇. Mentioned with 1030.

Mu yun chang 暮雲場 [1]
Minor place name. It is located somewhere near present-day Laos but specific details are lacking.

Mu zhou 睦州 [4]
Name of a *zhou* 州. It was founded under the Sui 隋, in 603. Its seat of administration was in Zhi shan 雉山. Tang 唐 moved the seat of administration to Jian de 建德. The administrative area corresponded to the present-day three cities and counties of Tong lu 桐廬, Jian de and Chun an 淳安 in Zhe jiang 浙江. Under Northern Song 宋, in 1121, the area became Yan zhou 嚴州. There were many mountains within its territories. With lacquer, bamboo and an abundance of trees. The rebellion led by Fang La 方臘 (died 1121) started in the area. Mentioned with 172, 313, 768, 1017.

-N-

Nan 南 [108 + 1]
□ Regional designation, South, in contradistinction to *bei* 北, "North." [108] Mentioned with 54, 70, 94, 101, 103, 117, 142, 144, 164, 198, 243, 290, 320, 332, 336, 344, 347, 358, 388, 413, 414, 415, 422, 429, 438, 442, 450, 470, 497, 501, 503, 518, 530, 537, 590, 596, 603, 606, 614, 618, 628, 633, 647, 660, 663, 667, 673, 685, 692, 694, 759, 768, 782, 925, 960, 971, 1004, 1038, 1064, 1065, 1087, 1148, 1158, 1194, 1204, 1219, 1222, 1245, 1248, 1256, 1257, 1264, 1272, 1275, 1296, 1297, 1305, 1316, 1340, 1342, 1358, 1369, 1381, 1386, 1388, 1398, 1400, 1419, 1439, 1447, 1460, 1475, 1479, 1486, 1490, 1499.
□ Name of a *zhou*. [1] The reference is to Nan kang zhou 南康州. It was established under Tang 唐, in 627. Its seat of administration was in present-day De

qing 德慶 county in Guang dong 廣東. The administrative area included the territories of the cities and counties of De qing, Yu nan 郁南, and Yun fu 雲浮. It was eliminated in 637. Mentioned with 535.

Nan an 南安 [1 + 1]
□ Name of a commandery. [1] It was established by Eastern Han 漢, in 188, by splitting Han yang 漢陽 commandery. Its seat of administration was in San tai xiang 三台鄉, located southeast of present-day Long xi 隴西 county in Gan su 甘肅. Its jurisdiction corresponded to the eastern part of Long xi county and the territories of Ding xi 定西 city and Wu shan 武山 county in present-day Gan su. It was abolished under Sui 隋, at the beginning of the *kai huang* 開皇 reign period (581 – 600). Mentioned with 249.
□ Name of an administrative unit. [1] It was established as Nan an army, Nan an jun 南安軍, by Northern Song 宋, in 990. Its seat of administration was in present-day Da yu 大余 county in Jiang xi 江西. The territory administered comprised the watersheds of the Zhang shui 章水 and Shang you shui 上猶水 in present-day Jiang xi. In 1277, under Yuan 元, its status was raised to be Nan an lu 南安路. Mentioned with 348.

Nan bang zhu guo 南邦諸國 [1]
This is a regional name. It refers generally to a strip of present-day Southeast Asia. Mentioned with 106.

Nan cheng 南城 [1]
This is an error for Nan yue 南越. See → Nan yue.

Nan chu 南楚 [5]
Regional name. The term corresponds to the central portion of present-day An hui 安徽, all of Jiang xi 江西 and the eastern parts of Hu nan 湖南 and Hu bei 湖北. Mentioned with 442, 782, 850, 877, 1004.

Nan dan 南丹 [1]
Name of a *zhou* 州. See → Nan dan zhou 南丹州. Mentioned with 951.

Nan dan zhou 南丹州 [2]
Name of a *zhou* 州. It was established under Northern Song 宋, in 974. Its seat of administration was in present-day Ba e 巴峨 village, located northeast of Yue li xiang 月里鄉 which in turn is located northwest of Nan dan 南丹 county in Guang xi 廣西. In 1107, the *zhou* was changed to be Guan zhou 觀州. In 1110, it again became Nan dan zhou. Under Yuan 元, in 1276, the seat of administration was moved to the present Nan dan county. Under Ming 明, in 1395, the *zhou* was eliminated. Instead, a Nan dan guard was established. In 1404, Nan dan zhou was reestablished. In 1924, it became Nan dan county. Mentioned with 970, 1366.

Nan di 南地 [7]
General regional name. It refers in general to the South. Mentioned with 29, 195, 314, 415, 996, 1241, 1399.

Nan en zhou 南恩州 [5]
Name of a *zhou* 州. It was established by Northern Song 宋, in 1048, by changing the name of En zhou 恩州. Its seat of administration was in present-day Yang

jiang 陽江 city in Guang dong 廣東. The territory administered comprised the three present-day cities of En ping 恩平, Yang jiang 陽江 and Yang chun 陽春 in Guang dong. Under Yuan 元, in 1276, it become Nan en lu 南恩路. In 1282, it was again Nan en zhou. It was abolished under Ming 明, in 1369. Mentioned with 112, 144, 248, 294, 1044.

Nan fan 南番 [27]

Regional name. It refers to the maritime region of Southeast Asia and countries with which China had an ocean contact. Mentioned with 14, 104, 110, 226, 330, 478, 493, 603, 738, 748, 794, 807, 840, 898, 945, 1140, 1236, 1248, 1264, 1340, 1384, 1386, 1440, 1467, 1515.

Nan fan zhu guo 南番諸國 [6]

Name of a region. See → Nan fan 南番. Mentioned with 197, 480, 680, 887, 1246.

Nan fang 南方 [124]

Regional name referring to the Chinese South. Mentioned with 74, 94, 126, 161, 168, 175, 206, 222, 234, 254, 285, 294, 298, 300, 316, 317, 323, 347, 364, 372, 381, 412, 467, 474, 493, 495, 515, 541, 572, 573, 602, 610, 631, 632, 644, 647, 656, 671, 692, 694, 760, 763, 768, 787, 793, 799, 806, 810, 814, 833, 846, 850, 861, 882, 892, 944, 954, 960, 963, 968, 984, 995, 1006, 1007, 1013, 1014, 1017, 1030, 1038, 1041, 1067, 1091, 1094, 1106, 1110, 1117, 1197, 1201, 1222, 1226, 1238, 1241, 1243, 1252, 1272, 1287, 1289, 1291, 1294, 1295, 1296, 1298, 1307, 1340, 1377, 1378, 1399, 1401, 1409, 1410, 1415, 1420, 1475, 1482, 1492, 1497, 1516, 1518, 1526, 1528, 1529, 1538, 1575.

Nan guang 南廣 [1]

Regional name. It is a general reference to the present-day Ling nan 嶺南 area. Mentioned with 1429.

Nan hai 南海 [1 + 5 + 82 + 5 + 1 + 11 + 10]

□ Regional name. [1] It refers to the areas occupied by various nationalities in the South.

□ Regional name. [5] It refers exclusively to the present-day Ling nan 嶺南 region. Mentioned with 777, 930, 1076, 1335.

□ Regional name. [82] The reference is to the South China Sea. Mentioned with 43, 80, 82, 94, 127, 133, 138, 169, 175, 217, 232, 243, 267, 302, 318, 346, 347, 376, 393, 396, 398, 400, 401, 405, 409, 421, 424, 438, 464, 478, 501, 506, 518, 531, 591, 608, 621, 656, 674, 716, 772, 824, 840, 847, 855, 892, 894, 919, 945, 961, 1012, 1021, 1030, 1044, 1056, 1078, 1084, 1101, 1123, 1170, 1194, 1264, 1273, 1294, 1297, 1341, 1356, 1389, 1421, 1422, 1455, 1463, 1467, 1489, 1508, 1515, 1517, 1576.

□ Regional name. [5] It refers to the area south of the Western Ocean, that is, present-day Qing hai hu 青海湖/Kokonor lake. Mentioned with 1335.

□ Name of an ocean district. [1] It refers to the Ocean east of China. Mentioned with 1030.

□ Name of a commandery. [11] It was established by Qin 秦, in 214 BCE. Its seat of administration was in present-day Guang zhou 廣州 city in Guang dong 廣東 province. Later, during the Qin and during the Han 漢, the area became part of Nan yue 南越. It was reestablished under Western Han, in 111 BCE, after it destroyed Nan yue. Its jurisdiction corresponded to the area south of the Weng jiang 滃江 and Da luo 大羅 mountains, the delta of the Pearl River and the area east of the watershed of the Sui jiang 綏江. Later, its territories were reduced. Under Sui 隋, in 589, it was eliminated but, in 607, it was reestablished by renaming Fan zhou 番州. Its seat of administration was in present-day Guang zhou city. Under Tang 唐, in 621, it became Guang zhou but, in 742, it was changed to be Nan hai commandery. It again became Guang zhou in 758. Mentioned with 80, 110, 113, 376, 405, 427, 685, 790, 1335, 1467.

□ Regional name. [10] It refers to a strip of present-day Southeast Asia and its littoral and even as far as the Indian Ocean region. Mentioned with 11, 49, 511, 680, 708, 775, 961, 1030, 1086, 1264.

Nan hai huo zhou 南海火洲 [1]

Regional name. It refers to the volcanic, that is, *huo shan* 火山, islands in a strip of present-day Southeast Asia. Mentioned with 487.

Nan hai zhu guo 南海諸國 [3]

Regional designation. See under → Nan hai 南海. Mentioned with 187, 480, 843.

Nan he xian 南河縣 [3]

Name of a county. It was established under Tang 唐, in 622. Its seat of administration was in present-day Gu cheng 古城 town, located southeast of Lu chuan 陸川 county in Guang xi 廣西. In 773, it was put under Shun zhou 順州. Under Northern Song 宋, in 972, it was abolished. Mentioned with 428.

Nan huang 南荒 [1]

Regional name. It refers to the distant regions of the south. Mentioned with 1341.

Nan jian 南劍 [1]

Name of a *zhou* 州. It was established by Northern Song 宋, in 979. Its seat of administration was in present-day Nan ping 南平 city. The territory administered corresponded to the present-day cities and counties of Nan ping, San ming 三明, Jiang le 將樂, Shun chang 順昌, Sha xian 沙縣, You xi 尤溪, Yong an 永安 and Da tian 大田, in Fu jian. Under the Yuan 元, in 1278, its status was raised to Nan jian lu 南劍路. Mentioned with 535.

Nan jiang 南江 [1]

Reference to a river in the south. Details of its exact location are lacking. Mentioned with 1105.

Nan jing 南京 [1]

Name of a capital city. Under the Jin 金, in 1153, Bian jing 汴京 was changed to be Nan jing. Its seat of administration was in present-day Kai feng 開封 city in He nan 河南. In 1214, then Jin emperor Xuan zong 宣宗 left Zhong du 中都, a city located just southwest of present-day Beijing 北京, and fled south to this Nan jing. It was abolished after the fall of Jin. Mentioned with 733.

Nan jun 南郡 [6]

Name of a commandery. It was established by Qin 秦, in 278 BCE. Its seat of administration was in present-day Ji nan cheng 紀南城, located northwest of the former Jiang ling 江陵 county seat, in the Jing zhou 荊州 district of Jing zhou city in Hu bei 湖北. Later, it was moved to the old Jiang ling county seat in Jing zhou district of present-day Jing zhou city. Under Western Han 漢, the administrative area of the commandery corresponded in Hu bei to an area extending from Xiang fan 襄樊 city and the area of Nan zhang 南漳 county toward the South, from Song zi 松滋 county and Gong an 公安 county toward the North, from Hong hu 洪湖 city toward the West, and from Li chuan 利川 city and the area of Wu shan 巫山 in Chong qing 重慶 toward the East. It was eliminated under Sui 隋, in 581, but, in 605, reestablished. Tang 唐 changed the commandery to be Jing zhou. Mentioned with 258, 442, 723, 1443, 1532.

Nan kang 南康 [6]

Name of a commandery. See → Nan kang jun 南康郡. Mentioned with 348, 957, 1105, 1435.

Nan kang jun 南康軍 [2]

Administrative unit. It was established under Northern Song 宋, in 982. Its seat of administration was in present-day Xing zi 星子 county in Jiang xi 江西. The territory administered corresponded to the counties of Xing zi, Yong xiu 永修 and Du chang 都昌 in Jiang xi. Under Yuan 元, during the *zhi yuan* 至元 reign period (1264 – 1294), the status of the area was raised to a *lu* 路. Mentioned with 644, 890.

Nan kang jun 南康郡 [2]

Name of a commandery. It was established under Western Jin 晉, in 282. Its seat of administration was at a location northeast of present-day Yu du 于都 county in Jiang xi 江西. Under Eastern Jin, in 349, the seat of administration was moved to a point southwest of present-day Gan zhou 贛州 city in Jiang xi. In 411, it was moved to a point northeast of the present Gan zhou city. During Jin times, the administrative area of the commandery corresponded to the region of Nan kang 南康, Gan xian 贛縣, Xing guo 興國, and Ning du 寧都 in the South of present-day Jiang xi. In 420, under Liu Song 劉宋, it was changed to be Nan kang country/domain. At the beginning of the *yong ming* 永明 reign period (483 – 493) of Southern Qi 齊, it again became Nan kang commandery. Under Liang 梁, in 552, the seat of administration was moved to a point southwest of Gan zhou. Under Sui 隋, in 589, it was changed to establish Qian zhou 虔州 but, in 609, the area again became Nan kang commandery. Under Tang 唐, in 622, the area was changed to be Qian zhou. Later, the seat of administration was moved to present-day Gan zhou city. In 742, it again became Nan kang commandery but, in 758, it was changed again to be Qian zhou. Mentioned with 288.

Nan liang jun 南涼郡 [1]

This is a common referent for → Gao liang jun 高涼郡. Mentioned with 316.

Nan man 南蠻 [1]

Name for "southern aboriginals" tribal groups. In ancient times, the term was a general one for the minority groups of China's South. Mentioned with 1353.

Nan ping cheng 南平城 [1]
Name of a city. It was located southwest of present-day Turfan city in Xin jiang 新疆. Mentioned with 174.

Nan pu 南浦 [1]
Minor place name located outside the southern gate of present-day Pu cheng 浦城 county in Fu jian 福建. Mentioned with 1014.

Nan qiu cun 南丘村 [1]
Name of a village located on the outskirts of present-day Peng lai 蓬萊 city in Shan dong 山東, but further details are lacking. Mentioned with 361.

Nan shan 南山 [1 + 7 + 5]
□ Name of a mountain. [1] It is Qing long 青龍 mountain of present-day Liu bu 柳埠 town, Li cheng 歷城 district in Ji nan 濟南 city in Shan dong 山東. Mentioned with 474.
□ Name of a mountain. [7] Further details are not available. Mentioned with 689, 760, 782, 809, 933, 1250.
□ Name of mountains. [5] They are also called Zhong nan shan 終南山 and Zhong nan shan 中南山. The mountains in question are the Qing ling 秦嶺 mountain range of Shaan xi 陝西. Mentioned with 311, 633, 660, 1275, 1475.

Nan tian zhu 南天竺 [1]
This is a regional name and refers to the countries of Southern India, Tian zhu 天竺. India was divided into five parts: East, South, West, North and Central. "Southern India," also known as the South Indian states, referred to some tiny kingdoms located south of the Deccan Plateau in the south-central part of the Indian sub-continent. Mentioned with 670.

Nan tu 南土 [14]
Regional name. It is a general reference to the China South. Mentioned with 114, 126, 298, 314, 522, 547, 873, 942, 980, 1110, 1420.

Nan xi 南息 [1]
This is an error of the BCGM authors for Nan en 南恩. See → Nan en zhou 南恩州.

Nan xiong 南雄 [1]
Name of a *fu* 府. It was established by Northern Song 宋, in 971, by changing the name of Xiong zhou 雄州. Its seat of administration was in the present-day Nan xiong 南雄 city in Guang dong 廣東. Because there was a Xiong zhou in He bei 河北, it was named Nan xiong. Its jurisdiction corresponded to the territories of the two present-day counties of Nan xiong and Shi xing 始興 in Guang dong. Under Yuan 元, in 1278, the area became Nan xiong lu 南雄路. Under Ming 明, in 1368, it was changed to Nan xiong fu 南雄府. In 1806, the area became the Nan xiong directly administered *zhou*, Nan xiong *zhi li zhou* 南雄直隸州. In 1811, it was again promoted to be Nan xiong fu. In 1812, the area was again changed to be Nan xiong zhou 南雄州. In 1919, it became Nan xiong county. Mentioned with 1040.

Nan yang 南陽 [21]

Name of a commandery. It was established under Warring States Qin 秦, in 272 BCE. Its seat of administration was in present-day Nan yang city in He nan 河南. Its jurisdiction under Western Han 漢 corresponded in present-day He nan to an area extending from Tong bai 桐柏 county toward the West, from Dan jiang kou 丹江口 city in Hu bei 湖北 toward the East, from Lu shan 魯山 county in He nan toward the South, and from Deng zhou 鄧州 city in He nan and from Guang shui 廣水 city in Hu bei toward the North. Western Jin 晉 changed the area into Nan yang country and reduced the area of its jurisdiction. Under Liu Song 劉宋, the area again became Nan yang commandery. Under Sui 隋, in 581, the area was changed to be Deng zhou but, in 605, under Tang 唐 it was again made Nan yang commandery. The seat of administration was moved to Deng zhou city. In 619, under Tang, it became Deng zhou again but, in 742, again became Nan yang commandery. It was changed to be Deng zhou again in 758. Mentioned with 298, 376, 474, 575, 707, 750, 787, 988, 1065, 1068, 1406, 1482, 1485, 1509, 1532, 1551, 1577.

Nan ye xi 南野溪 [1]

Name of a river. It is also called the Nan ye shui 南野水, and is located northwest of present-day Nan kang 南康 city in Jiang xi 江西. Mentioned with 1435.

Nan yi 南夷 [2]

Regional name in early times designating the minority peoples of the South. It also referred to regions distant on the frontiers of the South. Mentioned with 1188, 1506.

Nan yin du 南印度 [1]

Regional name. This is another term for → Nan tian zhu 南天竺, "Southern India." India was divided into five parts: East, South, West, North and Central. "Southern India," also known as the South Indian states, Nan yin du zhu guo 南印度諸, referred to some tiny kingdoms located south of the Deccan Plateau in the south-central part of the Indian sub-continent. Mentioned with 945.

Nan yin du jing 南印度境 [1]

Regional name. See → Nan yin du 南印度. Mentioned with 680 and 945.

Nan yue 南越 [8]

Name of an early country. Originally this was a regional term for the areas occupied by the ancestral Yue 越 people in Fu jian 福建 and related areas. During Western Han 漢 times, in 203, the Qin 秦 official Zhao Tuo 趙佗 (230 – 137) established himself as king of Nan Yue, in this case still located in southeast China. In 196 BCE, the Han government sent Lu Jia 陆賈 (ca. 240 – 170) to recognize him as king. Zhao later, during the reign of Empress Lü Zhi 吕雉 (241 – 180), declared himself the emperor of Nan yue. His capital was in what is now Guang zhou 廣州 in Guang dong 廣東. This kingdom or empire included the area of the three present-day provinces of Guang dong, Guang xi 廣西 and Hai nan 海南, and the northern part of present-day Vietnam. The area was conquered by

Han, in 111 BCE, and the kingdom destroyed. Mentioned with 135, 234, 287, 380, 501, 585, 961, 1329.

Nan yue 南粵 [2]
This term is the same as → Nan yue 南越. Mentioned with 54, 113.

Nan yue 南岳 [1]
Name of a mountain. This is one of the "Five Peaks," wu yue 五岳. It is Tian zhu shan 天柱山 mountain located south of present-day Qian shan 潛山 county in An hui 安徽. Mentioned with 1157, 1469.

Nan yue 南嶽 [1]
Name of a mountain. See → Nan yue 南岳.

Nan yue shan 南越山 [1]
Name of a mountain. Details are lacking. Mentioned with 362.

Nan zhao 南詔 [4]
Name of an early kingdom. Its original name was Meng she zhao 蒙舍詔, and it constituted one of the six Zhao 詔 existing during the Tang 唐 period in the Er hai 洱海 region. Its seat of administration was at a location 34 *li* northwest of the Wei shan yi hui 巍山彝回 independent county of the Wei mountain Li 彝 people Muslims in present-day Yun nan 雲南. During the *kai yuan* 開元 reign period (713 – 741) of early Tang times, Pi Luoge 皮羅閣 (died 748) unified the six Zhao and moved the seat of administration to present-day Tai he 太和 village, located 10 *li* north of Da li 大理 city in Yun nan. In 738, the ruler of Nan Zhao was enfeoffed by Tang as King of Yun nan. Later he made Yang ju mie 陽苴咩 city (this is the former Da li city 26 *li* north of present-day Da li city in Yun nan) as his western capital, and made Tuo dong 拓東 city (this is present-day Kun ming 昆明 city in Yun nan) as his eastern capital. The territories of Nan zhao included the entire province of Yun nan, the area in Si chuan 四川 south of the Da du he 大渡河, the western part of Gui zhou 貴州 and parts of Burma, Thailand, Laos and Vietnam. In 795, Tang established a Yun nan Pacification Commission, Yun nan an fu si 雲南安撫司. In 902, Nan zhao was destroyed by aristocrat Zheng Maisi 鄭買嗣 (861 – 909). Mentioned with 10, 404, 794.

Nan zheng 南鄭 [3]
This is the name of a county. It was established by Warring States Qin 秦 and was located two *li* east of present-day Han zhong 漢中 city in Shaan xi 陝西. Under Western Wei 魏, in 554, it was changed to be Guang yi 光義 county. Under Sui, in 583, it again became Nan zheng county. Under Southern Song 宋, in 1219, the seat of administration was moved to present-day Han zhong city. Mentioned with 1449, 1485.

Nan zhong 南中 [17 + 1 + 3]
□ Regional name. [17] It corresponds to the area in Si chuan 四川 south of the Da du he 大渡河, and the two provinces of Yun nan 雲南 and Gui zhou 貴州. Three Kingdoms Shu Han 蜀漢 made the Ba Shu 巴蜀 area its base and its lands were south of Ba Shu, thus the name. Mentioned with 182, 283, 300, 499, 740, 780, 838, 951, 953, 986, 1000, 1010, 1054, 1105, 1107, 1185, 1331.

□ Regional name. [1] It refers to the Chinese South. Mentioned with 1461.
□ Regional name. [4] It refers to the Ling nan 嶺南 area. Mentioned with 65, 255, 489, 1283.

Nan zhong ba jun 南中八郡 [1]
Combined regional name. This corresponds to the area south of the Da du he 大渡河 in Si chuan 四川 and the two provinces of Yun nan 雲南 and Gui zhou 貴州. Mentioned with 1128.

Nan zhong zhou jun 南中州郡 [1]
Combined regional name referring to the Chinese South. Mentioned with 558.

Nan zhou 南州 [1]
Regional name. It refers to the Chinese South and in particular to the Ling nan 嶺南 area. Mentioned with 1427.

Nei huang 內黄 [1]
Name of a county. It was established under Western Han 漢. Its seat of administration was in present-day Gu 故 village located northeast of Tang yin 湯陰 county in He nan 河南. During Eastern Wei 魏, at the beginning of the *tian ping* 天平 reign period (729 – 749), the county was eliminated. It was reestablished under Sui 隋, in 586. Northern Song 宋 moved the seat of administration to present-day Nei huang county. Mentioned with 1092.

Nei xiang 內鄉 [2]
Name of a county. It was established under Sui 隋, in 583, by changing the name of Zhong xiang 中鄉 county to avoid a taboo. Its seat of administration was in present-day Xi xia 西峽 county in He nan 河南. Jin 金 moved the seat of administration to present-day Nei xiang county in He nan. Mentioned with 707, 1379.

Ni bo luo guo 尼波羅國 [1]
This is the name of an ancient country written in various ways (Ni po luo 泥婆羅; Ni ba la 尼八剌) in addition to the above. This is certainly Nepal. Mentioned with 108.

Ni shan 泥山 [1]
Name of a town. It was established under Northern Song 宋, and came under Ping yang 平陽 county. This is present-day Yi shan 宜山 town, located 30 *li* east of Cang nan 蒼南 county in Zhe jiang 浙江. Mentioned with 940.

Ning 寧 [1]
Name of a *zhou*. See under → Ning zhou 寧州. Mentioned with 535.

Ning bo 寧波 [1]
Name of a *fu*. It was founded under Ming 明, in 1381, by changing the name of Ming zhou 明州. Its seat of administration was in present-day Ning bo 寧波 city in Zhe jiang 浙江. The territory administered comprised the cities and counties of Ning bo, Yin zhou 鄞州, Ci xi 慈溪, Feng hua 奉化 and Xiang shan 象山, as well as the Zhou shan 舟山 archipelago, in Zhe jiang. It was abolished in 1912. Mentioned with 815.

Ning guo 寧國 [2]

Name of a *fu* 府. It was established under Southern Song 宋, in 1166, by raising Xuan zhou 宣州 to the status of Ning guo fu 寧國府. Its seat of administration was in present-day Xuan cheng 宣城 city in An hui 安徽. The territory administered comprised the present-day cities and counties of Xuan zhou, Ning guo, Nan ling 南陵, Jing xian 涇縣, Jing de 旌德 and Huang shan 黃山 in An hui. Under Yuan 元, in 1277, the area became Ning guo lu 寧國路. At the beginning of Ming 明, it again became Ning guo fu. Ning guo fu was abolished in 1912. Mentioned with 641.

Ning pu 寧浦 [1]

Name of a commandery. It was established under Western Jin 晉, in 286, by converting the He pu shu guo *du wei* 合浦屬國都尉, "Commandant for the [Tribal] Nations under He pu." Its seat of administration was at a location on the southern bank of the Yu jiang 鬱江, 7 *li* southwest of present-day Heng 橫 county in Guang xi 廣西. The territory administered comprised the present territory of Heng xian county in Guang xi. Mentioned with 787.

Ning xia 寧夏 [3]

Name of a *fu* 府. It was established under Ming 明, in 1370, by changing the name of Ning xia lu 寧夏路. It was subordinate to the Gan su Branch Secretariat, Gan su *xing sheng* 甘肅行省. The seat of administration was at present-day Yin chuan 銀川 city in Ning xia 寧夏. Its administrative territory comprised the area along the banks of the Yellow River in the northwestern part of Ning xia. In 1372, it was abolished but, in 1393, it was changed to establish a Ning xia guard. Under the Qing 清, in 1724, it was again made a *fu*. In 1913, it was abolished. Mentioned with 445, 738, 1335.

Ning xiang 寧鄉 [1]

Name of a county. It was established under Southern Qi 齊. Its seat of administration was at a location on the outskirts of present-day Luo ding 羅定 city in Guang dong 廣東. Mentioned with 983.

Ning zhou 寧州 [8 + 2]

□ Name of a *zhou* 州. [8] It was founded, in 271, by splitting Yi zhou 益州. Its seat of administration was in Jin cheng 晉城, located 32 *li* northeast of present-day Jin ning 晉寧 county in Yun nan 雲南. The territory administered was somewhat greater than present-day Yun nan, but did not include the Yun nan Northeast. In 282, Ning zhou was abolished and made part of Yi zhou. A Nan yi jiao wei 南夷校尉, "Southern Barbarians Commandant," was established to protect the area. In 303, Ning zhou was reestablished and its jurisdiction expanded. It comprised the area of the two present-day provinces of Yun nan and Gui zhou 貴州. Under Liu Song 劉宋, the seat of administration was moved to present-day San cha 三岔, 14 *li* north of Qu jing 曲靖 city in Yun nan. Southern Qi 齊 moved the seat of administration to present-day Jiu cheng 舊城, located 3 *li* southwest of Lu Liang 陸良 county in Yun nan. Western Wei 魏 changed the name of the *zhou* to Nan ning zhou 南寧州. Mentioned with 461, 493, 535, 666, 818, 995, 1264, 1289, 1375.

□ Name of a *zhou*. [2] It was established under Western Wei 魏, in 554, by changing the name of Bin zhou 豳州. Its seat of administration was in present-day Ning xian 寧縣 county in Gan su 甘肅. Under Sui 隋, in 605, it was changed to Bei di 北地 commandery but under Tang 唐, in 618, it again became Ning zhou. In 742, its name was changed again to Peng yuan 彭原 commandery but, in 758, it again became Ning zhou. The territory administered was reduced, and by and large it did not exceed the present-day boundaries of Gan su. Mentioned with 1413.

Niu tou shan 牛頭山 [1]
Name of a mountain. It is also called Niu jiao 牛角 mountain. It is situated at Utchat on the banks of the Karakash river, located in Xin jiang 新疆 southwest of present-day Khotan (He tian 和田) city. Mentioned with 1406.

Niu yang zhi shan 杻陽之山 [1]
This is a place name from the *Shan hai jing* 山海經, "Classic of Mountains and Seas." Additional details are lacking. Mentioned with 1315.

Niu zhu ji 牛渚磯 [1]
Name of a mountain. It is also called Niu zhu shan 牛渚山 and Cai shi shan 采石山. This was a quarry located southwest of present-day Ma an shan 馬鞍山 city in An hui 安徽. Mentioned with 1264.

Nü chuang zhi shan 女床之山 [1]
Place name from the *Shan hai jing* 山海經, "Classic of Mountains and Seas." Details are lacking. Mentioned with 285.

Nü gua 女瓜 [1]
A region in the Southwest. Details are lacking. Mentioned with 1467.

Nü guo 女國 [1 + 1]
□ Name of an ancient country, the country of the female king. [1] This is generally taken as referring to the early Yamato in Kyushu in Japan. Mentioned with 1271.
□ This is the name of an ancient tribe. [1] A geographical location is lacking. Mentioned with 1532

Nü ji zhi shan 女幾之山 [2]
Place name from the *Shan hai jing* 山海經, "Classic of Mountains and Seas." Details are lacking. Mentioned with 543, 966.

Nü zhen 女真 [1]
Ethnic name. There are many transcription variants, such as Lü zhen 慮真,Nü zhi 女直, Nü zhi 女質 and Zhu li zhen 朱里真. These are the Mo he 靺鞨 peoples of Tang 唐 times that were called Nü zhen 女真 beginning with the Five Dynasties period. They resided in Northeast Manchuria and adjacent parts of Siberia, along the Song hua jiang 松花江 and the lower watershed of the Hei long jiang 黑龍江, down to the sea. Mentioned with 215.

Nü zhen di mian 女真地面 [1]
Regional name. It generally refers to the area occupied by the Nü zhen 女真 tribes. Mentioned with 397.

Nü zhi 女直 [3]
This is another name for the → Nü zhen 女真. This may be written so due to a Liao 遼 taboo, but most likely this is simply another transliteration of the tribal name. Mentioned with 824, 1205, 1363.

-O-

Ou yue 甌越 [1]
Name used in antiquity in referring to early tribal peoples in the South. Originally, the Ou yue were a kind of Yue 越. During Qin 秦 and Han 漢 times, they were spread out in a strip of the Ou jiang 甌江 watershed in the southern part of present-day Zhe jiang 浙江. During the time of Emperor Hui 惠 (210 – 188) of Western Han, the chief of the Ou yue was enfeoffed as Dong hai wang 東海王 with a capital at Dong ou 東甌, thus the name "The Yue of Ou" applied to the group. Mentioned with 254.

-P-

Pan hou zhi shan 潘侯之山 [1]
Mountain name found in the *Shan hai jing* 山海經, "Classic of Mountains and Seas." Details are lacking. Mentioned with 747

Pan pan guo 盤盤國 [2]
Also: Pan pan 槃槃, this is an ancient name for a kingdom located on the eastern coast of the isthmus of the Malay peninsula, across from the Gulf of Siam. The area once maintained an active communication with China. Mentioned with 1030, 1139.

Pan yu 番禺 [5]
Name of a county. It was founded under Qin 秦, in 214 BCE, after the conquest of Lu liang di 陸梁地 of the Nan yue 南越 area. It was administered by Nan hai 南海 commandery and from what is now Canton city in Guang dong 廣東. In 1933, the administrative seat was moved to Xin zao 新造. In 1945, administration was moved to Shi qiao 市橋 town. Mentioned with 585, 1036.

Pan zhou 潘州 [2]
Name of a *zhou* 州. It was founded under Tang 唐, in 634. Its seat of administration was in present-day Gao zhou 高州 city in Guang dong 廣東. It was abolished, in 643, but reestablished in 650. Its administrative area corresponded to the present-day cities and counties of Gao zhou, Mou ming 茂名, Dian bai

雷白 and Wu chuan 吳川 in Guang dong. Under Northern Song 宋, in 972, the *zhou* was abolished. Mentioned with 428, 1028.

Pei 沛 [1]

Regional name. It can either be the Pei country of Western Jin 晉 or Pei county under its control.

□ For Pei country see the entry ' Pei guo 沛國.

□ Name of a county. It was established by Qin 秦, and put under Si shui 泗水 commandery. Its seat of administration was in present-day Pei xian 沛縣 county in Jiang su 江蘇. Under Western Han 漢 , it was subordinated to Pei commandery and, under Eastern Han, it was subordinated to Pei country/domain. Under Liu Song 劉宋, it came under Pei commandery. It was eliminated under Northern Qi 齊. Under Sui 隋, in 596, it was reestablished and put under Xu zhou 徐州. At the beginning of the *da ye* 大業 reign period (605 – 618), it came under Peng cheng 彭城 commandery. Under Tang 唐, it was subordinated to Xu zhou. Jin 金 put it under Teng zhou 滕州. In 1235, under the early Mongols, its seat of administration was in Teng zhou. In 1252, it was subordinated to Teng zhou. In 1265, under Yuan 元, it was eliminated and its territory was combined with Feng xian 豐縣 county. It was reestablished the next year, subordinate to Ji zhou 濟州. At the beginning of Ming 明, it was subordinated to Xu zhou, but Qing 清 put it under Xu zhou fu 徐州府. In 1781, because of the Yellow River flooding, the seat of administration was moved to the Qi shan 栖山 embankment, southwest of the present county. In 1851, the seat of administration was again transferred to present-day Wei shan 微山 county in Shan dong 山東. In 1862, it was transferred to the present-day Pei xian county. Mentioned with 633.

Pei guo 沛國 [2]

Name of a country/domain. It was founded by Eastern Han 漢, in 44, by changing Pei 沛 commandery. Its seat of administration was in the present-day Xiang shan 相山 district northwest of Huai bei 淮北 city in An hui 安徽. Its administrative area comprised present-day Su zhou 宿州 city, Xiao 蕭 county, Ling bi 靈壁 county, Bo zhou 亳州 city and Gu zhen 固鎮 county of Ban bu 蚌埠 city, Wu he 五河 county, Huai bei city and Sui xi 濉溪 county in An hui, Pei xian county and Feng xian 豐縣 county in Jiang su 江蘇, and Yong cheng 永城 city in He nan 河南. Three Kingdoms Wei 魏 moved the seat of administration to present-day Pei county in Jiang su 江蘇. Western Jin 晉 returned it to the old seat. Later, it was again made a commandery. Mentioned with 206.

Peng cheng 彭城 [0 + 12 + 1]

□ Name of a county. Established by Southern Dynasties' Liang 梁, and put under Dong peng cheng 東彭城 commandery. Its seat of administration was in the outskirts of present-day Guan yun 灌雲 county in Jiang su 江蘇. Under Eastern Wei 魏, in 549, it was changed to An le 安樂 county.

□ Name of a commandery. [12] It was established by Western Han 漢, in 69 BCE, by changing the name of Chu zhou 楚州. Its seat of administration was in present-day Xu zhou 徐州 city in Jiang su 江蘇. Its administrative area comprised present-day Xu zhou city, Tong shan 銅山 county, the southeast part of

Pei xian 沛縣 county, the northwestern part of Pei zhou 邳州 city in Jiang su, the eastern portion of Sui xi 濉溪 county in An hui 安徽, and the area of Wei shan 微山 county in Shan dong 山東. In 49 BCE, the area again became Chu 楚 country. Under Eastern Han, in 88, it was changed to Peng cheng 彭城 country/domain. Under Liu Song 劉宋, in 421, it again became Peng cheng commandery. It was abolished as a commandery under Sui 隋, at the beginning of the *kai huang* 開皇 reign period (601-620), but restored in 608. Under Tang 唐, in 621, it was again changed to be Xu zhou. In 742, it was changed to Pen cheng commandery and, in 758, it was changed again to be Xu zhou. Mentioned with 222, 272, 462, 733, 941, 949, 1017, 1175, 1393, 1417, 1435, 1478.

□ Name of a county. [1] It was established under Qin 秦, and subordinated to Si shui 泗水 commandery. Its seat of administration was in present-day Xu zhou city in Jiang su. After the fall of Qin, Xiang Yu 項羽 (232 – 202) established himself in the area as hegemon of Western Chu 楚. His capital was there. Western Han put the county under Chu country. It became Xu zhou under Liu Song and later Peng cheng commandery. Sui left it under Peng cheng commandery, but Tang put it under Xu zhou. Under Tang and during the Five Dynasties, the area was divided into Wu ning Army Military Commissioner, Wu ning *jun jie du shi* 武寧軍節度使, and Gan hua Army Military Commissioner, Gan hua *jun jie du shi* 感化軍節度使. Under Yuan 元, in 1265, it was eliminated and its territory became part of Xu zhou. Mentioned with 864, 1037.

Peng jia shan 蓬葭山 [1]

Name of a mountain. Details are lacking. Mentioned with 1260.

Peng lai 蓬萊 [2]

Name of a mountain. This is one of three legendary mountains found in the Eastern Ocean. Mentioned with 895, 1301.

Peng lai shan 蓬萊山 [1]

Name of a mountain. It is north of the present-day Xin hui 新會 district of Jiang men 江門 city in Guan dong 廣東. Mentioned with 627.

Peng lai xian 蓬萊縣 [2]

Name of a county. It was established under Tang 唐, in 707, by dividing up Huang xian 黃縣 county. It was administered by Deng zhou 登州, with the seat of administration located at present-day Peng lai 蓬萊 city in Guang dong 廣東. During Ming 明 and Qing 清, the area was put under Deng zhou fu 登州府. In 1991, the county was changed into a city. Mentioned with 361, 474.

Peng xi 蓬溪 [2]

Name of a county. It was established under Tang 唐, in 742, by changing the name of Tang xing 唐興. It was placed under Sui ning 遂寧 commandery. Its seat of administration was in present-day Peng xi 蓬溪 county in Si chuan 四川. Under Ming 明, in 1377, it was eliminated and made part of Sui ning county. Three years later, Peng xi county was restored. It has continued to the present.

Peng xian 彭縣 [1]

Name of a county. It was established under Ming 明, in 1377, by reducing the status of Peng zhou 彭州. It was put under Cheng du fu 成都府. Its seat of administration was in present-day Peng zhou city in Si chuan 四川. It was eliminated under Qing 清, in 1688, but restored again in 1728. In 1993, the county was changed into a city. Mentioned with 473.

Piao guo 剽國 [1]

Name of an early country. Identical with Piao guo 驃國. It was located in Burma along the Irrawaddy River. Mentioned with 245.

Ping gu 平谷 [1]

Name of a county. It was established under Western Han 漢, and put under Yu yang 漁陽 commandery. Its seat of administration was in Cheng zi zhuang 城子莊, located 20 *li* northwest of present-day Ping gu 平谷 district in Bei jing 北京 city. It was eliminated under Western Jin 晉, but was later reestablished. It was abolished under Northern Wei 魏, in 446. The present Ping gu district was reestablished by Yuan 元, in 1276. Mentioned with 900, 1071.

Ping jiang 平江 [1]

□ Name of a county. It was established by Five Dynasties' Chu 楚 by changing the name of Chang jiang 昌江 county, and put under Yue zhou 岳州. Its seat of administration was in the present-day Ping jiang county in Hu nan 湖南. Under Yuan 元, in 1295, its status was raised to be Ping jiang zhou 平江州. Under Ming 明, in 1370, it was again changed to be a county, and put under Yue zhou fu 岳州府.

□ Name of a *fu*. It was established under Northern Song 宋, in 1113, by raising the status of Su zhou 蘇州. Its seat of administration was in present-day Su zhou city in Jiang su 江蘇. Its administrative area comprised present-day Su zhou city, Chang shu 常熟 city, Kun shan 崑山 city, and Wu jiang 吳江 city in Jiang su, and the northwestern part of Shang hai 上海 city. Under Yuan 元, in 1276, it was changed to be Ping jiang lu 平江路, and put under Zhe jiang Branch Secretariat, Zhe jiang *xing sheng* 浙江行省. At the beginning of Ming 明, it was changed to be Su zhou fu 蘇州府. Mentioned with 315.

Ping mian 平緬 [1]

Name of a *lu* 路. It was established under Yuan 元, in 1276, and put under Yun nan Branch Secretariat, Yun nan *xing sheng* 雲南行省. Its seat of administration was in present-day Long chuan 瀧川 county in Yun nan 雲南. The territory administered comprised more or less Long chuan county in modern Yun nan and parts of Burma. It was abolished at the beginning of Ming 明. Mentioned with 794.

Ping nan xian 平南縣 [1]

Name of a county. It was established under Tang 唐, in 633. Its seat of administration was in present-day Ping nan 平南 county in Guang xi 廣西. Mentioned with 991.

Ping quan 平泉 [1]
This is the villa of Tang 唐 poet and writer Li Deyu 李德裕 (787 – 849/850), located at present-day Liang cun gou 梁存溝, north of Yi chuan 伊川 county in He nan 河南.

Ping shi 平氏 [1]
Name of a county. It was established under Western Han 漢, and put under Nan yang 南陽 commandery. Its seat of administration was in present-day Ping shi 平氏 town located northwest of Tong bai 桐柏 county in He nan 河南. Western Jin 晉 put it under Yi yang guo 義陽國. It was abolished under Liu Song 劉宋, but reestablished under Southern Qi 齊, in 487, and subordinated to Nan yi yang 南義陽 commandery. Under Northern Song 宋, it was abolished in 972. Mentioned with 1509.

Ping shou 平壽 [1]
Name of a county. It was established under Western Han 漢, and put under Bei hai 北海 commandery. Its seat of administration was located southwest of present-day Wei fang 濰坊 city in Shan dong 山東. It was eliminated under Northern Qi 齊, in 556, but restored under Tang 唐, in 619, and subordinated to Wei zhou 濰州. Four years later it was abolished. Mentioned with 787.

Ping xian 平縣 [1]
Name of a county. Specific information on its location is lacking. Mentioned with 126.

Ping yang 平陽 [2 + 4]
□ Name of a county. [2] It was founded by the state of Jin 晉, around 514 BCE. Its seat of administration was in present-day Jin dian 金殿 town, located 18 *li* southwest of Lin fen 臨汾 city in Shan xi 山西. It was eliminated under Northern Wei 魏, in 445. A Ping yang county was reestablished, in 487. Under Sui 隋, in 581, it was changed to be Ping he 平河 county. Mentioned with 444, 1034.
□ Administrative unit. [4] It was established under Northern Song 宋, in 1116, by raising the status of Jin zhou 晉州 and establishing Ping yang fu 平陽府. Its seat of administration was in Lin fen city in modern Shan xi. The territory administered comprised the present-day cities of Lin fen and Huo zhou 霍州, and the present-day counties of Hong tong 洪洞, Xiang fen 襄汾, Fu shan 浮山, Fen xi 汾西, An ze 安澤 and Gu xian 古縣 in Shan xi. At the beginning of Yuan 元, the area became Ping yang lu 平陽路 and, in 1305, it was changed to be Jin ning lu 晉寧路. Under Ming 明, in 1368, it was changed to Ping yang fu 平陽府. Its administrative area was expanded to include a region in the Southwest of present-day Shan xi extending from Shi lou 石樓, the area south of Ling shi 靈石 county, An ze 安澤, and Yuan qu 垣曲 county toward the West. The administrative unit was abolished in 1912. Mentioned with 444, 861, 862.

Ping yi 馮翊 [1]
Name of a commandery. See → Ping yi jun 馮翊郡 Mentioned with 532.

Ping yi jun 馮翊郡 [1]
Name of a commandery. It was established as Zuo ping yi 左馮翊 under Western Han 漢, in 104 BCE, by changing the name of Nei shi 内史. Its seat of administration was located northwest of present-day Xi an 西安 city in Shaan xi 陝西. Its administrative territory comprised in Shaan xi at the middle and lower watershed of the Luo he 洛河 river an area extending from the Wei he 渭河 river toward the North and from the Jing he 涇河 river toward the East. Eastern Han moved the seat of administration to a point southwest of present-day Gao ling 高陵 county. Three Kingdoms Wei 魏 removed the character *zuo* 左, "left" from the name, and changed it to be Ping yi commandery. Its seat of administration was in present-day Da li 大荔 county in Shaan xi. Northern Wei 魏 administered it from the present-day Gao ling 高陵 county, and its administrative area was reduced in size. It was abolished under Northern Zhou 周. Sui 隋 reestablished it, in 607, in the present Da li county. Tang 唐, in 618, changed it to Tong zhou 同州, but in 742 again changed it to Ping yi commandery. In 758, it was again changed to Tong zhou. Mentioned with 594.

Ping zhou 平州 [1 + 1]
□ Name of a *zhou* 州. [1] Details are lacking. Mentioned with 126.
□ Name of a *zhou*. [1] It was established under Northern Wei 魏, in 407. Its seat of administration was located north of present-day Lu long 盧龍 county in He bei 河北. Tang 唐 moved the seat of administration to the present-day Lu long county. The administrative area of the *zhou* corresponded to the area from the Tu he 徒河 watershed toward the East and from the Great Wall toward the South. Liao 遼 put it under Nan jing 南京 circuit. In 1215, the Mongols changed it to Xing ping fu 興平府. Mentioned with 931.

Po li 頗黎 [1]
Name of an early country. Alternative writings Po li 婆里 and Suo li 娑里. This may be Sāri, a city now the capital of Iran's Mazandaran province. Mentioned with 104 See also under → Po ling guo 頗陵國.

Po ling guo 頗陵國 [1]
Name of an early country. This is apparently Bolor in India near Nepal. See also under Po li 頗黎, which may be a variant of this place name. Bolor is itself a variant of the word giving rise to the Chinese word for glass, *bo li* 玻璃. Mentioned with 103.

Po lü guo 婆律國 [2]
Name of an early country. Alternative writing: Bo lü 波律. It also occurs apparently as Bo lü 波律, and is believed by some to be a variant of Po li 婆利. This is present-day Barus/Baros on the West coast of Sumatra of Indonesia. Mentioned with 680.

Po luo men 婆羅門
Name used by the BCGM authors to refer to India possibly including Sri Lanka. See → Po luo men guo 婆羅門國.

Po luo men guo 婆羅門國 [9]

Name used by the BCGM authors to refer to India possibly including Sri Lanka, and probably representing the word Brahman, pfiualamun. Mentioned with 14, 485, 614, 852, 853, 854, 1169, 1279, 1359.

Po yang 鄱陽 [3]

□ Name of a county. It was created under Western Han by changing the name of Fan yang 番陽 county. It was put under Yu zhang 豫章 commandery. Its seat of administration was in present-day Gu xian du 古縣渡 town, located northeast of Po yang county in Jiang xi 江西. Under Three Kingdoms' Wu 吳, the seat was moved to the present Po yang county.

□ Name of a commandery. It was established under Eastern Han 漢, in 210, when Sun Quan 孫權 (182 – 252) divided Yu zhang 豫章 commandery. Its seat of administration was in the present Po yang county. In 245, under Three Kingdoms' Wu 吳, the seat of administration was moved to the old city of Wu rui 吳芮. Its administration covered the eastern bank of Lake Po yang and the area of Jin xian 進賢 county in the East, and the watersheds of the Xin jiang 信江, and Le an jiang 樂安江 (other than Wu yuan 婺源 county) in Jiang xi 江西. Jin 晉 moved the administration to Shi men jie 石門街 town located north of modern Po yang county. Liu Song 劉宋 restored the present Po yang county as the seat of administration. Sui 隋 abolished it, in 589. But later, in 605, reestablished Po yang 鄱陽 commandery by changing the name of Rao zhou 饒州. It was continued to be administered from Po yang county. At the beginning of Tang 唐, the name was changed again to be Rao zhou. In 742, it was changed again to be Po yang commandery. It again became Rao zhou, in 758. Yuan 元 changed the area to be Rao zhou lu 饒州路. In 1361, this was changed to Po yang fu 鄱陽府, but this was subsequently changed to Rao zhou fu 饒州府. Mentioned with 840, 896, 1375.

Pu 蒲 [1]

Name of a *zhou* 州. See → Pu zhou 蒲州. Mentioned with 1318.

Pu ban xian 蒲坂縣 [1]

Name of a county. It was established under Qin 秦, and put under He dong 河東 commandery. Its seat of administration was in present-day Pu zhou 蒲州 town, located southwest of Yong ji 永濟 city in Shan xi 山西. Western Han 漢 changed this to be Pu fan 蒲反 county, but Eastern Han restored it as Pu ban 蒲坂 county. Under Sui 隋, in 596, the seat of administration was moved to a point east of Pu zhou town. In 606, it was abolished and made part of He dong county. Mentioned with 324.

Pu ding fen si 普定分司 [1]

This is the name of a military affairs unit. It was established under Ming 明, in 1382, and subordinated to the Si chuan Regional Military Commission, Si chuan *du si* 四川都司. Its seat of administration was in present-day An shun 安順 city in modern Gui zhou 貴州. In 1438, it was changed and subordinated to the Gui zhou administration. During the *cheng hua* 成化 reign period (1465 – 1487), the An shun zhou 安順州 administration was moved to Pu ding wei cheng 普定衛城. In 1672, it became Pu ding 普定 county. Mentioned with 1061.

Pu man 蒲蠻 [1]

Regional name of a settlement of minority nationalities. The administrative territory comprised present-day Chang ning 昌寧 county, Feng qing 鳳慶 county and Yun xian 雲縣 county in Yun nan 雲南. In 1327, a Shun ning fu 順寧府 was established here. Its seat of administration was in present-day Feng qing county in Yun nan. In 1382, it became Shun ning zhou 順寧州. In 1384, its status was raised to be a *fu* 府. It was put under the Yun nan 雲南 Provincial Administration Commission, Yun nan *bu zheng si* 雲南布政司. Qing 清 put it under Yun nan province. Its seat of administration was in Shun ning county as the *fu* seat. It was abolished in 1913. Mentioned with 896

Pu tian 莆田 [2]

Name of a county. It was founded under Sui 隋, in 589, by separating the Pu tian area from Nan an 南安 county. It was put under Quan zhou 泉州. Its seat of administration was located southeast of present-day Pu tian city in Fu jian. In 590, it was abolished, but reestablished under Tang 唐, in 622, under Feng zhou 豐州. The seat of administration was moved to the present-day Pu tian city. Mentioned with 674, 1532.

Pu yang 濮陽 [1]

Name of a feudal country. It was founded by Western Jin 晉, in 277, by changing the name of Dong 東 commandery. It was put under Yan zhou 兗州. Its seat of administration was in Pu yang county at a point located southwest of present-day Pu yang county in He nan 河南. Its administrative area comprised Hua xian 滑縣 county, and the cities and counties of Pu yang and Fan xian 范縣 in modern He nan, and Yun cheng 鄆城 and Juan cheng 鄄城 in Shan dong 山東. At the end of Western Jin, the area was changed to be Pu yang commandery. Under Northern Wei 魏, it was subordinated to Si zhou 司州. The seat of administration was moved to Jiu cheng 舊城 town, located north of present-day Juan cheng county in Shan dong. At the beginning of Sui 隋, it was abolished. Mentioned with 635.

Pu yang xian 濮陽縣 [1]

Name of a county. It was established by Qin 秦. Its seat of administration was in Gu xian 故縣 village, located 16 *li* southwest of present-day Pu yang 濮陽 county in He nan 河南. Under Five Dynasties' Jin 晉, in 939, the seat of administration was moved to De sheng cheng 德勝城, located 5 *li* southeast of the present-day Pu yang county. It was put under Chan zhou 澶州. In 1077, under Northern Song 宋, the seat of administration was moved to Pu yang county, but later the county was put under Kai de fu 開德府. Under Ming 明, in 1369, the county became part of Kai zhou 開州. The present-day Pu yang county was established, in 1914, by changing the name of Kai xian 開縣 county. Mentioned with 311.

Pu zhou 蒲州 [10]

Name of a *zhou* 州. It was established by Northern Zhou 周, in 558, by changing Tai zhou 泰州. Its seat of administration was in present-day Pu zhou town, located 24 *li* southwest of Yong ji 永濟 city in Shan xi 山西. Its administrative area included present-day Yong ji city, Wan rong 萬榮 county, Lin yi 臨猗 county and Rui cheng 芮城 county in Shan xi. In 607, the *zhou* became He dong 河東 commandery. In 618, it was reestablished and administered from Lin jin 臨晉 town, located 40 *li* southwest of Lin yi county in Shan xi. In 620, the seat of administration was moved to Pu zhou town, located southwest of present-day Yong ji city. In 720, its status was raised to be He zhong fu 河中府, but again changed to be Pu zhou the same year. In 742, it was changed to be He dong commandery. In 758, it again became Pu zhou. In 760, its status was raised to be He zhong fu. Under Jin 金, in 1128, it was changed to be Pu zhou. In 1149, it again became He zhong fu. Under Ming 明, in 1369, Pu zhou was reestablished, but under Qing 清, in 1728, its status was raised to be Pu zhou fu. In 1912, the *fu* 府 was split up, and Yong ji county was retained. In 1993, it became Yong ji city. Mentioned with 178, 186, 1014, 1254, 1519.

-Q-

Qi 岐 [1]
Name of a *zhou* 州. See under → Qi zhou 岐州. Mentioned with 1008.

Qi 齊 [18 + 2 + 4]
□ Name of an area. [18] The reference is to the watershed of the Yellow River north of Tai shan 泰山 mountain in Shan dong 山東 and the area of the Jiao dong 膠東 peninsula. This is the Qi state of the Warring States period. During Han 漢 times and subsequently, the area continued to be called Qi. Mentioned with 10, 22, 64, 147, 320, 356, 690, 735, 856, 867, 883, 955, 1105, 1210, 1242, 1323, 1380, 1519.
□ Name of a feudal state. [2] It was enfeoffed to Lü shang 呂尚 (fl 11th c. BCE) at the beginning of Western Zhou 周. Its first capital was at Ying qiu 營丘, located at the old city 50 *li* southeast of present-day Chang le 昌樂 county in Shan dong 山東 (according to another tradition it was the former city of Lin zi 臨淄 north of the present-day Lin zi district of Zi bo 淄博 city). Hu gong 胡公, in 862 BCE, moved the capital to Bo gu 薄姑. This is present-day Bo gu city 薄姑城, located 15 *li* northeast of Bo xing 博興 county in Shan dong. Later, Xian gong 獻公 (died 651 BCE) moved the capital to Lin zi. This is the former city of Lin zi located north of present-day Lin zi district in Zi bo city. During the Spring and Autumn Period, Huan gong 桓公 of Qi (died 643 BCE) was the first hegemon. During the Warring States period, Qi was one of the "seven powerful states," *qi xiong* 七雄. Qi was destroyed by Qin 秦, in 221 BCE. Mentioned with 269, 711.
□ Name of a *zhou* 州. [4] See → Qi zhou 齊州. Mentioned with 38, 381, 980, 1087.

Qi 蘄 [8]
Name of a *zhou* 州. See → Qi zhou 蘄州. Mentioned with 29, 120, 865, 1004, 1354, 1444.

Qi an 齊安 [1]
Name of a commandery. It was founded under Tang 唐 by changing the name of Huang zhou 黃州. Its seat of administration was in the present-day Xin zhou 新洲 district in Hu bei 湖北. At the beginning of the *qian yuan* 乾元 reign period (758 - 760), it became Huang zhou again. Mentioned with 1446.

Qi dan 契丹 [3]
Regional name. The Qi dan, also known as Khitan, were originally inhabitants of the northern grasslands, and later founders of the Liao 遼 dynasty. They controlled a huge territory north of Shan xi 山西 and the Northern part of He bei 河北, the region to the East of the Altai Mountain Range, south of the Cherlen river. In later times, this region was called Qi dan. Mentioned with 584, 1296, 1340.

Qi di 齊地 [1]
Name of a region. See under → Qi 齊.

Qi di 蘄地 [1]
Place name. It refers to → Qi zhou 蘄州. Mentioned with 29.

Qi dong 齊東 [1]
Regional name. It refers to the Yellow River watershed north of Tai shan 泰山 mountain in Shan dong 山東, and the eastern part of the Jiao dong 膠東 peninsula.

Qi fu lu 乞弗虜 [1]
Name of a region inhabited by minority nationalities. It was located somewhere in the present-day northwest of China, but details are lacking. Mentioned with 1116.

Qi ge shan 祈閣山 [1]
Name of a mountain. Located in the vicinity of present-day Chang de 常德 city in Hu nan 湖南. Mentioned with 1134.

Qi gui 齊歸 [1]
Place name. It is present-day Zhang ming 彰明 town located south of Jiang you 江油 city in Si chuan 四川. Mentioned with 322.

Qi guo 齊國 [5]
Name of a feudal country/domain from Qin 秦 and Han 漢 times. It was established at the transition from the Qin to the Han period by Xiang Yu 項羽 (232 - 202), with its capital located north of present-day Lin zi 臨淄 district of Zi bo 淄博 city of Shan dong 山東. Western Han changed the country to a commandery in 110 BCE, but Eastern Han reestablished the country, and combined it with Qing zhou 青州. During Eastern Jin 晉, the area was changed to be a commandery. Mentioned with 191, 631, 1216, 1480, 1578.

Qi jun 齊郡 [1]
Name of a commandery. It was established by Western Han 漢 by changing the name of Lin zi 臨淄 commandery. Its seat of administration was at a location north of present-day Lin zi district of Zi bo 淄博 city. Its administrative area

comprised the present-day Zi bo city, Qing zhou 青州 city, Lin qu 臨朐 county and Guang rao 廣饒 county in Shan dong 山東. Subsequently, the area became Qi 齊 country but, in 110 BCE, it again become a commandery. Eastern Han reestablished it to be a country. Eastern Jin once again changed it to be a commandery. Northern Wei 魏 moved the seat of administration to the present-day Qing zhou city. Sui, at the beginning of the *kai huang* 開皇 reign period (581 – 600), abolished the commandery. Mentioned with 706.

Qi li zhou 七里洲 [1]

This is a sand island in the middle of the Yang zi, north of present-day Jiu jiang 九江 city in Jiang xi 江西. Mentioned with 789.

Qi lian shan 祁連山 [1]

Name of a mountain. Another name is Tian shan 天山. It is located south of present-day Jiu quan 酒泉 city in Gan su 甘肅. However, in a broader meaning the term refers to mountainous regions in the border areas in the western portion of Gan su and the northeastern portion of Qing hai 青海 province. Mentioned with 1108.

Qi lu 齊魯 [5]

Combined regional name. Qi 齊 refers to the watershed of the Yellow River north of the Tai shan 泰山 mountain in Shan dong 山東, and the area of the Jiao dong 膠東 peninsula. This was the territory of Qi 齊 in Warring States times. During Han 漢 times and thereafter, the area continued to be called Qi 齊. Lu 魯 refers to the watersheds of the Wen 汶, Si 泗, Yi 沂 and Shu 沭 rivers south of the Tai shan 泰山 in Shan dong. During Qin 秦 and Han times and thereafter, the area continued to be called Lu. Later, the term Qi and Lu combined referred to the area of the Shan dong peninsula. Mentioned with 123, 355, 580, 786, 1371.

Qi men 祁門 [2]

Name of a county. It was founded under Tang 唐, in 766, by changing the name of Chang men 閶門 county. It was subordinated to She zhou 歙州. Its seat of administration was in Shi shan wu 石山塢, located west of present-day Qi men county in An hui 安徽. In 770, the county was moved to its present administrative seat.

Qi men 蘄門 [1]

Minor place name. Further details are lacking. Mentioned with 768

Qi shan 齊山 [6]

Name of a mountain. It refers to the Qi shan located 30 *li* south of present-day Zhao yuan 招遠 city in Shan dong 山東. Mentioned with 1017, 1254, 1344, 1430.

Qi shui 淒水 [1]

This is a river name from the *Shan hai jing* 山海經, "Classic of Mountains and Seas." Further details are lacking. Mentioned with 73.

Qi shui 蘄水 [1]

Name of a county. It was founded by Tang 唐, in 742, by changing the name of Lan xi 蘭溪 county. It was put under Qi chun 蘄春 commandery. Its seat of administration was in present-day Xi shui 浠水 county in Hu bei 湖北. In 1933, it was changed to be Xi shui county. Mentioned with 1564.

Qi ting 岐亭 [1]
This is a minor place name. Qi ting is located west of present-day Ma cheng 麻城 city in Hu bei 湖北. Mentioned with 1238.

Qi xian 蘄縣 [1]
Name of a county. It was established by Qin 秦, and subordinated to Si shui 泗水 commandery. Its seat of administration was in Qi xian 蘄縣 town, located 40 *li* south of present-day Su zhou 宿州 City in An hui 安徽. In 548, under Eastern Wei 魏, it was changed to be Qi cheng 蘄城 county. Under Sui 隋, in 583, it again became Qi county. It was abolished by Yuan 元, in 1265. Mentioned with 1084.

Qi xu 齊徐 [1]
Combined place name. It more or less corresponds to the lower watersheds of the Yellow River and the Huai 淮 including the Shan dong 山東 peninsula and the plain north of the Huai. Mentioned with 1004.

Qi yan 齊兗 [1]
Combined place name. It refers to the area of the Shan dong 山東 peninsula. Mentioned with 1137.

Qi yang 蘄陽 [1]
Minor place name. It is located at the place where the Yang zi and the Qi shui 蘄水 come together, south of present-day Qi chun 蘄春 county in Hu bei 湖北. It was called Qi yang because it was located north of the Qi shui.

Qi yang xian 祁陽縣 [2]
Name of a county. It was established under Three Kingdoms' Wu 吳 by breaking up Quan ling 泉陵 county. It was subordinate to Ling ling 零陵 commandery. Its seat of administration was in present-day Jin lan 金蘭 town, located 22 *li* southeast of Qi dong 祁東 county in Hu nan. Sui 隋 eliminated the county. Tang 唐 reestablished it, in 621, but put it under Yong zhou 永州. Its seat of administration was in present-day Lao shan wan 老山灣, located 10 *li* southwest of Qi yang county in Hu nan 湖南. Under Ming 明, in 1452, its administrative seat was moved to Qi yang county. Mentioned with 1058.

Qi yun 齊鄆 [1]
Combined place name. Qi zhou 齊州 and Yun zhou 鄆州 are two *zhou* 州 that during Northern Song 宋 times were subordinate to the eastern and western *lu* 路 around the capital. The scope of the territory included the present Ji nan 濟南 city, Yu cheng 禹城 city, Zhang qiu 章丘 city, Ji yang 濟陽 county, Ping yin 平陰 county, Dong ping 東平 county, Yang gu 陽穀 county and Shou zhang 壽張 county. Mentioned with 1155, 1573.

Qi zhou 岐州 [2]
Name of a *zhou* 州. It was established under Northern Wei 魏, in 487. Its seat of administration was at a location 5 *li* east of present-day Feng xiang 鳳翔 county in Shaan xi 陝西. Its administrative area corresponded to the present-day cities and counties of Zhou zhi 周至, Lin you 麟游, Long xian 隴縣, Bao ji 寶雞 and

Tai bai 太白 in Shaan xi. Under Sui 隋, in 581, the seat of administration was moved to Yong 雍 county. In 607, it was changed to Fu feng 扶風 commandery but under Tang 唐, in 618, it again became Qi zhou. In 742, it was again changed to Fu feng commandery. In 757, it was changed to establish Feng xiang fu 鳳翔府. Mentioned with 167, 907.

Qi zhou 齊州 [14]

Name of a *zhou* 州. It was established under Northern Wei 魏, in 469. Its seat of administration was in present-day Ji nan 濟南 city in Shan dong 山東. Its administrative area corresponded to present-day Ji nan city, Zi bo 淄博 city, Chang qing 長清 district, Qi he 齊河 county, Yu cheng 禹城 city, Lin yi 臨邑 county, Ji yang 濟陽 county, Zou ping 鄒平 county, Zhang qiu 章丘 city and Huan tai 桓台 county in Shan dong. At the beginning of the *da ye* 大業 reign period of Sui 隋, in 605, it was changed to Qi 齊 commandery but, in 618, under Tang 唐, it was again changed to Qi zhou. Under Northern Song 宋, in 1116, its status was raised to be Ji nan fu 濟南府. Mentioned with 70, 191, 272, 474, 510, 614, 683, 718, 1344.

Qi zhou 蘄州 [17 + 1]

□ Name of a *zhou* 州. [17] It was established by Southern Dynasties' Chen 陳 by changing the name of Luo zhou 羅州. Its seat of administration was in Luo zhou city, located 6 *li* northwest of Qi chun 蘄春 county in Hu bei 湖北. Under Sui 隋, in 607, it was changed to be Qi chun commandery. Tang 唐 changed it back to Qi zhou. Its administration included the cities and counties of Qi chun, Xi shui 浠水, Luo tian 羅田, Ying shan 英山, Huang mei 黃梅 and Wu xue 武穴 in modern Hu bei. Under Southern Song 宋, in 1263, the seat of administration was moved to Qi zhou town located southwest of modern Qi chun county. Yuan 元 raised the status of the area to be Qi zhou lu 蘄州路. At the beginning of Ming 明, it was changed to be Qi zhou fu 蘄州府 but, in 1376, it was made Qi zhou again. In 1912, the *zhou* became a county. Mentioned with 29, 233, 303, 573, 707, 768, 865, 945, 986, 1241, 1251, 1450, 1463.

□ Place name. [1] This was a city in Warring States Chu 楚. It is now Qi xian 蘄縣 town, located 14 *li* south of Su zhou 宿州 city in An hui 安徽. Mentioned with 1084.

Qi zhou wei 蘄州衛 [1]

Name of guard. It was established under Ming 明, in 1379, and subordinated to the Hu guang 湖廣 administration. Its seat of administration was located west of present-day Qi zhou 蘄州 town, located southwest of Qi chun 蘄春 county in Hu bei 湖北. It was abolished in the late Qing 清 period. Mentioned with 322.

Qian 虔 [1]

Name of a *zhou* 州. It was established by Sui 隋, in 589. Its seat of administration was at a location southwest of present-day Gan zhou 贛州 in Jiang xi 江西. In 607, it was changed to be Nan kang 南康 commandery. Under Tang 唐, in 622, it again became Qian zhou 虔州. During the *zhen guan* reign period (627–649), the seat of administration was moved to present-day Gan zhou city. Under Southern Song 宋, in 1153, it was changed to be Gan zhou. Mentioned with 389.

Qian 黔 [11 + 2]

□ Name of a *zhou* 州. [11] See → Qian zhou 黔州. Mentioned with 31, 58, 129, 337, 346, 456, 774, 806, 1264, 1441.

□ Regional name. [2] It is the northeastern section of present-day Gui zhou 貴州. During Warring States and Qin 秦 times, it was under Qian zhong 黔中 commandery. Tang 唐 put it under Qian zhong dao 黔中道, and today this is used as an abbreviation for Gui zhou. Mentioned with 29, 953.

Qian ling 乾陵 [1]

Name of an imperial mausoleum. This was the joint burial site of Li Zhi 李治, i.e., Tang emperor Gao zong 唐高宗 (628 – 683), and Empress Wu Ze tian 武則天 (624 - 705) of Wu Zhou 武周 dynasty. It is on Liang 梁 mountain, located 18 *li* northwest of present-day Qian 乾 county in Shaan xi 陝西. In 1961, it was established as a national noteworthy cultural protection site. Mentioned with 20.

Qian nan 黔南 [2]

Name of a *lu* 路. It was established under Northern Song 宋, in 1107, by splitting the western *lu* of Guang nan 廣南. Its seat of administration was located south of the present-day Rong shui miao 融水苗 Autonomous County in modern Guang xi 廣西. Its administrative area comprised in present-day Guang xi an area extending from the San jiang Dong 三江侗 Autonomous County and Liu zhou 柳州 city toward the West, from He chi 河池 city toward the East, and from Xin cheng 忻城 county toward the North. In 1109, it was combined with Guang xi, and became Guang xi qian nan lu 廣西黔南路. In 1110, the old name was restored as Guang nan xi lu 廣南西路. Mentioned with 511, 1316.

Qian shan 前山 [1]

Mountain name from the *Shan hai jing* 山海經, "Classic of Mountains and Seas." Details are lacking. Mentioned with 1504.

Qian shan 鉛山

See → Yan shan 鉛山

Qian shan xian 鉛山縣.

See → Yan shan xian 鉛山縣

Qian tang 錢塘 [8]

Name of a county. See → Qian tang xian 錢塘縣. Mentioned with 186, 381, 1017, 1162, 1168, 1407, 1420.

Qian tang xian 錢塘縣 [1]

Name of a county. It was established during the Southern Dynasties period by changing the name of Qian tang 錢唐 county. Its seat of administration was in present-day Hang zhou 杭州 city in Zhe jiang 浙江. In 1912, it was combined with Ren he 仁和 county to make Hang 杭 county. Mentioned with 1017.

Qian wei 犍為 [2 + 4]

□ Name of a county. [2] It was established by Sui 隋, in 583. Its seat of administration was on the eastern shores of the Min jiang 岷江 river, located 15 *li* southeast of present-day Qian wei county in Si chuan 四川. Under Five Dynasties' Jin 晉, in 936, the seat of administration was moved to the present Qian wei county.

Under Northern Song 宋, in 1011, the administration was moved to Qing xi 清溪 town, located south of the modern Qian wei county. In Ming 明 times, during the *hong wu* 洪武 reign period (1368 – 1398), the administration was moved to Qian wei county. Mentioned with 866.

□ Name of a commandery. [4] It was established under Western Han 漢, in 135 BCE. Its seat of administration was located west of present-day Zun yi 遵義 city in Gui zhou 貴州. The territory administered comprised in present-day Si chuan 四川 an area extending from the Jian yang 簡陽 and Peng shan 彭山 counties toward the South, and from Guang xi toward the North, as well as most of Gui zhou. In 130 BCE, the seat of administration was moved to the borders of present-day Yun lian 筠連 county in Si chuan. In 86 BCE, the administration was moved to a point southwest of present-day Yi bin 宜賓 city in Si chuan and, under Eastern Han, in 107, the seat of administration was moved to a point east of present-day Peng shan county in Si chuan. The commandery was abolished under Liang 梁 of the Southern Dynasties. Mentioned with 322, 782, 994.

Qian yang 黔陽 [1]

Name of a county. The county was founded under Northern Song 宋, in 1080, and subordinated to Yuan zhou 沅州. Its seat of administration was in present-day Qian cheng 黔城 town in Hong jiang 洪江 city in Hu nan 湖南. In 1922, the area was directly subordinated to Hu nan province. In 1949, the seat of administration was moved to An jiang 安江 town. In 1997, it was combined with Hong jiang county-rank city. Mentioned with 768.

Qian yang xian 汧陽縣 [2]

Name of a county. It was established under Northern Zhou 周, in 570. It was administered by Qian yang 汧陽 commandery. The seat of administration was at a location 40 *li* northwest of present-day Qian yang 千陽 county in Shaan xi 陝西. Subsequently, the commandery was abolished. The county was subordinated to Long zhou 隴州. In 575, the seat of administration was moved to a location 5 *li* northwest of Qian yang county. Under Ming 明, in 1548, the seat of administration was moved to Qian yang county, and the area was put under Feng xiang fu 鳳翔府. In 1928, it was directly subordinated to Shaan xi province. In 1964, the name was changed to Qian yang 千陽 county. Mentioned with 1051, 1056.

Qian zhong 黔中 [2 + 4]

□ Name of a commandery. [2] It was established under Warring States Chu 楚. During the Qin 秦 era, the seat of administration was in present-day Chang de 常德 city in Hu nan 湖南. The administrative area comprised the watersheds of the Yuan shui 沅水 and Li shui 澧水 in Hu nan 湖南, the watershed of the Qing jiang 清江 in Hu bei, the Qian jiang 黔江 watershed in Chong qing 重慶, and the northeastern portion of Gui zhou 貴州. Western Han 漢 changed the area to be Wu ling 武陵 commandery. Mentioned with 585, 1375.

□ Name of a commandery. [4] See Qian zhong jun 黔中郡. Mentioned with 29, 273, 528, 1103.

Qian zhong jun 黔中郡 [1]

Name of a commandery. It was founded under Tang 唐, in 742, by changing the name of Qian zhou 黔州. Its seat of administration was in present-day Peng shui 彭水 county of Chong qing 重慶 municipality. Its administration corresponded to the present-day districts and counties of Peng shui and Qian jiang 黔江 of You yang 酉陽 and in Gui zhou 貴州 to parts of the counties of Yan he 沿河 and Wu chuan 務川. In 758, it again became Qian zhou. Later, for many years, the old name continued in use. Mentioned with 399.

Qian zhou 乾州 [2]

Name of a *zhou* 州. It was established by Tang 唐, in 894. Its seat of administration was in present-day Qian xian 乾縣 county in Shaan xi 陝西. Its administration included the counties of Qian xian, Wu geng 武功, Zhou zhi 周至 and Li quan 禮泉 in Shaan xi. Later, its administration was reduced, and the *zhou* was abolished under Northern Song 宋, in 1072. In 1103, a Li zhou 醴州 was established where the old *zhou* was. Under Jin 金, in 1151, Qian zhou was reestablished. In 1913, it was reduced to Qian county. Mentioned with 20.

Qian zhou 黔州 [4]

Name of a *zhou* 州. It was founded under Northern Zhou 周, in 575, by changing the name of Feng zhou 奉州. Its seat of administration was in Yu shan 郁山 town, located northeast of present-day Peng shui 彭水 county in Chong qing 重慶 city. Under Sui 隋, in 583, Peng shui county was changed to Fu guo 附郭 county and, shortly thereafter, in 607, it became Qian an 黔安 commandery. Under Tang 唐, in 618, it was again changed to be Qian zhou. In 630, the seat of administration was moved to the present-day Peng shui county. Its administration comprised the territories of the modern Peng shui county and the district of Qian jiang 黔江. Southern Song 宋, in 1228, raised the status of the area to be Shao qing fu 紹慶府. Mentioned with 202, 483, 552, 1049.

Qiang 羌 [8]

Ancient name of a probably Tibetan-speaking minority nationality. They were spread about the Chinese Northwest, in what is now Gan su 甘肅, Chuan xi 川西 and Qing hai 青海. Mentioned with 298, 331, 387, 495, 660, 869, 960, 986.

Qiang dao 羌道 [2]

Name of a county. It was established under Western Han 漢, and subordinated to Long xi 隴西 commandery. Its seat of administration was located northwest of present-day Zhou qu 舟曲 county in Gan su 甘肅. It was abolished under Western Jin 晉. Mentioned with 1014, 1029.

Qiang di 羌地 [2]

Regional name. See → Qiang 羌. Mentioned with 249, 738.

Qiang li 羌里 [2]

Regional name. Its exact location remains to be determined. Mentioned with 1014.

Qiang long 羌隴 [1]
Combined place name. The term refers to the border region where present-day Gan su 甘肅 connects to Si chuan 四川. Mentioned with 1433.

Qiang zhong 羌中 [1]
Name of a region. See under → Qiang 羌. Mentioned with 249.

Qiao 譙 [1]
Regional name. Reference is either to Qiao country during Western Jin 晉, or a county subordinate to it.
□ Name of a country/domain. It was established under Three Kingdoms Wei 魏, in 220, by changing the name of Qiao commandery. Its seat of administration was in present-day Bo zhou 亳州 city in An hui 安徽. Its administration covered the cities and counties of Xiao xian 蕭縣, Ling bi 靈璧 and Wu he 五河 in An hui, and Lu yi 鹿邑 and Yong cheng 永城 in He nan.
□ Name of a county. It was established by Qin 秦 through changing Jiao yi 焦邑, and subordinated to Si shui 泗水 commandery. It was administered in present-day Bo zhou city in An hui. Under Eastern Jin 晉, in 338, it was changed to be Xiao huang 小黃 county. Under Sui 隋, in 607, it again became Qiao county. At the beginning of the *hong wu* 洪武 reign period (1368 – 1398) of the Ming 明, it was abolished. Its territory became part of Bo zhou. Mentioned with 633.

Qiao jun 譙郡 [1]
Name of a commandery. It was established during Eastern Han 漢 by splitting Pei guo 沛國. Its seat of administration was in present-day Bo zhou 亳州 city in An hui 安徽. During Three Kingdoms Wei 魏, in 220, it was changed to Qiao 譙 country/domain. Subsequently, it again became a commandery, and was put under Yu zhou 豫州. Under Western Jin 晉, it again became Qiao 譙 country. Under Liu Song 劉宋, the seat of administration was moved to Lao meng qiang si 老蒙墻寺, located 22 *li* north of present-day Shang qiu 商丘 city in He nan 河南. Under Northern Wei 魏, it was subordinated to Yan zhou 兗州. It was abolished under Northern Qi 齊. Mentioned with 648.

Qiao nan 嶠南 [1]
Regional name. It refers to the Ling nan 嶺南 area. That is present-day Guang dong 廣東, Guang xi 廣西 and Hai nan 海南 provinces, and the northern part of Vietnam. Mentioned with 94.

Qiao shan 喬山 [3]
Name of a mountain. This is Qiao 橋 mountain located north of present-day Huang ling 黃陵 county in Shaan xi 陝西. Mentioned with 687, 867.

Qie mi shan 且彌山 [1]
Name of a mountain. It is one of the volcanic mountains located in the Tian shan 天山 range west of present-day Turfan in Xinjiang 新疆. Mentioned with 1030.

Qin 秦 [33 + 5]
□ Regional name. [33] It is the region in Shaan xi 陝西 within the passes, *guan zhong* 關中, the area north of the Qin ling 秦嶺 mountain range up to Shaan bei

陝北. The area gets its name from the Warring States state of Qin, located in the area. Mentioned with 72, 199, 285, 322, 478, 502, 562, 566, 614, 620, 635, 735, 741, 825, 839, 899, 908, 1065, 1105, 1171, 1219, 1254, 1275, 1380, 1390, 1410, 1499, 1565.
□ Name of a *zhou* 州. [5] See → Qin zhou 秦州. Mentioned with 468, 660, 741, 802, 908.

Qin di 秦地 [5]
Regional name. See under → Qin 秦. Mentioned with 456, 899, 911, 1462.

Qin guan 秦關 [1]
Name of a pass. This is Han gu 函谷 pass. It was established during the Warring States period by Qin 秦. It was located at a point 30 *li* northeast of present-day Ling bao 靈寶 city in He nan 河南. All that survives is the gate to the pass. Mentioned with 735.

Qin jin 秦晉 [1]
Regional name. It refers to the southwestern portion of present-day Shan xi 山西, and the "Shaan xi region between the passes", Shaan xi guan zhong 陝西關中 area. Mentioned with 1340.

Qin ling 秦嶺 [2]
Name of a mountain range. Also called the Nan shan 南山. The mountains are located in the southern section of present-day Shaan xi 陝西, and are the boundary mark between North and South in China. Still another name is Bei ling 北嶺, „Northern Range." Mentioned with 908.

Qin long 秦隴 [6]
Regional name. It refers to the middle northern part of present-day Shaan xi 陝西 and the middle eastern part of present-day Gan su 甘肅. Mentioned with 188, 194, 196, 249, 385, 620.

Qin ning xian 秦寧縣 [1]
Name of a county. This should be → Tai ning 泰寧 county.

Qin shan 秦山 [1]
Name of a place. The reference is from the *Shan hai jing* 山海經, "Classic of Mountains and Seas," but details are lacking. Mentioned with 888.

Qin shui 沁水 [1]
Name of a river. It is also called the Shao shui 少水. This is the Qin he 沁河 river in the southeastern part of present-day Shan xi 山西. Its sources come from Er lang shen gou 二郎神溝 on Mian shan 綿山 mountain, north of Qin yuan 沁源 county. It flows south through the counties of An ze 安 澤 , Qin shui and Yang cheng 陽城. It flows further south and enters the border of Ji yuan 濟源 city in He nan 河南. After flowing east, it enters the Yellow River at a point south of Wu zhi 武陟 county. Mentioned with 1062.

Qin ting 秦亭 [3]
Name of a minor place. It is in the area of present-day Long xi 隴西 county in Gan su 甘肅. Mentioned with 620.

Qin zhong 秦中 [5]

Regional name. Reference is to the middle south area of Shaan xi 陝西 province. This was Qin 秦 territory during the Spring and Autumn and the Warring States period, thus the name: "Within Qin." Mentioned with 216, 378, 495, 907, 1473.

Qin zhou 欽州 [2]

Name of a *zhou* 州. It was founded under Sui 隋, in 598, and administered from present-day Jiu long 久隆 town, located 30 *li* northeast of Qin zhou city in Guang xi 廣西. Its administrative area included Qin zhou and the area of Ling shan 靈山 county in Guang xi. During the reign period *da ye* 大業 (605 – 615) of the Sui 隋, and during the reign periods *tian bao* 天寶 (742 – 756) and *zhi de* 至德 (756 – 758) of the Tang 唐, the *zhou* was periodically changed to be Ning Yue 寧越 commandery. Under Tang 唐, in 621, it again became Qin zhou. In 742, it was changed to Zhu yue 宁越 commandery. In 758, it again became Qin zhou. Under Northern Song 宋, in 1023, the seat of administration was moved to the old *zhou* ruins west of modern Ling shan county. Southern Song moved the seat of administration to modern Qin zhou city. Under Yuan 元, in 1280, it became Qin zhou lu 欽州路. Mentioned with 144, 376.

Qin zhou 沁州 [2 + 3]

□ Name of a *zhou* 州 [2]. It was founded under Sui 隋, in 596. Its seat of administration was in present-day Qin yuan 沁源 county in Shan xi 山西. In 606, it was eliminated. Under Tang 唐, in 618, it was restored, and its seat of administration was once again in present-day Qin yuan county. Its administration included present-day Qin yuan county and the northern part of An ze 安澤 county in Shan xi. In 981, under Northern Song 宋, it was abolished. Mentioned with 931, 1032.

□ Name of a *zhou* 州 [3]. It was founded by Jin 金, in 1128, by changing Wei sheng 威勝 army. Its seat of administration was in present-day Qin xian 沁縣 county in Shan xi. Its administration included the present-day counties of Qin yuan, Qin xian and Wu xiang 武鄉 in Shan xi. Yuan 元 put it under Jin ning lu 晉寧路. Ming 明 and Qing 清 made it a directly administered *zhou*, *zhi li zhou* 直隸州. In 1912, it became Qin county. Mentioned with 461, 931.

Qin zhou 秦州 [16]

Name of a *zhou* 州. It was founded under Western Jin 晉, in 269. Its seat of administration was at a location east of present-day Gan gu 甘穀 county in Gan su 甘肅. It was abolished, in 282, but reestablished, in 286. The seat of administration was moved to present-day Tian shui 天水 city in Gan su. The territory administered comprised an area reaching in Gan su from Ding xi 定西 city and Jing ning 靜寧 county toward the South, and from Qing shui 清水 county toward the West. It reached in Shaan xi 陝西 from Feng 鳳 county and Lue yang 略陽, in Si chuan 四川 from Ping wu 平武 and Jiu Zhai gou 九寨溝, and in Qing hai 青海 from the Yellow River toward the South, and from Gui de 貴德 county toward the East. The territory was later reduced. Under Sui 隋, the area became Tian shui 天水 commandery. Under early Tang 唐, it again became Qin zhou. In 734, the seat of administration was moved to a location northwest of present-day Qin an 秦安 county in Gansu. In 742, the seat was moved back to the present Tian shui city. After 762, the area was lost to the Tibetans. It was recovered, in 849, and the seat of administration was again placed at Tian shui city. In 1913, it was reduced to be Tian shui county. Mentioned with 45, 199, 289, 314, 468, 607, 620, 650, 687, 727, 986, 1014, 1091, 1255, 1275, 1308.

Qin zhou 勤州 [1]

Name of a *zhou* 州. It was founded under Tang 唐, in 621. Its seat of administration was at a location northeast of Yang chun 陽春 city in modern Guang dong 廣東. It was eliminated the next year but reestablished in 697. It was again eliminated during the *chang an* 長安 reign period (701 – 704). It was reestablished in 730. Its seat of administration was in Fu lin 富霖 town, located southwest of present-day Yun fu 雲浮 city in Guang dong. In 742, the area was changed to be Yun fu commandery but, in 758, became Qin zhou. The seat of administration was at the time transferred to a location northeast of present-day Yang chun city. The administrative area of the *zhou* comprised the area connecting the present-day cities of Yang chun and Yun fu in Guang dong. The *zhou* was eliminated under Northern Song 宋, in 973. Mentioned with 428.

Qing 青 [9 + 1]

□ One of the nine ancient *zhou*. [9] There is a Qing zhou 青州 in the *Book of History's* "Yu gong 禹貢," "Tribute of Yu 禹," and its scope is the northern part of Shan dong 山東 from Bo hai 渤海 to Tai shan 泰山 mountain. Subsequently, the name came to designate the area. Mentioned with 10, 639, 690, 733, 856, 877, 1004, 1087, 1443.

□ Name of a *zhou* 州 [1]. See → Qing zhou 青州. Mentioned with 781.

Qing cheng shan 青城山 [4]

Name of a mountain. It was located 30 *li* southwest of present-day Du jiang yan 都江堰 city in Si chuan 四川. During Tang 唐 times, the mountain was one of the four great scenic mountains in Jian nan 劍南 circuit. In China, it is a famous Daoist scenic spot. Mentioned with 631, 1163, 1301, 1430.

Qing dui 青堆 [1]

Minor place name. It is positioned in the vicinity of present-day Zhang ming 彰明 town, south of Jiang you 江油 city in Si chuan 四川. Mentioned with 322.

Qing he 清河 [1]

Name of an administrative unit. Perhaps it is Qing he commandery or Qing he county.

□ Name of a commandery, established at the beginning of Western Han 漢. Its seat of administration was located southeast of present-day Qing he county in He bei 河北. Its administration comprised present-day Qing he county, a part of both Zao qiang 棗強 county and Nan gong 南宮 city in He bei, as well as Lin qing 臨清 city, Xia jin 夏津 county, Wu cheng 武城 county and parts of Gao tang 高唐 county and Ping yuan 平原 county in present-day Shan dong 山東. During the reign of Emperor Huan di 桓帝 (132 – 168) of Eastern Han, the area

was changed to be Qing he country/domain, and the seat of administration was moved to a point northeast of present-day Lin qing city in Shan dong. Under Three Kingdoms' Wei 魏, the area again became Qing he commandery. It was Qing he country under Western Jin 晉 and was administered from a point east of Lin qing city. After that, the territory of the former commandery was reduced. Northern Wei 魏 changed it back again to be Qing he commandery. It was abolished under Sui 隋, at the beginning of the *kai huang* 開皇 reign period (581–600). Later, during the *da ye* 大業 reign period (605 – 616) of Sui and during the *tian bao* 天寶 (742 – 755) and *zhi de* 至德 (756 – 757) reign periods of Tang 唐, Bei zhou 貝州 was periodically changed to be Qing he commandery.
□ Name of a county. It was established under Three Kingdoms Wei 魏 and was under the administrative control of Qing he commandery. Its seat of administration was located northeast of present-day Lin qing city in Shan dong. Northern Qi 齊 changed it to Bei qiu 貝丘 county. Mentioned with 1532.

Qing liang si 清涼寺 [1]
Name of a temple. It was located within Qing liang 清涼 valley, 80 *li* northeast of present-day Wu tai 五台 county in Shan xi 山西. It was established during the reign of Emperor Xiao wen di 孝文帝 (467 – 499) under Northern Wei 魏. It was renovated under Yuan 元, in 1342. The temple has Qing liang stone. Mentioned with 553.

Qing lin hu 青林湖 [1]
Name of a lake. This is the Qing lin hu of Guang ji 廣濟 county which existed during the Ming dynasty, located at present-day Mei chuan 梅川 town, 62 *li* north of Wu xue 武穴 city in Hu bei 湖北. Mentioned with 573.

Qing liu 清流 [2]
Name of a county. It was established under Sui 隋, in 598, by changing the name of Xin chang 新昌 county. Its seat of administration was at present-day Chu zhou 滁州 city in An hui 安徽. At the beginning of Ming 明, it was abolished, and the area became part of Chu zhou. Mentioned with 338, 931.

Qing qi 青齊 [1]
Combined place name. It refers to the Yellow River watershed north of Tai shan 泰山 mountain in Shan dong 山東 and the region of the Jiao dong 膠東 peninsula. Mentioned with 863.

Qing qiu zhi shan 青丘之山 [1]
Name of a mountain from the *Shan hai jing* 山海經, "Classic of Mountains and Seas." Details are lacking. Mentioned with 440.

Qing xi 青溪 [1]
Name of a county. It is also written Qing xi 清溪 county. It was founded under Tang 唐, in 805, by changing the name of Huan chun 還淳 county to avoid a taboo. It was put under Mu zhou 睦州. Its seat of administration was at a location near to Nan shan 南山 island of Qian dao 千島湖 lake, west of present-day Chun an 淳安 county in Zhe jiang 浙江. Under Northern Song 宋, in 1121, it was changed to be Chun hua 淳化 county. Mentioned with 1063.

Qing yang 慶陽 [2]
Name of a *fu* 府. It was established under Northern Song 宋, in 1125, by changing the name of Qing zhou 慶州. Its seat of administration was in present-day Qing yang 慶陽 city in Gan su 甘肅. During Ming 明 and Qing 清, its administration corresponded to Qing yang city and the present-day counties of Ning xian 寧縣, Huan xian 環縣, He shui 合水, Hua chi 華池 and Zheng ning 正寧 in Gan su. In 1913, it was abolished. Mentioned with 554, 1289.

Qing yi 青衣 [1]
Name of a county. It was established by Western Han 漢, in 201 BCE, and put under Shu 蜀 commandery. Its seat of administration was in present-day Lu shan 蘆山 county in Si chuan 四川. According to another tradition, its seat of administration was located north of present-day Ming shan 名山 county. Under Eastern Han, in 133, the area became Han jia 漢嘉 county. Mentioned with 538.

Qing yi xian 青衣縣 [1]
Name of a county. It was founded under Sui 隋, in 589, by changing the name of E mei 峨眉 county. It was administered by Jia zhou 嘉州 and had its administrative seat in present-day Le shan 樂山 city in Si chuan 四川. In 590, the name was changed to Long you 龍遊 county. Mentioned with 538.

Qing yuan 慶遠 [1]
Name of a *fu* 府. It was established under Southern Song 宋, in 1265, by raising the status of the princely residence of Emperor Du zong 度宗, Qing yuan 慶遠 army. Its seat of administration was at present-day Yi zhou 宜州 city in Guang xi 廣西. Its administration comprised Yi zhou, as well as the present-day cities and counties of Xin cheng 忻城, He chi 河池, Nan dan 南丹, Tian e 天峨, Feng shan 鳳山, Dong lan 東蘭 and Huan jiang 環江 in Guang xi, and Li bo 荔波 in Gui zhou 貴州. Under Yuan 元, in 1279, the area became Qing yuan lu 慶遠路. During early Ming 明, in 1370, the area again became Qing yuan fu 慶遠府. It was abolished in 1913. Mentioned with 540.

Qing zhou 青州 [19 + 3 + 8 + 2]
□ Name of a *zhou* 州. [19] It was established under Western Han 漢, and constituted one of the 13 Regional Inspector Divisions, *shi san ci shi bu* 十三刺史部. Its administration comprised in present-day Shan dong an area extending from De zhou 德州 city and Qi he 齊河 county toward the East, from the Ma jia he 馬頰河 toward the South, from Ji nan 濟南 city, Lin qu 臨朐 county, An qiu 安丘 city, Gao mi 高密 city, Lai yang 萊陽 city, Qi xia 棲霞 city and Ru shan 乳山 city toward the North and toward the East, and in present-day He bei 河北 Wu qiao 吳橋 county. Eastern Han moved the administration to a point north of present-day Lin zi 臨淄 district of Zi bo 淄博 city in Shan dong. Eastern Jin 晉 moved the seat of administration to present-day Qing zhou city. Under Sui 隋, in 607, it became Bei hai 北海 commandery. Tang 唐 again made it Qing zhou. Jin 金 changed it to Yi du fu 益都府. In 1986, Yi du 益都 county was changed to Qing zhou city. Mentioned with 36, 131, 269, 272, 324, 474, 578, 619, 819, 904, 1037, 1158, 1292, 1484.

□ Name of a *fu* 府. [3] It was established under Ming 明, in 1367, by changing Yi du lu 益都路. It was subordinated to the Branch Secretariat for Shan dong 山東 and other Places, Shan dong deng chu *xing zhong shu sheng* 山東等處行中書省. Its territory of administration corresponded in present-day Shan dong to an area extending from Bo xing 博興 county, Yi yuan 沂源 county and Meng yin 蒙陰 county toward the East, and from Chang le 昌樂 county, An qiu 安丘 city and Zhu cheng 諸城 city toward the West, as well as the region of the southern and northern coast. Qing 清 put the *fu* under Shan dong province, with a reduced administration. It was abolished in 1913. Mentioned with 285, 903, 1338.

□ Name of a *zhou*. [8] Under Liu Song 劉宋, during the *tai shi* 泰始 reign period (465 – 471), it was combined with Ji zhou 冀州, and the name was moved to a portion of the territory of Yun tai 云臺 mountain east of present-day Lian yun gang 連雲港 city in Jiang su 江蘇. After the rebellion of General Hou Jing 侯景 (died 552) against the Liang 梁, the territory became part of Eastern Wei 魏, and Qing zhou was changed to Hai zhou 海州. Mentioned with 70, 666, 733, 1017, 1254, 1430, 1443, 1449.

□ Name of a *zhou*. [2] It was one of the ancient nine *zhou*. Ancient Qing zhou comprised the northern part of Shan dong province from modern Bo hai 渤海 to Tai shan 泰山 mountain. Mentioned with 1538, 1551.

Qiong 瓊 [2]

Name of a *zhou* 州. It was established under Tang 唐, in 631, by splitting Ya zhou 崖州. Its seat of administration was at present-day Jiu zhou 舊州 town, located southeast of Qiong shan 瓊山 district in Hai kou 海口 city in Hai nan 海南. It was eliminated, in 639, but was subsequently restored. Under Northern Song 宋, in 1071, the seat of administration was moved to Qiong shan district. The administrative area corresponded to present-day Hai kou city, the Qiong shan district, Qiong hai 瓊海 city and the counties of Ding an 定安, Cheng mai 澄邁 and Lin gao 臨高 in Hai nan province. Under Yuan 元, in 1329, the area became the Qian ning Tribal Pacification Commission, Qian ning *jun ming an fu si* 乾寧軍民安撫司. Under Ming 明, in 1368, it was changed to Qiong zhou fu 瓊州府. In 1369, it again became Qiong zhou but, the next year, its status was raised to be a *fu* 府 again. Mentioned with 144, 1057.

Qiong po sai jiang 邛婆塞江 [1]

Name of a river. No further information is available. Mentioned with 559.

Qiong zhou 瓊州 [2]

Name of a *fu* 府. It was established under Ming 明, in 1368, by changing the name of Qian ning Tribal Pacification Commission, Qian ning *jun min an fu si* 乾寧軍民安撫司. It was put under Guang dong 廣東 province. Its seat of administration was in present-day Qiong shan 瓊山 district of Hai kou 海口 city of Hai nan 海南 province. In 1369, it again became Qiong zhou. In 1370, its status was raised to be a *fu* again. Its administrative area included the territory of modern Hai nan 海南 province. It was abolished in 1911. Mentioned with 556, 1355.

Qiong zhou 邛州 [6]

Name of a *zhou*. It was established under Southern Dynasties' Liang 梁. Its seat of administration was located 55 *li* southeast from present-day Qiong lai 邛崍 city in Si chuan 四川. Under Sui 隋, in 606, it was abolished. It was restored again under Tang 唐, in 618. In 657, the seat of administration was moved to the present-day Qiong lai city. Its administration comprised the present-day cities and counties of Qiong lai, Da yi 大邑 and Pu jiang 蒲江 in Si chuan. Under Ming 明, in 1376, the *zhou* was demoted to be Qiong 邛 county. In 1483, its status was raised to be a directly administered *zhou*, *zhi li zhou* 直隸州. In 1913, the area became Qiong lai county. Mentioned with 183, 284, 524, 736, 768, 1220.

Qiu chi 仇池 [3]

Name of a city. It was located in the Nan luo 南洛 river valley in present-day Xi he 西和 county in Gan su 甘肅. Mentioned with 173, 202, 1307.

Qiu ci guo 龜茲國 [1]

Name of an ancient country in the western regions. It was a part of present-day Kuqa/Ku che 庫車, in Xin jiang 新疆. Mentioned with 1050.

Qu 衢 [2]

Name of a *zhou* 州. See → Qu zhou 衢州. Mentioned with 121, 871.

Qu jiang 曲江 [1]

Name of a town. It was established under Northern Song 宋, and put under Feng cheng 豐城 county. This is present-day Qu jiang town, located north of Feng cheng city in Jiang xi 江西. Mentioned with 1014.

Qu ren xian 朐腮縣 [1]

Name of a county. It was established under Western Jin 晉 by changing the name of Qu ren 朐忍 county. Its seat of administration was at present-day San ba xiang 三壩鄉, located east of Yun yang 雲陽 county in Chong qing 重慶 city. Northern Zhou 周 changed it to Yun an 雲安 county. Mentioned with 1335.

Qu shan 朐山 [1]

Name of a mountain. It is located 2 *li* southeast of present-day Lin qu 臨朐 county in Shan dong 山東. Mentioned with 677.

Qu shan 區山 [1]

Name of a mountain. It is located east of present-day Liang cheng 兩城 town of Dong gang 東港 district of Ri zhao 日照 city in Shan dong 山東. Mentioned with 1250.

Qu tan 曲灘 [2]

This is a general reference to an accumulation where the river is fast flowing and moves dirt and silk which accumulates on the river bed to form something like a sand bank. Mentioned with 1234.

Qu zhou 衢州 [1]

Name of a *zhou* 州. It was established under Tang 唐, in 621, by dividing Wu zhou 婺州. It was administered in present-day Qu zhou city in Zhe jiang 浙江. In 623, it was eliminated. It was restored in 686. In 742, it was changed to be Xin an 信安 commandery. In 758, it again became Qu zhou. Under Yuan 元, in 1276, it became Qu zhou lu 衢州路. Mentioned with 3.

Qu zhou 渠州 [2]

Name of a *zhou* 州. It was established under Southern Dynasties' Liang 梁, in 537. Its seat of administration was in present-day Qu 渠 county in Si chuan 四川. Under Sui 隋, in 607, it was changed to be Tan qu 宕渠 commandery. Under Tang 唐, in 618, it again became Qu zhou. Its administrative area comprised present-day Qu county, Da zhu 大竹 county, Lin shui 鄰水 county and the territory of Guang an 廣安 city in Si chuan 四川. Under Northern Song 宋, in 969, it was divided and Guang an army was established. Its territory was smaller. Under Southern Song, its administrative area was greatly expanded. In 1255, the seat of administration was moved to Li yi 禮義 mountain, 60 *li* northeast of present-day Qu county. Yuan 元 restored the old seat of administration. Under Ming 明, in 1376, it was demoted to be Qu county. Mentioned with 736.

Quan 全 [1]

Name of a zhou 州. See → Quan zhou 全州. Mentioned with 780.

Quan zhou 泉州 [2 + 2]

□ This is the name of a *zhou* 州. [2] Under Tang 唐, in 700, Wu rong zhou 武榮州 was established. In 711, the name was changed to Quan zhou. Its seat of administration was in present-day Quan zhou city in Fu jian 福建. Its administration comprised in present-day Fu jian the watersheds of the Jin jiang 晉江 and the Mu lan xi 木蘭溪, the area of Lake Peng 澎 , the city of Xia men 廈門, Tong an 同安 district and Jin men 金門 county. After the Five Dynasties period, its northwestern part including De hua 德化 county and its southwestern part Chang tai 長泰 county were separated off, and put under Zhang zhou 漳州. Mentioned with 809, 925.

□ Name of a *fu* 府. [2]. It was founded under Ming 明, in 1368, by changing Quan zhou lu 泉州路 into a *fu*. It was put under Fu jian 福建 province. Its seat of administration was in present-day Quan zhou city. Its administrative area comprised the watershed of the Jin jiang 晉江, the Peng hu 澎湖 peninsula and Xia men 廈門 city, the Tong an 同安 region, and the counties of Jin men 金門 and De hua 德化, in Fu jian. It was abolished in 1913. Mentioned with 9, 1246.

Quan zhou 全州 [2]

Name of a *zhou* 州. It was established under Five Dynasties' Jin 晉, in 939, by splitting Yong zhou 永州. Its seat of administration was at present-day Quan zhou in Guang xi 廣西. During Song 宋, its administrative area comprised the two counties of present-day Quan zhou and Guan yang 灌陽, in Guang xi. Under Yuan 元, in 1277, it became Quan zhou lu 全州路. Under Ming 明, in 1368, it was changed to Quan zhou fu 全州府. In 1376, it was demoted again to be Quan zhou, and put under present-day Yong zhou fu 永州府 in Hu guang 湖廣. In 1394, it was put under Gui lin fu 桂林府 in Guang xi 廣西. In 1912, it was changed to be Quan 全 county. In 1959, it became Quan zhou county. Mentioned with 817, 1329.

Que shan 鵲山 [1]

Name of a mountain. It is also called Peng shan 蓬山 or Peng que shan 蓬鵲山. It is located 62 *li* west of present-day Nei qiu 內丘 county in He bei 河北. Mentioned with 1344.

-R-

Ran mang yi 冉駹夷 [2]

Name of a Han 漢 dynasty minority tribe. They were spread over the regions of the southwest. Mentioned with 689, 747.

Rang cheng 穰城 [1]

Place name. It is present-day Deng zhou 鄧州 city in He nan 河南. Mentioned with 1567.

Rao 饒 [6]

See → Rao zhou 饒州. Mentioned with 75, 121, 535, 595, 1375.

Rao yang jun 饒陽郡 [1]

Name of a commandery. It was founded under Tang 唐, in 742, by changing the name of Shen zhou 深州. Its seat of administration was in present-day Shen zhou city in He bei 河北. The territory administered comprised the area of Shen zhou and the cities and counties of Rao yang 饒陽, Xin ji 辛集 and An ping 安平 in present-day He bei. In 758, it again became Shen zhou. Mentioned with 544.

Rao zhou 饒州 [6 + 2]

□ Name of a *zhou* 州 mentioned by that name or as Rao 饒. [6] It was established under Sui 隋, in 589. Its seat of administration was in present-day Po yang 鄱陽 county in Jiang xi 江西. Its administrative area extended to the watersheds of the Po jiang 鄱江 and of the Xin jiang 信江 in modern Jiang xi, beyond Wu yuan 婺源 and Yu shan 玉山. Later, at the beginning of the *da ye* 大業 reign period (605 – 616) of Sui, and during the *tian bao* 天寶 (742 – 755) and *zhi de* 至德 (756 – 757) reign periods of Tang 唐, the area periodically became Po yang commandery. Under Yuan 元, in 1277, its status was raised to be Rao zhou lu 饒州路. Mentioned with 24, 1140, 1173, 1375, 1412, 1420.

□ Name of a *fu* 府. [2] It was established under Ming 明, and subordinated to the Jiang xi 江西 province. Its seat of administration was in present-day Po yang 鄱陽 county in Jiang xi. Its territory of administration corresponded to present-day Po yang, Yu gan 余干, Yu jiang 余江, Wan nian 萬年, De xing 德興 and Le ping 樂平 in Jiang xi. It was abolished in 1912. Mentioned with 24, 1375.

Ren he xian 仁和縣 [1]

Name of a county. It was founded under Northern Song 宋 by renaming Qian jiang 錢江 county. It, with Qian tang 錢塘 county, was one of the suburbian counties of Hang zhou 杭州. Its seat of administration was in present-day Hang zhou city in Zhe jiang 浙江. In 1912, it was combined with Qian tang county to be Hang xian 杭縣 county. Mentioned with 1030.

Ri ben guo 日本國 [1]
Ancient name of a country, Japan. Mentioned with 738.

Ri nan 日南 [8]
Name of a commandery. It was founded under Western Han 漢, in 111 BCE. Its seat of administration was at the confluence of the Quảng Trị and Cam Lộ rivers northwest of Quảng Trị in Tỉnh Quảng Trị province in Vietnam. Its administration comprised the central part of modern Vietnam in the North to Hoành mountain and in the South to the region of Đại Lĩnh. After Southern Qi 齊, the commandery was abolished. Mentioned with 94, 259, 400, 1138, 1248, 1366, 1406.

Ri zhu 日鑄 [1]
Name of a mountain range. It is located 55 *li* southeast of present-day Shao xing 紹興 city in Zhe jiang 浙江. In ch. 1 of his *Gui tian lu* 歸田錄, Ouyang Xiu 歐陽修 (1007 – 1072) referred to it as Ri zhu 日注. Mentioned with 768.

Rong 容
See → Rong zhou 容州.

Rong 榮 [2]
Name of a *zhou* 州, established under the Tang 唐, in 618, and governed from Gong jing 貢井, located 10 *li* 里 west of present-day Zi gong 自貢 city in Si chuan 四川. In 623, the seat of administration was moved to a point west of present-day Rong xian 榮縣 county in modern Si chuan. In 651, the seat of administration was moved to the present-day Rong xian county. The administrative area comprised the present-day cities and counties of Zi gong, Rong xian county and Wei yuan 威遠, in Si chuan. Under Southern Song 宋, during the *shao xi* 紹熙 (1190-1194) period, the status of the area was raised to Shao xi fu 紹熙府. Later, between 1253-1258, the *fu* 府 was abolished. It was reestablished at the end of Yuan 元, but was again demoted to be Rong xian county under Ming 明, in 1376. Mentioned with 1054.

Rong 融
See → Rong zhou 融州. Mentioned with 1063, 1329.

Rong 戎 [7 + 4]
□ General designation. [7] It refers to areas of minority peoples settlement. Mentioned with 14, 34, 660, 1097, 1192, 1304, 1551.
□ Name of a *zhou* 州. [4] See → Rong zhou 戎州. Mentioned with 9, 1057, 1097, 1339.

Rong cheng xian 戎成縣 [1]
Name of a county. It was established by Tang 唐 and administered from Rong xu 戎圩 town, this is present-day Long xu 龍圩 town of Cang wu 蒼梧 county in Guang xi 廣西. It was abolished under Northern Song 宋, in 1071.

Rong guan 容管 [1]
This is an abbreviation for the Rong zhou Area Command, Rong zhou *du du fu* 容州都督府. It was established during the *kai yuan* 開元 reign period (713 – 741) of Tang 唐. Its seat of administration was in present-day Bei liu 北流 county in Guang xi 廣西. Its administrative area comprised some ten *zhou* 州 with a territory equivalent to the southeast section of present-day Guang xi and a strip of the western part of present-day Guang dong 廣東. It was later abolished. Mentioned with 909.

Rong nan 容南 [1]
Name for a Tang 唐 period region. It refers to the Southeast of present-day Guang xi 廣西. Mentioned with 817.

Rong xian 戎縣 [1]
Name of a county. This is an error for → Rong cheng 戎成 county. Mentioned with 520.

Rong xian 融縣 [2]
Name of a county. It was founded under Ming 明, in 1377, by demoting Yong zhou 融州. It was subordinated to Liu zhou fu 柳州府. Its seat of administration was in present-day Rong shui 融水 county in Guang xi 廣西. In 1966, it was changed to be the Rong shui Miao 苗 Autonomous County. Mentioned with 698.

Rong zhou 戎州 [6]
Name of a *zhou* 州. It was established under Southern Dynasties' Liang 梁, in 544. Its seat of administration was in present-day An bian 安邊 town, located west of Yi bin 宜賓 county in Si chuan 四川. Its administrative area comprised the southern part of modern Si chuan, the northeastern part of Yun nan 雲南, and a strip of the border zone of northwestern Gui zhou 貴州. At the beginning of Tang 唐 and later, during the *chang qing* reign period (821 – 824), the seat of administration was twice moved to Li zhuang 李莊, located 60 *li* southeast of the present Yi bin county. In 843, it was moved to Jiu zhou ba 舊州垻, located 6 *li* northwest of the modern Yi bin city. In 1114, under Northern Song, the area became Xu zhou 敘州. Mentioned with 19, 39, 129, 524, 555, 819.

Rong zhou 容州 [5]
Name of a *zhou* 州 (referred to by that name or simply as Rong 容). It was founded under Tang 唐, in 634. Its seat of administration was in present-day Bei liu 北流 county located in Guang xi 廣西. Its administrative area comprised present-day Bei liu and Rong 容 county in Guang xi. Later the seat was transferred to the present Rong xian county. At the beginning of Yuan 元, it became Rong zhou lu 容州路. Afterwards, it again became Rong zhou. During early Ming 明, it was changed to be Rong county. Mentioned with 362, 432, 550, 909, 1257.

Rong zhou 融州 [2]
Name of a *zhou* 州 (referred to by that name or simply as Rong 融). It was founded under Sui 隋, in 598, by changing the name of Dong ning zhou 東宁州. Its seat of administration was in present-day Rong shui 融水 county in Guang

xi 廣西. Its territory of administration comprised Rong shui county, and the present-day counties of Luo cheng 羅成, Rong an 融安 and San jiang 三江 in Guang xi. It was eliminated, in 606, but restored under the Tang 唐, in 621. Under Ming 明, in 1377, it was changed to be Rong xian county. Mentioned with 1063, 1329.

Rou zhi guo 月氏國 [1]
Name of an ancient country in the West. It originally was part of a minority nationaly in the Northwest, inhabiting the He xi/Gan su corridor, He xi zou lang 河西走廊. Pressed by the Xiong nu, they moved westward into the Amur river region of Central Asia. Mentioned with 282.

Ru nan 汝南 [1]
Name of a commandery. See → Ru nan jun 汝南郡. Mentioned with 575, 612, 637, 1210, 1262, 1446, 1449, 1497, 1532.

Ru nan jun 汝南郡 [3]
Name of a commandery. It was established under Western Han 漢, in 203 BCE. Its seat of administration was at a location southwest of present-day Shang cai 上蔡 county in He nan 河南. Its administration comprised in present-day He nan the area between the Ying he 穎河 and the Huai he 淮河 river, and an area reaching from the west side of Jing Guang 京廣 railroad toward the East, and in An hui 安徽 from the Ci he 茨河 and Xi fei he 西淝河 rivers toward the West, as well as from the Huai 淮 river toward the North. During Eastern Han, the seat of administration was moved to a point north of present-day Ping yu 平輿 county in He nan. Under Three Kingdoms Wei 魏, the seat of administration was moved to present-day Xi 息 county in He nan. Under Eastern Jin 晉, it was moved to the present-day Ru nan 汝南 county in He nan. Under Sui 隋, in 581, it was abolished. It was reestablished, in 607, by changing the name of Cai zhou 蔡州. Under Tang 唐, at the beginning of the *wu de* 武德 reign period (618 – 626), it was changed to Yu zhou 豫州. In 742, it was again changed to be Ru nan commandery. In 758, it was changed to Yu zhou. Mentioned with 648, 1253, 1449.

Ru zhou 汝州 [1]
Name of a *zhou* 州. It was founded under Sui 隋, in 606, by changing the name of Yi zhou 伊州. Its seat of administration was at present-day Ru zhou city in He nan 河南. Its administrative area comprised the two present-day cities of Ru zhou and Ping ding shan 平頂山, and the present-day counties of Ru yang 汝陽, Jia xian 郟縣, Bao feng 寶豐, Xiang cheng 襄城, Ye xian 葉縣 and Lu shan 魯山 in He nan. In 607, it was changed to be Xiang cheng commandery. Under Tang 唐, in 634, it was again established by changing the name of Yi zhou. Its seat of administration was at present-day Ru zhou city. Under Ming 明, in 1476, its status was raised to Ru zhou directly administered *zhou*, *zhi li zhou*. In 1913, the *zhou* was abolished and became Lin ru 臨汝 county the next year. Mentioned with 51.

Rui zhou lu 瑞州路 [1]
Name of a *lu* 路. It was founded, in 1277, by raising the status of Rui zhou 瑞州. Its seat of administration was in present-day Gao an 高安 city in Jiang xi 江西.

Its administrative area consisted of the present-day cities and counties of Yi feng 宜豐, Shang gao 上高 and Gao an 高安 in Jiang xi 江西. Under Ming, in 1369, it was changed to be Rui zhou fu 瑞州府.

Run 潤

See → Run zhou 潤州.

Run zhou 潤州 [10]

Name of a *zhou* 州. It was founded under Sui 隋, in 586. Its seat of administration was in present-day Zhen jiang 鎮江 city in Jiang su 江蘇. Its administrative area comprised present-day Nan jing 南京, and the counties of Ju rong 句容, Zhen jiang, Dan tu 丹徒, Dan yang 丹陽 and Jin tan 金壇 in Jiang su. It was eliminated in 607. It was reestablished under Tang 唐, in 620. In 742, it was changed to Dan yang commandery. In 758, it again became Run zhou. Under Northern Song 宋, in 1113, it was changed to Zhen jiang fu 鎮江府. Mentioned with 19, 52, 53, 78, 361, 508, 644, 905.

-S-

Sa ma er han 撒馬兒罕 [2]

Name of an ancient city in Central Asia, the present-day Samarqand in Uzbekistan. Ancient Greek sources refer to it as Marcanda. Semescant is a Turkic spelling found in Yuan 元 sources. The *Shi ji* 史記, "Historical Records," the *Han shu* 漢書, "Book of Han Dynasty,", the *Wei lüe* 魏略, "Account of Wei Dynasty," and the *Jin shu* 晉書, "Book of Jin Dynasty,", refer to it as Kang ju 康居 territory. The *Wei shu* 魏書, „Book of Wei Dynasty," refers to it as Xi wan jin 悉萬斤. The *Xi yu ji* 西域記, "Records of Western Territories," refers to it as Sa mo jian 颯秣建, the *Jing xing ji* 經行記 refers to it as Sa mo jian 薩末鞬, and the *Xin Tang shu* 新唐書, "New Book of Tang Dynasty," refers to it as both Kang guo 康國, Kang country, and Sa mo jian 薩末鞬, identifying it as Kang ju Area Command, Kang ju *du du fu* 康居都督府. The *Liao shi* 遼史, "History of Liao Dynasty," refers to it as Xun si gan 尋思干, identifying it as He zhong fu 河中府. The *Yuan shi* 元史, "History of Yuan Dynasty," too, names it Xun si gan 尋思干, and also Xue mi si gan 薛迷思干. The *Ming shi* 明史, "History of Ming Dynasty," refers to it as Sa ma er han 撒馬兒罕, and identifies it as the ancient capital of Kang ju 康居/Kan guo 康國. Mentioned with 174, 334.

Sai bei 塞北, "North of the barriers" [7]

Regional name. The term refers to regions extending from the outer Great Wall toward the North, including the present-day Inner Mongolia Self-Government region, the northern part of Gan su 甘肅 and of the Ning xia 寧夏 Muslim Nationality Self-governing Region, and areas north of the outer Great Wall in He bei 河北. Mentioned with 504, 1187, 1192, 1226, 1231, 1242, 1290.

Sai lan di fang 賽藍地方 [1]

Name of an ancient city in Central Asia: Sairam. It was located 30 English miles east of the present-day Kazakhstan city of Shymkent, capital of Southern Kazakhstan Oblast. The name is transliterated in Chinese sources in various ways, e.g., Sai lan 賽蘭 in the *Yuan shi* 元史 and in the *Ming shi* 明史, and in the latter also as Sai yi 賽夷. Mentioned with 1480.

Sai shang 塞上 [2]

Regional name. Reference is to the border area within and without the northern Great Wall. Mentioned with 404, 1109.

Sai wai 塞外 [4]

Regional name. It also is referred to as Sai bei 塞北, and encompasses the present-day Inner Mongolia Self-Government region, the northern part of Gan su 甘肅, and the Ning xia 寧夏 Muslim Nationality Self-Governing Region, as well as areas north of the outer Great Wall in He bei 河北. Mentioned with 420, 1253, 1364, 1433.

San cang 三蒼 [1]

This term is not a place name but the name of a book.

San fo qi 三佛齊 [8]

Name of an early country, the great trade emporium of Śrīvijaya. See → San fo qi guo 三佛齊國. Mentioned with 11, 14, 700, 855, 1124, 1139.

San fo qi guo 三佛齊國 [2]

Name of an early country, in varying transcriptions (San fo qi 三佛臍, San fu qi 三弗齊, Fo qi 佛齊, San fo guo 三佛國) referring to the various trading emporiums of Śrīvijaya the current version of which, in Song 宋 times, was the dominant Malayan trading state in Sumatra for a long time until ultimately replaced by Malacca during Ming 明 times. Śrīvijaya originally had its capital at Palembang on Sumatra. In Song times it was moved to Jami. In Ming times it was moved back to Palembang again. Mentioned with 1196, 1205.

San fu 三輔 [9]

Regional name. Western Han 漢, in 155 BCE, divided the *nei shi* 內史, "Region of the Internal Official," to become *zuo nei shi* 左內史 and *you nei shi* 右內史. These two and the Ranking Middle Authority, *zhu jue zhong wei* 主爵中尉 (in 144 BCE, this became a Ranking General Authority, *zhu jue du wei* 主爵都尉) jointly administered Chang an 長安 city. Its territory of administration included all the territory of the capital. Hence it was known collectively as the San fu 三輔, "Three Territories." In 104 BCE, under Emperor Wu di 武帝, the left and right *nei shi* and the *zhu jue du wei* were changed respectively to the Jing zhao yin 京兆尹, "Region of the Capital Governor," Zuo peng yi 左馮翊 and You fu feng 右扶風. Their territory of administration corresponded to the region of central Shaan xi 陝西. Later, although there were changes in the administrative divisions right up to the Tang 唐 period, the area was customarily called the San fu. Mentioned with 311, 579, 623, 740, 1033, 1469, 1478, 1519.

San jiao yi 三交驛 [1]
Minor place name. Located south of Zhou zhi 周至 county in Shaan xi 陝西. Mentioned with 1201.

San qin 三秦 [1]
Regional name. After the fall of Qin 秦, Xiang Yu 項羽 (232 – 202) divided the former Qin territory in the Guan zhong 關中 area into three parts and made the turncoat Qin General Zhang Han 章邯 (died 205 BCE) to be king of Yong 雍. He was to be in charge of the central part of present-day Shaan xi 陝西, the area from Xian yang 咸陽 toward the West, and the eastern part of Gan su 甘肅. Sima Xin 司馬欣 (died 204 BCE) became the king of Sai 塞, with charge of the western part of present-day Shaan xi from Xian yang to the east, and Dong Yi 董翳 (died 204 BCE) became Zhai 翟 king, with charge of the territory of the northwestern part of present-day Shaan xi. Together these areas were the San Qin, "Three Qin." Mentioned with 631.

San shan 傘山 [1]
Name of a mountain. Its name is also written San zi 傘子山. It is located northeast of present-day Sui ning 遂寧 city in Si chuan 四川. Mentioned with 1036.

San shou guo 三首國 [1]
Legendary name. It is from the *Shan hai jing* 山海經, "Classic of Mountains and Seas." Further details are unavailable. Mentioned with 1532.

San wei 三危 [2]
Name of a mountain. The reference in pre-Qin 秦 sources is an empty reference but later there was found a real San wei 三危 mountain located southeast of present-day Dun huang 敦煌 city in Gan su 甘肅. Alternative tradition places it northwest of Long xi 隴西 county in Gan su. Mentioned with 333, 1555.

San yuan xian 三原縣 [1]
Name of a county. It was established under Northern Wei 魏, in 446. Its seat of administration was at a location north of Cuo e 嵯峨 mountain, east of present-day Chun hua 淳化 county in Shaan xi 陝西. In 528, the seat was moved to a location northwest of the present-day San yuan 三原 county. Under Tang 唐, in 621, it was eliminated. It was reestablished in 623. Its seat of administration was at a location 30 *li* northeast of present-day San yuan county. It was abolished again in 627. At the same time, Hua chi 華池 county had its name changed to San yuan county. Its seat of administration was in Ren cheng 任城, located south of Qing shui yu 清水峪, and northwest of the present county. Under Northern Song 宋, in 976, the seat of administration was moved to a location northeast of the present-day county near the tomb of the Tang emperor Gao zu 唐高祖 (566 – 635). Under Yuan 元, in 1287, the seat of administration was moved to present-day San yuan county.

Sha 沙 [1]
Name of a *zhou* 州. See → Sha zhou 沙州. Mentioned with 738.

Sha lu hai ya 沙鹿海牙 [1]
Name of a city in Central Asia. The ruins are located on the right bank of the Syr-darya in present-day Uzbekistan. Mentioned with 14.

Sha mo zhu di 沙漠諸地[1]
Name of a region. The name is a general reference to the "desert and waste areas" in the North of China. Mentioned with 464.

Sha xian 沙縣 [1]
Name of a county. It was founded under Sui 隋, at the beginning of the *kai huang* 開皇 reign period (581-600). Its seat of administration was in Jiu xian 舊縣 located east of present-day Sha 沙 county in Fu jian 福建. In 596, the county was eliminated. It was reestablished under Tang 唐, in 621. Later, it was combined with Jian an 建安 county. In 655, it was reestablished by splitting Jian an county. In 884, the administration was moved to the present seat. Mentioned with 288.

Sha yuan 沙苑 [8]
Regional name. It is located some 40 *li* southeast of present-day Da li 大荔 county in Shaan xi 陝西. Mentioned with 125, 272, 532, 733, 1221.

Sha yuan he 沙苑河 [1]
Name of a river. This is the Yellow River located on the eastern side of present-day Sha yuan 沙苑 some 40 *li* southeast of Da li 大荔 county in Shaan xi 陝西. Mentioned with 733.

Sha zhou 沙州 [5]
Name of a *zhou* 州. It was founded under Tang 唐, in 633. Its seat of administration was at a location west of present-day Dun huang 敦煌 city in Gan su 甘肅. In 742, it became Dun huang commandery. In 758, it again became Sha zhou. Its territory of administration comprised the area from present-day Dun huang city in Gan su toward the West, up to the region of Luo bu bo 羅布泊 and Qie mo 且末 county in present-day Xin jiang 新疆. In 776, the area was lost to the Tibetans. It was recovered in 851. Later the *zhou* was abolished. Under Yuan 元, in 1277, the *zhou* was reestablished. In 1280, its status was raised to Sha zhou lu 沙州路. Mentioned with 274, 449, 695, 931, 1335.

Shaan 陝 [5 + 10 + 2]
□ Administrative unit [5] See under ' Shaan xi 陝西 [5]. Mentioned with 199, 322, 361, 801, 1040.
□ Name of a *zhou* 州. [10] See → Shaan zhou 陝州. Mentioned with 22, 31, 421, 473, 495, 639, 1067, 1096, 1367, 1417, 1449.
□ Name of an administrative unit. [2] See under ' Shaan xi 陝西 [39]. Mentioned with 247, 557.

Shaan fu 陝府 [1]
Administrative unit. This is the Shaan zhou Area Command, Shaan zhou *zong guan fu* 陝州總管府. It was established under Tang 唐, in 618, and its administrative area corresponded to the San men 三門 gorges, and the cities and counties of Shaan xian 陝縣, Luo ning 洛寧, Mian chi 澠池, Ling bao 靈寶 and Yi

yang 宜陽 in present-day He nan 河南. In 627, it was dissolved. In 742, it was reestablished to be Shaan 陜 commandery. Mentioned with 186.

Shaan luo 陜洛 [1]

Regional term. This is a combined name of Shaan zhou 陜州 and Luo 洛. This corresponds to a region including the present-day San men 三門 gorges in He nan 河南 and Luo yang 洛陽 city. Mentioned with 1096.

Shaan xi 陜西 [39 + 5 + 1]

□ Name of a *lu*. [39] It was founded under Northern Song 宋, in 997, as Shaan xi lu 陜西路. Its seat of administration was in present-day Xi an 西安 city in Shaan xi 陜西. Its territory of administration extended in present-day Shaan xi from the Qin ling 秦嶺 mountain range toward the North, and in Ning xia 寧夏 from the Great Wall toward the South, along with the southwestern part of Shan xi 山西, the northwestern part of He nan 河南, and the southeastern part of Gan su 甘肅. Later people called the area Shaan 陜. Jin 金 reorganized the area as the five *lu* 路 of Qin feng 秦鳳. Mentioned with 52, 56, 188, 199, 202, 203, 211, 324, 338, 361, 369, 389, 437, 461, 462, 473, 499, 620, 653, 665, 748, 764, 801, 811, 871, 893, 911, 934, 986, 995, 1122, 1140, 1175, 1215, 1254, 1324, 1340, 1392, 1428.

□ Name of an administrative area. [5] It was founded by Ming 明, in 1376, when a Shaan xi Provincial Administration Commission, Shaan xi *bu zheng shi si* 陜西布政使司, was established. It had two *shi* 使, "officials," a left and a right one, and was administered from present-day Xi an 西安 city in Shaan xi 陜西. Its territory of administration comprised the three present-day provinces of Shaan xi, Ning xia 寧夏 and Gan su 甘肅, and the eastern part of Qing hai 青海. In 1663, under Qing 清, the provinces of Shaan 陜 and Gan 甘 were split off. Mentioned with 361, 449, 619, 1230, 1334.

□ Name of a Branch Secretariat, *xing sheng* 行省. [1] It was established under Yuan 元 in 1286. Its seat of administration was in present-day Xi an city in Shaan xi. Its territory of administration included the whole province of present-day Shaan xi, the eastern portion of Gan su, the southern portion of Ning xia and part of Inner Mongolia. Under Ming, in 1376, the area became the Provincial Administration Commission for Shaan xi and other places, Shaan xi deng chu *cheng xuan bu zheng shi si* 陜西等處承宣布政使司. Mentioned with 461.

Shaan zhou 陜州 [6]

Name of a *zhou* 州. It was established under Northern Wei 魏, in 487. Its seat of administration was in the old city of Shaan xian 陜縣, located west of present-day San men xia 三門峽 city in He nan 河南. Its territory of administration included in present-day He nan 河南 the cities and counties of San men xia, Shaan xian 陜縣, Luo ning 洛寧, Mian chi 澠池, and Ling bao 靈寶, and in Shan xi 山西 the cities and counties of Yun cheng 運城, Ping lu 平陸 and Rui cheng 芮城. In 494, it was eliminated. It was reestablished at the beginning of the *tian ping* 天平 reign period (534 – 547) of Eastern Wei. It was eliminated at the beginning of the *da ye* 大業 reign period (605 – 618) of Sui 隋. It was reestablished under Tang 唐, in 618. In 742, it was changed to be Shaan 陜 commandery. In 758, it again was made Shaan zhou 陜州. Under the Qing 清, in 1724, its status was raised to the Shaan zhou directly administered *zhou*, *zhi li zhou* 直隸州. In 1913, it became Shaan county. Mentioned with 20, 186, 365, 473, 905.

Shan 剡 [1]

Name of a county. It was established during Western Han 漢. Its seat of administration was at a location southwest of present-day Sheng zhou 嵊州 city in Zhe jiang 浙江. Under Three Kingdoms' Wu 吳, the administration was moved to present-day Sheng zhou city. In 1121, the county became Sheng county.

Shan dan wei 山丹衛 [1]

Name of a guard. It was established under the Ming 明, in 1390. Its seat of administration was in present-day Shan dan 山丹 county in Gan su 甘肅. Its territory of administration included the territory of present-day Shan dan county in Gan su. Under Qing 清, in 1724, it was demoted to be Shan dan county. Mentioned with 1335.

Shan dong 山東 [8 + 7 + 2 + 1]

□ Name of a province. [8] It was established under the Ming 明, in 1368. Its seat of administration was in present-day Qing zhou 青州 city in Shan dong 山東. In 1378, the seat of administration was moved to present-day Ji nan 濟南 city. Later, the province was changed to become the Shan dong Provincial Administration Commission, Shan dong *bu zheng shi si* 山東布政使司. Its territory of administration corresponded to the present-day province of Shan dong. Mentioned with 268, 474, 566, 738, 776, 976, 1023, 1057.

□ Regional name. [7] It refers in general to the area east of Tai hang 太行 mountain. Mentioned with 117, 562, 600, 1038, 1238, 1264, 1449, 1480.

□ Regional name. [2] It refers in general to the area east of Hua 華 mountain or Xiao 崤 mountain. Mentioned with 115, 1264.

□ Regional name. [1] Under Eastern Jin 晉 the Three Wu 吳 area extending toward the East from Ju qu 句曲 mountain/Mao 茅 mountain belonged to Shan dong 山東. This corresponds to an area in today's Jiang su 江蘇 extending from the Tai hu 太湖 lake toward the East and the North, and the northern part of Zhe jiang 浙江. Mentioned with 1316.

Shan dou 山都 [1]

Name of a county. It was established by Qin 秦. Its seat of administration was at a location north of the present-day Xiang zhou 襄州 district of Xiang yang 襄陽 city in Hu bei 襄陽. Eastern Han 漢 moved the seat of administration to a location southeast of present-day Gu cheng 穀城 county in Hu bei. Northern Zhou 周 abolished it and made it part of An yang 安養 county. Mentioned with 628.

Shan nan 山南 [3 + 21 + 3]

□ Name of a location but the reference south of the mountain(s) is somewhat vague as a place name. [3] Further details are unavailable. Mentioned with 650, 730, 1158.

□ Name of a circuit. [21] This is the Shan nan 山南 circuit established under Tang 唐, in 627. It was one of ten such circuits that the entire country was divided into. Its territory of administration comprised an area extending in present-day Si chuan 四川 from the Jia ling 嘉陵 watershed toward the East, in Shaan xi 陝西 from the Qin ling 秦嶺 mountain range, and in Gan su 甘肅 from Pan zhong 潘塚 mountain toward the South, including in He nan 湖南 the area southwest of Fu niu 伏牛 mountain, and in Hu bei 湖北 from Yun shui 涓水 toward the West, and in Hu nan 湖南 the area north of the Yang zi from Chong qing 重慶 city to Yue yang 岳陽 city. Mentioned with 51, 123, 178, 317, 322, 502, 644, 653, 687, 714, 768, 797, 863, 973, 1033, 1034, 1172, 1238, 1273, 1407.

□ Regional name. [3] It refers to the area south of the Qin ling 秦嶺 mountain range. Mentioned with 578, 1099.

Shan rong 山戎 [1]

Name of a minority tribe, also known as Bei rong 北戎, "Northern Rong." This was one of the Yi 夷 countries during the Spring and Autumn period, covering the northern part of present-day He bei 河北. Mentioned with 1206.

Shan xi 剡溪 [1]

Name of a watershed. This is one of the affluents of the Cao e jiang 曹娥江 in present-day Zhe jiang 浙江 province. Mentioned with 1471.

Shan xi 山西 [4 + 2]

□ Name of a province-level administrative region. [4] It was established under Ming 明, in 1369. Its seat of administration was in present-day Tai yuan 太原 city in Shan xi 山西. Its territory of administration corresponded to present-day Shan xi province. In 1376, the area was changed to a Shan xi Provincial Administration Commission, Shan xi *bu zheng shi si* 山西布政使司. Mentioned with 566, 702, 1037, 1532.

□ Name of an administrative region. [2] Yuan 元 established a Pacification Office for the He dong and Shan xi Circuits, He dong shan xi dao *xuan wei si* 河東山西道宣慰司. This corresponded to the present-day Shan xi 山西 province. Mentioned with 461, 1150.

Shan yang 山陽 [3 + 3]

□ General reference. [3] The southern part of a mountain is yang 陽, and this is a general reference to the southern face of a mountain. Mentioned with 829, 1072, 1178, 1445, 1524.

□ Name of a commandery. [3] It was established under Han Wu di 漢武帝, in 136 BCE, by changing the name of Shan yang 山陽 country. Its seat of administration was at a location 60 *li* south of present-day Ju ye 巨野 county in Shan dong 山東. Its administrative territory comprised an area in present-day Shan dong extending from Ju ye toward the South, from Cheng wu 成武 and Cao 曹 county toward the East, from Shan 單 county toward the North, and from Yu tai 魚臺 toward the West, as well as the cities of Zuo cheng 鄒城 and Yan zhou 兗州. During Western Jin 晉, it was changed to Gao ping 高平 country. Mentioned with 631.

Shan yin 山陰 [2 + 7]

□ Name of a county. [2] It was established by Qin 秦. Its seat of administration was in Shao xing 紹興 city in present-day Zhe jiang 浙江. It got its name from being north of Kuai ji 會稽 mountain. Under Eastern Han 漢, in 129, it was put under the control of Kuai ji commandery. It was eliminated under Sui 隋, in 589. It was restored under Tang 唐, in 624. In 1912, it was combined with Kuai ji county to form Shao xing 紹興 county. Mentioned with 785.

□ Designation of a position. [7] The northern face of a mountain is *yin* 陰. This is a general reference to the northern face of a mountain. Mentioned with 154, 365, 635, 640, 867, 1010, 1374.

Shan zhou 剡州 [1]

Name of a *zhou* 州. This is Sheng zhou 嵊州. It was established under Tang 唐, in 621. Its seat of administration was in present-day Sheng zhou city in Zhe jiang 浙江. Its territory of administration comprised the two present-day counties of Sheng zhou and Xin chang 新昌 in Zhe jiang. Mentioned with 1017.

Shan zhou 單州 [1]

Name of a *zhou* 州. It was established during the *guang qi* reign period (885 – 888) of Tang 唐. It was administered from a location south of present-day Shan 單 county in Shan dong 山東. Later, it became Hui zhou 輝州, and the seat of administration was moved to present-day Dang shan 碭山 county in An hui 安徽. In 924, it was again made Shan zhou, and administered as before from Shan county in Shan dong. Under Song 宋, the territory of administration corresponded in Shan dong to the area of Shan county, Cheng wu 成武 and Yu tai 魚台 and in An hui 安徽 Dang shan county. In 1369, the area became Shan county. Mentioned with 687.

Shang 商 [7]

Name of a *zhou* 州. See → Shang zhou 商州. Mentioned with 38, 107, 381, 457, 654, 660.

Shang cai 上蔡 [3]

Name of a county. See → Shang cai 上蔡 county. Mentioned with 272, 605, 1529.

Shang cai xian 上蔡縣 [1]

Name of a county. It was founded under Sui 隋, in 607. Its seat of administration was in present-day Shang cai 上蔡 county in He nan 河南. Mentioned with 1003.

Shang cheng 商城 [1]

Name of a county. It was established under Northern Song 宋, in 960. Its seat of administration was at a location west of present-day Shang cheng 商城 county in He nan 河南. In 997, it was abolished and combined with Gu shi 固始 county. It was reestablished under Ming 明, in 1475, but its seat of administration was moved to the present Shang cheng county. Mentioned with 1289.

Shang dang 上黨 [27]

Name of a commandery. See → Shang dang jun 上黨郡. Mentioned with 6, 111, 131, 261, 426, 485, 575, 599, 648, 687, 931, 1067, 1109, 1158, 1313, 1462, 1531.

Shang dang jun 上黨郡 [1]

Name of a commandery. It was established by Warring States Han 韓. During Qin 秦 and Han 漢, the seat of administration was at a location southwest of present-day Chang zi 長子 county in Shan xi 山西. Its territory of administration amounted to the southeastern part of present-day Shan xi. At the end of Eastern Han, the seat of administration was moved to present-day Gu yi 故驛 village, 35 *li* north of the Chang zhi 長治 city. Western Jin 晉 moved the administration to 古城 village, located 40 *li* northeast of the present Lu cheng 潞城 county. Northern Wei 魏 again established the administration at the present-day Gu yi village. Its territory of administration was reduced, and included the present-day Chang zi city and the counties of Tun liu 屯留, Chang zi 長子, Lu cheng 潞城, Ping shun 平順, Hu guan 壺關 and An ze 安澤. Under early Sui 隋, at the beginning of the *kai huang* 開皇 reign period (581-600), it was eliminated. It was restored at the beginning of the *da ye* 大業 reign period (605-618). The seat of administration was moved to present-day Chang zhi city. Under Tang 唐, in 618, it was changed to be Lu zhou 潞州. At the beginning of the *tian bao* 天寶 reign period (742 – 756), it again became Shang dang 上黨 commandery. In 758, it again was changed to Lu zhou. Mentioned with 223.

Shang gu 上谷 [3]
Name of a commandery. It was established by Warring States Yan 燕. Under Qin 秦, the administrative seat was located at a location southeast of present-day Huai lai 懷來 county in He bei 河北. Its territory of administration corresponded in present-day He bei 河北 to an area extending from Zhang jia kou 張家口 city and Xiao wu tai 小五台 mountain toward the East, from Chi cheng 赤城 county and Yan qing 延慶 county in Bei jing 北京 city toward the West, and from Nei chang cheng 內長城 and Chang ping 昌平 district toward the North. Northern Wei 魏 abolished it. Mentioned with 53, 740, 1262.

Shang jun 上郡 [4 + 1]
□ Name of a commandery. [4] It was established by Wei Wen hou 魏文侯 (died 396 BCE) of the Warring States period. During the Qin 秦 period, the seat of administration was located near Yu he bao 魚河堡, 70 *li* southeast of present-day Liu lin 榆林 city in Shaan xi 陝西. During Western Han 漢, the administrative area corresponded to the northern section of present-day Shaan xi and parts of the Uxin-Banner, 烏審旗, in Inner Mongolia. It was abolished under Eastern Han, in 215. Mentioned with 324, 687, 1392, 1548.
□ Regional name. [1] The reference is to the northern border areas of Shaan xi 陝西. Mentioned with 195.

Shang lin yuan 上林苑 [1]
Name of an old palace park. It was established by Qin 秦, when the Qin capital was at Xian yang 咸陽. The park is located north of Zhong nan 終南 mountain and south of the Wei shui 渭水 which is located west of present-day Xi an 西安 city in Shaan xi 陝西. The area was abandoned and overgrown by early Western Han 漢. During the time of Emperor Wu di 武帝 (156 – 87) it was restored and enlarged, its circumference reaching more than 200 *li*. Later it was abandoned. Mentioned with 804.

Shang long dong 上龍洞 [1]
Name of a mountain grotto. It is on Mao 茅 mountain in the southwestern part of present-day Jiang su 江蘇. Mentioned with 1351.

Shang luo 上洛 [2]
Ancient place name. It is also given as Shang luo 上雒. This was a city in Jin 晉 during the Spring and Autumn period. This is the present-day Shang zhou 商州 district of Shang luo 商洛 city in Shaan xi 陝西. Mentioned with 129, 1456.

Shang luo 商洛
See → Shang luo shan 上洛山.

Shang luo jun 上洛郡 [1]
Name of a commandery. It was established under Western Jin 晉, in 266. Its seat of administration was in the present-day Shang zhou 商州 district of Shang luo 商洛 city in Shaan xi 陝西. Its territory of administration comprised the upper reaches of the Dan jiang 丹江 river in present-day Shaan xi, and the area of the upper reaches of the Luo 洛 river northwest of Xiong er 熊耳 mountain in He nan 河南. Later, its administrative area was reduced. It was eliminated under Sui 隋, in 583. At the beginning of the *da ye* 大業 reign period (605 – 618), Shang zhou was changed to be Shang luo commandery. Under Tang 唐, in 618, the area again became Shang zhou. In 742, the area again become Shang luo commandery. In 758, it was changed to be Shang zhou. Mentioned with 129.

Shang luo shan 上洛山 [1]
Name of a mountain. In this case the character *shang* 上 is a phonetic mistake for Shang 商. Shang luo 上洛 mountain is thus Shang luo 商洛 mountain. See → Shang luo shan 商洛山. Mentioned with 1215.

Shang luo shan 商洛山 [2]
Name of a mountain. It is located in present-day Shang luo 商洛 city in Shaan xi 陝西. The mountain area extends across the present-day districts and counties of Shang zhou 商州, Luo nan 洛南, Dan feng 丹鳳 and Shan yang 山陽. Mentioned with 459, 1251.

Shang luo xian 上洛縣 [1]
Name of a county. It was established by Three Kingdoms Wei 魏. Its seat of administration was in the Shang zhou 商州 district of present-day Shang luo 商洛 city in Shaan xi 陝西. Western Jin 晉 put it under Shang luo commandery. Northern Wei 魏 put it under Luo zhou 洛州. Northern Zhou 周 put it under Shang zhou 商州. Sui 隋 put it under Shang luo 上洛 commandery. Tang 唐 again put it under Shang zhou. In 742, its administration was transferred to Shang luo commandery. In 758, it was changed again and put under Shang zhou. Yuan 元 abolished the county. Mentioned with 204.

Shang qing feng 上清峰 [1]
Name of a mountain peak. It is one of the mountain peaks of the Meng 蒙 mountains of the present-day border region west of Ming shan 名山 county in Si chuan 四川 with Ya an 雅安 city. Mentioned with 124.

Shang rao 上饒 [5]

Name of a county. See → Shang rao xian 上饒縣. Mentioned with 595, 859, 866, 1014, 1171.

Shang rao xian 上饒縣 [1]

Name of a county. It was established by Three Kingdoms' Wu 吳. Its seat of administration was in Tian jin qiao 天津橋, located northwest of present-day Shang rao 上饒 city in Jiang xi 江西. Western Jin 晉 eliminated it. Southern Dynasties Liu Song 劉宋 reestablished it. Sui 隋 eliminated the county. Under Tang 唐, in 621, it was reestablished. In 624, it was eliminated again. In 758, at the time that it was reestablished, it was put under Xin zhou 信州. Yuan 元 created a Xin zhou lu 信州路 to administer it. Under Ming 明, in 1370, the seat of administration was moved to the present Shang rao city. In 1949, its status was changed to city rank. Mentioned with 552.

Shang ru shan 商汝山 [1]

This should be a combination of Shang zhou 商州 and Ru zhou 汝州 rationalized to be a mountain name. See → Shang zhou 商州 and → Ru zhou 汝州 for details on these places. Mentioned with 986.

Shang shan 商山

Name of a mountain. This is Shang luo 商洛 mountain, also known as Di mai shan 地脈山 and Chu shan 楚山. It is located one *li* south of present-day Xi shang 西商 town in Dan feng 丹鳳 county in Shaan xi 陝西. Mentioned with 1519.

Shang yu 上虞 [1 + 1]

□ Name of a county. [1] It was established by Qin 秦 and subordinated to Kuai ji 會稽 commandery. Its seat of administration was in present-day Shang yu city in Zhe jiang 浙江. It was abolished under Sui 隋, in 589. It was reestablished under Tang 唐, in 785. In 822, the seat of administration was moved to Feng hui 豐惠 town, located 26 *li* southeast of the present-day Shang yu city. In 1954, the seat of administration was moved to Bai guan 百官 town. Mentioned with 261.

□ This is another name for Yu guo 虞國. [1] It was located northeast of present-day Ping lu 平陸 county in Shan xi 山西. Mentioned with 261.

Shang yuan 上元 [1]

Name of a county. It was established in 761, in the second year of the *shang yuan* 上元 reign period, by Tang 唐 and it was named after that reign period. Its seat of administration was in present-day Nan jing 南京 city in Jiang su 江蘇. In 887, it was put under Sheng zhou 昇州. In 1912, it was combined with Jiang ning 江寧 county. Mentioned with 735.

Shang yuan 上苑 [2]

Name of the park of an old palace. See → Shang lin yuan 上林苑.

Shang zhou 商州 [19]

Name of a *zhou* 州. It was established under Northern Zhou 周, in 578. Its seat of administration was in present-day Shang luo 商洛 city in Shaan xi 陝西. Its territory of administration corresponded to an area extending in present-day Shaan xi from the Qin ling 秦嶺 mountain range toward the South, and from the Xun he 旬河 (other than Xun yang 旬陽 county) toward the East, and included also in present-day Hu bei 湖北 Shang jin 上津 town in Yun xi 鄖西 county. During the *da ye* 大業 (605 – 618) reign period of the Sui, and the *tian bao* 天寶 (742 – 756) and *zhi de* 至德 (756 – 758) reign periods of the Tang 唐, the area periodically became a commandery. Under the Ming 明, in 1374, it was demoted to be a county. In 1477, its status was raised to a *zhou*. In 1725, its status was raised to a directly administered *zhou, zhi li zhou* 直隸州. In 1913, it was changed to be Shang 商 county. Mentioned with 202, 228, 261, 437, 660, 908, 986, 1091, 1215, 1251, 1255, 1417, 1463, 1470, 1476, 1532.

Shao 韶 [1]
Name of a *zhou* 州. See under → Shao zhou 韶州. Mentioned with 1063.

Shao 邵 [1]
Name of a *zhou*. It was founded under Tang 唐, in 636. Its administrative seat was at present-day Shao yang 邵陽 city in Hu nan 湖南. Its territory of administration included the Zi shui 資水 watershed south of present-day Ling shui jiang 冷水江 city in Hu nan. At the beginning of the *tian bao* 天寶 reign period (742 – 756) of Tang, the area became Shao yang commandery. At the beginning of the *qian yuan* 慶元 reign period (758 – 760), it became Shao zhou 邵州. Under Five Dynasties' Jin 晉, during the *tian fu* 天福 reign period (936 – 943), Chu 楚 changed it to be Min zhou 敏州. Under Han 漢, it again became Shao zhou. Under Southern Song 宋, in 1225, its status was raised to Bao qing fu 寶慶府. Mentioned with 202.

Shao ling 邵陵 [3]
Name of a commandery. During the *tai kang* 太康 reign period (280-289) of Western Jin 晉, its name was changed to Zhao ling 昭陵 commandery out of a taboo avoidance in respect of Sima Zhao 司馬昭 (211-265). Its seat of administration was in present-day Shao Yang 邵陽 city in Hu nan 湖南. Its territory of administration comprised the Zi shui 資水 watershed south of present-day Ling shui jiang 冷水江 city in Hu nan. It was abolished under Sui 隋, in 589. Mentioned with 107, 217.

Shao shi 少室 [14]
Name of a mountain. See under → Shao shi zhi shan 少室之山. Mentioned with 275, 299, 322, 810, 1003, 1061, 1063, 1168, 1250, 1435, 1469.

Shao shi shan 少室山
See under → Shao shi zhi shan. 少室之山.

Shao shi zhi shan 少室之山 [6]
Name of a mountain. It is located northwest of present-day Deng feng 登封 city in He nan 河南. It marks the western part of the Song 嵩 mountains. Mentioned with 62, 164, 230, 369, 605.

Shao wu 紹武 [1]
This is an error for Shao wu 邵武. See → Shao wu 邵武. Mentioned with 1028.

Shao wu 邵武 [1 + 1]

□ Name of an administrative area. [1] See → Shao wu jun 邵武軍. Mentioned with 1028.

□ Name of a *fu* 府. [1] It was established under Yuan 元, in 1367. Its seat of administration was in present-day Shao wu city in Fu jian 福建. Its territory of administration included the present-day cities and counties of Shao wu, Guang ze 光澤, Tai ning 泰宁 and Jian ning 建宁 in Fu jian. It was abolished in 1913. Mentioned with 1028.

Shao wu jun 邵武軍 [1]

Administrative unit. It was founded under Northern Song 宋, in 980, by raising the status of Shao wu 邵武 county of Jian zhou 建州. Its seat of administration was in present-day Shao wu city. Its territory of administration comprised the present-day cities and counties of Shao wu in Fu jian, Guang ze 光澤, Tai ming 泰寧 and Jian ning 建寧 in Fu jian 福建. Under Yuan 元, in 1276, the status of the area was raised to be Shao wu lu 邵武路. Mentioned with 1091.

Shao xing 紹興 [1]

Name of a *fu* 府. It was established under Southern Song 宋, in 1131. Its seat of administration was in present-day Shao xing 紹興 city in Zhe jiang 浙江. The territory administered comprised the watersheds of the Pu yang jiang 浦陽江 (other than Pu jiang 浦江 county) and of the Cao e jiang 曹娥江, and the western portions of the two present-day cities of Yu yao 余姚 and Ci xi 慈溪 in Zhe jiang. Under Yuan 元, in 1276, the area was changed to be Shao xing lu 紹興路. In 1366, it became Shao xing fu 紹興府. It was abolished in 1912. Mentioned with 365.

Shao yang 韶陽 [1]

Regional name. It refers to the area south of Shao shi 韶石 mountain of Shao guan 韶關 city in present-day Guang dong 廣東. Mentioned with 939.

Shao yang shan 燒羊山 [1]

Name of a mountain. It is located east of Turfan city in Xinjiang. Mentioned with 1335.

Shao yang zhi shan 少陽之山 [1]

This is a place name from the *Shan hai jing* 山海經, "Classic of Mountains and Seas." Details are lacking. Mentioned with 191.

Shao zhou 韶州 [3 + 7]

□ Name of a *fu* 府. [3] It was established under Ming 明, in 1368. Its seat of administration was in present-day Shao zhou 韶州 city in Guang dong 廣東. The territory administered comprised the present-day cities and counties of Shao guan 韶關, Qu jiang 曲江, Ying de 英德, Weng yuan 翁源, Ru yuan 乳源, Ren hua 仁化 and Le chang 樂昌 in Guang dong. The *fu* was abolished in 1912. Mentioned with 303, 789, 1454.

□ Name of a *zhou* 州. [7] It was founded under Sui 隋, in 589. Its seat of administration was west of the Wu shui 武水, located 10 *li* south of present-day Shao guan 韶關 city in Guang dong 廣東. It was eliminated in 591. It was reestablished under Tang 唐, in 627. In 742, it was changed to be Shi xing 始興 commandery. In 758, it was named Shao zhou again. Its territory of administration included in Guang dong the area extending toward the North from Ru yuan 乳源, Qu jiang 曲江 and Weng yuan 翁源. Under Yuan 元, in 1278, it was changed to be Shao zhou lu 韶州路. Mentioned with 324, 376, 428, 717, 1063.

She 歙 [3]
Name of a *zhou*. See → She zhou 歙州. Mentioned with 79, 189, 1485.

She yang 射陽 [1]
Name of a county. It was established by Western Han 漢. Its seat of administration was in present-day She yang 射陽 town, located northeast of Bao ying 寶應 county in Jiang su 江蘇. The county was eliminated during the Three Kingdoms period. It was reestablished under Western Jin 晉, in 280. In 413, Eastern Jin eliminated the county again. It was reestablished at the end of Sui 隋. In 624, it was again eliminated under Tang 唐. It was reestablished in 1942, and persists to the present. Mentioned with 1250.

She zhou 歙州 [4]
Name of a *zhou* 州. It was established under Sui 隋, in 589. Its seat of administration was in Wan an 萬安 town, located 10 *li* east of present-day Xiu ning 休寧 county in An hui 安徽. At the end of Sui, the seat of administration was moved to present-day She 歙 county in An hui. Its territory of administration comprised the watershed of the Xin an jiang 新安江 and present-day Qi men 祁門 county in An hui, and present-day Wu yuan 婺源 in Jiang xi 江西. During the *da ye* 大業 (605 – 618) reign period of the Sui, and the *tian bao* 天寶 (742 – 756) and *zhi de* 至德 (756 – 758) reign periods of the Tang 唐, the area was temporarily changed to be Xin an 新安 commandery. Under Northern Song 宋, in 1121, it was changed to be Hui zhou 徽州. Mentioned with 456, 556, 742, 864.

Shen 申 [2]
Name of a *zhou* 州. See → Shen zhou 申州. Mentioned with 973, 1034.

Shen mu xian 神木縣 [1]
Name of a county. It was established under Yuan 元, in 1269. Its seat of administration was at a location 3 *li* east of present-day Shen mu 神木 county in Shaan xi 陝西. Under Ming 明, in 1443, the seat of administration was moved to present-day Shen mu county. Mentioned with 126.

Shen zhou 申州 [4]
Name of a *zhou* 州. It was established by Northern Zhou 周. Its seat of administration was in present-day Xin yang 信陽 city in He nan 河南. Under Sui 隋, in 606, it was changed to Yi zhou 義州. Under Tang, in 621, it was changed to Shen zhou 申州. Its territory of administration corresponded to present-day Xin yang city in He nan. In 742, the area became Yi yang 義陽 commandery. In 758, it again became Shen zhou. Under Northern Song 宋, in 976, it became Yi yang army. Mentioned with 31, 797, 1142, 1250.

Shen zhou 深州 [2]

Name of a *zhou* 州. It was founded under Sui 隋, in 596. Its seat of administration was in present-day An ping 安平 county in He bei 河北. At the beginning of the *da ye* 大業 reign period (605 – 618) of Sui 隋, it was abolished. It was reestablished in 621. That same year, the seat of administration was moved to present-day Rao yang 饒陽 county. In 643, it was eliminated. It was reestablished in 713. Its seat of administration was in present-day Jiu zhou 舊州 village, located west of Shen zhou city. Its territory of administration included present-day Shen zhou and the counties and cities of An ping, Rao yang and Xin ji 辛集 in He bei. Under Northern Song 宋, in 987, the seat of administration was moved to a location south of the present Shen zhou city. Under Ming 明, in 1412, the seat of administration was moved to the present Shen zhou city. Mentioned with 544, 1057.

Sheng nan 勝南 [1]

This term is not a place name. The original passage notes that medicinals produced in one area are superior (*sheng* 勝) to those produced in another (i.e., the south). The reference is associated with the production of products 275.

Shi 施 [2 + 1]

□ Name of a *zhou* 州. [2] See under → Shi zhou 施州. Mentioned with 58, 456.
□ Name of a guard. [1] See under → Shi zhou 施州. Mentioned with 585.

Shi an 始安 [5]

Name of a commandery. It was established under Three Kingdoms' Wu 吳, in 265. Its seat of administration was in present-day Gui lin 桂林 city in Guang xi 廣西. Its territory of administration comprised the Li jiang 漓江 watershed between Gui lin and Ping le 平樂 and Yong fu 永福 county in present-day Guang xi. Liu Song 劉宋 changed it to be Shi jian guo 始建國. Qi 齊 restored Shi an commandery. At the beginning of the *da ye* 大業 reign period (605 – 618) of Sui 隋, Gui zhou was changed to be Shi an commandery. Under Tang 唐, in 621, it was again changed to be Gui zhou. At the beginning of the *tian bao* 天寶 reign period (742 – 756), it became Shi an commandery. In 757, it was renamed as Jian ling 建陵 commandery. Mentioned with 380, 474.

Shi cheng 石城 [3 + 1]

□ Name of a county. [3] It was established by Western Han 漢. Its seat of administration was in present-day Shi cheng 石城 village of Guan kou xiang 灌口鄉, located 70 *li* southwest of Chi zhou 池州 city in An hui 安徽. Western Jin 晉 put it under Xuan cheng 宣城 commandery. Southern Dynasties' Liang 梁 put it under Nan ling 南陵 commandery. It was abolished under Sui 隋, in 589. Mentioned with 629, 660, 1178.
□ Name of a *xiang* 鄉 or sub-administrative unit. [1] It was located somewhere in the area of Jing men 荊門, Dang yang 當陽 and Sha yang 沙洋 of present-day Hu bei 湖北. Further details are unavailable. Mentioned with 178.

Shi cui zhi shan 石脆之山 [1]

Name of a mountain from the *Shan hai jing* 山海經, "Classic of Mountains and Seas." Further details are unavailable. Mentioned with 191.

Shi cui zhi shan 石翠之山 [1]

Name of a mountain from the *Shan hai jing* 山海經, "Classic of Mountains and Seas." Further details are unavailable. Mentioned with 1526.

Shi feng 始豐 [1]

Name of a county. It was founded under Western Jin 晉, in 280. Its seat of administration was in present-day Tian tai 天台 county in Zhe jiang 浙江. It was eliminated under Sui 隋, in 589. It was restored under Tang 唐, in 621. It was again eliminated in 625. It was restored, in 634, and put under Tai zhou 台州. Under Tang 唐, in 675, it was changed to be Tang xing 唐興 county. Mentioned with 635.

Shi men 石門 [2 + 1 + 1]

□ Name of a county. [2] It was founded under Tang 唐, in 618. Its seat of administration was at a location north of present-day Chun hua 淳化 county in Shaan xi 陝西. In 627, it was changed to be Yun yang 雲陽 county. Mentioned with 285, 1307.

□ Name of a county. [1] It was established under Liu song 劉宋. Its seat of administration was in the outskirts of the present-day Yang xi 陽西 or Dian bai 電白 county in Guang dong. Sui 隋 abolished it. Mentioned with 1307.

□ Name of a county. [1] It was founded under Northern Wei 魏, in 448. Its seat of administration was in present-day Shi men xiang 石門鄉, located 40 *li* northwest of Wu du 武都 district in Long nan 隴南 city in Gan su 甘肅. Western Wei changed it to be An yu 安育 county. Mentioned with 285.

Shi mo shan 石墨山 [1]

Name of a mountain. It is located two *li* southwest of present-day Yi yang 宜陽 county in He nan 河南. Mentioned with 1051.

Shi xing 始興 [11]

Name of a commandery. It was founded by Three Kingdoms' Wu 吳, in 265. Its seat of administration was in a place below Lian hua 蓮花 mountain range, southeast of present-day Shao guan 韶關 city in Guang dong 廣東. Under Liu Song 劉宋, in 472, it was changed to be Guang xing 廣興 commandery. Southern Qi 齊 again made it Shi xing commandery. Its territory of administration comprised in present-day Guang dong an area extending from Qing yuan 清遠, Fo gang 佛岡 and Weng yuan 翁源 toward the North. It was eliminated under Sui 隋, in 589. Under Tang 唐, in 742, it was reestablished as Shao zhou 韶州. Its seat of administration was at a location west of the Wu shui 武水, one *li* west of present-day Shao guan city in Guang dong. In 758, the area again became Shao zhou. Mentioned with 21, 122, 376, 594, 595, 1020, 1063, 1307, 1389, 1402.

Shi zhou 十洲 [1]

Legendary place name. In real terms it refes to the islands of Zu zhou 祖洲, Ying zhou 瀛洲, Xuan zhou 玄洲, Yan zhou 炎洲, Chang zhou 長洲, Yuan zhou 元洲, Liu zhou 流洲, Sheng zhou 生洲, Feng lin zhou 鳳麟洲 and Ju ku zhou 聚窟洲 in the ocean. Further details are unavailable.

Shi zhou 石州 [4]

Name of a *zhou* 州. It was founded under Northern Zhou 周, in 577. Its seat of administration was in present-day Li shi 離石 city in Shan xi 山西. Its territory of administration comprised the districts and counties of Li shi, Zhong yang 中陽, Liu lin 柳林, Lin xian 臨縣 and Fang shan 方山 in Shan xi. The *zhou* was eliminated under Sui 隋, in 607. It was reestablished under Tang 唐, in 618. Under Ming 明, in 1567, it was changed to be Yong ning zhou 永寧州. Mentioned with 620, 1032, 1191, 1258.

Shi zhou 施州 [20 + 3]

□ Name of a *zhou* 州. [20] It was established under Northern Zhou 周, in 574. Its seat of administration was in present-day En shi 恩施 city in He bei 湖北. At the beginning of the *da ye* 大業 reign period (605 – 618) of Sui 隋, the area became Qing jiang 清江 commandery. At the beginning of Tang 唐, it again became Shi zhou. In 742, it was changed to Qing hua 清化 commandery. In 758, it again became Shi zhou. Its territory of administration comprised in the Northwest of present-day Hu bei 湖北 an area extending from the counties of Wu feng 五峰 and Jian shi 建始 toward the West. At the beginning of the *hong wu* 洪武 reign period (1368 – 1398) of Ming 明, the *zhou* was abolished. It was restored in 1381. In 1390, it was abolished again and made part of the Shi zhou guard. Mentioned with 69, 246, 260, 370, 435, 468, 551, 571, 704, 725, 1019, 1185, 1284, 1316, 1333, 1361, 1362, 1368, 1507.

□ Name of a guard. [3] It was established under Ming 明, in 1381. Its seat of administration was in present-day En shi 恩施 city in Hu bei 湖北. Under Qing 清, in 1728, it became En shi county. Mentioned with 503, 511, 588.

Shi zi guo 師子國 [1]

This is an old name for Srilanka or Ceylon, the "country of lions." Mentioned with 961.

Shou 壽 [3]

Name of a *zhou* 州. See → Shou zhou 壽州. Mentioned with 78, 1446, 1523.

Shou chun 壽春 [2]

Name of a *fu* 府. It was founded under Northern Song 府, in 1116, by raising the status of Shou zhou 壽州. Its seat of administration was in Feng tai 鳳臺 county in present-day An hui 安徽. The administrative area comprised the counties of Feng tai 鳳臺 in An hui, Huo qiu 霍邱, and Shou 壽. Jin 金 changed it to be Shou zhou. Under Southern Song, in 1162, An feng 安豐 army was raised in status to be Shou chun fu 壽春府. Its seat of administration was in An feng pu 安豐鋪 located southwest of present-day Shou county in An hui. In 1167, the seat of administration was moved to Shou chun county, and it was changed to be An feng army. At the beginning of Ming 明, the area again became Shou chun fu. It was subsequently changed to be Shou zhou. Mentioned with 871, 1274.

Shou yang 壽陽 [1]

Name of a county. It was established under Eastern Jin 晉 by Emperor Xiao Wu di 孝武帝 (448 – 464) by changing the name of Shou chun 壽春. Its seat of administration was in present-day Shou 壽 county in An hui 安徽. Under Liu Song 劉宋, in 462, it was changed back to be Shou chun county. Mentioned with 47.

Shou yang 首陽 [1]

Name of a mountain. It is also called Shou shan 首山 and Lei shou shan 雷首山. It is in the South of present-day Pu zhou 蒲州 town located southwest of Yong ji 永濟 city in Shan xi 山西. Mentioned with 324.

Shou yang shan 首陽山 [1]

Name of a mountain. It is located in present-day Xiang tang gou 享堂溝 village in Lian feng xiang 蓮峰鄉, located southeast of Wei yuan 渭源 county in Gan su 甘肅. Mentioned with 1199.

Shou zhou 壽州 [3]

Name of a *zhou* 州. It was founded under Sui 隋, in 589. Its seat of administration was in present-day Shou 壽 county in An hui 安徽. In 607, it was changed to Huai nan 淮南 commandery. In 620, under Tang 唐, it again became Shou zhou. Its territory of administration corresponded to Shou county and the present-day cities and counties of Lu an 六安, Huo shan 霍山 and Huo qiu 霍邱 in An hui. Under Five Dynasties' Zhou 周, in 956, the seat of administration was moved to present-day Feng tai 鳳臺 county in An hui. Under Northern Song 宋, in 1116, its status was raised to Shou chun fu 壽春府. Jin 金 demoted it to be Shou zhou. It was eliminated under Yuan 元, in 1277, but later restored. In 1912, it became Shou county. Mentioned with 768, 1020, 1446.

Shu 舒 [6]

Name of a *zhou* 州. See → Shu zhou 舒州. Mentioned with 29, 52, 381, 873, 1324, 1485.

Shu 蜀 [77 + 12 + 25]

□ Name of a large administrative area. [77] This is another name for Si chuan 四川 and refers to Si chuan province. Mentioned with 29, 34, 82, 114, 134, 159, 188, 199, 254, 285, 290, 322, 344, 347, 367, 396, 448, 453, 456, 501, 520, 550, 566, 585, 588, 595, 637, 639, 674, 724, 744, 768, 806, 825, 857, 883, 908, 948, 950, 953, 958, 975, 995, 1028, 1036, 1047, 1060, 1064, 1100, 1168, 1185, 1213, 1242, 1310, 1339, 1410, 1471, 1475, 1490, 1494, 1499, 1516, 1526.

□ Regional name. [12] This was a designation for the ancient country of Shu during Qin 秦 and Han 漢 times. It was located in the western part of the present-day Si chuan 四川 basin. Mentioned with 159, 254, 768, 1096, 1097, 1206, 1214, 1241, 1330, 1437.

□ Name of a *zhou* 州. [25] See → Shu zhou 蜀州. Mentioned with 66, 99, 129, 188, 208, 218, 346, 389, 585, 660, 674, 768, 774, 781, 848, 864, 1092, 1204, 1264, 1308, 1407, 1441, 1446, 1493.

Shu bei 蜀北 [1]

Regional name. It refers to the northern part of the province of Si chuan 四川. Mentioned with 599.

Shu chuan 蜀川 [16]
Name of a region, one generally referring to Si chuan 四川. Mentioned with 66, 188, 221, 344, 437, 509, 636, 740, 789, 974, 995, 1096, 1098, 1279, 1407.

Shu dao 蜀道 [7]
Name of a traffic region. The original meaning referred to the traffic road stretching in early times through the Qin ling 秦嶺 mountain range to Shu 蜀 and the territories encountered along the way. Mentioned with 322, 456, 685, 1105, 1168, 1289, 1350.

Shu di 蜀地 [9]
Regional name. The term refers to present-day Si chuan 四川. Mentioned with 188, 275, 313, 381, 950, 982, 1308, 1425.

Shu du 蜀都 [2]
Name of an ancient capital. This was the ancient capital of Shu 蜀, referring to the present-day city of Cheng du 成都 in Si chuan 四川. Mentioned with 453, 456.

Shu han 蜀漢 [9]
Name of an ancient region. In 221, Liu Bei 劉備 proclaimed himself emperor in Cheng du 成都, calling his dynasty Han 漢. The histories wrote Shu han 蜀漢. The regime controlled present-day Si chuan 四川, most of Yun nan 雲南, all of Gui zhou 貴州 and a section of the Han zhong 漢中 watershed in Shaan xi 陝西 and the Bai long jiang 白龍江 watershed in Gan su 甘肅. Later periods have continued to refer to the region controlled by that dynasty as Shu han. Mentioned with 130, 249, 324, 328, 461, 557, 995, 1262, 1435.

Shu jiang 蜀江 [1]
Name of a watershed. It is, as the name implies, within Si chuan 四川. Mentioned with 1551.

Shu jiao 蜀徼 [1]
Regional name. See → Shu xi jiao wai 蜀西徼外. Mentioned with 490.

Shu jun 蜀郡 [33]
Name of a commandery. It was established by Warring States Qin 秦. Its seat of administration was in present-day Cheng du 成都 city in Si chuan 四川. Its Western Han 漢 territory corresponded to an area extending in Si chuan from Song pan 松潘 toward the South, from Bei chuan 北川, Peng xian 彭縣 and Hong ya 洪雅 toward the West, from E bian 峨邊 and Shi mian 石棉 toward the North, and from Qiong lai 邛崍 mountain and Da du he 大渡河 toward the East. Furthermore, from the region between the Da du he and the Ya long jiang 雅礱江, and Kang ding 康定 toward the South, and from Mian ning 冕寧 toward the North. Under Eastern Han, in 25, when Gongsun Shu 公孫述 (died 36 CE) occupied Shu, it was changed to be Cheng du yin 成都尹. In 36, it was changed back to be Shu 蜀 commandery. Its territory of administration was reduced. Under Western Jin 晉, in 289, the area was changed to be Cheng du country but later again became Shu commandery. In 605, under Sui 隋, it again became Shu commandery. Under Tang 唐, in 618, the area became Yi zhou 益

州. In 742, it again became Shu commandery. In 757, the area became Cheng du fu 成都府. Mentioned with 26, 29, 82, 122, 129, 155, 165, 188, 200, 453, 456, 461, 468, 476, 520, 557, 866, 868, 895, 1054, 1096, 1104, 1126, 1268, 1289, 1331, 1345, 1359, 1384.

Shu kui 蜀夔 [1]
Combined regional name. It refers to the province of Si chuan 四川 and the Chong qing 重慶 municipality. Mentioned with 1460.

Shu le 疏勒 [1]
Name of an ancient country. It was one of the thirty-six countries of the Han 漢 era western regions. Its capital was Kashgar city in present-day Xin jiang 新疆. Under Tang 唐, at the beginning of the *zhen guan* 貞觀 reign period (627 – 649), a Shu le garrison was established as one of the four garrisons pacifying the West. Mentioned with 1406.

Shu shan 蜀山 [1]
Name of mountains. The term refers to the mountains of the Si chuan 四川 region. Mentioned with 1171.

Shu tu 蜀土 [1]
Regional name used by the BCGM authors in referring to Si chuan 四川. Mentioned with 322.

Shu xi 蜀西 [1]
Regional name used by the BCGM authors in referring to the western portion of Si chuan 四川. Mentioned with 1481.

Shu xi jiao wai 蜀西徼外 [2]
Regional name. It refers to the Kang ding 康定 and A ba 阿壩 districts of the western part of Si chuan 四川. Mentioned with 296, 581.

Shu xiang 蜀鄉 [1]
Regional name. It indicates Si chuan. Mentioned with 883.

Shu you 蜀右 [1]
Regional name. It refers to the province of Si chuan 四川. Mentioned with 254.

Shu zhong 蜀中 [54]
Regional name. It refers in general to Si chuan 四川. Mentioned with 53, 107, 114, 122, 134, 145, 188, 199, 249, 395, 396, 410, 461, 469, 473, 501, 519, 535, 537, 558, 588, 644, 674, 675, 676, 716, 733, 774, 861, 943, 1020, 1030, 1036, 1057, 1096, 1182, 1235, 1279, 1289, 1308, 1318, 1339, 1425, 1467, 1482, 1486, 1488.

Shu zhou 蜀州 [1]
Name of a *zhou* 州. It was founded by Tang 唐, in 686. Its seat of administration was in present-day Chong zhou 崇州 city in Si chuan 四川. The territory administered comprised the present-day city and county of Chong zhou and Xin jin 新津 in Si chuan. In 742, it was changed to be Tang an 唐安 commandery. In 758, it again became Shu zhou. Under Southern Song 宋, in 1144, its status was raised to Chong qing 重慶 army. Mentioned with 674.

Shu zhou 舒州 [2]

Name of a *zhou* 州. It was founded under Tang 唐, in 621. Its seat of administration was in Qian shan 潛山 county in An hui 安徽. Its territory of administration comprised the present-day cities and counties of An qing 安慶, Huai ning 懷寧, Qian shan, Yue xi 岳西, Su song 宿松, Tai hu 太湖, Wang jiang 望江, Tong cheng 桐城 and Zong yang 樅陽 in An hui. Under Southern Song 宋, in 1147, the area became An qing 安慶 army. Mentioned with 20, 1217.

Shuang jing 雙井 [1]

Minor place name. The reference is to the present-day Shuang jing west of Xiu shui 修水 county in Jiang xi 江西. Mentioned with 768.

Shuang shui 瀧水 [1]

Name of a county. It was founded under Sui 隋, in 598. Its seat of administration was at a location 100 *li* south of present-day Luo ding 羅定 city in Guang dong 廣東. Under Yuan 元, in 1304, the seat of administration was moved to Luo ding city. In 1577, its status was raised to Luo ding zhou 羅定州. Mentioned with 983.

Shuang zhou 瀧州 [1]

Name of a *zhou* 州. It was established under Southern Dynasties' Liang 梁. Its seat of administration was at a location 100 *li* south of present-day Luo ding 羅定 city in Guang dong 廣東. At the beginning of the *da ye* 大業 reign period (605 – 618) of Sui 隋, it was changed to Yong xi 永熙 commandery. Under Tang 唐, in 621, it again became Long zhou. Its territory of administration comprised the territory within the borders of present-day Luo ding city in Guang dong. Under Northern Song 宋, in 973, it was abolished. Mentioned with 1521.

Shun an jun 順安軍 [2]

Name of an administrative unit, an army. It was founded under Northern Song 宋, in 992. Its seat of administration was in Guan cheng 關城, located southwest of present-day An xin 安新 county in He bei 河北. In 997, it was moved to present-day Jiu cheng 舊城 town, located 25 *li* east of Gao yang 高陽 county. Jin 金 abolished it. Mentioned with 291, 1278.

Shun chang 順昌 [1]

Name of a county. It was established under Five Dynasties' Min 閩, in 933. Its seat of administration was in present-day Shun chang 順昌 county in Fu jian 福建. Mentioned with 1262.

Shun qing 順慶 [1]

Name of a *fu* 府. It was established under Southern Song 宋, in 1227. Its seat of administration was at a location north of present-day Nan chong 南充 city in Si chuan 四川. In 1249, the seat of administration was moved to Qing ju 青居 town, located south of the present Nan chong city. Later it was eliminated. Under Yuan 元, in 1278, it was reestablished. In 1283, it was changed to Shun qing lu 順慶路. Under Ming 明, in 1371, it was again changed to Shun qing fu. The seat of administration was moved to Nan chong city. Its territory of administration corresponded to an area in present-day Si chuan extending from Yi long 儀隴 and

Xi chong 西充 toward the South, and from Yue chi 岳池, Guang an 廣安 and Lin shui 鄰水 toward the North,. It was abolished in 1913. Mentioned with 1096.

Shun tian fu 順天府 [1]

Name of a *fu* 府. It was founded under Ming 明, in 1403. Its seat of administration was in present-day Bei jing 北京 city. Its territory of administration corresponded to an area in He bei 河北 extending from the Great Wall toward the South, from the Western mountains toward the East, from Zun hua 遵化 and Feng nan 豐南, toward the West, and from the Ju ma 拒馬 river, the Da qing 大清 river and the Hai 海 river toward the North. The *fu* was abolished in 1914. Mentioned with 111.

Shun yang xian 順陽縣 [1]

Name of a county. It was established under Eastern Han 漢. Its seat of administration was at a location south of Xi chuan 淅川 county in present-day He nan 河南. Southern Qi 齊 changed it to be Cong yang 從陽 county. Later, it again became Shun yang county. Northern Zhou 周 eliminated it and made it a part of Qing xiang 清鄉 county. At the beginning of the *kai huang* 開皇 reign period (581-600) of Sui 隋, it was reestablished, and the seat of administration was moved to a location 30 *li* west of the present-day Deng zhou 鄧州 city. Under Tang 唐, in 623, it was eliminated. It was restored under Northern Song 宋, in 981. Jin 金 eliminated it and later reestablished it. Yuan 元 finally eliminated it. Mentioned with 1379.

Shun zheng 順政 [1]

Name of a county. It was founded under Sui 隋, in 598. Its seat of administration was in Lue yang 略陽 county in present-day Shaan xi 陝西. Southern Song 宋 changed the name of the county to Lue yang county. Mentioned with 520.

Shun zheng jun 順政郡 [1]

Name of a commandery. It was established by Western Wei 魏. Its seat of administration was in present-day Lue yang 略陽 county in Shaan xi 陝西. The territory administered comprised the area of present-day Lue yang county. Under Sui 隋, in 583, it was eliminated. In 607, it was reestablished. Under Tang 唐, in 618, it was changed to be Xing zhou 興州. In 742, it was changed again to be Shun zheng 順政 commandery. In 758, it was changed to be once more Xing zhou. Mentioned with 575.

Shun zhou 順州 [2]

Name of a *zhou* 州. It was established under Tang 唐, in 773. Its seat of administration was at a location 40 *li* south of present-day Lu chuan 陸川 county in Guang xi 廣西. Its territory of administration corresponded to the southern portions of present-day Lu chuan county. It was abolished under Northern Song 宋, in 972. Mentioned with 428.

Si 泗 [4]

Name of a *zhou*. See → Si zhou 泗州. Mentioned with 541, 877, 1323, 1523.

Si an 思安 [1]

Name of a tea market. It was established by Northern Song 宋. Its seat of administration was at a location 50 *li* west of present-day Da yi 大邑 county in Si chuan 四川. It produced a large amount of tea and was called the Si an tea market. Under Yuan 元, it was abolished. Mentioned with 768.

Si chuan 四川 [11 + 3]

□ Name of an administrative unit. [11] Under Ming 明, in 1376, a Si chuan Provincial Administration Commission, Si chuan *bu zheng shi si* 四川布政使司, was established. Its seat of administration was in present-day Cheng du 成都 in Si chuan. Its territory of administration comprised an area in present-day Si chuan extending from the Bai 白 river, the Qiong lai 邛崍 mountain and Da liang 大涼 mountain toward the East, from Min 岷 mountain and Da ba 大巴 mountain toward the South, in present-day Yun nan 雲南 from Dong chuan 東川 toward the North, as well as Wei ning 威寧 in present-day Gui zhou 貴州, and the region extending from Zun yi 遵義 and Weng an 甕安 toward the North. Under Qing 清, in 1645, the area became Si chuan province. Mentioned with 160, 569, 686, 778, 1018, 1057, 1096, 1166, 1499.

□ Name of a *lu*. [3] At the beginning of Northern Song 宋, the old Shu 蜀 territory of the Five Dynasties period was dived into the two *lu* 路 of Chuan 川 and Xia 峽, more or less corresponding in present-day Si chuan to the area northeast of the Da du he 大渡河, and in present-day Shaan xi 陝西 to Han zhong 漢中. In 1001, the territory was divided into the four *lu* of Yi zhou 益州, Li zhou 利州, Zi zhou 梓州 and Kui zhou 夔州. These were collectively called "The four *lu* of Chuan and Xia," Chuan Xia *si lu* 川峽四路, shortly: Si chuan. Mentioned with 110, 183, 1057.

Si diao 斯調 [1]

Name of an ancient country. See → Si diao guo 斯調國. Mentioned with 775.

Si diao guo 斯調國 [1]

Name of an ancient country. According to one tradition it was located on Sri lanka, and according to another on Java. Mentioned with 775.

Si hui xian 四會縣 [1]

Name of a county. It was established by Qin 秦. Its seat of administration was in present-day Si hui 四會 city in Guang dong 廣東. In 1933, it was changed to be Si hui city. Mentioned with 428.

Si ming 四明 [9]

Place name. It refers to the Ning bo fu 寧波府 of Ming 明 and Qing 清 times. The region includes within its boundaries the Si ming mountain range, thus the name. This area corresponds to present-day Ning bo 寧波 city in Zhe jiang 浙江. Mentioned with 3, 309, 756, 1015, 1036, 1105.

Si ming shan 四明山 [2]

Name of a mountain range. It is in the eastern part of Zhe jiang 浙江. It is the range that divides the waters of the Yang zi and the Cao e jiang 曹娥江. It stretches through the present-day cities and city territories of Yu yao 余姚, Yin zhou 鄞州, Feng hua 奉化, Sheng zhou 嵊州 and Shang yu 上虞 in Zhe jiang. Mentioned with 561, 797.

Si yang 四陽 [1]
Possibly a regional name. Located in present-day Gan su 甘肅 but this may be an error. Mentioned with 199.

Si zhou 泗州 [1]
Name of a *zhou* 州. It was established under Northern Zhou 周, in 580. Its seat of administration was in the old walled city of former Zheng lou xiang, Zheng lou xiang gu cheng 鄭樓鄉古城, located northwest of present-day Si yang 泗陽 county in Jiang su 江蘇. It was eliminated at the beginning of the *da ye* 大業 reign period (605 – 618) of Sui 隋. It was reestablished under Tang 唐, in 621. In 735, the seat of administration was moved to a location northwest of present-day Xu yi 盱眙 county in Jiang su. Its territory of administration comprised in present-day Jiang su the cities and counties of Su qian 宿遷, Pi zhou 邳州, Sui ning 睢寧, Si yang 泗陽, Lian shui 漣水, Guan nan 灌南 and Si hong 泗洪, and in An hui 安徽 Si xian 泗縣. In 742, it was changed to be Lin huai 臨淮 commandery. In 758, it again became Si zhou. In 1680, under Qing 清, the *zhou* city fell into Hong ze 洪澤 lake. Its administration was relocated to present-day Xu yi county. In 1724, its status was raised to a directly administered *zhou, zhi li zhou* 直隸州. In 1777, the seat of administration was moved to Si 泗 county in An hui. It was abolished in 1912. Mentioned with 1417.

Si zhou 司州 [1]
Name of a *zhou* 州. Three Kingdoms' Wei 魏 referred to a Metropolitan Commandant Region, *si li xiao wei bu* 司隸校尉部 as Si zhou. Western Jin 晉 formally established the name. Its seat of administration was in Han wei gu cheng 漢魏古城, located northeast of present-day Luo yang 洛陽 in He nan 河南. The territory administered comprised the western part of present-day He nan, the northwestern part of present-day Shan xi 山西 and He bei 河北, and the Shang luo 商洛 mountain region in Shaan xi 陝西. At the end of the *yong jia* 永嘉 reign period (307 – 313) it was eliminated. Shi le 石勒 (274-333) of Later Zhao 趙 of the Sixteen Kingdoms reestablished it. Shi hu 石虎 (295-349), Northern Wei 魏 and Eastern Wei all temporarily changed it to Luo zhou 洛州. It was divided under Eastern Jin during the *yong he* 永和 reign period (345 – 356). Under Northern Wei, in 493, and under Western Wei, it was changed to Si zhou. Northern Qi 齊 made it Luo zhou. Mentioned with 474.

Song 淞 [1]
Name of a river. See → Song jiang 淞江. Mentioned with 598.

Song 宋 [4]
Name of one of the feudal states. After the eastern campaign of Zhou gong 周公 (died 1105 BCE), Song was established by enfeoffing Wei Ziqi 微子啟 at Shang qiu 商丘 in He nan 河南 which he used to found the Song state. It embraced the eastern part of He nan and the nearby areas of Jiang su 江蘇, An hui 安徽 and Shan dong 山東. During the Spring and Autumn period, Song and Chu 楚

fought for hegemony and Song Xiang gong 襄公 (died 637 BCE) was defeated by Chu Cheng wang 楚成王 (died 628 BCE). The power of Song was greatly reduced. During Warring States time, the Duke of Song established himself as a king and moved his capital to present-day Xu zhou 徐州 city in Jiang su. In 286, Song was annihilated by Qi 齊. Mentioned with 272, 417, 665, 1242.

Song gao 嵩高 [10]
Name of a mountain. See → Gao shan 嵩山. Mentioned with 123, 237, 275, 525, 644, 810, 995, 1105, 1149.

Song gao shan 嵩高山 [2]
Name of a mountain. See → Gao shan 嵩山. Mentioned with 230, 1250.

Song jiang 淞江 [2]
Name of a river. This is the Wu song jiang 吳淞江. It has its sources in Lake Tai hu 太湖 lake in Jiang su 江蘇, and flows to Shang hai 上海 city there pouring into the Yang zi. Mentioned with 723.

Song li shan 宋里山 [2]
Name of a mountain. It is located west of present-day Xu zhou 徐州 city in Jiang su 江蘇. Mentioned with 1039, 1234.

Song pan 松潘 [1]
Name of a guard. In 1379, the two guards of Song zhou 松州 and Pan zhou 潘州 were established. Subsequently they were united to become Song pan guard. Its seat of administration was in present-day Song pan county in Si chuan 四川. Its administrative area comprised the counties of Song pan, Jiu zhai gou 九寨溝, Ruo er gai 若爾蓋, Hong yuan 紅原, Ma er kang 馬爾康 and Hei shui 黑水 in present-day Si chuan, and a region southeast of Die bu 迭部 county in present-day Gan su 甘肅. In 1387, it was changed to Song pan Office of a Tribal Command Administration for Song Pan and other Places, Song pan deng chu *jun min zhi hui shi si* 松潘等處軍民指揮使司, and in 1563 it became Song pan guard again. Under Qing 清, in 1731, it was changed to be Song Pan subprefecture, Song pan ting 松潘聽. Mentioned with 1481.

Song shan 嵩山 [11]
Name of mountains. It is the middle range of the traditional Five Ranges. Its ancient names were Song gao 嵩高, Wai fang 外方 and Da shih 大室. It is located to the north of present-day Deng feng 登封 city in He nan 河南. Mentioned with 230, 311, 428, 455, 1155, 1234, 1250, 1469, 1485, 1573.

Song yang 松陽 [1]
Name of a county. It was founded under Eastern Han 漢, in 199. Its seat of administration was in present-day Gu shi 古市 town, located 24 *li* northwest of Song yang 松陽 county in Zhe jiang 浙江. Under Sui 隋, in 589, it was eliminated. In 592, it was reestablished. During the *zhen yuan* 貞元 reign period (785 – 805), the seat of administration was moved to the present-day Song yang county. In 910, Wu yue 吳越 changed it to be Chang song 長松 county. Under later Jin 晉, in 939, it was changed to be Bai long 白龍 county. Under Northern Song 宋, in 999, it was again made Song yang county. Mentioned with 485.

Song yang 嵩陽 [1]
Regional name. The term refers to the area south of the Song shan 嵩山 mountains in present-day Deng feng 登封 city. Mentioned with 866.

Song yang xian 松楊縣 [1]
Name of a county. Song yang 松楊 is an alternative writing of Song yang 松陽. See → Song yang 松陽. Mentioned with 1113.

Song yue 嵩岳 [1]
Name of a mountain range. These are the Song shan 嵩山 mountains located northwest of present-day Deng feng 登封 city in He nan 河南. Mentioned with 1014.

Song zhou 松州 [3]
Name of a *zhou* 州. It was established under Tang 唐, in 618. Its seat of administration was in present-day Song pan 松潘 county in Si chuan 四川. In 742, it became Jiao chuan 交川 commandery. In 758, it became Song zhou again. At its height, the *zhou* included most of the territory of the present-day self-governing *zhou* of the A ba 阿壩 Tibetan nationality of Si chuan and a region of Jiu zhi 久治 and Ma qu 瑪曲 of Qinghai. In 763, the area became part of Tibet. It was reestablished under Yuan 元. It was then administered from Song pan county in present-day Si chuan. Under Ming 明, in 1387, it was abolished. Mentioned with 199, 337, 387.

Su 蘇 [2]
Name of a *fu* 府. See under → Su zhou 蘇州. Mentioned with 323, 598.

Su fang guo 蘇方國 [1]
Name of an ancient country. The reference is to the present-day South China Sea, but details are not available. Mentioned with 1123.

Su he guo 蘇合國 [1]
Name of an ancient country. Its location is unknown. Mentioned with 1124.

Su men da la guo 蘇門答剌國 [1]
Name of an ancient country, apparently a transcription of the Sanskrit word for "ocean", Samudra. Here it refers to a region on the northern shore of the Indonesian island of Sumatra. Mentioned with 671.

Su shen guo 肅慎國 [2]
Name of an ancient tribe. Its name is also written Xi shen 息慎. In pre-Qin 秦 times, it occupied a strip of the present-day Ji lin 吉林 and the Hei long 黑龍 river. From Han 漢 on, the area was called Yi lou 挹婁. Mentioned with 1041, 1497.

Su shui 涑水 [1]
Name of a river. It is located to the northeast of present-day Nan zhang 南漳 county in Hu bei 湖北. Its present name is Nan qu 南渠, "Southern Canal." Mentioned with 1079.

Su zhou 肅州 [2 + 4]

□ Name of a guard [2]. It was established under Ming 明, in 1394. Its seat of administration was in present-day Jiu quan 酒泉 city in Gan su 甘肅. Its territory of administration comprised the three cities and counties of Jia yu guan 嘉峪關, Jin ta 金塔 and Jiu quan in Gan su, and the western part of the Gan nan 甘南 Yugur nationality self-government county. In 1724, it was abolished. Mentioned with 1040, 1130.

□ Name of a *zhou* 州 [4]. It was established under Sui 隋, in 602. Its seat of administration was in present-day Jiu quan 酒泉 city in Gan su 甘肅. It was eliminated at the beginning of the *da ye* 大業 reign period (605 – 618) of Sui 隋. It was reestablished under Tang 唐, in 619. Its administrative territory comprised an area in present-day Gan su extending from the Shu le 疏勒 river to the East, and from Gao tai 高臺 county toward the West. In 742, it was changed to be Jiu quan commandery. In 758, it was changed to be Su zhou. Under Yuan 元, in 1270, it was raised to the status of Su zhou lu 肅州路. Mentioned with 41, 496, 934.

Su zhou 宿州 [1]

Name of a *zhou* 州. It was established under Tang 唐, in 809. Its seat of administration was in present-day Si 泗 county in An hui 安徽. Later, the seat of administration was moved to present-day Fu li 符離 town north of Su zhou city in An hui province. The *zhou* was eliminated in 809. It was reestablished in 833. The seat of administration was moved to present-day Su zhou city. The territory of administration of the *zhou* comprised the present-day cities and counties of Su zhou, Gu zhen 固鎮, Si xian 泗縣, Ling bi 靈璧 and Sui xi 濉溪 in An hui. Yuan 元 put the *zhou* under Gui de fu 歸德府. Ming 明 and Qing 清 put it under Feng yang fu 鳳陽府. In 1912, the *zhou* was reduced to a county. Mentioned with 1532.

Su zhou 蘇州 [5 + 6]

□ Name of a *zhou* 州. [5] It was established under Sui 隋, in 589. Its seat of administration was at a location east of Heng 横 mountain located southwest of present-day Su zhou 蘇州 city in Jiang su 江蘇. Under Tang 唐, in 624, the seat of administration was moved to Su zhou city. Its territory of administration included in present-day Jiang su an area extending from the Wu zhong 吴中 district, the Xiang cheng 相城 district and Chang shu 常熟 city toward the East, and in Zhe jiang from Tong xiang 桐鄉 and Hai yan 海鹽 toward the North, and part of the Shang hai 上海 city mainland. After Five Dynasties' Jin 晉, its administrative area was reduced to the part of Jiang su mentioned above and the two districts of Jia ding 嘉定 and Bao shan 寶山 in Shang hai. Under Northern Song 宋, in 1113, the status of the area was raised, and it became Ping jiang fu 平江府. Mentioned with 562, 578, 823, 1250.

□ Name of a *fu* 府. [6] It was established at the beginning of Ming 明. Its seat of administration was in present-day Su zhou 蘇州 city in Jiang su 江蘇. Its territory of administration comprised the present-day cities and districts and counties of Su zhou, Chang shu 常熟, Kun shan 昆山, Wu jiang 吳江, Wu zhong 吳

中 and Xiang cheng 相城, as well as the northwest portion of present-day Shang hai 上海 city. It was abolished in 1912. Mentioned with 100, 566, 631, 1087, 1287.

Suan zao xian 酸棗縣 [2]

Name of a county. It was established by Qin 秦. Its seat of administration was at a location 15 *li* southwest of present-day Yan jin 延津 county in He nan 河南. Under Northern Wei 魏, in 494, the seat of administration was moved to a location 15 *li* north of present-day Yan jin county. Northern Qi 齊 abolished it. The county was reestablished by Sui 隋, in 586. The seat of administration moved to the present-day Yan jin county. Under Northern Song 宋, in 1117, it was changed to be Yan jin county. Mentioned with 1122.

Sui 綏 [1]

Name of a *zhou* 州. It was established under Western Wei 魏, in 552. Its seat of administration was at a location 50 *li* southeast of present-day Sui de 綏德 county in Shaan xi 陝西. Its territory of administration comprised the counties of Sui de, Qing jian 清澗, Zi chang 子長, Zi zhou 子洲, Mi zhi 米脂, Jia xian 佳縣 and Wu bao 吳堡, and the eastern part of Heng shan 橫山 county, and the southern part of Yu lin 榆林 city in present-day Shaan xi. Under Sui 隋, in 605, it was changed to Shang zhou 上州. Two years later, in 607, a Diao yin 雕陰 commandery was established. Under Tang 唐, in 620, Sui zhou 綏州 was established again. In 628, the seat of administration was moved to present-day Sui de county. Its territory of administration was reduced and comprised only the three counties of Sui de, Wu bao and Qing jian and parts of the territories of the counties of Zi chang and Zi zhou. In 742, it was changed to be Shang commandery. In 758, it again became Sui zhou. It was abolished in 1069. Mentioned with 893.

Sui 隨 [5]

Name of a *zhou* 州. See → Sui zhou 隨州. Mentioned with 78, 973, 980, 1238, 1446.

Sui 遂 [1]

Name of a *zhou* 州. It was established under Northern Zhou 周, in 557. Its seat of administration was in present-day Sui ning 遂寧 city in Si chuan 四川. Its territory of administration comprised the present-day cities and counties of Sui ning and Peng xi 蓬溪, in present-day Si chuan, and present-day Tong nan 潼南 in Chong qing 重慶 city. Northern Song 宋 changed it to be Sui ning fu 遂寧府 in 1115. Mentioned with 535.

Sui ding xian 綏定縣 [1]

Name of a county. It was established by Liu Song 劉宋, but details on its location are lacking. It should have been located in a strip of Yang jiang 陽江 city in Guang dong 廣東. Sui 隋 abolished it. Mentioned with 1238.

Sui jun 隨郡 [1]

Name of a commandery. It was established under Southern Qi 齊. Its seat of administration was in present-day Sui zhou 隨州 city in Hu bei 湖北. Its territory of administration comprised the two cities of Sui zhou and Guang shui 廣水 in Hu bei. It was abolished under Sui, in 581. Mentioned with 986.

Sui ning 遂寧 [1 + 1]

□ Name of a commandery. [1] It was established under Sui 隋, in 607. Its seat of administration was in present-day Sui ning city in Si chuan 四川. Its territory of administration comprised the present-day city and county of Sui and Peng xi 蓬溪 in Si chuan, and present-day Tong nan 潼南 in Chong qing 重慶 city. The area became Sui zhou 遂州 under Tang 唐, in 618. In 742, it was changed to be Sui ning commandery. It again became Sui zhou in 758. Mentioned with 1036, 1092.

□ Name of a county. [1] It was established under Ming 明, in 1376. Its seat of administration was in present-day Sui ning city in Si chuan. It 1985, it became Sui ning city. Mentioned with 1036.

Sui yang 睢陽 [1]

Name of a county. It was established by Qin 秦. Its seat of administration was at a location one *li* south of the present-day Sui yang district of Shang qiu 商丘 city in He nan 河南. Under Sui 隋, in 598, it was changed to Song cheng 宋城 county. Jin 金, in 1200, restored the old Sui yang. Under Southern Song 宋, in 1228, it was again changed to be Song cheng county. Yuan 元 changed it back to Sui yang county. At the beginning of Ming 明, it was abolished. Mentioned with 631.

Sui zhou 隨州 [2]

Name of a *zhou* 州. It was established under Western Wei 魏, in 554. Its seat of administration was in present-day Sui zhou city in Hu bei 湖北. Its territory of administration comprised the boundaries of the two present-day cities of Sui zhou and Zao yang 棗陽 in Hu bei. During the *da ye* 大業 (605 – 618) reign period of the Sui, and the *tian bao* 天寶 (742 – 756) and *zhi de* 至德 (756 – 758) reign periods of the Tang 唐, the area periodically became Han dong 漢東 commandery. Under Yuan 元, in 1276, the seat of administration was moved to Da hong 大洪 mountain, located southwest of the present Sui zhou city. Not long after, it was moved back to Sui zhou city. In 1912 the area became a county. Mentioned with 203, 986.

-T-

Tai 台 [3]

Name of a *zhou* 州. See → Tai zhou 台州. Mentioned with 323, 1057.

Tai bai shan 太白山 [4]

Name of a mountain. This is the principal peak of the Qin ling 秦嶺 mountain range in Shaan xi 陝西. It is located to the southeast of present-day Tai bai 太白 county. The high point of the range is 3767 meters. The mountains are rugged and eternally snow covered. Mentioned with 109, 185, 1030.

Tai cang 太倉 [1]
Name of a *zhou* 州. It was founded under the Ming 明, in 1497, and subordinated to Su zhou fu 蘇州府. Its seat of administration was in present-day Tai cang city in Jiang Su 江蘇. In 1993, it was changed to be Tai cang city. Mentioned with 805.

Tai gu 太谷 [1]
Minor place name. It is located west of present-day Tai gu county in Shan xi 山西. Mentioned with 702.

Tai hang 太行 [3]
Name of mountains. See → Tai hang shan 太行山. Mentioned with 132, 931.

Tai hang shan 太行山 [8]
Name of mountains. Originally the term referred to a single mountain, located in the present-day He nan 河南 and Shan xi 山西 boundary area. Later the term gradually expanded in meaning towards the North and became the name of a whole mountain range at the boundary between present-day Shan xi and He bei 河北. Mentioned with 359, 857, 862, 1210, 1350, 1516, 1524.

Tai he 太和 [1]
Name of a mountain. See → Tai he shan 太和山. Mentioned with 349.

Tai he shan 太和山 [7]
Name of a mountain. This is the famous Daoist scenic spot Wu dang 武當 mountain, located southwest of present-day Dan jiang kou 丹江口 city in Hu bei 湖北. Legend has it that the mountain has palaces of immortals. Zhen wu 真武 received the words of the Yuan jun 元君 and went wandering to look at this mountain, and he changed the name to Tai he 太和. Later people said that no one less than Xuan wu 玄武 could have "matched" it and changed its name to Wu dang mountain. Mentioned with 349, 354, 570, 622, 876, 1496.

Tai hu 太湖 [1]
Name of a lake. This is the present-day Tai hu lake situated in between Jiang su 江蘇 and Zhe jiang 浙江. Its water surface is part of Jiang su and it is the third largest fresh water lake in China. Mentioned with 880.

Tai hua 太華 [1]
Name of a mountain. See → Tai hua shan 太華山. Mentioned with 311.

Tai hua shan 太華山 [2]
Name of a mountain. It is Hua shan 華山, located 10 *li* south of present-day Hua yin 華陰 city in Shaan xi 陝西. An alternative name is Xi yue 西岳. To the west there is a Shao Hua shan 少華山, "Small Hua mountain," thus the name: "Eminent Hua mountain." Mentioned with 1426, 1497.

Tai ning xian 泰寧縣 [1]
Name of a county. It was founded under Northern Song 宋, in 1086, by changing the name of Gui hua 歸化 county. It was put under Shao wu 邵武 army. Its seat of administration was in present-day Tai ning 泰寧 county in Fujian 福建.

Tai qing gong 太清宮 [1]

Minor place name. It is located 10 *li* east of present-day Lu yi 鹿邑 county in He nan 河南. Mentioned with 298.

Tai shan 太山 [66]

Name of a mountain. This is Tai shan 泰山. It is located north of present-day Tai an 泰安 city in Shan dong 山東. It is also called Dong yue 東岳, Dai shan 岱山, and Dai yue 岱岳. Mentioned with 20, 47, 131, 175, 185, 195, 203, 275, 311, 319, 338, 456, 474, 500, 538, 609, 620, 644, 653, 675, 714, 789, 859, 880, 922, 1030, 1033, 1043, 1063, 1109, 1125, 1134, 1140, 1155, 1207, 1217, 1250, 1322, 1328, 1344, 1378, 1393, 1417, 1430, 1448, 1456, 1521, 1573.

Tai shan 泰山 [8]

Name of a mountain. One of the "Five Mountain Ranges," wu yue 五岳. It is located north of present-day Tai an 泰安 city in Shan dong 山東. It is also called Dong yue 東岳. Mentioned with 832, 908, 931, 1157, 1308, 1323, 1392, 1469.

Tai wu 太吳 [3]

Name of a district. This is the place where Tai bo 太伯 of Wu 吳, the founder of the Spring and Autumn period's state of Wu 吳, is said to have lived. Therefore it was called Tai wu. It was located approximately in the southern part of present-day Jiang su 江蘇. Mentioned with 616.

Tai ye chi 太液池 [1]

Name of a palace ground. The pond was dug out to the North of Jian zhan gong 建章宮 palace under Western Han, in 110 BCE. It was located within the present-day ruins of the Han era Chang an 長安 city northwest of present-day Xi an 西安 city in Shaan xi 陝西. Mentioned with 387.

Tai yuan 太原 [5 +6 + 1 +2]

□ Name of a governmental unit. [5]. Which government unit was meant remains uncertain. The possibilities include:

A) A commandery that was established during the Warring States period under Zhuang Xiang wang 莊襄王 (281-247) of Qin 秦, in 246 BCE. Its seat of administration was at a location southwest of present-day Tai yuan city. Under Qin, its administrative area included in present-day Shan xi 山西 Wu tai 五臺 mountain and an area extending from Guan cen 管涔 mountain toward the South, and from Huo 霍 mountain toward the North. From Han 漢 times on, its size was reduced. Emperor Wen 文 (202 – 157) of Han changed it into a country, but soon the area was made a commandery again. Jin 晉 also made it a country, but Northern Wei 魏 made it a commandery again. Its territory of administration comprised the middle part of Shan xi between present-day Yang qu 陽曲, Jiao cheng 交城, Ping yao 平遙 and He shun 和順. Under Sui 隋, in 583, it was changed to be Bing zhou 并州. In 607, it became Tai yuan commandery. Under Tang 唐, in 618, it was again changed to be Bing zhou.

B) A country/domain founded by Emperor Wen (202 – 157) of Han who changed the name of Tai yuan commandery. Its territory of administration comprised the middle part of Shan xi between present-day Yang qu, Jiao cheng, Ping yao and

He shun. Consequently, it became a commandery again. Western Jin made it a country, but Northern Wei made it a commandery. Mentioned with 675, 1157, 1171, 1532.

□ Name of a *fu* 府. [6] It was founded under Tang 唐, in 723, by raising the status of Bing zhou 并州. Its seat of administration was in present-day Jin yuan 晉源 town, located southwest of Tai yuan city. Its administrative territory comprised an area in present-day Shan xi of the middle reaches of the Fen shui 汾水 extending from Yang qu toward the South, and from Wen shui 文水 toward the North, as well as Yang qu city, and the counties of Ping ding 平定, Shou yang 壽陽, Xi yang 昔陽 and Yu xian 盂縣. During Song tai ping xing guo 宋太平興國 (976 – 984), the *fu* was changed to be Bing zhou. The seat of administration was moved to Tai yuan city. During the *jia you* 嘉佑 reign period (1056 – 1063), Tai yuan fu 太原府 was restored. At the beginning of the Yuan 元 dynasty, it was changed to be Tai yuan lu 太原路. During the *da de* 大德 reign period (1135 – 1139), the name was changed to Ji ning lu 冀寧路. Ming 明 restored the name as Tai yuan fu. It was abolished in 1912. Mentioned with 34, 464, 698, 861, 890, 1258.

□ Name of a *lu* 路. [1] It was founded by the Mongol conquerors in 1216, by changing Tai yuan fu. In 1305, under Yuan, it became Ji ning lu. Ming restored Tai yuan fu. Mentioned with 862.

□ Name of a county. [2] It was established under Sui 隋, in 590, by changing the name of Jin yang 晉陽 county. Its seat of administration was at a location southwest of present-day Tai yuan 太原 city. During Song tai ping xing guo 宋太平興國, in 979, after the suppression of Northern Han 漢, it was changed to Ping jin 平晉 county. Under Ming 明, in 1375, it was again named Tai yuan. In 1914, the name was changed to be Jin yuan 晉源. Mentioned with 1140, 1242.

Tai zhou 泰州 [3]

Name of a *zhou* 州. It was established under Five Dynasties' Southern Tang 唐, in 937. Its seat of administration was in present-day Tai zhou 泰州 city in Jiang su 江蘇. Its territory of administration comprised the present-day cities of Tai zhou, Jiang yan 姜堰, Ru gao 如皋, Tai xing 泰興 and Xing hua 興化 in Jiang su. Under Yuan 元, in 1277, it became Tai zhou lu 泰州路. In 1284, it was again made Tai zhou. It was subordinated to Yang zhou lu 揚州路 with reduced territories. Under Ming 明 and Qing 清, the area became an "attached *zhou*" *san zhou* 散州. In 1912, it became Tai 泰 county. Mentioned with 546, 1273, 1318.

Tai zhou 台州 [15]

Name of a *zhou* 州. Abbreviated: Tai 台 (this is not a simplified writing of Tai 臺). It was established under Tang 唐, in 622. Its seat of administration was in Lin hai 臨海 city in present-day Zhe jiang 浙江. Its territory of administration comprised the totality of Tai zhou city, and the two counties of Ning hai 寧海 and Xiang shan 象山 in Zhe jiang. Under Yuan 元, in 1277, the area became Tai zhou lu 台州路. Ming 明 changed it to Tai zhou fu 台州府. It was abolished in 1912. Mentioned with 31, 37, 400, 416, 508, 578, 891, 1020, 1164, 1170, 1257, 1420, 1510, 1568.

Tan 潭 [1]

Name of a *zhou* 州. See → Tan zhou 潭州. Mentioned with 981.

Tan chang 宕昌 [6]

Name of a region. It is the basin of the Xi han shui 西漢水 and the Bai long jiang 白龍江 in the south of present-day Gan su 甘肅. Mentioned with 461, 599, 620, 1289, 1307.

Tan ya 檀崖 [1]

Minor place name. It was located somewhere in the territory of present-day Nan an 南安 city in the southern part of Fu jian 福建, but the exact location is uncertain. Mentioned with 298.

Tan yu shan 檀嵎山 [1]

Name of a mountain. The mountain is located within the borders of Gao mi 高密 city in Shan dong 山東. Mentioned with 648.

Tan zhou 宕州 [4]

Name of a *zhou* 州. It was established under Northern Zhou 周, in 566. Its seat of administration was at a location southeast of Tan chang 宕昌 county in Gan su 甘肅. The territory administered comprised the two counties of Tan chang and Zhou qu 舟曲 in Gan su. In 607, the *zhou* was abolished. It was reestablished in 618. Its seat of administration was at a location southwest of present-day Tan chang county in Gan su. In 627, the administration was moved to the northern bank of the Bai long jiang 白龍江, northwest of Zhou qu 舟曲 county in Gan su. In 742, the area became Huai dao 懷道 commandery. In 758, it again became Tan zhou. Later the area was conquered by the Tibetan Empire. Mentioned with 188, 199, 345, 1307.

Tan zhou 檀州 [1]

Name of a *zhou* 州. It was established under Sui 隋, in 596. Its seat of administration was at a location northeast of present-day Mi yun 密雲 county of Bei jing 北京 city. Under Tang 唐, in 618, the seat of administration was moved to the present Mi yun county. The administration comprised the present-day districts and counties of Mi yun, Huai rou 懷柔 and Ping gu 平谷 of Bei jing city. At the beginning of Jin 金 rule, the *zhou* was eliminated. It was reestablished by the Mongols, in 1215. Yuan 元 put it under Da du lu 大都路. Ming 明, in 1368, abolished it. Mentioned with 931.

Tan zhou 潭州 [1]

Name of a *zhou* 州. It was founded under Sui 隋, in 589, by changing the name of Xiang zhou 湘州. Its seat of administration was in present-day Chang sha 長沙 city in Hu nan 湖南. Its territory of administration comprised the present-day cities and counties of Chang sha, Zhu zhou 株洲, Xiang tan 湘潭, Yi yang 益陽, Liu yang 瀏陽, Xiang xiang 湘鄉 and Li ling 醴陵 in Hu nan. Five Dynasties' Chu 楚 changed the *zhou* to be Chang sha fu 長沙府. Northern Song 宋 again changed it to be Tan zhou. Its territory of administration was expanded. Under Yuan 元, in 1277, it became Tan zhou lu 潭州路. Mentioned with 314.

Tang 唐 [4]
Name of a *zhou* 州. It was established under Tang 唐, in 626. Its seat of administration was in present-day Mi yang 泌陽 county in He nan 河南. Its territorial administration corresponded to the present-day counties of Mi yang, Tang he 唐河, Fang cheng 方城, She qi 社旗 and Tong bai 桐柏 in He nan. In 906, it became Mi zhou 泌州. The seat of administration was moved to present-day Tang he county. Under Five Dynasties' Tang it again became Tang zhou 唐州. Later Jin 晉 also changed it to Mi zhou. Later Han 漢 restored the name Tang zhou. Under Ming 明, in 1380, it was demoted again to be Tang county. Mentioned with 72, 1238, 1400, 1459.

Tang luo 溏濼 [1]
Name of a body of water. The term refers to the lakes of different extensions in the northern part of the He bei 河北 plateau. Mentioned with 1467.

Tang luo jie he 塘濼界河 [1]
Name of various ponds and lakes stretched like a belt. It refers to the border river between Northern Song 宋 and Liao 遼 formed by ponds and lakes in the northern portion of the He bei 河北 plateau. Mentioned with 291.

Tang shan xian 唐山縣 [1]
Name of a county. It was founded during the *da ding* 大定 reign period (1161 – 1189) of Jin 金 when Yao shan 堯山 county was changed to Tang shan 唐山 county to avoid a taboo of a Jin ruler. Its seat of administration was in Yao shan xiang 鄉山鄉, located southwest of Long yao 隆堯 county in He bei 河北. It was eliminated under Yuan 元, in 1265. Later, it was reestablished. In 1928, the name was changed again to Yao shan county. Mentioned with 1532.

Tang shao shan 堂少山 [1]
Name of a mountain. It is within the boundaries of present-day Ba zhou 巴洲 village of Ba zhou xiang 巴洲鄉 of Xi yang 昔陽 county of Shan xi 山西. Mentioned with 1375.

Tang xian 唐縣 [1]
Name of a county. It was founded by Ming 明, in 1380, by changing the name of Tang zhou 唐州. It was put under Nan yang fu 南陽府. Its seat of administration was in present-day Tang he 唐河 county in He nan 河南. Mentioned with 707.

Tang yin 湯陰 [1]
Name of a county. It was established under Sui 隋, in 586. Its seat of administration was at a location east of present-day Tang yin county in He nan 河南. At the end of the *da ye* 大業 reign period (605 – 618) it was eliminated. Under Tang 唐, in 627, it was restored. The seat of administration was moved to the present Tang yin county. At the end of Yuan 元, it was eliminated. It was reestablished under Ming 明. The county has continued up to the present. Mentioned with 3.

Tao yang 洮陽 [1]
Name of a county. It was established under Emperor Jin Hui di 晉惠帝 (259-307), and put under Di dao 狄道 commandery. Its seat of administration was in present-day Lin zhang 臨潭 county in Gan su 甘肅. Later the area was taken

over by the peoples of the Jiang 羌 nationality. It was abolished at the beginning of the *kai huang* 開皇 reign period (581-600) of Sui 隋 era. Mentioned with 461.

Teng zhou 藤州 [2]

Name of a *zhou* 州. It was founded under Sui 隋, in 590. Its seat of administration was at a location northeast of present-day Teng 藤 county in Guang xi 廣西. Its territory of administration corresponded to the area of present-day Teng county. Under Ming 明, in 1377, it was reduced to be Teng county. Mentioned with 1041, 1532.

Tian di zhi shan 天帝之山 [1]

Place name from the *Shan hai jing* 山海經, "Classic of Mountains and Seas." Further details are lacking. Mentioned with 247.

Tian fang guo 天方國 [3]

Name of an ancient country. It is also called Tian fang 天房 and Tian tang 天堂. Originally the term applied to Mecca city. Later, the meaning was expanded to cover the territories of the Arabic empires of Western history. The term may be a variant transcripton of Tian fang 天房, "House of Heaven," this referring to the ka'ba or "House of God" in Mecca which Muslims pray facing towards. Mentioned with 2, 280, 796.

Tian lou shan 天婁山 [1]

Name of a mountain. It is located in Zheng an 正安 city in Gui zhou 貴州. Mentioned with 1250.

Tian mu shan 天目山 [2]

Name of a mountain. This is Tian mu 天目 mountain found within the borders of present-day Lin an 臨安 city in Zhe jiang 浙江. Its ancient name was Fou yu shan 浮玉山. This is the mountain range that divides the Yang zi from the Qian tang jiang 錢塘江. The mountains are divided into a Dong tian mu 東天目, "Eastern Tian mu," mountain and a Xi Tian mu 西天目, „Western Tian mu," mountain. The former is located in present-day Mei jia 梅家 village of Tai hu yuan 太湖源 town in Lin an city. The latter is located 31 km west of present-day Lin an city in Zhe jiang. Long wang 龍王 mountain is the highest peak at 1587 m. Mentioned with 225, 797.

Tian shui 天水 [2]

Name of a commandery. It was founded under Western Han 漢, in 114 BCE. Its seat of administration was in present-day Tong wei 通渭 county in Gan su 甘肅. The administrative area included the counties of Tong wei, Jing ning 靜寧, Qin an 秦安, Ding xi 定西, Qing shui 清水, Zhuang lang 莊浪, Gan gu 甘谷 and Zhang jia chuan 張家川, and the northwest portion of Tian shui city in Gan su. Under Eastern Han, in 74, it became Han yang 漢陽 commandery. At the same time, the seat of administration was moved to a location south of Gan gu county in Gan su. Under Three Kingdoms Wei 魏, the area again became Tian shui commandery. Western Jin 晉 moved the seat of administration to Tian shui city. The administrative area of the commandery under Northern Wei 魏 corresponed to the present-day cities and counties of Tian shui, Qin an 秦安 and

Gan gu. The commandery was abolished under Sui 隋, in 583. During the *da ye* 大業 reign period of Sui, and during the *tian bao* 天寶 (742-756) and *zhi de* 至德 (756-758) reign periods of Tang 唐, Qin zhou 秦州 was periodically changed to be Tian shui commandery. Mentioned with 908, 1428.

Tian tai 天台 [9]
Name of a county. It was founded by Five Dynasties' Liang 梁, in 908, by changing the name of Tang xing 唐興 county. This is the present-day Tian tai 天台 county in Zhe jiang 浙江. Mentioned with 19, 485, 809, 1015, 1189, 1257, 1277, 1308.

Tian tai shan 天台山 [9]
Name of a mountain. It is Tian tai mountain located north of present-day Tian tai county in Zhe jiang. Mentioned with 59, 130, 181, 309, 458, 874, 891, 912, 1048.

Tian zhu 天竺 [8]
Name of an ancient country. This is India. See → Tian zhu guo 天竺國. Mentioned with 206, 368, 542, 799, 945, 1170, 1420.

Tian zhu guo 天竺國 [3]
Name of an ancient country. This is a name for India and designates India and the other countries of the subcontinent centering on India. Mentioned with 14, 895, 1489.

Tian zhu zhu guo 天竺諸國 [1]
This is a name for "the various countries of India." It designates India and the other countries of the subcontinent centering on India. Mentioned with 144.

Ting shan 亭山 [1]
Name of a county. It was established under Sui 隋, in 586. Its seat of administration was at a location east of Ji 雞 mountain located 40 *li* southwest of present-day Xiu hui 繡惠 town, and southwest of Zhang qiu 章丘 city in Shan dong 山東. Under Tang 唐, in 820, it was combined with Zhang qiu county. Mentioned with 191.

Tong 通 [3]
Name of a *zhou* 州. It was founded by Five Dynasties' Zhou 周, in 958. Its seat of administration was in present-day Nan tong 南通 city in Jiang su 江蘇. The administrative area of the *zhou* corresponded to an area extending from the Yang zi in Jiang su toward the North, and from Tai xing 泰興 and Ru gao 如皋 toward the East. Under Northern Song 宋, in 1023, the *zhou* was changed to be Chong zhou 崇州. In 1033, it again became Tong zhou. Under Qing 清, in 1724, the status of the *zhou* was raised to be a directly administered *zhou*, *zhi li zhou* 直隸州. Because Shun tian fu 順天府 already had a Tong zhou 通州, it was usually called Nan tong zhou 南通州. Mentioned with 790, 1057, 1318.

Tong 同 [2]
Name of a *zhou* 州. See → Tong zhou 同州. Mentioned with 126, 1340.

Tong an 同安 [1]
Name of a county. It was established under Western Jin 晉, in 282. Its seat of administration was in the Tong an district of Xia men 廈門 city in Fu jian 福建. It

was abolished at the end of Western Jin. It was reestablished under Five Dynasties' Min 閩, in 939. In 1996 the county became a district.

Tong bai 桐柏 [3]
Name of a mountain. See → Tong bai shan 桐柏山. Mentioned with 203, 233.

Tong bai shan 桐柏山 [1]
Name of a mountain. It is located southwest of present-day Tong bai 桐柏 county in He nan 河南. Mentioned with 1177.

Tong cheng xian 通城縣 [1]
Name of a county. It was founded under Northern Song 宋, in 1072, and is the present-day Tong cheng 通城 county in Hu bei 湖北. Mentioned with 757.

Tong chuan 潼川 [1]
Name of a *zhou* 州. It was established under Ming 明, in 1376, by demoting Tong chuan fu 潼川府. It was put under the Si chuan Provincial Administration Commission, Si chuan *bu zheng shi si* 四川布政使司, for administration. It was administered from present-day San tai 三台 county in Si chuan 四川. Its territory of administration comprised the middle watershed of the Fu jiang 涪江, an area in Si chuan extending from the Zhong jiang 中江 and Yan ting 鹽亭 toward the South, and from An yue 安岳 and Tong nan 潼南 toward the North. Under Qing 清, in 1734, its status was raised to Tong chuan fu 潼川府. Mentioned with 1096.

Tong guan 銅官 [3]
Name of a mountain. From the Southern Dynasties period on, "Copper Administrations," *tong guan*, to manage copper mining were set up at various places, for example, at Tong ling 銅陵 in An hui 安徽, at Wang cheng 望城 in Hu nan 湖南 and at Qiong lai 邛崍 in Si chuan 四川. Further details are unavailable. Mentioned with 122, 595, 1134.

Tong ling xian 銅陵縣 [1]
Name of a county. It was established under Five Dynasties and Ten Countries' Southern Tang 唐, in 951. Its seat of administration was in present-day Tong ling 銅陵 city in An hui 安徽. In 1958, the county was changed to be Tong ling city. Mentioned with 695.

Tong lu 桐廬 [1]
Name of a county. It was established under Three Kingdoms' Wu 吳, in 226. Its seat of administration was at a location 25 *li* west of present-day Tong lu county in Zhe jiang 浙江. It was eliminated in 589. It was restored in 602, and persists until the present. Mentioned with 1497.

Tong shan 銅山 [2]
Name of a mountain. The name is a reference to some mountain producing copper. Mentioned with 1180, 1535.

Tong zhou 同州 [10]
Name of a *zhou*. It was founded by Western Wei, in 554. Its seat of administration was in present-day Da li 大荔 county in Shaan xi 陝西. It was eliminated under

Sui 隋, in 607. It was restored under Tang 唐 in 618. Its territory of administration comprised the present-day counties and cities of Da li, He yang 合陽, Han cheng 韓城, Cheng cheng 澄城 and Bai shui 白水 in Shaan xi. Under Qing 清, in 1735, its status was raised to Tong zhou fu 同州府. Mentioned with 222, 272, 461, 532, 733, 816, 1258.

Tong zhou 通州 [1]
Name of a *zhou* 州. It was established under Western Wei 魏, in 553. Its seat of administration was in present-day Da chuan 達川 city in Si chuan 四川. Its territory of administration corresponded to the present-day counties and cities of Da chuan, Da xian 達縣, Xuan han 宣漢, Kai jiang 開江 and Wan yuan 萬源 in Si chuan, and Cheng kou 城口 in Chong qing 重慶 city. Under Northern Song 宋, in 965, it became Da zhou 達州. Mentioned with 1359.

Tu bo 吐番 [1]
Regional name. This is Tibet. Tu bo, ultimately from Tibetan Bod (Pöd), "Tibet," is the most common Tang 唐 and Song 宋 Dynasty term for Tibet. Mentioned with 319.

Tu fan 土番 [3]
Regional name. The name refers to present-dayTu lu fan 吐魯番, Turfan, in Xin jiang 新疆. Mentioned with 188, 639, 1192.

Tu huo luo 吐火羅 [1]
Name of an ancient country. This was a state established by the Da rou zhi 大月氏 during Han 漢 and Wei 魏 times, and located in present-day Central Asia. The state had various names later, including Da xia 大夏, Kushan/Gui shuang 貴霜 and Yan da 嚈噠. The area was later conquered by the Turks. Mentioned with 1196.

Tu jue 突厥 [1]
Name of a tribe. See → Tu jue guo 突厥國. Mentioned with 1187.

Tu jue guo 突厥國 [1]
Name of an ancient country. In 552, it was founded as the Tu jue 突厥, the Tfiutkyat, led by Tu men 土門, also known as Bumin Qaghan (died 552), overthrew the power of their Avar masters and their ruler made himself qaghan of a new empire, the Köke Türk Empire. During Sui 隋 times, in 583, the empire fell into two parts due to internal divisions, an eastern and a western empire. The Western Tfiutkyat were particularly powerful during early Tang 唐, but later became divided themselves and grew weak. The eastern Tfiutkyat controlled a strip of territory located south of the Central Asian deserts. In 745, the empire was destroyed by the Uighurs and most of the Tfiutkyat came under the Uighurs. Some moved to Central Asia, and some went south and came under Tang dynasty control. Mentioned with 1205.

Tu ling 荼陵 [1]
This is an error for → Cha ling 茶陵.

Tu yu hun 吐谷渾 [2]

Name of a tribal group, and of a geographic territory. Originally the term referred to a branch of the Xian bei 鮮卑 nomadizing northwest of present-day Ling hai 淩海 city in Liao ning 遼寧. At the end of Western Jin 晉, the leader of the tribe, known as the Tu yu hun 吐谷渾, led it west to an area between Gan su 甘肅 and Qing hai 青海 and called himself Qaghan. He situated his capital at a place northwest of present-day Gong he 共和 county in Qing hai. The territory of administration of the Tu yu hun state reached an extension of about 3000 *li* east and west and more than a thousand *li* south and north. This corresponded to much of present-day Qing hai and the northwestern part of Si chuan 四川. The Tu yu hun were defeated during Sui 隋 times and destroyed during Tang 唐 times. The Tu yu hun people were dispersed. Mentioned with 799, 1242.

Tuo 沱 [1]

Name of a river. It is also called the Tuo jiang 沱江. Its upper reaches are the present Bai tiao he 柏條河 and the Pi he 毗河. From Du jiang yan 都江堰 city it separates from the Min jiang 岷江 and flows east. The lower reaches is called Tuo jiang which below present-day Jin tang 金堂 flows south to Lu zhou 瀘州 city and enters the Yang zi. Mentioned with 1096.

Tuo shan 橐山 [1]

Name of a mountain. This is a great mountain in the northern part of the Qin ling 秦嶺 mountain range, east of present-day Hua 華 county in Shaan xi 陝西. It reaches 1200 *m* above sea level. Mentioned with 1339.

-W-

Wai fan 外番 [1]

General reference to "foreign countries." Mentioned with 1091.

Wai guo 外國 [6]

General reference to "foreign countries." Mentioned with 186, 799, 890, 1115, 1246, 1289.

Wan an 萬安 [2]

Name of an administrative area. Northern Song 宋, in 1074, changed Wan an zhou 萬安州 to Wan an army. It was administered in present-day Wan ning 萬寧 county in Hai nan 海南 province. Its territory of administration corresponded to the two present-day counties of Wan ning and Ling shui 陵水 in Hai nan. Under Ming 明, in 1368, it was changed to be Wan zhou 萬州. Mentioned with 144.

Wan zhou 萬州 [6]

Name of a *zhou* 州. It was established under Tang 唐, in 634. It was administered in the city district of present-day Wan zhou district of the Chong qing 重慶 municipality. Its territory of administration comprised today's Wan zhou district, and Liang ping 梁平 county. Under Ming 明, in 1373, it was changed to Wan 萬 county. Mentioned with 127, 468, 566, 956, 1091.

Wang chu shan 望楚山 [1]
Name of a mountain. It is located southwest of Xiang yang 襄陽 city in present-day Hu bei 湖北. Its original name was Ma an 馬鞍 mountain. In Liu Song 劉宋 times its name was changed to Wang chu shan. Mentioned with 275.

Wang wu 王屋 [1]
Name of a mountain. See → Wang wu shan 王屋山. Mentioned with 1134.

Wang wu shan 王屋山 [6]
Name of a mountain. It is located 90 *li* northwest of present-day Ji yuan 濟源 city in He nan 河南. The mountain borders in the North at Yang cheng 陽城 county in Shan xi 山西. Mentioned with 381, 857, 1241, 1407, 1445, 1516.

Wei 威
Name of a *zhou* 州 see → Wei zhou 威州.

Wei 衛 [1 + 2]
□ Name of an ancient area. [1] The reference is to the Spring and Autumn period country of Wei. The kernel of this state lay in a strip of present-day Shang qiu 商丘 in He nan 河南. Mentioned with 856.
□ Name of a *zhou* 州. [2] See → Wei zhou 衛州. Mentioned with 1289, 1478.

Wei 魏 [4]
This is a regional name used with Wei di 魏地. The term refers to the former lands of the Wei country of pre-Qin 秦 times. See → Wei guo 魏國. Mentioned with 417, 434, 1242.

Wei cheng 渭城 [2]
Name of a county. It was founded under Western Han 漢, in 114 BCE, by changing Xin cheng 新城 county. It was subordinated to You fu feng 右扶風. Its seat of administration was in the region of present-day Yao dian 窯店 town located northeast of Xian yang 咸陽 city in Shaan xi 陝西. Eastern Han eliminated the county and made it part of Chang an 長安 county. Mentioned with 222.

Wei di 魏地
See → Wei 魏

Wei guo 魏國 [1]
Name of a region. It referred to the former land of Wei 魏 country of the pre-Qin 秦 period. After the division of Jin 晉 into three parts, Wen hou 文侯 of Wei (died 396 BCE) established his capital at An yi 安邑 (present-day Yun cheng 運城 city in Shan xi 山西). Hui wang 惠王 (400 – 319) moved the capital to Da liang 大梁 (this is present-day Kai feng 開封 city in He nan 河南). The administration comprised the southwestern part of present-day Shan xi 山西, and a region in the northern and eastern parts of He nan. Mentioned with 1509.

Wei jun 魏郡 [3]
Name of a commandery. It was founded by Western Han 漢, in 195 BCE. Its seat of administration was in present-day Ye cheng 鄴城 town, located southwest of

Lin zhang 臨漳 county in He bei 河北. Its territory of administration comprised in present-day He bei Da ming 大名, Ci xian 磁縣, She xian 涉縣, Wu an 武安, Lin zhang 臨漳, Fei xiang xian 肥鄉縣, Wei xian 魏縣, Qiu xian 邱縣, Cheng an 成安, Guang ping 廣平 and Guan tao 館陶, in present-day He nan 河南 Hua xian 滑縣, Jun xian 浚縣 and Nei huang 內黃, and in present-day Shan dong 山東 the region of Kuan xian 冠縣. Western Jin 晉 subordinated the commandery to Si zhou 司州. Northern Wei 魏, in 401, put it under Xiang zhou 相州. Eastern Wei established its capital there, and changed it to be Wei yin 魏尹. Northern Qi 齊 changed the *zhou* to be Qing du yin 清都尹. At the beginning of the *da ye* 大業 reign period (605 – 618) of Sui 隋, the seat of administration was moved to the present An yang 安陽 city. Tang 唐, at the beginning of the *wu de* 武德 reign period (618 – 626), changed the *zhou* to be Xiang zhou. Mentioned with 453, 1071. 1532.

Wei qiang shan 韋羌山 [1]

Name of a mountain. It is located west of present-day Xian ju 仙居 county in Zhe jiang 浙江. Mentioned with 1277.

Wei sheng jun 威勝軍 [1]

Name of an administrative unit, an army. It was established under Northern Song 宋, in 978. Its seat of administration was in present-day Qin 沁 county in Shan xi 山西. Its territory of administration comprised the present-day counties of Qin xian 沁縣, Wu xiang 武鄉 and Qin yuan 沁源 in Shan xi. In 1128, the area became Qin zhou 沁州. Mentioned with 1334.

Wei shui 渭水 [1]

Name of a river. This is the Wei 渭 river. This is the largest river in the Guan zhong 關中 area. It has its springs in the East of present-day Gan su 甘肅, in a mountain called "Common cave of Bird and Rodent" (Niao shu tong xue 鳥鼠同穴) in antiquity. It flows eastward to pass north of Chang an 長安 city. After taking up the Jing he 涇河, it continues to flow east and enters the Yellow River at present-day Chao yi 朝邑 town in Da li 大荔 county in Shaan xi 陝西. In ancient times, the Wei shui had a much greater flow volume. Later, due to destruction of the forests of the loess plateau and the grass steppes, water volume gradually decreased and the bed of the river moved towards the north. Because the water of the ancient Wei shui was turbid and because the water of the Jing he was clear, where the two rivers came together there was the remarkable phenomenon of a "clearly visible separation of Jing [he] and Wei [shui]," 涇渭分明. Mentioned with 516.

Wei xing 魏興 [5]

Name of a commandery. It was established under Three Kingdoms Wei 魏 by changing the name of Xi cheng 西城 commandery. It was put under Jing zhou 荊州. Its seat of administration was on the northern bank of the Han shui 漢水, located 4 *li* northwest of present-day An kang 安康 city in Shaan xi 陝西. Its territory of administration corresponded to an area extending in present-day Shaan xi from the counties of Shan yang 山陽, Zuo shui 柞水 and Ning shaan 寧陝 toward the South, from the two counties of Shi quan 石泉 and Zi yang

紫陽 toward the East, from the counties of Lan gao 嵐皋, Ping li 嵐皋 and Bai he 白河 toward the North, and in present-day Hu bei 湖北 from the counties of Yun 鄖 and Yun xi 鄖西 toward the West. Later, the seat of commandery administration was repeatedly moved. During the *yong jia* 永嘉 reign period (307-313), it was settled at the present-day An kang city. Western Wei 魏, in 552, put it under Dong liang zhou 東梁州. In 554, it was put under Jin zhou 金州. Under Sui 隋, in 583, the commandery was abolished. Mentioned with 879, 1218, 1305, 1435, 1532.

Wei zhou 渭州 [2]

Name of a *zhou* 州. It was founded under Northern Wei 魏, in 530. It was named after the Wei shui 渭水. Its seat of administration was at a location 5 *li* southeast of present-day Long xi 隴西 county in Gan su 甘肅. Its territory of administration comprised the present-day counties of Long xi, Wei yuan 渭源, Zhang xian 漳縣, Ding xi 定西 and Wu shan 武山 in Gan su. From the *bao ying* reign period (762 – 763) of Tang 唐 on, the area fell to the Tibetans. In 809, a separate Wei zhou 渭州 was established in Ping liang 平涼 county in Yuan zhou 原州. In 880, this was also destroyed by the Tibetans, but the area was recovered in 851. During Northern Song 宋 times, its administrative area comprised the present-day cities and counties of Ping Liang 平涼, Hua ting 華亭 and Chong xin 崇信 in Gan su, and Jing yuan 涇源 in Ning xia 寧夏. Jin 金 changed the *zhou* to be Ping liang fu 平涼府. Mentioned with 650, 1201.

Wei zhou 衛州 [1]

Name of a *zhou* 州. It was founded by Northern Zhou 周, in 578. Its seat of administration was in present-day Qi men 淇門 ford located southwest of Jun 浚 county in He nan 河南. During Tang 唐, in 627, the seat of administration was moved to the present Wei hui 衛輝 city. At the beginning of the *da ye* 大業 (605 – 618) reign period of the Sui 隋, and during the *tian bao* 天寶 (742 – 756) and *zhi de* 至德 (756 – 758) reign periods of the Tang, the area periodically became Ji 汲 commandery. Its territory of administration during Song 宋 comprised the present-day cities and counties of Wei hui, Xin xiang 新鄉, Hui xian 輝縣, Jun xian 浚縣, Qi xian 淇縣 and Hua xian 滑縣 in He nan. In 1260, under Qubilai, the status of the area was raised to be Wei hui lu 衛輝路. Mentioned with 258.

Wei zhou 維州 [1]

Name of a *zhou* 州. It was founded under Tang 唐, in 624, and is named after Jiang wei 姜維 city. Its seat of administration was in present-day Xue cheng 薛城 town, located 36 *li* northeast of Li 理 county in Si chuan 四川. Its administrative territory comprised the area of present-day Li county in Si chuan. The area is near to Tibet. It is the gateway to western Si chuan. In 763, the area fell to Tibet and Wei zhou became Wu you 無憂 city. Under Northern Song 宋, in 1036, the area was changed to be Wei zhou 威州. Mentioned with 557.

Wei zhou 威州 [2]

Name of a *zhou* 州. It was founded under Northern Song 宋, in 1036, by changing the name of Wei zhou 維州. Its seat of administration was in present-day Xue cheng 薛城 city, located 36 *li* northeast of Li 理 county in Si chuan 四川.

Under the Ming 明, in 1435, its seat of administration was moved to Wen chuan 汶川 county in Si chuan. Under Qing 清, in 1727, the *zhou* was abolished. Mentioned with 561, 585.

Wen 溫 [7]
Name of a *zhou*. See → Wen zhou. Mentioned with 278, 323, 328, 359, 994, 1057, 1248.

Wen 汶 [1]
Name of a river. This is the Da wen 大汶 river in the southwestern part of Shan dong 山東. It has its sources north of present-day Lai wu 萊蕪 city in Shan dong. It flows southwest through Tai an 泰安 city and Ning yang 寧陽 county to Dai cun 戴村 dam in Dong ping 東平 county. In ancient times, from there on down the Wen shui 汶水 flowed westward through the South of Dong ping county and to a location southeast of Liang 梁 mountain where it entered the Ji shui 濟水. After Ming 明 built the Dai cun dam, it contained the Wen shui so that it would flow south and enter the Nan wang 南旺 lake, in order to increase canal water. After that, its western flow became smaller. At the end of Qing 清, the water transport of grain to the capital was stopped, and the main stream of the Wen in the West poured into Dong ping lake and in the North into the Yellow River. Mentioned with 422.

Wen quan xian 溫泉縣 [1]
Name of a county. It was established under Tang 唐, in 620, and was named because of the "warm springs," *wen quan* 溫泉, facing it on the south. It was under Bei wen zhou 北溫州. Its seat of administration was in present-day Wen quan xiang 溫泉鄉, located 45 *li* northeast of Jiao kou 交口 county in Shan xi 山西. In 627, it was subordinated to Xian zhou 隰州. Northern Song 宋 took over the county. It was abolished under Qubilai khan, in 1266. Mentioned with 695.

Wen shan 汶山 [7]
Name of a mountain. This is Min shan 岷山 mountain in the northwestern part of present-day Si chuan 四川. According to *Yuan he jun County Annals*, *Yuan he jun xian zhi* 元和郡縣志, *juan* 32, Mao zhou 茂州, "Wen shan is Min shan." Qian Daxin 錢大昕 (1728 – 1804) suggested that because of a lack of light labials in ancient Chinese, the words Wen 汶 and Min 岷 were pronounced identically. Mentioned with 188, 219, 324, 348, 368, 473, 701.

Wen shan jun 汶山郡 [1]
Name of a commandery. It was established under Western Han 漢, in 111 BCE. Its seat of administration was at a location north of present-day Mao 茂 county. Its territory of administration corresponded to an area in present-day Si chuan 四川 extending from Qiong lai 邛崍 mountain toward the East, from Min 岷 mountain toward the South, included Bei chuan 北川 county and the area from Du jiang yan 都江堰 city toward the West. In 67 BCE, it was combined with Shu 蜀 commandery. Under Eastern Han, during the *jian an* 建安 reign period (196 – 220), Liu Bei 劉備 (161-223) reestablished it. It was administered from present-day Mian si 綿虒 town, located southwest of Wen chuan 汶川 county

in Si chuan. Under Northern Zhou, in 564, the seat of administration was moved to the present Wen chuan county. Under Sui 隋, in 607, it was moved to present-day Mao 茂 county. Under Tang 唐, in 618, it was changed to be Hui zhou 會州. Mentioned with 1289.

Wen xiang 閿鄉 [1]
Name of a county. It was established by Sui 隋, in 596, and subordinated to Shaan zhou 陝州. Its seat of administration was in present-day Wen di 文底, located northwest of Ling bao 靈寶 city in He nan 河南. At the beginning of the *hong wu* 洪武 reign period (1368 – 1398) of Ming 明, the seat of administration was moved to present-day Wen xiang 閿鄉, located northwest of Ling bao city. In 1954, it was abolished and made part of Ling bao county. Mentioned with 473.

Wen zhou 汶州 [1]
Name of a *zhou* 州. It was founded by Northern Zhou 周, in 564, by changing Liang sheng zhou 梁繩州. Its seat of administration was at a location northwest of present-day Mao 茂 county in Si chuan 四川. Its territory of administration comprised the present-day counties of Mao xian 茂縣, Wen chuan 汶川 and Bei chuan 北川 in Si chuan. Under Sui 隋, in 585, it was changed to be Shu zhou 蜀州. Mentioned with 199, 1289.

Wen zhou 文州 [4]
Name of a *zhou* 州. It was established under Northern Zhou 周, in 558. Its seat of administration was at a location southwest of present-day Wen 文 county in Gan su 甘肅. It was eliminated at the beginning of the *da ye* 大業 reign period (605 – 618) of Sui 隋. It was reestablished at the beginning of the *wu de* 武德 reign period (618 – 626) of Tang 唐. In 782, the seat of administration was moved to the present Wen county. The territory of administration comprised only a strip of present-day Wen county. Later following the *duan ping* 端平 reign period (1232 – 1234) of Song 宋, it was abolished. It was reestablished under Yuan 元. Ming 明, in 1371, reduced the *zhou* to a county. Its territory was between Long 隴 and Shu 蜀, in the rocky steep vallies with hanging paths. This is the shortcut for entering Shu. Mentioned with 285, 986, 1310, 1445.

Wen zhou 溫州 [4]
Name of a *zhou*. It was founded under Tang 唐, in 675, by dividing Kuo zhou 括州. Its seat of administration was in present-day Wen zhou city in Zhe jiang 浙江. It got its name from the Wen jiao 溫嶠 mountain range. Its territory of administration comprised Wen zhou city, along with the two present-day counties of Yong jia 永嘉 and Yue qing 樂清 in Zhe jiang, the Fei yun jiang 飛雲江 water course and the area south of it. Under Northern Song, in 1262, the status of the area was raised to be Rui an fu 瑞安府. The area corresponded to the southeast littoral. During Song 宋 and Yuan 元, a Maritime Administration, *shi bo si* 市舶司, was periodically established there. Mentioned with 323, 328, 578, 1020.

Wo 倭 [5]
Name of a foreign country, also mentioned as Wo guo 倭國. See → Wo guo.

Wo guo 倭國 [5]
Name of a country. This is an old name for Japan, specifically referring to the early Yamatai 邪馬臺國 and Yamato 大和國 states that occupied the region of present-day Nara. Mentioned with 493, 635, 953, 1080, 1390.

Wu 婺
→ Wu zhou 婺州.

Wu 吳 [60]
Regional name. The term is a general reference to a region covering the southern part of the present Jiang su 江蘇 region centered on the city of Su zhou 蘇州, Shang hai 上海 city and the northern part of Zhe jiang 浙江. Since this area was the central part of the state of Wu during the Spring and Autumn periods, it was also the administrative center of the Wu belonging to the Three Kingdoms period. Mentioned with 27, 100, 142, 159, 170, 171, 211, 326, 338, 409, 429, 456, 497, 519, 588, 602, 614, 615, 616, 630, 635, 690, 723, 781, 839, 848, 863, 908, 960, 1032, 1064, 1097, 1118, 1126, 1174, 1210, 1218, 1223, 1239, 1257, 1259, 1270, 1274, 1283, 1307, 1312, 1329, 1339, 1340, 1352, 1471, 1485, 1499, 1515.

Wu chang 武昌 [7 + 3]
□ Name of a commandery. [7] It was established by Three Kingdoms' Wu 吳, in 221,. Its seat of administration was in present-day E zhou 鄂州 city in Hu bei 湖北. Its territory of administration included the area south of the Yang zi in the eastern part of present-day Hu bei, the area east of Jia yu tong 嘉魚通 mountain, and areas such as Jiu jiang 九江 and Rui chang 瑞昌 in Jiang xi 江西. The commandery was abolished under Sui 隋, in 589. Mentioned with 75, 768, 1122, 1264, 1499, 1532.
□ Name of a county. [3] It was established under Three Kingdoms' Wu 吳, in 221. Its seat of administration was in present-day E zhou 鄂州 city in Hu bei 湖北. In 1913, the area was changed to Shou chang 壽昌 county. Mentioned with 82, 157, 1080.

Wu chang guo 烏場國 [1]
Ancient country of the western regions. It was located on the upper reaches of the Indus River in the Swat area. Mentioned with 1289.

Wu cheng 武城 [1]
Name of a place. Further details are lacking. Mentioned with 1279.

Wu cheng xian 烏程縣 [1]
Name of a county. It was established by Qin 秦 and put under Kuai ji 會稽 commandery. Its seat of administration was in present-day Xia gu cheng 下菰城, located 15 *li* south of Hu zhou 湖州 city in Zhe jiang 浙江. Under Eastern Han 漢, it was subordinated to Wu 吳 commandery. Three Kingdoms' Wu 吳 put it under Wu xing 吳興 commandery. Under Eastern Jin 晉, in 405, its seat of administration was moved to the city district of present-day Hu zhou city. Under Sui 隋, in 602, its seat of administration was at Hu zhou. Under Northern Song 宋, in 982, a Gui an 歸安 county was split off and established, and it and Wu cheng 烏城 county were both governed at Hu zhou. In 1225, it came under An ji

zhou 安吉州. Yuan 元 created a Hu zhou lu 湖州路 to administer it. Ming 明 and Qing 清 put it under a Hu zhou fu 湖州府. In 1912, it was combined with Gui an 歸安 county to create Wu xing 吳興 county. Mentioned with 1521.

Wu chu 吳楚 [1]

Combined regional name. It refers collectively to the watershed of the Yang zi river in the south. During Spring and Autumn times, Wu 吳 was situated along the lower reaches of the Yang zi, and Chu 楚 was situated along the middle and upper reaches of the Yang zi. Mentioned with 1004.

Wu dang 武當 [3]

Name of a mountain. See → Wu dang shan 武當山. Mentioned with 188, 876, 1435.

Wu dang shan 武當山 [3]

Name of a mountain. This is the Wu dang mountain located southwest of present-day Dan jiang kou 丹江口 city in Hu bei 湖北. This is a famous scenic spot for Daoism. Mentioned with 556. 1163, 1240.

Wu di 吳地 [5]

Name of a region. The reference refers to the ancient region of which the Wu 吳 state was the center. See → Wu. Mentioned with 64, 735, 883, 1064, 1262.

Wu du 武都 [24]

Name of a commandery and a county. It was established under Western Han 漢, in 111 BCE. Its seat of administration was in the Wu du county established by Western Han, located southwest of present-day Xi he 西和 county in Gan su 甘肅. The administration comprised much of present-day Long nan 隴南 city in Gan su, and Feng 鳳 county and Lue yang 略陽 in Shaan xi 陝西. Eastern Han moved the seat of the commandery to a location west of present-day Cheng 成 county in Gan su. Northern Wei 魏 changed the name of the commandary to be Yong du 永都, and abolished Wu du county. Mentioned with 82, 173, 202, 285, 298, 762, 765, 908, 1031, 1096, 1182, 1184, 1289, 1307, 1497.

Wu du 吳都 [2]

This refers to the capital city of pre-Qin 秦 era Wu 吳. It was located in present-day Su zhou city 蘇州 in Jiang su 江蘇. Mentioned with 587, 1219.

Wu gang zhou 武岡州 [2]

Name of a *zhou* 州. It was established under the Ming 明, in 1376, by changing the name of Wu gang fu 武岡府. It was put under Bao qing fu 寶慶府. Its seat of administration was in present-day Wu gang 武岡 city in Hu nan 湖南. Its territory of administration comprised the counties of Wu gang, Xin ning 新寧, Sui ning 綏寧 and Dong kou 洞口, and the area of the Cheng bu miao 城步苗 people self-governed county, all in present-day Hu nan. In 1913, the area was changed to be Wu gang county. Mentioned with 616, 1329.

Wu gong 武功 [2]

Name of a county. It was established by Warring States Qin 秦. Its seat of administration was in the southern bank of the Wei shui 渭水, located 40 *li* east of present-day Mei 眉 county in Shaan xi 陝西. The Qin and Western Han 漢

dynasties continued the county. Under Eastern Han, in 65, the seat of administration was moved to present-day Yong an 永安 village in the Yang ling 楊陵 district of Xian yang 咸陽 city in Shaan xi. The county was eliminated under Northern Wei 魏. It was reestablished under Northern Zhou 周, in 574. The seat of administration was moved to present-day Wu gong 武功 town, located northwest of Wu gong county in Shaan xi. Under Jin 金, in 1189, the area was changed to Wu ting 武亭 county. Yuan 元 restored Wu gong county. Ming 明 subordinated it to Xi an fu 西安府. Qing 清 changed this and subordinated the county to Qian zhou 乾州 directly administered *zhou* 州, *zhi li zhou* 直隸州. In 1961, the seat of administration was moved to its present-day venue in Pu ji 普集 town. Mentioned with 1308.

Wu gou shan 烏勾山 [1]

Name of a mountain. It is located within the boundaries of present-day Xun dian 尋甸 county in Yun nan 雲南. The exact location is unavailable. Mentioned with 795.

Wu ji guo 勿吉國 [1]

Name of a tribal group. In ancient times, it was positioned in the Chinese northeast and spread across the Song hua jiang 松花江 in the area north of Chang bai 長白 mountain in present-day Ji lin 吉林 province, and the area of the middle and lower watershed of the Hei long jiang 黑龍江. In the East, the group reached to the sea. One group of their later descendants were the Wan yan 完顏 tribe of the Nü zhen 女真 who were founders of the Jin 金 dynasty, and the Manchus founding the Qing 清 dynasty. Mentioned with 1339.

Wu jiang 吳江 [1]

Name of a county. Five Dynasties' Wu yue 吳越 established the county. It was administered in present-day Wu jiang 吳江 city in Jiang su 江蘇. In 1992, the status of the county was raised to be a city. Mentioned with 332.

Wu jun 吳郡 [3]

Name of a commandery. It was established by Eastern Han 漢, in 129, by dividing Kuai ji 會稽 commandery. Its seat of administration was in Wu 吳 county, the present-day Su zhou 蘇州 city in Jiang su 江蘇. Its administrative territory comprised an area south of the Yang zi in present-day Jiang su, the area east of Da mao 大茅 mountain, Shang hai 上海 city, and in Zhe jiang 浙江 the area extending from Chang xing 長興, Hu zhou 湖州 and Tian mu 天目 mountain toward the East, and the two banks of the Qian tang jiang 錢塘江 river below Jian de 建德 city. Its territory was reduced gradually after the Three Kingdoms period. In 589, under Sui 隋, the seat of administration was moved to a location five *li* east of Heng 横 mountain, located southwest of present-day Su zhou city. At the same time, the commandery became Su zhou. At the beginning of the *da ye* 大業 reign period (605 – 618) of Sui 隋, it again became Wu 吳 commandery. Under Tang 唐, in 621, it was changed to be Su zhou. In 624, the administration was returned to present-day Su zhou city. In 742, it was changed back to be Wu commandery. In 758, it again became Su zhou. Mentioned with 308, 1219, 1250.

Wu kuai 吳會 [1]

Name of an ancient region. The name refers to a region within present-day Jiang zhe 江浙. Because Eastern Han 漢 divided Qin kuai ji 秦會稽 commandery into Wu 吳 commandery and Kuai ji 會稽 commandery, later times referred to both of them as Wu kuai. Mentioned with 563.

Wu lao xian 無勞縣 [2]

Name of a county. It was established under Western Jin 晉 by Emperor Wu di 武帝 (236 – 290) by dividing up Bei ying 比景 county. It was put under Ri nan 日南 commandery. Its seat of administration was located in present-day Quảng Trạch in Quảng Bình province in Vietnam. It was abolished under Northern Qi 齊. Mentioned with 384, 1051.

Wu ling 武陵 [1]

Name of a commandery. See → Wu ling jun 武陵郡.

Wu ling 吳陵 [1]

Minor place name. This is the location of the mausoleum of Sun Jian 孫堅 (155 – 191) of Three Kingdoms' Wu 吳. It is located 15 *li* west of present-day Dan yang 丹陽 city in Jiang su 江蘇. Mentioned with 820.

Wu ling 五嶺 [2]

General designation for mountain ranges. These are the comparatively large five mountain ranges located at the borders of present-day Jiang xi 江西, Guang dong 廣東, Hu nan 湖南 and Guang xi 廣西. These are namely the Da yu ling 大庾嶺 (Mei ling 梅嶺), the Qi tian ling 騎田嶺, the Meng zhu ling 萌渚嶺, the Du pang ling 都龐嶺 and the Yue cheng ling 越城嶺 (Lao shan jie 老山界). Mentioned with 535, 1486.

Wu ling jun 武陵郡 [1]

Name of a commandery. It was established under Western Han 漢, when Qian zhong 黔中 commandery was renamed. Its seat of administration was at a location south of present-day Xu pu 溆浦 county in Hu nan 湖南. Its territory of administration comprised an area in present-day Hu nan extending from the the watershed of the Yuan jiang 沅江 toward the West, as well as the eastern part of Gui zhou 貴州 and the southeastern part of Chong qing 重慶 city, the southwestern part of Hu bei 湖北, and a corner of the northeastern part of Guang xi 廣西. Eastern Han moved the seat of administration to present-day Chang de 常德 city in Hu nan. Sui 隋, in 589, turned it into Lang zhou 朗州. At the beginning of the *da ye* 大業 (605 – 618) reign period of the Sui, and during the *tian bao* 天寶 (742 – 756) and *zhi de* 至德 (756 – 758) reign periods of the Tang 唐, the area periodically became Wu ling 武陵 commandery. It was abolished in 758. Mentioned with 1069.

Wu ling zhou 武陵洲 [1]

This is a designation for an island. It is located in the Yang zi at present-day Jiu jiang 九江 city in Jiang xi 江西. Mentioned with 323.

Wu meng shan 烏蒙山 [1]

Name of a mountain. It is Jiao zi 轎子 mountain located northeast of the Lu quan 祿勸 Yi 彝 people and Miao 苗 people self-governing county in present-day Yun nan 雲南. Mentioned with 1057.

Wu meng xia 烏蒙峽 [1]

Name of a gorge. It is more or less located in the northeastern part of present-day Yun nan 雲南. Mentioned with 943.

Wu ping 武平 [3]

Name of a commandery. It was founded by Three Kingdoms' Wu 吳, in 271. Its seat of administration was in Ping zhou 平州, located southeast of Vĩnh Phúc county in Vĩnh Phúc province in present-day Vietnam. Its territory of administration comprised the provinces of Vĩnh Phúc and Bac Thai in present-day Vietnam. Under Sui 隋, in 590, it was abolished. Mentioned with 135, 489, 534.

Wu shan 巫山 [1]

Name of a mountain. It is located in the eastern part of the present-day Chong qing municipality, Chong qing *zhi xia shi* 重慶直辖市. Da ba 大巴 mountain arises in the North, and the range moves northeast and southwest, and spreads out on the Chong qing and Hu bei 湖北 border, reaching more than 200 *km* in length. The height above sea level is 1000 to 2000 meters, and the Yang zi tunnels between the mountains forming the colorful and grand three gorges. The most beautiful among them are the 12 peaks of the Wu shan 巫山 mountains. Mentioned with 1307.

Wu sun guo 烏孫國 [1]

Name of an ancient Central Asian country from the Han 漢 and Tang era. Its seat of administration was at Chi gu cheng 赤谷城, the present-day Yshtyk in Kyrgyzstan. During its period of greatest power, the country controlled the watershed of the Yi li 伊犁 river and the Issyk Kul 伊塞克湖 lake area. The later Wu sun moved westward to the Cong ling 蔥嶺 mountains during the period of the Northern and Southern Dynasties, before finally disappearing through amalgamation with neighboring groups. Mentioned with 897.

Wu tai 五臺

→ Wu tai zhu shan 五臺諸山.

Wu tai shan 五臺山

→ Wu tai zhu shan 五臺諸山.

Wu tai zhu shan 五臺諸山 [9]

Name of a mountain group. The Wu tai 五臺 mountains are located at the northeast corner of present-day Wu tai county in Shan xi 山西. They are one of the four great mountains of Chinese Buddhism. The primary peak is Bei tai ding 北台頂, rising 3058 *m*. Mentioned with 132, 240, 417, 553, 859, 1150, 1277, 1279.

Wu tao shan 無桃山 [1]

Name of a mountain. Details are unavailable. Mentioned with 1308.

Wu wan 烏丸 [1]
Name of a people also called Wu huan 烏桓. They were a branch of the Eastern Hu 胡, and subordinate to the Xiong nu 匈奴. Their ancestral lands were in the southern part of the Da xing an 大興安 chain. But under Eastern Han 漢, they moved to within the passes. After Cao Cao 曹操 (155-220) attacked and subdued the Wu huan, most of them moved to → Zhong yuan 中原 and gradually became Chinese. Mentioned with 239.

Wu wei 武威 [3]
Name of a commandery. It was established under Western Han 漢, in 212 BCE. Its seat of administration was in present-day Wu wei 武威 city in Gan su 甘肅. Its territory of administration comprised the region of the eastern part of the He xi 河西 corridor. Under Tang 唐, in 758, the commandery was changed to be Liang zhou 涼州. Mentioned with 799, 1037, 1382.

Wu wei zhou 無為州 [1]
Name of a *zhou* 州. It was established under Yuan 元, in 1291. Its seat of administration was in present-day Wu wei 無為 county in An hui 安徽. Its territory of administration comprised the three present-day counties and cities of Wu wei, Lu jiang 廬江 and Chao hu 巢湖 in An hui. The *zhou* became a county in 1912. Mentioned with 285.

Wu xi 五溪 [4]
General designation for watersheds. The term refers to the five watercourses found within the confines of the ancient Chen zhou 辰州. These are the Xiong xi 雄溪, Men xi 樠溪, Wu xi 潕溪, You xi 酉溪 and the Chen xi 辰溪, all in the western part of present-day Hu nan 湖南. Mentioned with 202, 535, 1375.

Wu xi shi ku 舞徯石窟 [1]
Name of a rock cave. It is located in the central part of Quảng Bình province in present-day Vietnam. Mentioned with 384.

Wu xian 巫縣 [1]
Name of a county. It was established by Warring States' Qin 秦, in 277 BCE, by changing the name of Wu 巫 commandery of Chu 楚. It was subordinated to Nan 南 commandery. Its seat of administration was in present-day Wu shan 巫山 county in Chong qing 重慶. At the beginning of the *kai huang* 開皇 reign period (581 – 600) of Sui 隋, it was changed to Wu shan county. Mentioned with 1283.

Wu xing 吳興 [6]
Name of a commandery. See → Wu xing jun 吳興郡. Mentioned with 381, 677, 805, 871, 1521, 1566.

Wu xing jun 吳興郡 [1]
Name of a commandery. It was established by Three Kingdoms' Wu 吳, in 266, by dividing the two commanderies of Wu and Dan yang 丹陽. It was put under Yang zhou 揚州. Its seat of administration was at a location 15 *li* south of present-day Hu zhou 湖州 city in Zhe jiang. Its territory of administration corresponded to the Tiao xi 苕溪 watershed in the northern part of Zhe jiang 浙江,

and Yi xing 宜興 city in Jiang su 江蘇. Under Eastern Jin 晉, in 405, the seat of administration was moved to the city district of present-day Hu zhou city. The commandery was eliminated under Sui 隋, in 589. Under Tang 唐, in 742, Hu zhou was changed to be Wu xing 吳興 commandery, but this was abolished in 758. Mentioned with 1516.

Wu xu guo 烏許國 [1]
Name of an ancient western regions country. It was located on along the present Amu-darya. Mentioned with 352.

Wu yang 武陽 [1]
Name of a county. It was established by Qin 秦. Its seat of administration was at a location 15 *li* northeast of present-day Peng shan 彭山 county in Si chuan 四川. Southern Dynasties' Liang 梁 changed it to Qian wei 犍為 county. Mentioned with 1437.

Wu yang 吳揚 [1]
Combined regional name. It refers to a region in present-day Jiang su 江蘇 and southern part of An hui 安徽. During the Han 漢 periods, prior to Yang Xiong's 揚雄 (53 BCE – 18 CE) life time, Wu 吳 referred to the old Wu state of the Spring and Autumn period, and Yang 揚 referred to one of the then 13 Regional Inspector Divisions, the Yang zhou Regional Inspector Division, Yang zhou *ci shi bu* 揚州刺史部. Mentioned with 1004.

Wu yang 巫陽 [1]
Early place name. It is found in present-day Ba dong 巴東 county in Hu bei 湖北. Mentioned with 456.

Wu yu he 烏玉河 [1]
Name of a river. This is the Qaraqash ("Black Stone") river on the border of present-day Khotan (He tian 和田) and Pi shan 皮山 in Xin jiang 新疆. Also called *Hei yu he* 黑玉河, the "Black Jade river." Mentioned with 1406.

Wu yu zhi shan 務隅之山 [1]
Name of a mountain from the *Shan hai jing* 山海經, "Classic of Mountains and Seas." This is Fu yu 鮒鰅 mountain. It is located south of present-day Nei huang 內黃 county in He nan 河南. Mentioned with 293.

Wu yuan 五原 [2]
Name of a county. It was established by Western Wei 魏. Its seat of administration was in present-day Ding bian 定邊 county in Shaan xi 陝西. Northern Song 宋 abolished it. Mentioned with 368, 861.

Wu yuan cheng 五原城 [1]
Name of an ancient city. In ancient times, there were Wu yuan 五原 commandery cities in three places. The authors of the *BCGM* do not make clear which one they were referring to. The Wu yuan commandery cities of Western Han 漢 and Sui 隋 were administered from the Urad front banner of present-day Inner Mongolia (part in San ding zhang fang cun 三頂帳房村 located southeast of that banner and Tu cheng cun 土城村 located northwest of that banner). The

Wu yuan 五原 commandery cities of Western Wei 魏 were in present-day Ding bian 定邊 county of Shaan xi 陝西. Mentioned with 126.

Wu yue 五岳 [3]

This is a general name for ancient China's five great mountains. These are Dong yue Tai shan 東岳泰山 (located north of present-day Tai an 泰安 city in Shan dong 山東), Nan yue Heng shan 南岳衡山 (This was originally Tian zhu shan 天柱山 in present-day Qian shan 潛山 county in An hui 安徽, Emperor Wen 文 of Sui 隋 changed the point of sacrifice to a location northwest of present-day Heng shan 衡山 county in Hu nan 湖南), Xi yue Hua shan 西岳華山 (south of present-day Hua yin 華陰 city in Shaan xi 陝西), Bei yue Heng shan 北岳恒山 (originally located northwest of present-day Qu yang 曲陽 county in He bei 河北, but at the beginning of Qing 清 the sacrifice was changed to a location southeast of present-day Hun yuan 渾源 county in Shan xi 山西), and the Zhong yue Song shan 中岳嵩山 (north of present-day Deng feng 登封 city in He nan 河南). According to ancient tradition, during the time of Yao 堯 and Shun 舜, there were references to patrols of the Wu yue. However, Han 漢 Confucians drew a far-fetched analogy whereby the system of the Wu yue first started during the time of Han Emperor Wu 武 (140-87 BCE). Xuan zong 玄宗 of Tang 唐 and Zhen zong 真宗 of Song 宋 once enfiefed the Wu yue as princes. At the beginning of Ming 明, they were honored as beneficent spirits. Mentioned with 1029, 1469, 1485.

Wu yue 吳越 [14]

Regional name. It refers to the present Jiang zhe 江浙 area. The name was because during the Spring and Autumn Period the states of Wu 吳 and Yue 越 were centered in Su zhou 蘇州 city in present-day Jiang su 江蘇 and Shao xing 紹興 city in present-day Zhe jiang 浙江. The name is also associated with the Five Dynasties and Ten Countries' Wu yue country founded by Qian Liu 錢鏐 (852 – 932), which had its capital in present-day Hang zhou 杭州 city. The area controlled by it was located in the southern part of present-day Jiang su 江蘇, and included the area of present-day Shang hai 上海 city and the entire province of Zhe jiang, thus the reason the area was known as Wu yue. Mentioned with 160, 168, 303, 429, 572, 768, 769, 810, 1027, 1400, 1485, 1498, 1525, 1569.

Wu yue 吳粵 [1]

Regional name. This is a variant of → Wu yue 吳越. Mentioned with 550.

Wu zhong 吳中 [12]

Regional name . It refers to the land of Spring and Autumn period → Wu 吳. Mentioned with 70, 168, 225, 285, 364, 588, 723, 871, 949, 1241, 1378.

Wu zhou 婺州 [1]

Name of a *zhou* 州. It was founded by Sui 隋, in 589, by dividing Wu zhou 吳州. Its seat of administration was in present-day Jin hua 金華 city in Zhe jiang 浙江. Its territory of administration corresponded to the present-day cities and counties in the watersheds of the Jin hua jiang 金華江 and Qu jiang 衢江 in Zhe jiang 浙江. At the beginning of the *da ye* 大業 reign period (605 – 618) of Sui 隋,

it became Dong yang 東陽 commandery. Under Tang 唐, in 621, the area again became Wu zhou 婺州. In 686, and after its administration was reduced in size, it comprised the Jin hua watershed and the territories of the present-day county and city of Lan xi 蘭溪 and Pu jiang 浦江 in Zhe jiang. In 742, the area became Dong yang commandery. In 758, it again became Wu zhou. Under Yuan 元, in 1276, it became Wu zhou lu 婺州路. Mentioned with 508.

Wu zhou 梧州 [1]

Name of a *zhou* 州. It was established under Tang 唐, in 621. Its seat of administration was in present-day Wu zhou city in Guang xi 廣西. Its territory of administration comprised Wu zhou city and present-day Cang wu 蒼梧 county in Guang xi. Under Yuan 元, in 1279, the area became Wu zhou lu. Mentioned with 1446.

-X-

Xi 西 [8]

General geographical reference. The term refers to West China as it was during the Ming. Mentioned with 276, 298, 467, 660, 746, 838, 861, 1242.

Xi 奚 [2]

Tribal designation. The Xi were originally a branch of the Xiong nu 匈奴. During the Southern and Northern Dynasties period, they were called the Ku mo xi 庫莫奚. They were spread along the Rao le shui 饒樂水 (this is the watershed of the Shiramören of present-day Inner Mongolia). They were primarily nomadic pastoralists. During Sui 隋 and Tang 唐 times, they were called Xi. At the beginning of the *kai yuan* 開元 reign period (713 – 741), the chief leader of the Xi tribe, Li Dapu 李大酺, was enfeoffed as prince of Rao le 饒樂 commandery. During Liao 遼 times, many Xi were scattered about the area of Zhong jing 中京. Later, they were absorbed by the Khitan. Mentioned with 1351.

Xi an 西安 [1]

□ Name of a *fu* 府. Ming 明 established Xi an fu 西安府 in 1369. Its seat of administration was in present-day Xi an city in Shaan xi 陝西. Its territory of administration comprised the territory near to Xi an city. The *fu* was abolished in 1913.

□ Name of a county. It was established during the *xian tong* 咸通 reign period (860 – 874) of Tang 唐. Its seat of administration was in present-day Qu zhou 衢州 city in Zhe jiang 浙江. In 1912, it became Qu 衢 county. Mentioned with 695.

Xi an zhu jun 熙安諸郡 [1]

General designation for commanderies. During the Southern Dynasties and Sui 隋, the commanderies of Xi ping 熙平, Guang xi 廣熙, Yong xi 永熙, Song xi 宋熙 and Xin xi 新熙 were established in the western part of Guang dong 廣東. Also established were the commanderies of Xin an 信安 and Qi an 齊安. The seat of administration of Xi ping commandery was in present-day Lian zhou city in Guang dong. The seat of administration of Guang xi commandery was at a location south of present-day Luo ding 羅定 city in Guang dong. The seat of administration of Song xi commandery was in the Southwest of Gao ming district of present-day Fo shan city in Guang dong. The seat of administration of Xin an commandery was in present-day Zhao qing 肇慶 city in Guang dong. The seat of administration of Qi an commandery was to the North of present-day En ping 恩平 city in Guang dong. Mentioned with 1245.

Xi bei 西北 [7]
Directional name. It refers to the region of northwest China but with a very broad application. During Ming 明, the term primarily referred to the area administered by the Shaan xi Provincial Administration Commission, Shaan xi *bu zheng shi si* 陝西布政使司. This corresponds to the present-day provinces of Shaan xi 陝西, Gan su 甘肅 and Ning Xia 寧夏. Mentioned with 177, 191, 298, 447, 464, 724, 861, 986.

Xi bei fan jie 西北番界 [1]
Regional name. As used by Su Song 蘇頌蘇頌 (1020 – 1101), it referred to the border region in the northwest of Northern Song 宋 with Xi xia 西夏, by and large a territory comprising the eastern part of present-day Gan su 甘肅 and the western part of Shaan xi 陝西. Mentioned with 1192.

Xi bei fang 西北方 [1]
Positional term. See under → Xi bei 西北. Mentioned with 1452.

Xi bei zhou jun 西北州郡 [1]
General administrative designation. As used by Su Song 蘇頌蘇頌 (1020 – 1101), it refers to the various *zhou* 州 of the northwestern territory of the Northern Song 宋. This more or less corresponds to a region comprising the western part of present-day Shaan xi 陝西 and the eastern part of Gan su 甘肅. Mentioned with 1122.

Xi bian 西邊 [1]
General indication. In Ming 明 times, it referred to the border region of the west. Mentioned with 861.

Xi cheng 析城 [1]
Name of a mountain. This is Xi cheng shan 析城山 in present-day Yang cheng 陽城 county in Shan xi 山西. Mentioned with 1171.

Xi chuan 西川 [16]
□ This was a regional designation. During middle Tang 唐 times, Jian nan 劍南 was divided into Xi chuan 西川 and Dong chuan 東川. Xi chuan was administered from Cheng du 成都. Its territories comprised the Cheng du plateau and the area west and north, together with the area east of the Ya long jiang 雅礱江. At the end of Tang, Wang Jian 王建 (847 – 918) founded Former Shu 蜀 based on this area.
□ This was a regional designation. After Northern Song 宋 pacified Shu 蜀, it established Xi chuan lu 西川路 administered from the present-day Cheng du city. Its territory of administration corresponded to an area extending in present-day

Si chuan from Qiong lai 邛崍 mountain, Da xue 大雪 mountain and Da liang 大涼 mountain toward the East, from Jiang you 江油 and Bei chuan 北川 toward the South, and from Yan ting 鹽亭, Da zhu 大竹 and the area west of Yong chuan 永川 in Chong qing 重慶 toward the West. In 1001, the *lu* 路 was divided to form the two *lu* of Yi zhou 益州 and Zi zhou 梓州.

□ Name of a county. It was established under Three Kingdoms Wei 魏. Its seat of administration was at a location northwest of present-day Xun yi 旬邑 county in Shaan xi 陝西. It was abolished after Western Jin 晉.

These areas collectively were said to produce 3, 9, 188, 199, 202, 249, 285, 345, 443, 600, 728, 1242, 1289, 1392, 1459, 1526.

Xi dong 溪峒 [3]

General indication. It refers to the mountainous areas occupied by minority peoples. This is the area today occupied by the Dong 侗 nationality. Mentioned with 511, 1139, 1371.

Xi fan 西番 [30]

Regional name. During the Tang 唐, Song 宋, Yuan 元 and Ming 明 periods, the term referred to the ancient Tibetan empire, and occasionally to the areas occupied by the Tibetan tribes. It is present-day Tibet. Mentioned with 14, 73, 163, 174, 280, 334, 467, 493, 496, 509, 542, 738, 768, 862, 992, 1070, 1171, 1183, 1205, 1242, 1264, 1307, 1335, 1396, 1467, 1474, 1501.

Xi fang 西方 [14]

Regional indication. Some times it refers to the western part of Central China but other times it refers to Central Asia west of China. It also is a term that simply contrasts with what is east. Mentioned with 176, 581, 584, 660, 804, 1140, 1272, 1371, 1538, 1579.

Xi guo 西國 [18]

General regional reference. It designates, in the broadest sense, the territories of the so-called western regions countries. This includes the territories known in antiquity to exist west of Yu men guan 玉門關 and Yang guan 陽關. Mentioned with 5, 9, 14, 103, 104, 146, 151, 282, 314, 342, 433, 526, 738, 1124, 1146, 1193, 1253.

Xi guo zhu fan 西國諸番 [1]

General regional designation. This is a general reference to the tribal nations and countries known to exist in the West in early times. Mentioned with 15.

Xi guo zhu rong 西國諸戎 [1]

General regional designation. The term refers generally to the minority tribes known to live in the West in antiquity. Mentioned with 827.

Xi hai 西海 [4 + 1 + 3 + 1]

□ Theoretical place name. [4] It designates an imaginary ocean in the west. Further details require additional research. Mentioned with 282, 542, 1230, 1524.

□ Ancient name for a lake. [1] It refers to the Ju yan hai 居延海. This is located north of the present-day E ji na qi 額濟納旗 city (Marco Polo's Etzina) in Gan su 甘肅. Mentioned with 1335.

□ Name of an ancient lake. [3] This refes to the present-day Aral Sea in Central Asia. Mentioned with 680, 851, 1129.

□ Name of an ancient lake [1] The reference is to the present-day South China Sea. Mentioned with 946.

□ Name of an ancient body of water. [1] The reference is to the Qing hai 青海 lake. Mentioned with 245.

Xi he 西河 [1]

Name of a commandery. It was established under Western Han 漢. Its seat of administration was in the southeast boundary region of the present Ejin horo banner of Inner Mongolia. Its territory of administration comprised an area extending from present-day Ordos city in Inner Mongolia and Yi chuan 宜川 in Shaan xi 陝西 toward the North, and also the region extending from Shi lou 石樓 in Shan xi 山西 toward the North. Eastern Han moved the seat of administration to present-day Li shi 離石 county in Shan xi 山西. Three Kingdoms' Wei 魏 moved the seat of administration to present-day Fen yang 分陽 county in Shan xi 山西. The commandery was abolished at the beginning of Sui 隋. Mentioned with 361.

Xi hu 西胡 [7]

General reference. It refers to the area occupied by minority groups in the western regions. Mentioned with 114, 202, 799, 887, 937, 1206, 1303.

Xi hu 西湖 [1]

Reference to the name of a lake. This is the Xi hu of present-day Hang zhou 杭州.

Xi jian 西間 [3]

Regional name. Details are lacking. Mentioned with 456, 1117.

Xi jiao zhu zhou 西徼諸州 [1]

This is a combined regional name. It refers to the *zhou* of Wei 維 (Wei 威), Feng 奉, Gong 恭, Zhe 柘, Dang 當, Xi 悉, Yi 翼, Jing 靜, Ba 霸, Shi 時 and Tan 宕 established in the Si chuan 四川 plateau northwest of present-day Cheng du 成都 during Tang 唐 and Song 宋. Mentioned with 746.

Xi jing 西京 [2]

Name of an ancient capital. It was located in present-day Xi an 西安 city in Shaan xi 陝西. After Eastern Han 漢 moved the capital of Luo yang 洛陽, it called the old Western Han capital of Chang an 長安 Xi jing 西京. Under the Tang 唐, in 657, Luo yang became Dong du 東都 and Chang an was called Xi du 西都, also Xi jing. Mentioned with 338.

Xi liang 西涼 [4]

Regional name. It refers to a strip of Wu wei 武威 city in present-day Gan su 甘肅. Mentioned with 811, 730, 1335.

Xi liao ban 西遼坂 [1]

Minor place name located east of present-day Shi yan 十堰 city in Hu bei 湖北. The exact location remains to be determined. Mentioned with 1435.

Xi lu 西路 [1]
Abbreviated administrative name. This is → Guang nan xi lu 廣南西路. Mentioned with 350.

Xi luo 西洛 [6]
Reference to a place. It refers to the ancient capital of Luo yang 洛陽. Mentioned with 7, 428, 639, 785, 799, 1239.

Xi nan 西南 [6 + 1]
□ Regional name. [6] It refers to the Ming 明 southeast, namely Si chuan 四川, Gui zhou 貴州, Guang xi 廣西, and Yun nan 雲南. Mentioned with 14, 72, 388, 555, 1238, 1453.
□ Positional name but the application is uncertain. [1] Mentioned with 466.

Xi nan fan 西南番 [1]
General regional name. It refers to the minority peoples living in the Southwest. Mentioned with 840.

Xi nan guo ming 西南國名 [1]
This term is used once by the BCGM authors to explain the "Name of a country in the Southwest," Persia (Bo si 波斯), present-day Iran. Mentioned with 1.

Xi nan hai 西南海 [1]
Body of water "in the Southwest." Details are lacking. Mentioned with 325.

Xi nan hai yang 西南海洋 [1]
Name of a large body of water "in the Southwest." Details are lacing. Mentioned with 675.

Xi nan jiao wai 西南徼外 [2]
Regional name. It refers to the area occupied by the minority peoples of the southwest. Mentioned with 746, 1532.

Xi nan wai 西南外 [1]
This name is a permutation of → Xi nan jiao wai 西南徼外. Mentioned with 746.

Xi nan yi 西南夷 [7]
General name for a collection of tribal groups. It refers to the tribal groups spread about present-day Si chuan's 四川 western part during Western Han 漢 times as well as the minorities inhabiting a strip of Yun nan 雲南 and Gui zhou 貴州. These are principally the Ye lang 夜郎, Dian 滇, Qiong du 邛都, Sui 嶲, Kun ming 昆明, Zuo du 筰都, the Ran mang 冉駹 and Bai ma 白馬. They all had close economic and cultural relations with Ba guo 巴國 and Shu guo 蜀國. During Western Han, during the time of Emperor Wu 武, there was active management of the people of the Southwest. Seven base commanderies were established: Yue sui 越嶲, Shen li 沈黎, Wen shan 汶山, Qian wei 犍為, Zang ke 牂牁, Wu du 武都 and Yi zhou 益州. Mentioned with 111, 213, 288, 290, 541, 837, 1057.

Xi nan zhang hai 西南瘴海 [1]
Vague indication. It refers to the lakes and ponds and other bodies of water in the Southwest associated with malaria. Mentioned with 1171.

Xi nan zhu fan 西南諸番 [1]
Vague indication. It refers to the areas occupied by the minority peoples of the Southwest. Mentioned with 1139.

Xi nan zhu guo 西南諸國 [2]
Vague indication. It refers to the tribal peoples of the Southwest. Mentioned with 738, 812.

Xi ping shan 西平山 [1]
Name of a mountain. It is located somewhere in the southern part of present-day Jiang su 江蘇. Exact details are unavailable. Mentioned with 1039.

Xi qi dan 奚契丹 [1]
Combined tribal designation. Compare → Xi 奚 and → Qi dan 契丹. Mentioned with 619.

Xi qiang 西羌 [7]
Name of a tribal grouping, the "Western Qiang." This is an old name for Tibetan nomads and geographically refers generally to present-day Tibet and the territories of Gan su 甘肅, Qing hai 青海, Si chuan 四川 and Yun nan 雲南 inhabited by Tibetans. Mentioned with 188, 249, 324, 934, 1091, 1289, 1335.

Xi qiang bei di 西羌北地 [1]
This is a combined place name. See → Xi Qiang 西羌 and → Bei di 北地. Mentioned with 1335.

Xi rong 西戎 [34]
Name of a tribal group, the "Western Rong." In Chinese literature and other source material this is a referance to Tibet, namely present-day Tibet and the areas occupied by the various Tibetan ethnic groups. Mentioned with 11, 232, 285, 323, 480, 493, 509, 522, 535, 585, 811, 819, 838, 840, 923, 933, 982, 1036, 1042, 1088, 1129, 1158, 1196, 1206, 1252, 1289, 1307, 1335, 1341, 1370, 1425.

Xi rong jie 西戎界
→ Xi rong 西戎.

Xi shan 錫山 [1]
Name of a mountain. It is located southwest of present-day Yun xi 鄖西 county in Hu bei 湖北. Mentioned with 1218.

Xi shan 西山 [1 + 1 + 1]
□ Name of a place. [1] It is located west of present-day Bei jing 北京 city, and the term is a general designation for the mountains west of the city region. Mentioned with 1051.
□ Place name. [1] The reference is to various mountains in the southwestern part of present-day Si chuan 四川. Mentioned with 188.
□ Place name. [1] It is located west of the present-day Ya an 雅安 city in Si chuan 四川. Mentioned with 825.

Xi shu 西蜀
→ Xi shu zhou jun 西蜀州郡.

Xi shu zhou jun 西蜀州郡 [10]
General regional designation. It refers to the center part of present-day Si chuan 四川, centered about Cheng du 成都. The present Chong qing 重慶 city was the ancient Ba 巴, in the East. The given region was the ancient Shu 蜀 in the west. Thus the name. Mentioned with 249, 288, 689, 856, 994, 1149, 1163, 1171, 1406, 1482.

Xi tu 西土 [5]
Place name. This is a Buddhist name for India and, in terms of China, India is to the west. Mentioned with 284, 331, 691, 804, 1436.

Xi xi si 西溪寺 [1]
Name of a temple. It is in present-day Hang zhou 杭州 city in Zhe jiang 浙江. Mentioned with 1162.

Xi xia 西夏 [5]
Regional name. Ancient designation of a territory in the western section of present-day China. Mentioned with 746, 960, 1057, 1065, 1364.

Xi yang 西洋 [1]
Regional name. During Yuan 元 and Ming 明 times, it referred to the ocean from the Chinese Nan hai 南海 west and the lands located along the ocean. The term extended to the eastern part of Africa. All of this was Xi yang. Mentioned with 1386.

Xi yang 西陽 [1 + 1]
□ This was an enfeoffment of Xu Zhicai 徐之才 (492-572) under Northern Qi 齊 and is not a place name. [1] Such ranks were often divorced of actual territorial association under the Southern and Northern Dynasties.
□ Name of a commandery. [1] It was established under Eastern Jin 晉. Its seat of administration was at a location east of present-day Huang zhou 黃州 city in Hu bei 湖北. Its territory of administration under the Southern Dynasties comprised Huang zhou, and the cities and counties of Ma cheng 麻城, Xin zhou 新洲 and Xi shui 浠水 in present-day Hu bei. It was abolished during Sui 隋. Mentioned with 768.

Xi yi 西夷 [1]
General indication. It refers to the minority peoples, the Yi 夷, of west China. Mentioned with 82.

Xi yu 西域 [61]
Regional name. From Western Han 漢 on, this was a general designation for the area west of Yu men guan 玉門關. This had a broad and a narrow meaning. The area, in the narrow meaning, referred only to the area east of the Cong ling 蔥嶺, this focused primarily on present-day Xin jiang 新疆. In the broader meaning, all the contact areas associated with the Xi yu in a narrow sense, including present-day central Asia, west Asia, the Indian peninsula and the eastern part of Europe and north Africa were implied. After Xin jiang was established in 1884, this name gradually fell into disuse. Mentioned with 1, 7, 10, 14, 16, 72, 146, 206, 229, 280, 282, 368, 434, 441, 477, 487, 493, 494, 495, 496, 525, 542, 567, 605, 660, 775,

811, 817, 826, 843, 861, 862, 885, 982, 1002, 1030, 1096, 1119, 1124, 1131, 1143, 1147, 1158, 1241, 1272, 1279, 1450, 1480, 1482, 1485.

Xi yue 西岳 [1]
One of the traditional Five Ranges of China. This is Hua 華 mountain, located 10 *li* south of present-day Hua yin 華陰 city in Shaan xi 陝西. Mentioned with 1157.

Xi zhou 隰州 [2]
Name of a *zhou* 州. It was founded under Sui 隋, in 585, by changing the name of Xi fen zhou 西汾州. Its seat of administration was in present-day Xi 隰 county in Shan xi 山西. Its territory of administration comprised the present-day counties of Xi 隰, Shi lou 石樓, Jiao kou 交口, Yong he 永和, Pu xian 蒲縣 and Da ning 大寧 in Shan xi. Northern Song 宋 took it over but Ming 明 turned it into an "attached" *zhou*, *san zhou* 散州, without subordinate counties. In 1912, it was changed into a county. Mentioned with 695, 816.

Xi zhou 溪州 [1]
Name of a *zhou* 州. It was established under Tang 唐, in 691. Its seat of administration was in present-day Lao si cheng 老司城, located southeast of Yong shun 永順 county in Hu nan 湖南. The territory administered comprised the present-day counties of Yong shun, Bao jing 保靖, Gu zhang 古丈 and Long shan 龍山 in Hu nan 湖南. Under Five Dynasties' Jin 晉, in 940, the seat of administration was moved to present-day Hui xi ping 會溪坪, located northeast of Gu zhang county. It was then called Xia xi zhou 下溪州. It was abolished at the beginning of Yuan 元. Mentioned with 202.

Xi zhou 西州 [1]
Name of a *zhou* 州. It was founded under Tang 唐, in 640. It was established after the Gao chang 高昌 country of the Qu 麴 family was destroyed. Its seat of administration was in the old city of Gao chang, located some 40 *li* east of present-day Turfan city in Xin jiang 新疆. Its territory of administration included the present Turfan city in Xin jiang and the area of Shan shan 鄯善 county. In 742, this area became Jiao he 交河 commandery. In 758, it again became Xi zhou. Later the area was lost to Tibet. Mentioned with 1370.

Xi zhou 巂州 [3]
Name of a *zhou* 州. It was established under Sui, in 537. Its seat of administration was in present-day Xi chang 西昌 city in Si chuan 四川. Its administrative territory covered an area extending in Si chuan from Yue xi 越西 and Mei gu 美姑 toward the South, from the Jin sha 金沙 river toward the West and toward the North, and from Jin ping shan 錦屏山 and the Yan jing he 鹽井河 toward the East. Under Tang 唐, in 757, the area was conquered by Tibet. It was recovered in 797. In 831, the area was conquered by Nan Zhao 南詔, and in the next year the seat of administration was moved to present-day Lu gu 瀘沽 town south of Mian ning 冕寧 county in Si chuan 四川. In 861, this was occupied by Nan Zhao, and a Jian chang fu 建昌府 was established in its place. Mentioned with 30, 819, 895.

Xia 峽 [4]

Name of a *zhou* 州. See → Xia zhou 峽州. Mentioned with 99, 674, 864, 1096.

Xia guo 夏國 [1]

Name of an administrative unit. It refers historically to the Xi xia 西夏 state, founded by the Dong xiang 黨項 Li Yuanhao 李元昊 (1003-1048). The capital was in Xing qing fu 興慶府 (present-day Yin chuan 銀川 city in Ning xia 寧夏). At the time of the greatest extend of its borders, Xi xia reached the Yu men guan 玉門關 in the west, and it went north into what is now the Ejin banner in Inner Mongolia and the area of Hou tao 後套. In the South, its territories reached the Qi lian 祁連 mountains, and in the East, with the Great Bend of the Yellow River, the area reached Heng shan 橫山 in the North of Shaan xi 陝西, bordering on Song 宋 and Jin 金. This is an area covering present-day Ning xia and the Ordos plateau in the Inner Mongolia, as well as the Alashan plateau and the He xi 河西 corridor of Gan su 甘肅. Xi xia was annihilated by Cinggis-qan in 1227. Mentioned with 811.

Xia pi 下邳 [1]

Could be either of the following.

□ Name of a commandery. It was established toward the end of Eastern Han 漢. Its seat of administration was at a location east of Gu pi 古邳 town northwest of present-day Sui ning 睢寧 county in Jiang su 江蘇. Its territory of administration comprised Su qian 宿遷, Pi zhou 邳州, Shu yang 沭陽, Si yang 泗陽, Si hong 泗洪, Lian shui 漣水, Sui ning 睢寧 and Xu yi 盱眙 in Jiang su. It was abolished at the beginning of Sui 隋.

□ Name of a county established by Qin 秦. It was administered from Gu pi town located northwest of present-day Sui ning 睢寧 county in Jiang su 江蘇. Ming 明 combined this with Pi zhou 邳州. Mentioned with 66.

Xia shan 峽山 [1]

General allusion to a place name. The reference is to the mountain region of the Three Gorges on the Yang zi. Mentioned with 768.

Xia zhong 峽中 [1]

Regional allusion. It points to an area of the Three Gorges of the Yang zi. Mentioned with 825.

Xia zhou 硤州 [4]

Alternative writing of → Xia zhou 峽州. Mentioned with 258, 381, 443, 768.

Xia zhou 峽州 [7]

Name of a *zhou* 州. It was established as Xia zhou 硤州 by Northern Zhou 周. Its seat of administration was at a location northwest of present-day Yi chang 宜昌 city in Hu bei 湖北. Its territory of administration comprised the present-day cities and counties of Yi chang, Zhi cheng 枝城, Chang yang 長陽 and Yuan an 遠安 in Hu bei. Under Tang 唐, in 635, the seat of administration was moved to Yi chang city. Northern Song 宋 changed Xia zhou 硤州 to be Xia zhou 峽州. The seat of administration and the territory of administration remained the same. Yuan 元 turned the area into Xia zhou lu 峽州路. Mentioned with 258, 261, 381, 468, 1063, 1241.

Xian ju 仙居 [1]
Name of a county. This is the present-day Xian ju county in Zhe jiang 浙江. It was established under Northern Song 宋, in 1007, by changing the name of Yong an 永安 county. It has been continued down to the present time. Mentioned with 1277.

Xian luo 暹羅 [4]
Name of a country. See → Xian luo guo 暹羅國. Mentioned with 511, 977, 1139, 1236.

Xian luo guo 暹羅國 [3]
This is an old name for Thailand. Originally there were the two countries of Xian 暹 and Luo hu 羅斛. The northern one was Xian, and it had its capital in what is now present-day Thailand at Sangkhalot. The southern was Luo hu, and it had its capital at Ban ta khli in present-day Thailand. Approximately during late Yuan 元 times, the two countries combined and the combination was called Xian luo hu 暹羅斛 country. Under Ming 明, in 1377 this was shortened to Xian luo 暹羅 country. Mentioned with 14, 81, 1123.

Xian shan 峴山 [1]
Name of a mountain. It is located south of present-day Xiang fan 襄樊 city in Hu bei 湖北. Mentioned with 1285.

Xian yang 咸陽 [10]
Name of an ancient capital city. The city was built under Qin 秦, in 350 BCE, and the Qin capital was transferred there. The area was established as Xian yang county. The name comes from the fact that the city was located south of the Jiu zong shan 九嵕山 mountains, north of the Wei shui 渭水, and in an area considered "yang" for both mountains and waters. After Qin Shi huang 秦始皇 destroyed the six coexisting countries, Xian yang became the capital of the entire nation. It was burned down by Xiang Yu 項羽 (233-202) at the end of Qin. The ruins are located in the area of Yao dian 窯店 town found 20 *li* northeast of present-day Xian yang city in Shaan xi 陝西. Part of the ruins of the city have been eroded by the Wei shui 渭水. Mentioned with 129, 222, 572, 927, 959, 1010, 1300, 1397.

Xian zhou 憲州 [1]
Name of a *zhou* 州. It was established under Tang 唐, in 889. Its seat of administration was in present-day Lou fan 婁煩 county in Shan xi 山西. Its territory of administration comprised present-day Lou fan county and the southeastern part of Jing le 靜樂 county in Shan xi. Under Northern Song 宋, in 1002, the seat of administration was moved to present-day Jing le county. Under Jin 金, in 1151, it was changed to Guan zhou 管州. Mentioned with 461.

Xiang 湘 [2]
Abbreviation of a place name. The reference is to Hu nan 湖南 province. Mentioned with 503, 1038, 1158, 1503.

Xiang 襄 [12]
Name of a *zhou*. See → Xiang zhou 襄州. Mentioned with 38, 79, 328, 369, 381, 541, 793, 848, 864, 1005, 1238, 1400.

Xiang dong 湘東 [2]
Regional abbreviation. It refers to the eastern part of Hu nan 湖南. Mentioned with 698, 1435.

Xiang guo si 相國寺 [1]
Name of a temple. This is the Da xiang guo 大相國 temple in present-day Kai feng 開封 city in He nan 河南. Mentioned with 733.

Xiang han 襄漢 [3]
Combined place name. It refers to present-day Xiang yang 襄陽 city in the northern part of He bei 湖北, and the Han shui 漢水 that flows through Xiang yang. Mentioned with 497, 752, 1311.

Xiang lin 象林 [1]
Name of a county. It was founded under Western Han 漢, and made a part of Ri nan 日南 commandery. Its seat of administration was near the Đà Nẵng Independent City in present-day Vietnam. It was eliminated under Eastern Han. It was reestablished under Western Jin 晉. Its seat of administration was moved north to a location near the old city of Hue. Eastern Jin later entered the area into Lin yi 林邑 country. Mentioned with 586.

Xiang ling 襄陵 [1]
Name of a county. It was established under Sui 隋, in 606. Its seat of administration was in Xian di 縣底 town, located 18 *li* southeast of present-day Lin fen 臨汾 city in Shan xi 山西. Northern Song 宋 moved the seat of administration to present-day Xiang ling 襄陵 town, located 33 *li* northwest of Xiang fen 襄汾 county in Shan xi. In 1954, the area was combined with Fen cheng 汾城 county to make Xiang fen 襄汾 county. Mentioned with 566.

Xiang mian 襄沔 [1]
Combined regional name. It refers to present-day Xiang yang 襄陽 city in the northern part of Hu bei 湖北 and that part of the Han shui 漢水 which flows through Xiang yang (this was anciently called the Mian shui 沔水).

Xiang nan 湘南 [1]
Abbreviation of a regional name. It refers to the southern part of present-day Hu nan 湖南. Mentioned with 173.

Xiang ning xian 鄉寧縣 [1]
Name of a county. It came into being due to changing the name of Chang ning 昌寧 county into Xiang ning xian 鄉寧縣 on account of a taboo related to the name of Li Guochang 李國昌 (died 887) under Five Dynasties' Tang 唐. It was put under Ci zhou 慈州. Its seat of administration was at a location southeast of present-day Xiang ning 鄉寧 county in Shan xi 山西. In 1051, the seat of administration was moved to the present Xiang ning county. In 1072, it was eliminated. Jin reestablished it, and put it under Ji zhou 吉州. Under Yuan 元, in 1266, it was eliminated, but later reestablished. Ming 明 and Qing 清 put it under Ping

yang fu 平陽府. In 1928, it was put directly under Shan xi province. Mentioned with 1037.

Xiang shan 象山 [1]
Name of a mountain. It is located 10 *li* northwest of Xiang shan 象山 county in Zhe jiang 浙江. Mentioned with 441.

Xiang shan si 湘山寺 [1]
Name of a temple. It is in the western part of present-day Quan zhou xian 全州縣 city in Guang xi. Mentioned with 1096.

Xiang shan xian 象山縣 [1]
Name of a county. It was established under Tang 唐, in 705, and put under Tai zhou 台州. Its seat if administration was at present-day Dan cheng 丹城 town at Xiang shan xian cheng 象山縣城 in Zhe jiang 浙江. In 764, it was changed and put under Ming zhou 明州. Southern Song 宋 subordinated it to Qing yuan fu 慶元府. Yuan 元 subordinated it to Qing yuan lu 慶元路. Ming 明 and Qing 清 put it under Ning bo fu 寧波府. Mentioned with 1153.

Xiang shan xian 湘山縣 [1]
Name of a county. Details are lacking. Mentioned with 1056.

Xiang shui 湘水 [2]
Name of a river. This is the Xiang jiang 湘江 in present-day Hu nan 湖南. It originates in the northeastern corner of Guang xi 廣西, passes through all of Hu nan, takes up the Zi jiang 資江, the Yuan jiang 沅江 and the Li jiang 澧江, and west of Chang sha 長沙 city it forms sand islets such as Ju zi zhou 橘子洲. The river then goes through Dong ting 洞庭 lake and enters into the Yang zi. Mentioned with 1329.

Xiang xiang xian 襄鄉縣 [1]
Name of a county. It was established under Eastern Han 漢 and put under Nan yang 南陽 commandery. Its seat of administration was at a location northeast of present-day Zao yang 棗陽 city in Hu bei 湖北. Under Western Jin 晉, it was eliminated. It was reestablished under Liu Song 劉宋, and put under Yi yang 義陽 commandery. In 465, it was put under He nan 河南 commandery. Northern Zhou 周 abolished it. Mentioned with 902.

Xiang yang 襄陽 [9]
Name with several possible applications.
□ Name of a commandery. It was established at the end of Eastern Han 漢. Its seat of administration was in present-day Xiang yang 襄陽 city in Hu bei 湖北. Its territory of administration comprised the present-day cities and counties of Xiang yang, Yi cheng 宜城 and Yuan an 遠安 in Hu bei. At the beginning of Tang 唐, the area was changed to Xiang zhou 襄州.
□ Name of a county. It was established by Western Han. Its seat of administration was in the present-day Xiang zhou 襄州 district in Xiang yang city of Hu bei. In 1951, the seat was moved to Fan cheng 樊城. In 2001, the county was eliminated and became an urban district. Mentioned with 186, 275, 453, 639, 737, 1234, 1285, 1294, 1509.

Xiang zhou 象州 [1]

Name of a *zhou* 州. It was founded under Sui 隋, in 591. Its seat of administration was in present-day Shang gu cheng 上古城 village located southeast of Xiang zhou county in Guang xi 廣西. Its territory of administration comprised the counties of Xiang zhou and Wu xuan 武宣 in Guang xi. Later, during Tang 唐, in 621, the seat of administration was moved to a location 30 *li* northwest of the present-day Xiang zhou county. In 639, the seat of administration was moved to a location northeast of the present Xiang zhou. In 776, it was moved to the county seat of Xiang zhou. In 1278, under Yuan 元, the status of the area was raised to be Xiang zhou lu 象州路. Later, during the *da de* 大德 reign period (1297 – 1307) of Yuan, it was demoted to be Xiang zhou, and put under Guang xi lu 廣西路. Under Ming 明 and Qing 清, the area was an "attached" *zhou*, *san zhou* 散州, and put under Liu Zhou fu 柳州府. In 1912, it was changed to be Xiang zhou county. Mentioned with 376.

Xiang zhou 襄州 [10]

Name of a *zhou* 州. It was founded by Western Wei 魏, in 554, by changing the name of Yong zhou 雍州. Its seat of administration was in present-day Xiang yang cheng 襄陽城, south of the Han shui 漢水 of Xiang fan 襄樊 city of Hu bei 湖北. Under Sui 隋, in 607, the area became Xiang yang 襄陽 commandery. Under Tang 唐, in 621, it again became Xiang zhou. Its territory of administration comprised Xiang fan, and the present-day cities and counties of Lao he kou 老河口, Xiang yang, Nan zhang 南漳, Yi cheng 宜城 and Gu cheng 谷城 in Hu bei. Mentioned with 51, 78, 148, 194, 272, 381, 666, 691, 947, 987, 1034, 1098.

Xiang zhou 湘州 [3]

Name of a *zhou* 州. It was established by Western Jin 晉, in 307, by splitting the two *zhou* of Jing 荊 and Guang 廣. Its seat of administration was in present-day Chang sha 長沙 city in Hu nan 湖南. Its territory of administration comprised the watersheds of the Xiang 湘 and the Zi shui 資水 in Hu nan, and of the Lu shui 陸水 in Hu bei 湖北. It was eliminated under Eastern Jin, in 328, but the *zhou* was reestablished under Liu Song 劉宋, in 422. The watershed of the Lu shui was cut off and made part of Ying zhou 郢州. Added was the upper watershed of the Xiang, the Li jiang 灕江 and the He jiang 賀江 in the northern portion of present-day Guang xi 廣西, and much of the watershed of the Bei jiang 北江 in the northern part of present-day Guang dong. During the eras of Liang 梁 and Chen 陳, the southern part of the territories of the *zhou* was cut off to establish the *zhou* of Heng 衡 and Dong heng 東衡 and Gui 桂. The administrative area of Xiang zhou became smaller. Under Sui 隋, in 589, the area became Tan zhou 潭州. Mentioned with 376, 474.

Xiang zhou 相州 [4]

Name of a *zhou* 州. It was established by Northern Wei 魏, in 401, by dividing up Ji zhou 冀州. Its seat of administration was in present-day Ye cheng 鄴城 town located southwest of Lin zhang 臨漳 county in He bei 河北. Under Northern Zhou 周, in 580, the seat of administration was moved to a location southwest of An yang 安陽 city in present-day He nan 河南. In 605, Sui 隋 changed Xiang zhou to be Wei 魏 commandery and moved the seat of administration to An yang city. Under Tang 唐, in 618, it again became Xiang zhou. Its territory of administration was an area extending in present-day He bei 河北 from in Ci 磁 county and Cheng an 成安 county toward the South, in He nan from Nei huang 内黄 county toward the West, from Yang yin 湯陰 county toward the North, and from Lin zhou 林州 city toward the East. Under Jin 金, in 1192, it became Zhang de fu 彰德府. Mentioned with 175, 871, 1004, 1532.

Xiao 蕭 [1]
Name of a municipality. It is located northwest of Xiao 蕭 county in present-day An hui 安徽. Mentioned with 1308.

Xiao gui xian 小桂縣 [1]
Alternative name of a county. This is Gui yang 桂陽 county. It was established under Western Han 漢. Its seat of administration was in present-day Lian zhou 連州 city in Guang dong 廣東. During Three Kingdoms' Wu 吳, it was subordinated to Shi xing 始興 commandery. Under Southern Dynasties' Liang 梁, in 507, it was put under Yang shan 陽山 commandery. Under Sui 隋, in 590, it was put under Lian zhou. At the beginning of the *da ye* 大業 reign period (605 – 618), it came under Xi ping 熙平 commandery. Under Tang 唐, in 621, it was again put under Lian zhou. In 742, it was put under Lian shan 連山 commandery. In 758, it was put under Lian zhou. Under Yuan 元, in 1280, the area was put under Lian zhou lu 元. In 1282, its status was raised to Gui yang zhou 桂陽州. Mentioned with 21.

Xiao huo shan 小霍山 [1]
Name of a mountain. It is located 50 *li* south of present-day Lu an 六安 city in An hui 安徽. Mentioned with 1469.

Xiao ping 小坪 [1]
Minor place name. It lies in the region of the Jiang you 江油 and Bei chuan 北川 in present-day northern Si chuan 四川. Mentioned with 322.

Xiao qiu 蕭丘 [1]
Name of a legendary island. It may have been located in the present-day South China Sea, Nan hai 南海, but details are lacking. Mentioned with 1341.

Xiao shan 蕭山 [1]
Name of a county. It was established under Tang 唐. in 742. Its seat of administration was in the Xiao shan 蕭山 district of present-day Hang zhou 杭州 city in Zhe jiang 浙江. Mentioned with 461.

Xie 解 [3]
Name of a *zhou* 州. See → Xie zhou 解州. Mentioned with 1318, 1519.

Xie chi 解池 [2]
This is a salt lake. It is located south of present-day Yun cheng 運城 city in Shan xi 山西. Mentioned with 1057, 1318.

Xie gu 斜谷 [1]

Name of a mountain valley, also the name of a pass and of a river. All are located southwest of present-day Mei 眉 county in Shaan xi 陕西. These areas are the northern tip of the Han 漢 and Tang 唐 era precepitous road (See → Bao xie dao 褒斜道) cutting through the Qin ling 秦嶺 mountain range. Mentioned with 1038.

Xie gu xi ling 斜谷西嶺 [1]

Name of a mountain range. The reference is to the Qin ling 秦嶺 mountain range west of → Xie gu 斜谷. Mentioned with 1308.

Xie zhou 解州 [7]

Name of a *zhou* 州. It was established under Five Dynasties' Han 漢, in 948. Its seat of administration was in present-day Xie zhou located 35 *li* southwest of Yun cheng 運城 city in Shan xi 山西. Under Northern Song 宋, the area of administration corresponded to present-day Yun cheng and Wen xi 聞喜 county in Shan xi. From Jin 金 times on, its administrative area was expanded to encompass the present-day counties of Xia xian 夏縣, Rui cheng 芮城 and Ping lu 平陸. Under the Jin, in 1220, the seat of administration was moved to the old Ping lu located southwest of the present-day Ping lu county. Under the Qing 清, in 1724, the status of the area was raised to being a directly administered *zhou*, *zhi li zhou* 直隸州, but its administrative area was reduced. In 1912, the area became Xie 解 county. Mentioned with 653, 1057, 1318, 1478.

Xin 信 [4]

See → Xin zhou 信州. Mentioned with 75, 535, 849, 1375.

Xin an 新安 [5 + 1]

□ Name of a commandery. [5] It was established by Western Jin 晉, in 280. Its seat of administration was at the present-day Qian dao hu 千島湖, "Thousand Islands Lake," in Zhe jiang 浙江. Its territory of administration comprised Huang shan 黃山 in present-day An hui 安徽, Wu yuan 婺源 in Jiang xi 江西, and Chun an 淳安 in Zhe jiang 浙江. Under Sui 隋, in 589, it was abolished. Mentioned with 47, 456, 735, 1228, 1274.

□ Name of a county. [1] It was established by Qin 秦. Its seat of administration was in present-day Shi he 石河 village west of Yi ma 義馬 city in He nan 河南. It was abolished under Sui 隋, in 604. In 607, it was reestablished by changing the name of Dong yuan 東垣 county. Its seat of administration was at a location east of present-day Xin an county in He nan. Under Tang 唐, in 627, the seat of administration was moved to present-day Xin an county. Mentioned with 50.

Xin cai 新蔡

Not a place name. Alternative term for *feng jue* 封爵, „to raise to nobility."

Xin cheng jun 新城郡 [1]

Name of a commandery. It was founded under Three Kingdoms Wei 魏, in 220, by changing the name of Fang ling 房陵 commandery. It was put under Jing zhou 荊州. Its seat of administration was in present-day Fang 房 county in Hu bei 湖北. The administrative area comprised present-day Fang county, Bao kang

保康 county and the northern part of the Lin 林 („forest") district of Shen nong jia 神農架 in Hu bei. Under Liu Song 劉宋, it was changed and subordinated to Liang zhou 梁州. Southern Qi 齊 changed it to be Nan xin cheng 南新城 commandery. Liang again made it Xin cheng 新城 commandery. Western Wei 魏 changed it to be Guang qian 光遷 county. Mentioned with 1147.

Xin du 信都 [2 + 1]

□ Name of a county. It was established under Western Han 漢. Its seat of administration was in present-day Ji zhou 冀州 city in He bei 河北. Under early Ming 明, it was abolished. Mentioned with 1014, 1443.

□ Name of a commandery. [1] See Xin du jun 信都郡. Mentioned with 1092.

Xin du jun 信都郡 [1]

Name of a commandery. It was founded under Sui 隋, in 607, by changing the name of Ji zhou 冀州. Its seat of administration was in present-day Ji zhou city in He bei 河北. Its administrative area comprised the present-day cities and counties of Ji zhou, Nan gong 南宮, Xin he 新河, Zao qiang 棗強, Wu yi 武邑, Heng shui 衡水 and Fu cheng 阜城 in He bei. At the beginning of Tang 唐, the area was changed back to be Ji zhou. In 742, Ji zhou was again changed to be Xin du 信都 commandery. In 758, it was abolished. Mentioned with 1484.

Xin gan 新淦 [1]

Name of a county. It was established under Western Han 漢. Its seat of administration was in present-day Zhang shu 樟樹 city in Jiang xi 江西. Sui moved the seat of administration, in 591, to present-day Xin gan 新干 county in Jiang xi 江西. In 1957, the *gan* 干 was changed to *gan* 淦. Mentioned with 44.

Xin luo 新羅

→ Xin luo guo 新羅國

Xin luo guo 新羅國 [24]

This is the early Korean kingdom of Silla, a powerful country that occupied the southeastern part of the Korean peninsula opposite to Paekchae on the other side and Koguryo in the north. Silla was supposedly founded in 57 BCE, but this is doubtful. It later became the most powerful of these three Korean kingdoms. It eventually conquered Paekche and Koguryo and briefly united the peninsula south of the Da tong jiang 大同江 river under its rule after a period of Tang 唐 occupation of the North. Its capital was at Gyeongju and the city was a true metropolis at its height. Silla was conquered by the new northern state of Koryo in 935. Mentioned with 26, 100, 157, 201, 395, 404, 412, 495, 519, 572, 608, 625, 886, 931, 1140, 1205, 1215, 1375, 1462.

Xin ning 新寧 [1]

Name of a county. It was established under Southern Song 宋, in 1155. Its seat of administration was at a location east of present-day Xin ning 新寧 county in Hu nan 湖南. Its administration was moved to the present site of administration under Ming 明, in 1451. Mentioned with 1435.

Xin ping xian 新平縣 [1]

Name of a county. It was created under Sui 隋, in 584, by changing the name of Bai tu 白土 county. It was a satellite county, *fu guo xian* 附郭縣, of Bin zhou 豳州. Its seat of administration was in present-day Bin 彬 county in Shaan xi 陝西. Under Tang 唐, the Bin 豳 became Bin 邠, and the area came under Bin zhou 邠州 administratively. Under Ming 明, in 1370, it was abolished and made part of Bin zhou 邠州. Mentioned with 347.

Xin xing xian 新興縣 [1]

Name of a county. It was established under Eastern Jin 晉, in 351, by dividing Lin yun 臨允 county. Its seat of administration was in present-day Xin xing 新興 county in Guang dong 廣東. Southern Qi 齊 changed it to be Xin cheng 新成 county. Liang 梁 restored the old name. Ming 明 and Qing 清 put it under Zhao qing fu 肇慶府. Mentioned with 772.

Xin yang 信陽

See → Xin yang zhou 信陽州

Xin yang zhou 信陽州 [3]

Name of a county. It was founded under Northern Song 宋, in 976, by changing the name of Yi yang 義陽 county. The purpose was taboo avoidance for Song Tai zong 太宗 (939 – 937). Its seat of administration was in present-day Xin yang 信陽 city in He nan 河南. In 1961, the seat of administration was moved to Ping qiao 平橋. Today, this is the Ping qiao district of Xin yang city. Mentioned with 614, 797, 1142.

Xin ye 新野 [1]

Name of a county. It was established under Western Han 漢. Its seat of administration was in Xin ye 新野 county in present-day He nan 河南. Mentioned with 1509.

Xin zhou 新洲 [1]

Name of a sand island. It was in the Yang zi north of present-day Nan jing 南京 city in Jiang su 江蘇. The island was a precursor of the Ba gua zhou 八卦洲. Mentioned with 668.

Xin zhou 信州 [26]

Name of a *zhou* 州. It was founded under Tang 唐, in 758, by splitting the four *zhou* of Rao 饒, Qu 衢, Jian 建 and Fu 撫. Its seat of administration was at present-day Tian jin qiao 天津橋, located northwest of Shang rao 上饒 city in Jiang xi. The administrative territory comprised an area in present-day Jiang xi 江西 extending from Gui xi 貴溪 toward the East, and from Huai yu 懷玉 mountain toward the South. Under Yuan 元, in 1277, its status was raised to Xin zhou lu 信州路. Mentioned with 119, 202, 292, 452, 552, 595, 706, 717, 749, 866, 991, 1014, 1080, 1156, 1327, 1465, 1518.

Xing gu 興古 [1]

Name of a commandery. It was established under Three Kingdoms Shu 蜀, in 225. Its seat of administration was at a location located northwest of present-day Yan shan 硯山 county in Yun nan 雲南. Its territory of administration comprised the southeastern portion of present-day Yun nan, the western portion of Guang xi 廣西, and Xing yi 興義 city in Gui zhou 貴州. Later, the seat of administration was moved a number of times. At the end of Southern Dynasties' Liang 梁, the area was abolished. Mentioned with 534.

Xing guo 興國 [4]
See → Xing guo zhou 興國州. Mentioned with 1523.

Xing guo zhou 興國州 [4]
Name of a *zhou* 州. It was established under the Ming 明, in 1376, and put under Wu chang fu 武昌府. Its seat of administration was in present-day Yang xin 陽新 county in Hu bei 湖北. Its territory of administration comprised more or less the present-day cities and counties of Yang xin, Huang shi 黃石, Da ye 大冶 and Tong shan 通山 in Hu bei. In 1912, it became Xing guo 興國 county. Mentioned with 29, 1051, 1437.

Xing hua 興化
See → Xing hua jun 興化軍.

Xing hua jun 興化軍 [3]
Name of an administrative area. It was founded under Northern Song 宋, in 979, by changing the name of Tai ping jun 太平軍. It was administered from the old Xing hua city located northeast of present-day Xian you 仙游 county in Fu jian 福建. Four years later, it was moved to present-day Fu tian 莆田 city in Fu jian. Its territory of administration corresponded to present-day Fu tian city and Xian you county. Under Yuan 元, in 1277, its status was raised to Xing hua lu 興化路. Mentioned with 324, 674.

Xing nan 滎南 [1]
Name of a region. It refers to the region south of Xing ze 滎澤. In essence this is the area of Xing yang 滎陽, Zheng zhou 鄭州, Xin mi 新密 and Xin zheng 新鄭 in present-day He nan 河南. Mentioned with 631.

Xing qing chi 興慶池 [1]
Name of a palace garden. This is one of the most famous palace gardens found in Tang 唐 Chang an 長安. Its ruins are found in the Xing qing 興慶 park in present-day Xi an 西安 city in Shaan xi 陝西. Mentioned with 1527.

Xing yang 滎陽 [2 + 2]
□ Name of a commandery. [2] It was established under Cao wei 曹魏, in 242. Its seat of administration was in present-day Gu xing 古滎 town located northwest of Zheng zhou 鄭州 city in He nan 河南. Its territory of administration comprised the present-day areas of Zheng zhou, Xing yang 滎陽, Zhong mou 中牟, Xin mi 新密 and Xin zheng 新鄭. Northern Qi 齊 abolished it. Mentioned with 474, 733.

□ Name of county. [2] It was founded by Qin 秦. Its seat of administration was in present-day Gu xing 古滎 town located northwest of Zheng zhou 鄭州 city in He nan 河南. Under Northern Wei 魏, in 495, the seat of administration was moved to present-day Xing yang 滎陽 city in He nan 河南. In 1994, the county was abolished and a city established. Mentioned with 733, 953.

Xing yuan 興元
See → Xing yuan fu 興元府

Xing yuan fu 興元府 [5]
Name of a *fu*. It was founded under Tang 唐, in 784. Its seat of administration was at a location east of present-day Han zhong 漢中 city in Shaan xi 陕西. Its territory of administration comprised present-day Han zhong city, and the present-day counties of Nan zheng 南鄭, Mian xian 勉縣 and Cheng gu 城固, all in Shaan xi. Under Southern Song 宋, in 1209, the seat of administration was moved to present-day Han zhong city. Yuan 元 changed the area to be Xing yuan lu 興元路. Under Ming 明, in 1370, it was again changed to be Xing yuan fu. Not long after that it became Han zhong fu 漢中府. Mentioned with 216, 524, 1017, 1305, 1324.

Xing zhou 興州 [1]
Name of a *zhou* 州. It was established under Western Wei 魏, in 554. Its seat of administration was in present-day Lue yang 略陽 county in Shaan xi 陕西. Its administrative territory comprised the area of the present-day Lue yang county. Under Sui 隋, at the beginning of the *da ye* 大業 reign period (605 – 618), the area was changed to be Shun zheng 順政 commandery. Under Tang 唐, in 618, it again became Xing zhou. In 742, it was changed to be Shun zheng commandery again. In 758, it again became Xing zhou. Under Southern Song 宋, in 1207, it was changed to be Mian zhou 沔州. Mentioned with 275.

Xing zhou 邢州 [1]
Name of a *zhou* 州. It was founded under Sui 隋, in 596. Its seat of administration was in present-day Xing tai 邢臺 city in He bei 河北. Its administrative territory comprised an area extending in present-day He bei from the counties of Ju lu 巨鹿 and Guang zong 廣宗 toward the West, from the Zhi he 泜河 toward the South, and from the Sha he 沙河 toward the North. Under Northern Song 宋, in 1119, its status was raised to Xin de fu 信德府. Jin 金 made it Xing zhou again. Under Yuan 元, in 1262, its status was raised to Shun de fu 順德府. Mentioned with 1344.

Xiong 雄 [1]
Name of a *zhou* 州. It was established under Five Dynasties' Zhou 周, in 959. Its seat of administration was in Xiong county in present-day He bei 河北. The administrative area comprised Xiong county and Rong cheng 容城 county in He bei. At the beginning of Ming 明, the *zhou* was made a county. Mentioned with 291.

Xiong er 熊耳
See → Xiong er shan 熊耳山

Xiong er shan 熊耳山 [6]
This is the name of a mountain. It is located to the southeast of present-day Lu shi 盧氏 county in He nan 河南. Mentioned with 722, 1111, 1114, 1395, 1528.

Xiong she xhan 熊舍山 [1]
Name of a mountain. This is a mistake for Xiong cang shan 熊蒼山. It is located in the region of present-day Yao an 姚安 and Da yao 大姚 in Yun nan 雲南. Mentioned with 1069.

Xiu 秀 [1]
Name of a *zhou* 州. It was established during the Five Dynasties period, in 939, by Wu yue 吳越. Its seat of administration was in present-day Jia xing 嘉興 city in Zhe jiang 浙江. Its territory of administration comprised the boundaries of present-day Jia xing city. In 1195, it was changed to be Jia xing fu 嘉興府. Mentioned with 1057.

Xiu chuan 秀川 [1]
This is another name for Xiu zhou 秀州. It refers to present-day Jia xing 嘉興 city in Zhe jiang 浙江. Mentioned with 1399.

Xiu jiang 修江 [1]
This is an error for → Xiu ren 修仁.

Xiu ren 修仁 [1]
This is the name of a county. It was founded under Tang 唐, in 821. Its seat of administration was in Lao xian 老縣 to the west of present-day Xiu ren town located southwest of Li pu 荔浦 county in Guang xi 廣西. Under Ming 明, in 1479, the seat was moved to present-day Xiu ren town. In 1951, it was eliminated. Mentioned with 1038.

Xiu shui 休水 [1]
Name of a river. It is located in a region comprising Deng feng 登封, Gong yi 鞏義 and Yan shi 偃師 in the western part of present-day He nan 河南. Mentioned with 1176.

Xu 徐 [6]
Name of a *zhou* 州. This was one of the nine *zhou* of early China as seen in the *Book of History's* "Yu gong 禹貢," "Tribute of Yu 禹." The *zhou* corresponded to the area south of Tai shan 泰山 in Shan dong 山東, and the region north of the Huai he 淮河 in Jiang su 江蘇 and An hui 安徽. Mentioned with 733, 867, 877, 1004, 1275, 1538.

Xu 徐
See → Xu zhou 徐州.

Xu jiang 盱江 [1]
Name of a river. This is in present-day Jiang xi 江西 the Fu he 撫河 river of Lin chuan 臨川 city and the Xu jiang of Nan cheng 南城 county. Mentioned with 415.

Xu pu 溆浦 [1]
Name of a county. It was founded under Tang 唐, in 621, and subordinated to Chen zhou 辰州. Its seat of administration was in present-day Xu pu 溆浦 county in Hu nan 湖南. Ming 明 and Qing 清 put it under Chen zhou fu 辰州府. Mentioned with 768.

Xu shan 續山 [1]

Name of a mountain. It is located in the region of present-day Zi bo 淄博 city in Shan dong 山東. Mentioned with 980.

Xu shan ting 徐善亭 [1]

Name of a pavilion. It is located within the area of present-day Nan yang 南陽 city in He nan 河南. Mentioned with 1406.

Xu wen xian 徐聞縣 [1]

Name of a county. It was established in 111 BCE and subordinated to He pu 合浦 commandery. Its seat of administration was at a location south of present-day Xu wen 徐聞 county in Guang dong 廣東. Under Yuan 元, in 1291, the administration was moved to the present-day Xu wen county. Under Ming 明, in 1462, the seat of administration was moved to present-day Hai an 海安 town southeast of Xu wen county. In 1501, it was moved back to Xu wen county. Mentioned with 1192.

Xu wu shan 徐無山 [1]

Name of a mountain. It is located east of present-day Zun hua 遵化 city in He bei 河北. Mentioned with 111.

Xu yi xian 盱眙縣 [1]

Name of a county. It was founded by Western Han 漢, and put under Lin huai 臨淮 commandery. Its seat of administration was in the foot of Xu yi 盱眙 mountain, 25 *li* northeast of present-day Xu yi 盱眙 county in Jiang su 江蘇. Under Eastern Jin 晉, in 411, the seat of administration was moved to the southeastern foot of Du liang 都梁 mountain, located 5 *li* northeast of present-day Xu yi county. Under Tang 唐, in 625, the seat of administration was moved to Xu yi county. Under Northern Song 宋, during the *jing de* 景德 reign period (1004 – 1007), the status of the county was reduced to being a town. Under Southern Song, it was again raised to be a county. The seat of administration was moved to the present-day Xu yi county. Mentioned with 616.

Xu zhou 敘州 [1]

Name of a *fu* 府. It was founded under Ming 明, in 1373. Its seat of administration was in present-day Yi bin 宜賓 city in Si chuan 四川. Its territory of administration comprised most of the areas of the two present-day cities of Yi bin and Zi gong 自貢. It was abolished in 1913. Mentioned with 1499.

Xu zhou 徐州 [8]

Name of a *zhou* 州. It was established by Liu Song 劉宋, in 421. Its seat of administration was in present-day Xu zhou city in Jiang su 江蘇. During Sui 隋, it was changed to be Peng cheng 彭城 commandery. Under Tang 唐, in 621, it became Xu zhou again. In 742, it was again changed to Peng cheng commandery. It again became Xu zhou, in 758. Under Yuan 元, in 1348, its status was raised to be Xu zhou lu 徐州路. Under Ming 明, it again became Xu zhou and was put under Feng yang fu 鳳陽府. Under Qing 清, in 1733, its status was raised to Xu zhou fu 徐州府. Mentioned with 175, 441, 523, 1017, 1030, 1039, 1234, 1446.

Xuan 宣 [4]
See → Xuan zhou 宣州. Mentioned with 79, 189, 202, 874.

Xuan cheng 宣城
See → Xuan cheng jun 宣城郡

Xuan cheng 宣城 [1]
Name of a county. It was established under Sui 隋, in 589. Its seat of administration was in present-day Xuan cheng 宣城 city in An hui 安徽. In 1987, it became Xuan zhou 宣州 city. In 2000, it was changed to be Xuan cheng city. Mentioned with 429.

Xuan cheng jun 宣城郡 [8]
Name of a commandery. It was founded under Western Jin 晉, in 281, by dividing Dan yang 丹陽 commandery, and put under Yang zhou 揚州. Its seat of administration was in present-day Xuan zhou 宣州 in An hui 安徽. Its administrative territory comprised an area extending in present-day An hui from the Yang zi toward the South and the East, as well as from the counties of Ning guo 寧國, Jing de 旌德, Huang shan 黃山 district and Shi tai 石台 toward the West and the North. Under Sui 隋, in 589, it was changed to be Xuan zhou. At the beginning of the *da ye* 大業 reign period (605 – 618), it was changed to Xuan cheng 宣城 commandery. Under Tang 唐, in 620, it again became Xuan zhou. In 742, it was changed to be Xuan cheng commandary. In 758, it again became Xuan zhou. The two Song 宋 dynasties turned Xuan zhou commandery into a commandery title of Xuan zhou, an empty name. Mentioned with 189, 456, 631, 785, 1020, 1390, 1391.

Xuan shan 玄山 [1]
Name of a mountain. It was documented in the *Zheng lei ben cao* 證類本草, *juan* 卷 10, *guan zhong* 貫眾, as located somewhere in the region of present-day Zi bo 淄博 city in Shan dong 山東. Mentioned with 369.

Xuan tu 玄菟 [1]
Name of a commandery. It was established under Western Han 漢, in 108 BCE. Its seat of administration was in present-day Hamhung city in Korea's Kyongsang-namdo. Its territory of administration comprised present-day Kyongsang-namdo, Kyongsang-bukdo, Ryanggang-do, Chagang-do as well as Kuan dian 寬甸 in China's Liao ning 遼寧 and area within Tong hua 通化 in Ji lin 吉林. Later the seat of administration was moved to Xin bin 新賓 and Fu shun 撫順 in Liao ning. Its territory of administration was gradually reduced, and eventually the commandery was abolished under Northern Wei 魏. Mentioned with 737.

Xuan weng zhi shan 懸甕之山 [1]
Name of a mountain. It is located southwest of present-day Tai yuan 太原 city in Shan xi 山西. Mentioned with 966.

Xuan zhou 宣州 [19]
Name of a *zhou* 州. It was founded by Sui 隋, in 589, after it pacified Chen 陳, by changing the name of Xuan cheng 宣城 commandery. Its seat of administration was in present-day Xuan zhou city in An hui 安徽. Its territory of admin-

istration corresponded to an area extending in Anhui from the Yang zi toward the South, from Jing de 旌德 county toward the North, and from Dong zhi 東至 county toward the East to the territory of Guang de 廣德 county. At the beginning of the *da ye* 大業 (605 – 618) reign period of the Sui, and during the *tian bao* 天寶 (742 – 756) and *zhi de* 至德 (756 – 758) reign periods of the Tang 唐, the area periodically became Xuan cheng commandery. Under Southern Song 宋, in 1166, its status was raised to Ning guo fu 寧國府. Mentioned with 79, 129, 189, 202, 298, 595, 635, 735, 768, 781, 785, 874, 941, 1015, 1485.

Xue shan 雪山 [1]

Name of a mountain. It is Qi lian 祁連 mountain in Gan su 甘肅. It is called "snow mountain" because the mountain peaks have snow all year around. Mentioned with 498.

Xun 潯 [1]

See → Xun zhou 潯州. Mentioned with 1427.

Xun 循 [1]

Name of a *zhou* 州. It was founded under Sui 隋, in 590. Its seat of administration was at a location 5 *li* northeast of present-day Hui zhou 惠州 in Guang dong 廣東. Its territory of administration comprised in present-day Guang dong the watershed of the Dong jiang 東江 extending from the Luo fu 羅浮 mountain toward the East, and the area west of the Luo he 螺河 and south of Jiu lian 九連 mountain to the ocean. At the beginning of the *da ye* 大業 (605 – 618) reign period of the Sui, the area was changed to be Long chuan 龍川 commandery. Under Tang 唐, in 622, it again became Xun zhou 循州. Southern Han 漢 of the Five Dynasties period changed it to be Zhen zhou 禎州. Mentioned with 1297.

Xun yang 潯陽 [1]

Administrative name.

□ The name of a county established by Tang 唐, in 621. It was administered in present-day Jiu jiang 九江 city in Jiang xi 江西. During the Five Dynasties period the area became De hua 德化 county.

□ The name of a commandery. It was founded under Tang, in 742, by changing the name of Jiang zhou 江州. Its seat of administration was in present-day Jiu jiang city in Jiang xi. Its administrative territory comprised an area extending toward the North from the two counties of Du chang 都昌 and De an 德安. In 758, it was changed to be Jiang zhou. Mentioned with 1570.

Xun yang jiang 潯陽江 [1]

Name of a river. It refers to that part of the Yang zi flowing through the territories of the ancient Xun yang 潯陽 county, located north of present-day Jiu jiang 九江 city in Jiang xi 江西. Mentioned with 789.

Xun zhou 循州 [1]

Name of a *zhou* 州. It was established under Five Dynasties' Southern Han 漢, in 917. Its seat of administration was at a location northwest of present-day Long chuan 龍川 county in Guang dong 廣東. During the Song 宋 era, its territory of administration comprised the present-day counties and cities of Long chuan,

He ping 和平, Xing ning 興寧, Wu hua 五華 and Lian ping 連平. Under Yuan 元, in 1276, the area became Xun zhou lu 循州路. Ten years later, the *lu* 路 was reduced to being Xun zhou again. Under Ming 明, in 1369, it was abolished. Mentioned with 1272.

Xun zhou 潯州 [2]

Name of a *zhou* 州. It was founded under Tang 唐, in 624. Its seat of administration was at a location 40 *li* northeast of present-day Gui ping 桂平 city in Guang xi 廣西. It was abolished again soon afterwards. Its territory of administration comprised the northern portions of Gui ping city in Guang xi. Later, the *zhou* was eliminated. In 633, the *zhou* was reestablished. The seat of administration was moved to a location 5 *li* west of Gui ping city. Under Yuan 元, in 1279, the area became Xun zhou lu 潯州路. Its territory of administration was increased in size. During Ming and Qing, it was Xun zhou fu 潯州府. Mentioned with 1138.

-Y-

Ya 崖 [1]

Name of a *zhou* 州. In the Canton area this character is also widely read as Yai. See → Ya zhou 崖州. Mentioned with 144.

Ya men shan 牙門山 [1]

This is another name for E mei shan 峨眉山. It is the E mei mountain located southwest of present-day E mei shan city in Si chuan 四川. Mentioned with 744.

Ya shan 丫山 [1]

Name of a mountain. It is said to be located in present-day Xuan cheng 宣城 city in An hui 安徽, but the precise location is unclear. Mentioned with 768.

Ya zhou 崖州 [2]

Name of a *zhou* 州. It was established under Northern Song 宋, in 972. Its seat of administration was in Ya cheng 崖城 town, located northwest of San ya 三亞 city in Hai nan 海南 province. Its territory of administration corresponded to present-day San ya city and parts of the counties of Bao ting 保亭 and Le Dong 樂東 in Hai nan province. In 1073, it was changed to Zhu ya jun 朱崖軍. Under Ming 明, in 1368, the name of Ji yang jun 吉陽軍 was changed to again establish a Ya zhou. Under Qing 清, in 1905, its status was raised to Ya zhou directly-administered *zhou*, *zhi li zhou* 直隸州. In 1912, the *zhou* became a county. Mentioned with 144, 1056.

Ya zhou 雅州 [14]

Name of a *zhou* 州. It was founded under Sui 隋, in 604. Its seat of administration was at a location west of present-day Ya an 雅安 city in Si chuan 四川. Its territory of administration comprised the present-day cities and counties of Ya an, Ming shan 名山, Ying jing 榮經, Tian quan 天全, Lu shan 蘆山 and Bao xing 寶興 in Si chuan. At the beginning of the *da ye* 大業 (605 – 618) reign period of the Sui, and during the *tian bao* 天寶 (742–756) and *zhi de* 至德 (756–758) reign periods of the Tang 唐, the area periodically became Lu shan 蘆山 commandery. Northern Song 宋 moved the seat of administration to present-day Ya an city. Under Qing 清, in 1729, the status of the area was raised to Ya zhou fu 雅州府. Mentioned with 333, 456, 520, 698, 716, 768, 825, 832, 866, 1030, 1237.

Yan 延 [3]

Name of a *zhou* 州. See → Yan zhou 延州. Mentioned with 464, 781, 871.

Yan 兗 [2 + 3]

□ Name of a *zhou* 州. [2] See under → Yan zhou 兗州. Mentioned with 1004, 1551.

□ Name of a *zhou*. [3] See under → Yan zhou 兗州. Mentioned with 637, 644, 1523.

Yan 燕 [9]

One of the 7 powerful states of the Warring States period. Yan was enfeoffed by Western Zhou 周 and its capital was located near Liu li he 琉璃河 town of the Fang shan 房山 district of present-day Bei jing 北京. Later, it was moved to the western corner of present-day Bei jing city. A secondary capital was at present-day Yi 易 county in He bei 河北. Its territory of administration comprised present-day Bei jing, Tian jin 天津, the northern section of He bei 河北 and the western portion of Liao ning 遼寧. In 222 BCE, Yan was annihilated by Qin 秦. The BCGM borrows the old name for this area. Mentioned with 881, 955, 1004, 1051, 1110, 1137, 1358, 1532.

Yan an fu 延安府 [1]

Name of a *fu* 府. It was created under Northern Song 宋, in 1089, by raising the status of Yan zhou 延州. Its seat of administration was in present-day Yan an 延安 city in Shaan xi 陕西. Its territory of administration comprised the present-day counties and cities of Yan an, Gan quan 甘泉, Yan chang 延長, Yan chuan 延川 and An sai 安塞 in Shaan xi, and the upper watersheds of the Yan he 延河 and Da li he 大理河 rivers. Yuan 元 changed the area to Yan an lu 延安路, and its administrative area was increased. Ming 明 and Qing 清 made it Yan an fu 延安府. In 1913, it was abolished. Mentioned with 126.

Yan bei 燕北 [1]

Regional name. The reference is to the area north of present-day Bei jing. 北京 Mentioned with 1406.

Yan chang 延長 [1]

Name of a county. It was founded under Tang 唐, in 764, by changing the name of Yan an 延安 county. It was put under Yan zhou 延州. Its seat of administration was in present-day Yan chang 延長 county in Shaan xi 陕西. Mentioned with 1040.

Yan cheng 鹽城 [1]

Name of a city. It is in present-day Yan yuan 鹽源 county in Si chuan 四川. Mentioned with 174.

Yan dao 嚴道 [2]
Name of a county. See → Yan dao xian 嚴道縣. Mentioned with 129, 595.

Yan dao xian 嚴道縣 [1]
Name of a county. It was established by Qin 秦, and put under Shu 蜀 commandery. Its seat of administration was in present-day Xing jing 滎經 in Si chuan 四川. According to one tradition, the seat was at present-day Gu cheng ping 古城坪, located 5 *li* west of Xing jing county. The county was abolished under Cheng Han 成漢 during the era of Sixteen Kingdoms. Mentioned with 129.

Yan jing 燕京 [4]
Alternative name. It refers to present-day Bei jing 北京 city. Mentioned with 807, 1110, 1119, 1242.

Yan ling 嚴陵 [1]
Minor place name. This is the Yan zi ling 嚴子陵 fishing terrace on the left bank of the Fu chun jiang 富春江, located southwest of present-day Tong lu 桐廬 county in Zhe jiang 浙江. Mentioned with 415.

Yan ling 延陵 [1]
Name of a town. This is Yan ling 延陵 town, located southwest of Dan yang 丹陽 city in Jiang su 江蘇. Mentioned with 1537.

Yan men 雁門 [4+ 6]
□ Name of a pass. [4] It is the Yan men guan 雁門關, located 32 *li* northwest of present-day Dai 代 county in Shan xi 山西. Mentioned with 556, 938.
□ Name of a commandery. [6] It was established by Warring States Zhao 趙. During Qin 秦 and Western Han 漢, its seat of administration was located south of present-day You yu 右玉 county in Shan xi 山西. Its territory of administration corresponded to an area extending in present-day Shan xi from the counties of He qu 河曲, Wu zhai 五寨 and Ning wu 寧武 toward the North, from Heng shan 恒山 mountain toward the West, and in Inner Mongolia from the Huang qi hai 黃旗海 sea and the Dai hai 岱海 toward the South. Eastern Han moved the seat of administration to present-day Xia guan cheng 夏關城, located 55 *li* southeast of Shuo zhou 朔州 city in Shan xi. Three Kingdoms' Wei 魏 moved the seat of administration to the ancient city located 10 *li* southwest of the present Dai 代 county. At the beginning of the *kai huang* 開皇 reign period (581 – 600), Sui 隋 abolished the commandery. Mentioned with 191, 716, 809, 934, 1336.

Yan qi guo 焉耆國 [1]
Name of a country in the western regions. It was one of the 36 countries of the western regions. The area was later conquered by the Uighurs. The name still persists and the inhabitants involved form a self-governing Hui 回 county in central Xin jiang 新疆. Mentioned with 720.

Yan shan 鹽山 [1 + 1]
□ This is the name of a mountain. [1] It is located northeast of the present Wen su 溫宿 county in Xin jiang 新疆. Mentioned with 1335.
□ Name of a county. [1] It was established under Sui 隋, in 598. Its seat of administration was in present-day Jiu cheng xiang 舊城鄉, located 30 *li* southwest

of Huang hua 黄驊 city in He bei 河北. Under Ming 明, in 1376, the seat of administration was moved to present-day Yan shan county. Mentioned with 1346.

Yan shan 弇山 [1]
Variant of a place name. It refers to present-day Tai cang 太倉 city in Jiang su 江蘇.

Yan shan 鉛山 [1]
Name of a county. See → Yan shan xian 鉛山縣. Mentioned with 1014.

Yan shan xian 鉛山縣 [2]
Name of a county. It was established under Five Dynasties' Tang 唐 by raising the status of Yan shan 鉛山 market and subordinated to Xin zhou 信州. Its seat of administration was in present-day Yong ping 永平 town, located southeast of Yan shan county in Jiang xi 江西. Southern Song 宋, during the *shao ding* 紹定 reign period (1228 – 1233), moved the seat of administration to a location north of present-day Yong ping town in Yan shan county. In 1292, Yuan 元 raised the status of the county to Yan shan zhou 州. In 1369, it was demoted to be a county and put under Gang xin fu 廣信府. The seat of administration was returned to present-day Yong ping town. In 1949, the seat of administration was moved to He kou 河口 town in the present Yan shan county. Mentioned with 1014, 1518.

Yan shou xian 延壽縣 [1]
Name of a county. It was established under Eastern Han 漢, and subordinated to Jiu quan 酒泉 commandery. Its seat of administration was at a location near the oil field southeast of present-day Yu men 玉門 city in Gan su 甘肅. Northern Wei 魏 abolished the county. Mentioned with 1040.

Yan sui 延綏 [1]
Name of a garrison. It was also called Yu lin 榆林 garrison. This was one of nine boundary points under Ming 明. It was initially administered from present-day Sui de 綏德 county in Shaan xi 陝西. In 1471, the seat of administration was moved to present-day Yu lin city in Shaan xi. The territory reached in the East to the Yellow River, and in the West to Ding bian 定邊 county. It was abolished under Qing 清 in 1724. Mentioned with 464.

Yan yu 兗豫 [1]
Combined place name. It is a combination of the name of Yan zhou 兗州 and Yu zhou 豫州 from the classic nine *zhou* 州 of early China. The area involved comprised the northwestern part of present-day Shan dong 山東, and the southern part of present-day He bei 河北.

Yan zhou 弇州 [1]
Variant of a place name. It refers to present-day Tai cang 太倉 city in Jiang su 江蘇.

Yan zhou 兗州 [3 + 3 + 1]
□ Name of a *fu* 府. [3] See under → Yan zhou fu 兗州府. Mentioned with 269, 1043, 1289.
□ Name of a *zhou* 州. [3] It was founded under Western Han 漢, in 106 BCE. It was one of the 13 Regional Inspector Divisions, *ci shi bu* 刺史部. It corre-

sponded more or less to the southwestern part of present-day Shan dong 山東 and the eastern part of present-day He nan 河南. There was an administrative center under Eastern Han, located southeast of present-day Ju ye 巨野 county in Shan dong. During Three Kingdoms Wei 魏 and during Jin 晉, the seat of administration was moved to a location 64 *li* west of present-day Yun cheng 鄆城 county in Shan dong. Later the administrative area of the *zhou* was gradually reduced. During Liu Song 劉宋, the seat of its administration was moved to Yan zhou city in present-day Shan dong. Under Ming 明, in 1385, the area became Yan zhou fu 兗州府. Mentioned with 57, 272, 345, 462, 579, 635, 672, 687, 931, 1033, 1316, 1334, 1371, 1417, 1430, 1449, 1538.

□ Name of a *zhou*. [1] This was one of the 9 traditional *zhou* of early China, as mentioned in the *Book of History's* "Yu gong 禹貢," "Tribute of Yu 禹." The area comprised the northwestern part of present-day Shan dong 山東 and the eastern part of present-day He bei 河北.

Yan zhou 嚴州 [1]

Name of a *zhou* 州. It was founded under Northern Song 宋, in 1121, by changing the name of Mu zhou 睦州. Its seat of administration was in Mei cheng 梅城 town, located 50 *li* northeast of Jian de 建德 city in present-day Zhe jiang 浙江. Its territory of administration comprised the present-day cities and counties of Jian de, Chun an 淳安 and Tong lu 桐廬 in Zhe jiang. Southern Song, in 1265, changed the *zhou* to Jian de fu 建德府. Mentioned with 1486.

Yan zhou 鹽州 [1]

Name of a *zhou* 州. It was founded by Western Wei 魏, in 554, by changing the name of Xi an 西安 zhou. Its seat of administration was in present-day Ding bian 定邊 county in Shaan xi 陝西. Its territory of administration comprised a region of the present Ding bian and of Yan chi 鹽池 in Ning xia 寧夏. At the beginning of the *da ye* 大業 (605 – 618) reign period of the Sui, and during the *tian bao* 天寶 (742 – 756) and *zhi de* 至德 (756 – 758) reign periods of the Tang 唐, the area periodically became a commandery. From the *jian zhong* 建中 reign period (780 – 783) on, the area was conquered by the Tibetans. Mentioned with 368.

Yan zhou 延州 [5]

Name of a *zhou* 州. It was established by Western Wei 魏, in 554, by changing the name of Dong xia zhou 東夏州. Its seat of administration was at a location near to Gan gu yi 甘谷驛 town located northeast of present-day Yan an 延安 city in Shaan xi 陝西. Its territory of administration corresponded to Yan an city, Yan chuan 延川 county, and much of Yan chang 延長 county in present-day Shaan xi. During the Tang 唐, in 618, the seat of administration was moved to the eastern bank of the Yan 延 river east of present-day Yan an city. Its territory of administration was quite large and reached to the present-day cities and counties of Yan an, An sai 安塞, Yan chang, Yan chuan 延川 and Zhi dan 志丹. Northern Song 宋, in 1047, moved the seat of administration to present-day Yan an city. In 1089, the status of the area was raised to be Yan an fu 延安府. Mentioned with 72, 781, 1040, 1250, 1258.

Yan zhou fu 兗州府 [1]

Name of a *fu* 府. It was created under Ming 明, in 1385, by raising the status of Yan zhou 兗州. It was put under Shan dong 山東 province. Its seat of administration was at present-day Yan zhou city in Shan dong. Its administrative territory comprised the areas between the present-day counties and cities of Ping yin 平陰, Yang gu 陽穀, He ze 菏澤, Cao xian 曹縣, Shan xian 單縣, Yu tai 魚台, Wei shan 微山, Tan cheng 郯城, Lin yi 臨沂 and Si shui 泗水 in Shan dong. Under Qing 清, the administration was reduced. In 1913, the *fu* was abolished. Mentioned with 268.

Yang 揚 [3 + 1 + 1]

□ Name of a *zhou* 州. [3] See under → Yang zhou 揚州. Mentioned with 635, 690, 1493.

□ Name of a *zhou*. [1] See under → Yang zhou 揚州. Mentioned with 793.

□ Name of a *fu* 府. [1] See under → Yang zhou 揚州. Mentioned with 637.

Yang cheng 陽城 [1 + 3 + 1]

□ Name of a county. [1] It was established by Qin 秦. Its seat of administration was in present-day Gao cheng 告成 town, located 24 *li* southeast of Deng feng 登封 city in He nan 河南. It was later eliminated under Western Jin 晉, but re-established under Northern Wei 魏. In 696, under Wu Ze tian 武則天, it was changed to Gao cheng county. In 705, it again became Yang cheng 陽城 county. In 706, it again became Gao cheng county but was later changed under Tang 唐 to Yang yi 陽邑 county. Under Five Dynasties' Tang, it became Yang cheng county again. Under Later Zhou 周 it was abolished. Mentioned with 1250.

□ Name of a county. [3] It was established under Tang 唐, in 742. Its seat of administration was in present-day Yang cheng county in Shan xi 山西. Under Jin 金, in 1223, the status of the area was raised to be Ji zhou 勣州. Yuan 元 reestablished Yang cheng county, and took over the seat of administration that still exists. Mentioned with 698, 1149, 1537.

□ Minor place name. [1] This is Yang cheng 陽城 town, located 40 *li* west of present-day Qing yuan 清苑 county in He bei 河北. Mentioned with 709.

Yang di 陽翟 [1]

Name of a county. It was established by Qin 秦. Its seat of administration was in present-day Yu zhou 禹州 city in He nan 河南. Ming 明 eliminated this county, and made it a part of Jun zhou 峻州. Mentioned with 1532.

Yang gu xian 陽谷縣 [1]

Name of a county. It was founded by Sui 隋, in 596. Its seat of administration was at a location 30 *li* northeast of present-day Yang gu 陽谷 county in Shan dong 山東. Under Northern Song 宋, in 1006, the administration was moved to Meng dian 孟店. This is the present seat of administration. Mentioned with 269.

Yang gu xian 陽穀縣 [1]

Name of a county. See → Yang gu xian 陽谷縣. Mentioned with 268.

Yang jiang xian 陽江縣 [1]
Name of a county. It was established at the end of Sui 隋. Its seat of administration was in present-day Yang jiang 陽江 city in Guang dong 廣東. In 1988, it was reestablished as a city. Mentioned with 1437.

Yang keng 陽坑 [1]
Minor place name. It is located in the region of Xuan cheng 宣城 city in present-day An hui 安徽. Mentioned with 768.

Yang po 陽坡 [1]
Minor place name. This is in present-day Xuan cheng 宣城 city in An hui 安徽. The exact location remains unclear. Mentioned with 768.

Yang pu 楊樸 [1]
Minor place name. It is located within the boundaries of present-day Si chuan 四川. Further details require additional research. Mentioned with 994.

Yang qi shan 陽起山 [1]
Name of a mountain. It is located in the region of Ji nan 濟南 city in present-day Shan dong 山東, but details are lacking. Mentioned with 1344.

Yang shan 陽山 [1 + 2]
□ Name of a mountain. [1] It is located in the vicinity of present-day Ping shi 平氏 town in the northwestern part of Tong bai 桐柏 county in He nan 河南. Mentioned with 1509.
□ Name of a mountain. [2] It is Lang 狼 mountain located northwest of the Yellow River bend in Inner Mongolia. Mentioned with 504, 1392.

Yang shan xian 陽山縣 [1]
Name of a county. It was established under Western Han 漢. Its seat of administration was in the North of the Nan lian 南連 river, located east of present-day Qing lian 青蓮 town east of Yang shan 陽山 county in Guang dong 廣東. Eastern Han combined it with Yin shan 陰山 county. Three Kingdoms' Wu 吳 reestablished it and administered the county from a location south of the Nan lian river in the present Yang shan county. Under Tang 吳, in 705, the seat of administration was moved to the present Yang shan county. Mentioned with 1521.

Yang xian 陽羨 [3]
Name of a county. [1] See → Yang xian xian 陽羨縣. Mentioned with 129, 768, 1532.

Yang xian xian 陽羨縣 [1]
Name of a county. It was established by Qin 秦. Its seat of administration was at a location south of present-day Jing xi 荊溪, located 5 *li* south of Yi xing 宜興 city in Jiang su 江蘇. Three Kingdoms' Wu 吳 moved the seat of administration to the present Yi xing city. Sui 隋, in 589, changed the area to Yi xing county. Mentioned with 805.

Yang zhou 洋州 [2]
Name of a *zhou* 州. It was established by Western Wei 魏. Its seat of administration was at a location southwest of present-day Xi xiang 西鄉 county in Shaan

xi 陝西. Its territory of administration comprised present-day Yang xian 洋縣, Xi xiang, Zhen ba 鎮巴 and Fo ping 佛坪 in Shaan xi. Under Sui 隋, in 607, the *zhou* was eliminated. It was restored under Tang 唐, in 618. Under Ming 明, in 1370, the area became Yang 洋 county. Mentioned with 31, 660.

Yang zhou 揚州 [4 + 2 + 4 + 2]

□ Name of a *zhou* 州. [4] It was founded under Sui 隋, in 589. Its seat of administration was in present-day Yang zhou 揚州 city in Jiang su 江蘇. Under Five Dynasties' Wu 吳 it was changed to Jiang du fu 江都府. Later Zhou 周, during the xian de 顯德 reign period (954 – 960), restored it as Yang zhou. Under Yuan 元, in 1277, its status was raised to Yang zhou lu 揚州路. Mentioned with 615, 987, 1110, 1178.

□ Name of a *zhou* 州. [2] It was founded under Western Han 漢. Its territory of administration covered the area to the South of the Huai shui 淮水 in present-day An hui 安徽 and to the Yang zi in Jiang su 江蘇, furthermore the three provinces of Jiang xi 江西, Zhe jiang 浙江 and Fu jian 福建, as well as the present-day counties and cities of Ying shan 英山, Huang mei 黃梅 and Guang ji 廣濟 in Hu bei, and Gu shi 固始 and Shang cheng 商城 in He nan 河南. During Eastern Han times, the seat of administration was moved to present-day He 和 county in An hui. At the end of Eastern Han the seat of administration was moved to Shou 壽 county and to a location northwest of present-day He fei 合肥 city in present-day An hui. Three Kingdoms Wei 魏 and Wu 吳, each established a Yang zhou. Wei administered its Yang zhou from Shou chun 壽春, and Wu from present-day Nan jing 南京 city. After Western Jin 晉 annihilated Wu, they were combined, but after that their administrative area was reduced. Under Sui 隋, in 589, the area became Jiang zhou 蔣州. In 605, it was eliminated. Under Tang 唐, in 620, the *zhou* was reestablished. In 624, it became Jiang zhou again only to be renamed Yang zhou again the next year. In 626, the seat of administration was moved to present-day Yang zhou city in Jiang su. Mentioned with 994, 1342.

□ Name of a *fu* 府. [4] It was established by the Ming 明 rebels under Yuan 元, in 1366. Its seat of administration was in present-day Yang zhou 揚州 city in Jiang su 江蘇. Its administrative territory comprised an area extending from the Yang zi river toward the North, from Bao ying 寶應 toward the South and from Yi zheng 儀征 toward the East in present-day Jiang su. It was abolished in 1912. Mentioned with 978, 1110, 1239, 1485, 1532.

□ Name of a *zhou* 州. [2] This was one of the nine *zhou* of early China as seen in the *Book of History's* "Yu gong 禹貢," "Tribute of Yu 禹," Mentioned with 1400, 1538.

Yang zi 揚子 [1]

Name of a river. From Sui 隋 and Tang 唐 times, the Yang zi, Chinese: Chang jiang 長江, was referred to as Yang zi jiang 揚子江 in the region of present-day Yi zheng 儀征 and Yang zhou 揚州 city in Jiang su 江蘇. Mentioned with 1551.

Yao 瑤 [1]
Regional name. It is a general reference to the area occupied by the Yao 瑤 peoples in the South of China. Mentioned with 1242.

Yao 耀 [2]
Name of a *zhou*. See → Yao zhou 耀州. Mentioned with 56, 1523.

Yao dong 瑤峒 [1]
Regional name. The reference is to the areas occupied by the Yao 瑤 people in present-day Guang xi 廣西. Mentioned with 474.

Yao shan 堯山 [1]
Name of a mountain. This is Yao wang shan 堯王山, located 8 *li* northwest of present-day Qing zhou 青州 city in Shan dong 山東. Mentioned with 706.

Yao shan 搖山 [2]
Place name from the 山海經, "Classic of Mountains and Seas," Details are lacking. Mentioned with 333.

Yao zhou 耀州 [1]
Name of a *zhou* 州. It was founded under Tang 唐, in 906. Its seat of administration was in present-day Tong chuan 銅川 city in Shaan xi 陝西. Under Five Dynasties' Liang 梁, the name was changed to Chong zhou 崇州. Under Later Tang 唐, in 923, the area became Yao zhou 耀州 again. In 1913, it was changed to Yao 耀 county. Mentioned with 1017.

Ye 冶 [1]
Name of a county. It was established under Western Han 漢, during the reign of Emperor Wu di 武帝 (156 – 87). Its seat of administration was at the foot of Jiu ye 舊冶 mountain in present-day Fu zhou 福州 city in Fu jian 福建. Eastern Han changed it to be Dong ye 東冶 county. Mentioned with 362.

Ye bei 掖北 [1]
Regional name. Ye xian 掖縣 is in present-day Lai zhou 萊州 city in Shan dong 山東, and Ye bei 掖北 should have been north of that. Further details are lacking. Mentioned with 474.

Ye bei shan 液北山 [1]
Name of a mountain. It is located north of present-day Lai zhou 萊州 city. Details are lacking. Mentioned with 463.

Ye bei xiang 液北鄉 [1]
No such place name is known although this is cited in the BCGM. See → Ye bei shan 液北山. Mentioned with 46.

Ye du 鄴都 [1]
Ancient capital. Five Dynasties' Tang 唐, in 923, changed Wei zhou 魏州 to be Xing tang fu 興唐府 and established the name Dong jing 東京, "Eastern Capital." In 925, Dong jing was changed to be Ye du. Its seat of administration was in present-day Da jie xiang 大街鄉, located northeast of Da ming 大名 county in He bei 河北. In 929, the capital was abolished. Under Later Jin 晉, in 937, the area was changed to Xing tang fu. In 938, Guang jin fu 廣晉府 became Ye du.

Under Later Han 漢, in 948, it was changed to be Da ming fu 大名府. Mentioned with 631.

Ye huo luo 葉火羅 [1]
Name of a country located in the western regions. This is actually an error for Tu huo luo 吐火羅. Mentioned with 814.

Ye jun 鄴郡 [1]
Name of a commandery. It was founded under Tang 唐, in 742. Its seat of administration was in present-day An yang 安陽 city in He nan 河南. Its territory of administration included the present-day cities and counties of An yang, He bi 鶴壁, Tang yin 湯陰, Lin zhou 林州 and Nei huang 內黃 in He nan, and Lin zhang 臨漳, Cheng an 成安 and Ci xian 磁縣 in He bei 河北. In 758, the area became Xiang zhou 相州. Mentioned with 648.

Ye xi 耶溪 [1]
Name of a small river. This is the Ruo ye xi 若耶溪 of present-day Shao xing 紹興 city in Zhe jiang 浙江. Mentioned with 1340.

Ye xian 掖縣 [3]
Name of a county. It was established under Western Han 漢. Its seat of administration was in Dong lai 東萊 commandery. Dong lai commandery was subordinate to the Qing zhou Regional Inspector Division, Qing zhou *ci shi bu* 青州刺史部. Its seat of administration was in present-day Lai zhou 萊州 city in Shan dong 山東. Eastern Han changed it to a feudal lord country. Later it again became a county. In 1988, Lai zhou city was established. Mentioned with 474.

Ye zhong 鄴中 [1]
Name of an ancient capital city. This is present-day Ye 鄴 town, located southwest of Lin zhang 臨漳 county in Hei bei 河北.

Yi 沂 [3]
Name of a *zhou* 州. See → Yi zhou 沂州. Mentioned with 579, 703, 1523.

Yi 宜 [3]
Name of a *zhou* 州. See → Yi zhou 宜州. Mentioned with 376, 1063. 1329.

Yi 益 [5]
Name of a *zhou* 州. See → Yi zhou 益州. Mentioned with 535, 596, 637, 675.

Yi bin 宜賓 [1]
Name of a county. It was established under Northern Song 宋, in 1114. Its seat of administration was at the Jiu zhou 舊州 embankment, located 6 *li* northwest of present-day Yi bin city in Si chuan 四川. Under Southern Song, in 1243, it was moved to Dong shan 東山, two *li* east of present-day Yi bin city. Under Yuan 元, in 1276, it was moved to the present-day Yi bin city. In 1951, the area became Yi bin city. Mentioned with 1499.

Yi chang 益昌 [1]
Name of a county. It was established by Southern Song 宋. Its seat of administration was in present-day Zhao hua 昭化 town, located 40 *li* southwest of Guang yuan 廣元 city in Si chuan 四川. Northern Wei changed Yi chang to

be Jing zhao 京兆 county. Northern Zhou 周 again made it Yi chang county. Five Dynasties' Tang 唐, in 925, changed it to be Yi guang 益光 county. Northern Song again made it Yi chang county. In 972, it was changed to be Zhao hua county. Mentioned with 1485.

Yi chun jun 宜春郡 [1]

Name of a commandery. It was founded under Sui 隋, in 607. Its seat of administration was in present-day Yi chun 宜春 city in Jiang xi 江西. Its territory of administration included Ping xiang 萍鄉 city, plus the Yuan shui 袁水 watershed extending from Xin yu 新余 toward the West in present-day Jiang xi. Under Tang 唐, in 621, the area became Yuan zhou 袁州. In 742, it was changed to be Yi chun commandery. In 758, it again became Yuan zhou. Mentioned with 1516.

Yi du 益都 [1]

Name of a county. It was established under Three Kingdoms' Wei 魏. Its seat of administration was at a location 10 *li* south of present-day Shou guang 壽光 city in Shan dong 山東. Under Northern Qi 齊, in 556, the seat of administration was moved to present-day Qing zhou 青州 city in Shan dong. In 1986, the county was changed to be Qing zhou city. Mentioned with 1037.

Yi du 宜都 [9]

Name of a commandery. It was established under Eastern Han 漢, in 209. Its seat of administration was on the northern bank of the Yang zi southeast of present-day Yi chang 宜昌 city in Hu bei 湖北. Its territory of administration under Western Jin 晉 included the two present-day cities of Yi chang and Zhi cheng 枝城, and the present-day counties of Yi chang 宜昌, Chang yang 長陽 and Wu feng 五峰 in Hu bei. Under Liu Song 劉宋 , the seat of administration was moved to present-day Yi du city in Hu bei. Under Sui 隋, in 587, it was abolished. Mentioned with 66, 130, 261, 273, 437, 629, 660, 809, 1168.

Yi feng xian 移風縣 [1]

Name of a county. It was established under Three Kingdoms' Wu 吳. Its seat of administration was on the southern bank of the Sông Mã River (Ma jiang 馬江) north of Thanh Hóa in Thanh Hóa province in present-day Vietnam. The county was abolished during the *tian bao* 天寶 reign period (742 – 756) of Tang 唐. Mentioned with 1515.

Yi ling 夷陵 [1]

Name of an ancient city. It is located on the northern bank of the Yang zi southeast of present-day Yi chang 宜昌 city in Hu bei 湖北. Mentioned with 1051.

Yi lou 挹婁 [1]

This group was originally named Su shen 肅慎. During Han 漢 and Jin 晉 times, they were called Yi lou. They were spread about north of the Chang bai 長白 mountains and the middle and lower ranges of the Song hua jiang 松花江 and the Hei long jiang 黑龍江. In the east, they came up against the ocean. From Han times on, they were subordinate to the Fu yu 扶餘. During Three Kingdoms Wei 魏 they traded with Wei. During Northern Wei 魏 they were called Wu ji 勿吉. Mentioned with 1406.

Yi luo 伊洛 [6]
Name of a region. This name refers to the combined watershed of the Yi shui 伊水 and the Luo shui 洛水 in the vicinity of the ancient capital Luo yang 洛陽 city. The Yi shui is a tributary of the Luo shui. It emerges from the northern foot of the Fu niu 伏牛 mountains in Luan chuan 欒川 county in He nan 河南 and flows northeast to south of Yan shi 偃師 county and then enters the Luo shui. Mentioned with 234, 277, 1008, 1225, 1294.

Yi men 夷門 [1]
Place name. This is an alternative designation for present-day Kai feng 開封 city. There is a Yi men 夷門 mountain in the northeastern corner of Kai feng city. Hence the Eastern gate of the Warring States' Wei capital Da liang 大梁 was called "Yi men." Mentioned with 1417.

Yi qing shan 義情山 [1]
Name of a mountain. It is located in the eastern part of Zhe jiang 浙江. Details are lacking. Mentioned with 1017.

Yi shi xian 猗氏縣 [3]
Name of a county. It was established under Western Han 漢. Its seat of administration was in present-day Tie jiang ying 鐵匠營 village, located 20 *li* south of Lin yi 臨猗 county in Shan xi 山西. Under Western Wei 魏, in 555, it was changed to Sang quan 桑泉 county. Northern Zhou 周 restored Yi shi xian. In 613, the seat of administration was moved to present-day Lin yi county. In 1954, it was combined with Lin jin 臨晉 county, and together they became Lin yi 臨猗 county. Mentioned with 361, 1443.

Yi shui 伊水 [1]
Name of a river. The Yi shui comes from the northern foot of the Fu niu 伏牛 mountains in Luan chuan 欒川 county in He nan 河南, and flows northeast to south of Yan shi 偃師 county and then enters the Luo shui. Mentioned with 81.

Yi wu 義烏 [1]
Name of a county. It was established under Tang 唐, in 624. Its seat of administration was in present-day Yi wu 義烏 city in Zhe jiang 浙江. In 1988, it was designated Yi wu city.

Yi yang 義陽 [6]
Name of a commandery. It was established by Three Kingdoms' Wei 魏. Its seat of administration was at a location south of Zao yang 棗陽 county in Hu bei 湖北. Its territory of administration included Xin yang 信陽 city, the two counties of Xin yang and Luo shan 羅山 and the eastern part of Tong bai 桐柏 county in He nan 河南, and the two cities of Sui zhou 隨州 and Guang shui 廣水 as well as a portion of Da wu 大悟 county in Hu bei. Later the commandery was eliminated. It was reestablished at the end of Eastern Jin 晉. Its seat of administration was moved to present-day Xin yang city in Hu nan. Southern Qi 齊 changed it to be northern Yi yang 義陽 commandery. Under Eastern Wei 魏, in 549, it became Yi yang commandery. Sui 隋, at the beginning of the *kai huang* reign period (581 – 600), abolished it. It was reestablished in 697. Its seat of administra-

tion was in present-day Xin yang in He nan. The area became Shen zhou 申州 under Tang 唐, and in 742 it was again changed to be Yi yang commandery, but changed back to Shen zhou again in 758. Mentioned with 203, 272, 986, 1142, 1250.

Yi yang 易陽 [1]

Name of a county. It was established under Western Han 漢. Its seat of administration was at a location southeast of present-day Yong nian 永年 county in He bei 河北. It was abolished early in Northern Wei 魏 but later, under Emperor Xiao wen di 孝文帝 (467 – 499), reestablished. The seat of administration was moved to Yong nian county. Under Sui 隋, in 586, it was changed to be Han dan 邯鄲 county. Mentioned with 1030.

Yi yang xian 宜陽縣 [1]

Name of a county. It was established by Warring States Han 韓. Its seat of administration was in Han cheng 韓城 town, located 48 *li* west of present-day Yi yang 宜陽 county in He nan 河南. Under Northern Zhou 周, in 558, the seat of administration was moved to Fu chang 福昌, located west of present-day Yi yang 宜陽 county. Under Tang 唐, in 619, the area was changed to be Fu chang county. Mentioned with 1051.

Yi yang xian 伊陽縣 [1]

Name of a county. It was founded by Tang 唐 in 712. Its seat of administration was in present-day Jiu xian 舊縣 town, located 48 *li* southwest of Song gao 嵩高 county in He nan 河南. Under Jin 金, in 1151, the seat of administration was moved to the present-day Song 嵩 county. It was abolished under Yuan 元 in 1266. Mentioned with 437.

Yi zhou 翼州 [1]

Name of a *zhou* 州. It was founded under Northern Zhou 周, in 566. Its seat of administration was in the old city of Die xi 疊溪, located south of present-day Jiao chang xiang 較場鄉, 120 *li* northwest of Mao 茂 county in Si chuan 四川. Its territory of administration comprised the northern part of Mao county along with parts of neighboring Song pan 松潘 and Hei shui 黑水 counties in Si chuan. Under Sui 隋, in 607, it was eliminated. Under Tang 唐, in 618, it was restored and, in 643, the seat of administration was moved to present-day Jiao chang xiang. In 672, the seat of government was moved to a location northwest of present-day Mao county, but in 675 it was returned to Jiao chang xiang northwest of present-day Mao county. In 742, the area became Lin yi 臨翼 commandery. In 758, it again became Yi zhou. Later the area was conquered by the Tibetans. Mentioned with 199.

Yi zhou 益州 [46]

Name of a *zhou* 州. It was established under Western Han 漢, in 106, and was one of the 13 Regional Inspector Divisions, *ci shi bu* 刺史部. Its administrative territory comprised an area extending in present-day Si chuan 四川 from the Zhe duo 折多 mountain, and in Yun nan 雲南 from the Nu 怒 mountain and from the Ai lao 哀牢 mountain toward the East, in Gan su 甘肅 from Wu du 武都 and Liang dang 兩當 and in Shaan xi 陝西 from the Qin ling 秦嶺 mountain range toward the South, and in Hu bei 湖北 from Yun 鄖 county, Bao kang 保康 and Gui zhou 貴州 toward the West. Wang Mang 王莽 (45 BCE – 23 CE) changed this to be Yong bu 庸部. Gongsun Shu 公孫述 (died 36 CE) changed it to be a Metropolitan Commandant, *si li xiao wei* 司隸校尉. Eastern Han made it Yi zhou again, administered from a location north of present-day Guang han 廣漢 city in Si chuan. During the *zhong ping* 中平 reign period (184 – 189), the seat of administration was moved to present-day Huang hu 黃滸 town, located northeast of the present De yang 德陽 city. During the *chu ping* 初平 reign period (190 – 193), it was again moved to Luo 雒 county. During the *xing ping* 興平 reign period (194 – 195), it was moved to present-day Cheng du 成都 city. After Eastern Han, its administration was reduced. Under Sui 隋, in 607, it was changed to become a subordinate (*shu* 屬) commandery. Under Tang 唐, in 618, it again became Yi zhou. In 742, it again became a subordinate commandery. In 757, its status was raised to Cheng du fu 成都府. Under Northern Song 宋, in 981, it was reduced to be Yi zhou. In 988, it was again changed to be Cheng du fu. In 994, it was again reduced to be Yi zhou. In 1059, it was again changed to Cheng du fu. The *zhou* boundaries included the Cheng du plateau. From Qin 秦 and Han on, the area was one of the most economically developed regions of China. Mentioned with 20, 60, 130, 140, 153, 188, 249, 285, 313, 362, 423, 440, 535, 538, 595, 602, 678, 697, 705, 717, 768, 789, 819, 828, 856, 864, 986, 990, 995, 1036, 1115, 1264, 1289, 1310, 1344, 1373, 1375, 1486.

Yi zhou 易州 [2]

Name of a *zhou* 州. It was founded under Sui 隋, in 581. Its seat of administration was in present-day Yi 易 county in He bei 河北. At the beginning of the *da ye* 大業 reign period (605 – 618) of Sui 隋, it was changed to be Shang gu 上谷 commandery. Under Tang 唐, in 621, it again became Yi zhou. In 742, it was again named Shan gu commandery. In 758, it was again renamed Yi zhou. Its territory of administration under Tang comprised an area extending in present-day He bei 河北 from Nei chang cheng 内長城 toward the South, from An xin 安新 and Man cheng 滿城 toward the North, and from the Southern Ju ma 拒馬 river toward the West. After Liao 遼 times, there were many changes and alternations. Under Qing 清, in 1733, the status of the area was raised to be a directly administered *zhou*, *zhi li zhou* 直隸州. Mentioned with 931.

Yi zhou 儀州 [2]

Name of a *zhou* 州. It was founded under Northern Song 宋, in 977, by changing the name of Yi zhou 義州 to Yi zhou 儀州 to avoid a taboo. It was administered in present-day Hua ting 華亭 county in Gan su 甘肅. Its territory of administration comprised Hua ting county in today's Gan su. Mentioned with 1406.

Yi zhou 宜州 [20]

Name of a *zhou* 州. It was established under Tang 唐, during the *qian feng* 乾封 reign period (666 – 668). Its seat of administration was in present-day Yi zhou city in Guang xi 廣西. Its territory of administration comprised most of Yi shan 宜山 county and the southwestern part of Luo cheng 羅城 county in present-day Guang xi. In 1265, under Southern Song 宋, its status was raised to

Qing yuan fu 慶元府. Mentioned with 20, 25, 202, 246, 253, 265, 376, 461, 462, 558, 835, 956, 965, 970, 1082, 1247, 1250, 1266.

Yi zhou 沂州 [4]

Name of a *zhou* 州. It was established under Northern Zhou 周, in 578. Its seat of administration was at a location 20 *li* west of present-day Lin yi 臨沂 city in Shan dong 山東. Its territory of administration comprised Xin tai 新泰, Lin yi 臨沂, Fei 費 county and Ping yi 平邑 in present-day Shan dong. Sui 隋 moved the seat of administration to Lin yi city. During the *da ye* 大業 (605 – 618) reign period of the Sui, and the *tian bao* 天寶 (742 – 756) and *zhi de* 至德 (756 – 758) reign periods of the Tang 唐, the area was temporarily changed to be Lang ya 琅琊 commandery. Its territory of administration comprised the present-day cities and counties of Lin yi, Zao zhuang 棗莊, Xin tai, Cang shan 蒼山, Fei county, Ping yi, Meng yin 蒙陰, Yi shui 沂水, Yi yuan 沂源 and Yi nan 沂南 in present-day Shan dong. In 1734, its status was raised to Yi zhou fu 沂州府. Mentioned with 474, 687, 738.

Yin 銀 [2]

Name of a *zhou*. See → Yin zhou. Mentioned with 126, 893.

Yin fan shan 隱蕃山 [1]

Name of a mountain. Details are lacking. Mentioned with 1042.

Yin ping 陰平 [2]

Name of a county. It was established under Eastern Jin 晉 transferring an old name to a new territory. The seat of administration was at location north of present-day Xiao xi ba 小溪垻 town northeast of Jiang you 江油 city in Si chuan 四川. The county was abolished after Southern Song. Mentioned with 495, 866.

Yin shan 陰山 [1]

Name of a mountain. This is the Yin shan located north of the Great Bend of the Yellow River (He tao 河套) in Inner Mongolia. Mentioned with 1325.

Yin xian 銀縣 [1]

Apparently the name of a county. Details unknown.

Yin zhou 銀州 [3]

Name of a *zhou* 州. It was established under Northern Zhou 周, in 563. Its seat of administration was in Da zhai liang 大寨梁 of Dang cha 党岔 town, located east of present-day Heng shan 衡山 county in Shaan xi 陜西. Its territory of administration comprised an area extending toward the North from Heng shan, Mi zhi 米脂 and Jia 佳 county in present-day Shaan xi. It was eliminated under Sui 隋, in 608, but restored under Tang 唐, in 628. In 742, it became Yin chuan 銀川 commandery. In 758, it again became Yin zhou. In 1081, under Northern Song 宋, it was reestablished. The following year, the seat of administration was moved to present-day Ma hu yu 馬湖峪, located northwest of Mi zhi county in Shaan xi. It was abolished in 1106. Mentioned with 126, 931.

Ying 英 [1]

Name of a *zhou* 州. See → Ying zhou 英州. Mentioned with 1063.

Ying 郢 [2]
Name of a *zhou* 州. See → Ying zhou 郢州. Mentioned with 72, 78.

Ying cheng 郢城 [1]
Name of an ancient city. This is the Xia kou cheng 夏口城 of Three Kingdoms' Wu 吳. It was located on She 蛇 mountain in the present-day Wu chang cheng 武昌城 district of Hu bei 湖北. Mentioned with 562.

Ying chuan 潁川 [5]
Name of a commandery. See → Yin chuan jun 潁川郡. Mentioned with 113, 575, 648, 1250, 1405.

Ying chuan jun 潁川郡 [1]
Name of a commandery. It was established under Qin 秦, in 230 BCE. Its seat of administration was in present-day Yu zhou 禹州 city in He nan 河南. Its administrative territory comprised an area extending in present-day He nan from Deng feng 登封 and Bao feng 寶豐 toward the East, from Wei shi 尉氏 and Yan cheng 郾城 toward the West, from Xin mi 新密 toward the South, and from Ye 葉 county and Fu yang 舞陽 toward the North. Under Western Han 漢, in 202 BCE, the area became Han guo 韓國. In 201 BCE, the area again became Ying chuan jun. In 221 CE, under Three Kingdoms Wei 魏, the seat of administration was moved to Gu cheng 古城 located 36 *li* east of present-day Xu chang 許昌 city in He nan. After Western Jin 晉, the commandery's administrative area was reduced. Northern Wei 魏 administered the area from a location northeast of present-day Chang ge 長葛 city in He nan. Under Eastern Wei 魏, in 549, the seat of administration was moved to present-day Xu chang city. Under Sui 隋, in 607, it was changed to Ying chuan commandery. At the beginning of Tang 唐, it was changed to Xu zhou. In 742, it again became Ying chuan 潁川 commandery. In 758, it was again changed to be Xu zhou 許州. Mentioned with 648.

Ying dao 營道 [1]
Name of a county. It was established by Western Han 漢. Its seat of administration was in Mang shui kou 莽水口 and Chao shui kou 巢水口, some 30 *li* southeast of present-day Ning yuan 寧遠 county in Hu nan 湖南. Sui 隋 moved the seat of administration to Ling dao gu cheng 泠道故城, some 40 *li* southeast of Ning yuan county. Under Tang 唐, in 621, the seat of administration was moved to Ying 營 mountain, 40 *li* from the present Dao 道 county. In 622, the area was administered by Nan ying zhou 南營州. In 742, it became Hong dao 弘道 county and the seat of administration was moved to the present-day Dao county. Song 宋 restored the name Ying dao county. Under Ming 明, in 1376, it was abolished and made part of Dao zhou 道州. Mentioned with 550.

Ying hou zhi shan 嬰侯之山 [1]
Place name from the *Shan hai jing* 山海經, "Classic of Mountains and Seas." Details are lacking. Mentioned with 299.

Ying shan 英山 [1]
Name of a mountain. It is located east of Ying shan 英山 county in present-day Hu bei 湖北. Mentioned with 768.

Ying tian fu 應天府 [1]

Name of a *fu* 府. It was founded by the Ming 明 rebels led by Zhu Yuan zhang 朱元璋 under Yuan 元, in 1356, by changing Ji qing lu 集慶路 and put under the Jiang nan Branch Secretariat, Jiang nan *xing zhong shu sheng* 江南行中書省. Its seat of administration was in present-day Nan jing 南京 city in Jiang su 江蘇. Its administrative territory comprised an area in present-day Jiang su extending from the Da mao 大茅 mountain south of the Yang zi river, and from Li yang 溧陽 toward the West, and Jiang pu 江浦 and Lu he 六合 county north of the Yang zi river in Jiang su. At the beginning of Ming, the capital was established here. In 1441, it was determined to be "Southern Capital", Nan jing 南京. Under Qing 清, in 1645, it became Jiang ning fu 江寧府.

Ying yang 潁陽 [1]

Name of a county. It was founded under Northern Wei 魏, in 467. Its seat of administration was in present-day Ying yang 潁陽 town, located 54 *li* west of Deng feng 登封 city in He nan 河南. Northern Zhou 周 abolished it. Tang 唐, in 727, reestablished the county by changing the name of Wu lin 武林 county. Jin 金 abolished it. Mentioned with 270.

Ying zhou 郢州 [1 + 1]

□ Name of a *zhou* 州. [1] It was established under Liu Song 劉宋, in 454. Its seat of administration was in present-day Wu chang cheng 武昌城 district in Wu han 武漢 city in Hu bei 湖北. Its territory of administration corresponded to Han jiang 漢江 watershed below Zhong xiang 鍾祥 city, the watershed of the Yang zi between Jian li 監利 and Yang xin 陽新 in present-day Hu bei, and the northern part of the Yuan jiang 沅江 watershed in Hu nan 湖南. After that it was gradually reduced. Under Sui 隋, in 589, the area was changed to be E zhou 鄂州. Mentioned with 1067.

□ Name of a *zhou*. [1] It was established under Western Wei, in 551. Its seat of administration was in Zhong xiang city in present-day Hu bei. Its territory of administration comprised the two present-day cities and counties of Zhong xiang and Jing shan 京山 in Hu bei. Under Sui 隋, at the beginning of the *da ye* 大業 reign period (605 – 618), the area became Jing ling 竟陵 commandery. At the beginning of Tang 唐, the old name of Ying zhou was restored. It was abolished in 627, but restored in 643. The seat of administration was moved to Jing shan county. At the beginning of the *tian bao* 天寶 reign period (742 – 756), it became Fu shui 富水 commandery. At the beginning of the *qian yuan* 乾元 reign period (758 – 760), the old name was restored and it was administered from present-day Zhong xiang city. Under Yuan 元, in 1278, it was changed to be An lu fu 安陸府. Mentioned with 817.

Ying zhou 營州 [1]

Name of a *zhou* 州. It was established under Northern Wei 魏, in 444. Its seat of administration was in present-day Chao yang 朝陽 city in Liao ning 遼寧. Its territory of administration comprised a region including the watersheds of the Da ling he 大凌河, the Xiao ling he 小凌河, the Liu gu he 六股河 and the Nu er he 女兒河 in southwest present-day Liao ning. At the end of the *yong an* 永

安 reign period (528 – 530), the *zhou* was abolished. It was reestablished under Eastern Wei, during the *tian ping* 天平 reign period (534 – 537). Subsequently, its administrative area was gradually reduced. It was abolished during the Sui 隋, at the beginning of the *da ye* 大業 reign period (605 – 618). It was reestablished at the beginning of Tang 唐. In 696, the area fell to the Khitan. In 699 the seat of administration was moved over by name to present-day Ji 薊 county in Tian jin 天津. In 717, the seat of administration was returned to Liu cheng 柳城, the present-day Long cheng 龍城. In 742, the area became Liu cheng commandery. In 758, it again became Ying zhou. Later, it was abolished. Mentioned with 1205.

Ying zhou 瀛洲 [1]
Legendary place name. Its location is unknown. Mentioned with 62.

Ying zhou 英州 [4]
Name of a *zhou* 州. It was established under Five Dynasties' Southern Han 漢, in 947. Its seat of administration was in present-day Ying de 英德 city in Guang dong 廣東. Its territory of administration corresponded to the territory of present-day Ying de city in Guang dong. In 1195, the status of the area was raised to be Ying de fu 英德府. Mentioned with 680, 1279, 1340.

Yong 邕 [2]
Name of a *zhou* 州. See → Yong zhou 邕州. Mentioned with 909, 1427.

Yong 雍 [3 + 1]
□ Name of a *zhou* 州. [3] See → Yong zhou 雍州 (1). Mentioned with 298, 1004, 1306.
□ Name of a *zhou* 州. [1] See → Yong zhou 雍州 (2). Mentioned with 1551.

Yong 永 [3]
Name of a *zhou* 州. See →*yong zhou* 永州. Mentioned with 56, 160, 474.

Yong chang 永昌 [9]
Name of a commandery. See → Yong chang jung 永昌郡. Mentioned with 292, 493, 794, 799, 1264, 1375, 1486.

Yong chang jun 永昌郡 [2]
Name of a commandery. It was founded under Eastern Han 漢, in 69. Its seat of administration was in present-day Cao jian 漕澗 town, located 70 *li* southwest of Yun long 雲龍 county in Yun nan 雲南. Its territory of administration comprised the broad area of present-day Dian xi 滇西 (western Yun nan) and Dian nan 滇南 (southern Yunnan). In the West it reached to Ba te kai 巴特開 mountain on the border with India and Myanmar. In the Southeast it reached to Ai lao 哀牢 mountain between the Li she 禮社 river and the Ba bian 把邊 river, and in the South ít included present-day Xi shuang ban na 西雙版納. After 76, the seat of administration was at present-day Jin ji 金雞 village, 22 *li* northeast of Bao shan 保山 city in Yun nan. Under Three Kingdoms' Shu 蜀, it was subordinated to the Lai xiang Commander-in-Chief, Lai xiang *du du* 庲降都督. In 225, its administrative area in the East no longer comprised the area of the Er hai 洱海. Under Western Jin 晉, in 271, it was subordinated to Ning zhou 寧州. In 299, the seat of administration was moved to the borders of the Wa 佤 nation-

ality independent county of the Yun nan Geng ma tai 耿馬傣 nationality. Under Southern Qi 齊, the administration was moved to Yong an 永安 county, the present-day location of which is unknown. At the end of Southern Dynasties' Liang 梁, it was abolished. Mentioned with 379, 1069.

Yong ji 雍冀 [1]
Combined regional designation. This is Yong zhou 雍州 and Ji zhou 冀州, both of pre-Qin 秦 times. Mentioned with 1538.

Yong jia 永嘉 [6+ 2]
□ Name of a county. [6] It was founded under Sui 隋, in 589. Its seat of administration was in present-day Wen zhou 溫州 city in Zhe jiang 浙江. In 1958, the seat of administration was moved to present-day Shang tang 上塘 town. Mentioned with 646, 1149, 1296, 1376, 1521.
□ Name of a commandery. [2] It was founded under Eastern Jin 晉, in 323. Its seat of administration was in present-day Wen zhou 溫州 city in Zhe jiang 浙江. Its territory of administration comprised present-day Wen zhou city, and the two present-day counties of Yong jia and Yue qing 樂清, as well as the region south of the watershed of the Fei yun 飛雲 river in Zhe jiang. The commandery was abolished under Sui 隋, in 589. Under Tang 唐, in 742, it was reestablished as Wen zhou. It was abolished in 758. Mentioned with 790.

Yong kang 永康 [1]
Name of a county. It was established under Three Kingdoms' Wu 吳, in 245. Its seat of administration was in present-day Yong kang 永康 city in Zhe jiang 浙江. In 1992, it was changed to be Yong kang city. Mentioned with 368.

Yong ning wei 永寧衛 [1]
Name of a guard. It was established under Ming 明, in 1371, and subordinated to the Gui zhou Regional Military Commission, Gui zhou *du si* 貴州都司. Its seat of administration was at present-day Xi cheng 西城 of Xu yong 敘永 county in Si chuan 四川. In 1612, it was transferred to the Si chuan Regional Military Commission, Si chuan *du si* 四川都司. Under Qing 清, in 1687, it was changed to be Yong ning 永寧 county. Mentioned with 569.

Yong shun 永順 [1]
This is the name of a Pacification Office, *xuan wei si* 宣慰司. It was established under Ming 明, in 1373. Its seat of administration was in Lao si cheng 老司城, located southeast of Yong shun county in present-day Hu nan 湖南. Under Qing 清, in 1726, Yong shun 永順 sub-prefecture was established. Mentioned with 511.

Yong xing 永興 [1]
Abridged name of a *lu*. See → Yong xing jun 永興軍. Mentioned with 314.

Yong xing jun 永興軍 [1]
Name of a *lu*. It was established under Northern Song, in 1072. Its seat of administration was in present-day Xi an 西安 city in Shaan xi 陝西. Its territory of administration comprised the East of present-day Gan su 甘肅, a large part of Shaan xi, the area extending toward the West from the San men 三門 gorge in

He nan, and the southwestern corner of Shan xi 山西. Jin 金 changed it to Jing zhao fu lu 京兆府路. Mentioned with 763, 1140.

Yong yang 永陽 [1]
Name of a commandery. It was established under Tang 唐, in 742. Its seat of administration was in present-day Chu zhou 滁州 city in An hui 安徽. Its territory of administration included the cities and counties of Chu zhou, Lai an 來安 and Quan jiao 全椒 in present-day An hui. In 758, the area became Chu zhou. Mentioned with 1092.

Yong zhou 雍州 [23 + 1]
□ (1) Name of a *zhou* 州. [23] It was founded under Eastern Han 漢, in 194. Its seat of administration was in present-day Wu wei 武威 city in Gan su 甘肅. In 213, the seat of administration was moved to a location north of present-day Xi an 西安 city in Shaan xi 陝西. All of the commanderies north of the Qin ling 秦嶺 mountain range and from Hong nong 弘農 toward the West were subordinated to it. Under Three Kingdoms' Wei 魏, its territory of administration comprised the Guan zhong 關中 plateau in present-day Shaan xi, the southeastern part of Gan su 甘肅, the southern part of Ning xia 寧夏 and a strip of Qing hai 青海 south of the Yellow River. Under Sui 隋, in 607, the *zhou* was abolished and Yong zhou 雍州 became Jing zhao 京兆 commandery. Its seat of administration was in the present Xi an city. Under Tang 唐, in 618, it became Yong zhou and its administration included the area extending from the Qin ling 秦嶺 mountain range toward the North, from Qian 乾 county toward the East, from Tong chuan 銅川 city toward the South, and from Wei nan 渭南 city toward the West in present-day Shaan xi. In 713, it was changed to be Jing zhao fu 京兆府. Mentioned with 6, 32, 68, 249, 311, 353, 557, 575, 599, 619, 693, 771, 895, 927, 941, 986, 1155, 1306, 1393, 1444, 1510, 1573.
□ (2) Name of a *zhou*. [1] It was one of the nine pre-Qin 秦 *zhou* and located in present-day Shaan xi 陝西 and Gan su 甘肅 and in the eastern part of Qing hai 青海. Mentioned with 1538.

Yong zhou 邕州 [10]
Name of a *zhou* 州. It was founded under Tang 唐, in 632. Its seat of administration was in present-day Ting zi jie 亭子街 on the south bank of the Yu jiang 郁江 at Nan ning 南寧 city in Guang xi 廣西. Its territory of administration comprised Nan ning city and the present-day counties of Yong ning 邕寧, Wu ming 武鳴, Long an 隆安, Da xin 大新, Chong zuo 崇左, Shang si 上思 and Fu sui 扶綏 in Guang xi. In 742, it became Lang ning 朗寧 commandery. In 758, it again became Yong zhou. Under Five Dynasties' Jin 晉, in 942, it was changed to be Xian zhou 諴州. Southern Han 漢 restored it to Yong zhou. Northern Song 宋 moved the seat of administration to present-day Nan ning city. Under Yuan 元, in 1279, the status of the *zhou* was raised to be Yong zhou lu 邕州路. In 1324, it was changed to Nan ning lu 邕州路. Mentioned with 202, 263, 296, 332, 362, 428, 468, 1091, 1257, 1518.

Yong zhou 永州 [4]

Name of a *zhou* 州. It was established under Sui 隋, in 589. Its seat of administration was at present-day Yong zhou city in Hu nan 湖南. Its territory of administration corresponded in present-day Hu nan to Yong zhou, Dong an 東安 and Qi yang 祁陽, and in present-day Guang xi 廣西 to the city and county of Quan zhou 全州 and Guan yang 灌陽. During the *da ye* 大業 reign period of Sui, and during the *tian bao* 天寶 (742-756) and *zhi de* 至德 (756-758) reign periods of Tang 唐, the area was periodically changed to be Ling ling 零陵 commandery. During the Five Dynasties period it was divided to create Quan zhou. Yuan 元 changed the area to be Yong zhou lu 永州路.

You 幽 [1]

Name of a *zhou* 州. See → You zhou 幽州. Mentioned with 188.

You jiang 右江 [1]

Name of a river; also You xi 右溪. It is located in the Western part of Guang xi 廣西 and is one of the sources of the Yu jiang 郁江. The primary source of the You jiang is the Tuo niang 馱娘 river which originates at Long shan 龍山 mountain in Guang nan 廣南 county of Yun nan 雲南 and which flows through Xi lin 西林 to Bai se 百色 city where it combines with the river Cheng bi he 澄碧河 and is first known as the You jiang river. It flows towards the southeast and at a location northwest of Nan ning 南寧 city, near Tong jiang 同江 village, it combines with the Zuo jiang 左江 river to create the Yu jiang. Mentioned with 717.

You xi zhi shan 遊戲之山 [1]

Name of a place from the *Shan hai jing* 山海經, "Classic of Mountains and Seas." Details are lacking. Mentioned with 299.

You yan 幽燕 [2]

Combined place name. It more or less indicates the area of present-day Bei jing 北京, the northern part of He bei 河北 and a strip of Liao ning 遼寧. Mentioned with 877, 1371.

You yang 酉陽 [1]

This name refers to Xiao you 小酉 mountain. It is located 20 *li* northwest of present-day Yuan ling 沅陵 county in Hu nan 湖南.

You zhou 幽州 [10 + 1]

□ Name of a *zhou* 州. [10] It was one of the 13 *Zhou* Regional Inspector Divisions, *zhou ci shi bu* 州刺史部, established by Han Wu di 漢武帝 (r. 140-87 BCE) during Western Han 漢. During Eastern Han, its seat of administration was located southwest of present-day Bei jing 北京 city. Its territory of administration comprised the present-day Bei jing, the northern part of He bei 河北, much of Liao ning 遼寧, the area north of the Hai he 海河 river at Tian jin 天津, and the Taetong watershed in Korea. Western Jin 晉 moved the seat of administration to present-day Zhuo zhou 涿州 city in He bei. Northern Wei 魏 moved the seat of administration to Ji 薊 county. At the beginning of the *da ye* 大業 reign period (605 – 618) of Sui 隋, it was changed to Zhuo 涿 commandery, but You zhou was reestablished under Tang 唐, in 618. Its territory of administration comprised the territories of present-day Bei jing and areas associated with it, such as Tong zhou 通州, the Fang shan 房山 district and Da xing 大興 county, as well as Wu qing 武清 district of Tian jin city, and in He bei the counties of Yi xian 易縣, Yong qing 永清 and An ci 安次. In 938, under Liao 遼, the area became You du fu 幽都府, with the designation Nan jing 南京, "Southern Capital." Mentioned with 145, 164, 713, 877, 880, 883, 931, 1242, 1266, 1292, 1346, 1371, 1380.

▫ Name of a *zhou*. [1] It was one of the pre-Qin 秦 nine *zhou*. It was located in the area of present-day Bei jing, the northern part of He bei and Liao ning. Mentioned with 1538.

Yu 虞 [1]
This is a Xia 夏 era feudal country. It was located near to Li lao jia xiang 李老家鄉, 22 *li* north of present-day Yu cheng 虞城 county in He nan 河南. Mentioned with 261.

Yu 渝 [3]
Name of a *zhou*. See → Yu zhou 渝州. Mentioned with 585, 674, 781.

Yu 豫 [1]
Name of a *zhou* 州. See → Yu zhou 豫州. Mentioned with 1551.

Yu 蔚 [1]
Name of a *zhou* 州. See → Yu zhou 蔚州. Mentioned with 1037.

Yu ci 榆次 [1]
Name of a county. It was established by Qin 秦. Its seat of administration was in the present-day Yu ci district of Jin zhong 晉中 city in Shan xi 山西. Northern Wei 魏 eliminated the county in 448. It was reestablished in 500. Northern Qi 齊 eliminated it. It was reestablished under Sui 隋, in 590. In 1983, it was combined with Yu ci city. Mentioned with 702.

Yu ci zhi shan 羭次之山 [1]
Place name from the *Shan hai jing* 山海經, "Classic of Mountains and Oceans." Further details require additional research. Mentioned with 262.

Yu er 語兒 [1]
Minor place name. This is present-day Yu er 御兒. It is located southeast of present-day Chong fu 崇福 town which in turn is located southwest of Tong xiang 桐鄉 city in Zhe jiang 浙江. Mentioned with 631.

Yu er 御兒
See → Yu er 語兒

Yu gan 餘干 [1]
Name of a county. It was established by Liu Song 劉宋. Its seat of administration was in present-day Yu gan county in Jiang xi 江西. Under Yuan 元, in 1295, its status was raised to Yu gan zhou 餘干州. At the beginning of the *hong wu* 洪武 reign period (1386 – 1398) of Ming 明, it again became a county. Mentioned with 1486.

Yu hang 餘杭 [1]
Name of a commandery. It was founded under Sui 隋, in 607 by changing Hang zhou 杭州. Its seat of administration was in present-day Hang zhou city in Zhe jiang 浙江. Its territory of administration comprised the present-day regions of Hang zhou, Yu hang, Fu yang 富陽, Hai ning 海寧 and Lin an 臨安. At the beginning of the *wu de* 武德 reign period (618 – 628) of Tang 唐, the commandery was changed to be Hang zhou again. In 742, it became Yu hang again. Eventually, in 758, it was reorganized to be Hang zhou.

Yu hang shan 餘杭山 [1]
Name of a mountain. It is located near the Tai hu 太湖 lake in the southern portion of present-day Jiang su 江蘇. Mentioned with 1250.

Yu he 玉河 [1]
Name of a river. This is the present-day He tian 和田 river in southwest Xin jiang 新疆 and the region toward the East and West. Mentioned with 1406.

Yu hua tai 雨花臺 [1]
Name of minor place. It is located beyond the Zhong hua 中華 gate, south of present-day Nan jing 南京 city in Jiang su 江蘇. Mentioned with 738.

Yu lei 玉壘 [1]
Name of a mountain. It is located in the northwest corner of present-day Du jiang yan 都江堰 city in Si chuan 四川. Mentioned with 768.

Yu lin 鬱林 [1]
Name of a *zhou*. See → Yu lin zhou 鬱林州. Mentioned with 817.

Yu lin gang 榆林港 [1]
Name of a harbor. It is located southeast of present-day San ya 三亞 city in present-day Hai nan 海南 province. Mentioned with 1056.

Yu lin jun 鬱林郡 [1]
Name of a commandery It was founded under Western Han 漢, in 111 BCE. Its seat of administration was in the old city located southwest of present-day Gui ping 桂平 county in Guang xi 廣西. Its territory of administration included an area extending in present-day Guang xi from San jiang 三江, Lu zhai 鹿寨 and Gui ping toward the West, and from Yong ning 邕寧, Shang xi 上思 and Ning ming 寧明 toward the North, as well as in present-day Gui zhou 貴州 a region of the Rong jiang 榕江 and of Cao Bằng province in Vietnam. Under Three Kingdoms' Wu 吳, in 263, it was put under Guang zhou 廣州, and its administrative area was reduced. Under Southern Chen 陳, the area was more or less focused on present-day Gui ping county, the area between the Liu wan da shan 六萬大山 mountain range and Da yao shan 大瑤山 mountain and the watershed of the Yu jiang 鬱江. It was abolished under Sui 隋, in 590. Mentioned with 1427.

Yu lin zhou 鬱林州 [1]
Name of a *zhou* 州. It was created under Tang 唐, in 666, by changing the name of Yu zhou 鬱州. Its seat of administration was at a location northeast of present-day Shi nan 石南 town, northwest of Yu lin 玉林 city in Guang xi 廣西. Its administrative territory comprised the area northwest of present-day Yu lin city,

and the area southeast of Gui gang 貴港 city in Guang xi province. Under Five Dynasties' Southern Han 漢, it was administered from the south bank of the Yu 鬱 River southeast of present-day Gui gang city. Under Northern Song 宋, in 972, it was moved again to Shi nan town, located northwest of present-day Yu lin city. In 996, it was moved to present-day Yu lin city. Under Qing 清, in 1725, its status was raised to directly administered *zhou, zhi li zhou* 直隸州. Mentioned with 474.

Yu men 玉門 [1]
This is a legendary place name.

Yu qian 於潛 [1]
Name of a county. [1] It was established by Eastern Han 漢. Its seat of administration was in Yu qian town, located 60 *li* west of Lin an 臨安 county in present-day Zhe jiang 浙江. In 1958, it was incorporated into Lin an. Mentioned with 298, 1182.

Yu qing xian 虞卿縣 [1]
Name as used by the BCGM authors it is an error for Yu xiang xian 虞鄉縣. This is the name of a county. It was established under Northern Zhou 周, in 561. Its seat of administration was in present-day Gu cheng 古城 village, located 20 *li* northeast of Yong ji 永濟 city in Shan xi 山西. Under Sui 隋, in 613, the seat of administration was moved to Xie zhou 解州, located 35 *li* southwest of present-day Yun cheng 運城 city in Shan xi 山西. Under Tang 唐, in 618, the area became Xie 解 county. Tang also established a Yu xiang county at Yu xiang 虞鄉 town, located 35 *li* east of present-day Yong ji city. In 648, this was combined with Xie county. In 691, it was reestablished. Under Yuan 元, in 1266, it was eliminated. It was reestablished under Qing 清, in 1730. In 1954, it was combined with Xie county to create Xie yu 解虞 county. Mentioned with 1014.

Yu shan 玉山 [1]
This is the name of a county. See → Yu shan xian 玉山縣. Mentioned with 849.

Yu shan 羽山 [1]
Name of a mountain. There are many places it could be and details are lacking. One tradition locates the mountain northwest of present-day Dong hai 東海 county in Jiang su 江蘇, a place on the border of Lin shu 臨沭 county in Shan dong 山東. Another tradition puts it 70 *li* northeast of present-day Tan cheng 郯城 county in Shan dong. Yet another tradition places it 30 *li* southeast of present-day Peng lai 蓬萊 city in Shan dong. Mentioned with 1532.

Yu shan xian 玉山縣 [1]
Name of a county. It was established under Tang 唐, in 695. Its seat of administration was in Dong jin qiao 津橋 of the Lin gang xiang 林崗鄉 station, located two *li* east of Yu shan 玉山 county in present-day Jiang xi 江西. Later it was moved to Yu shan county. Mentioned with 292.

Yu tian 玉田 [2]
Name of a county. See → Yu tian xian 玉田縣. Mentioned with 235.

Yu tian 於闐 [5]

Name of a county in the western regions. The name has undergone various permutations over time but this form renders an *Odan which is now Khotan, although the Han 漢 period Yu tian was on a slightly different site. See → Yu tian guo 于闐國. Mentioned with 1406.

Yu tian 于闐 [2]

Name of a county in the western regions. The name is a variant of Yu tian 於闐 and designates what is present-day Khotan. Mentioned with 62, 1192.

Yu tian guo 于闐國 [2]

Name of an ancient country in the western regions with various orthographic forms. This was one of the 36 countries of the western regions in Han 漢 times. The ruins of the old Khotan capital are the Yotkan ruins 20 *li* west of present-day He tian xian 和田縣 city in present-day Xin jiang 新疆. Mentioned with 895, 958.

Yu tian xian 玉田縣 [2]

Name of a county. It was established under Tang 唐, in 696. Its seat of administration was in present-day Yu tian 玉田 county in He bei 河北. Mentioned with 111.

Yu yang 漁陽 [1 + 1]

□ Name of a commandery. It was established by Yan 燕 during the Warring States period. Its seat of administration was located southwest of present-day Mi yun 密雲 county of Bei jing 北京 city. Its territory of administration comprised a region of present-day Yan shan 燕山 and the Jing jin 京津 plain. During the era of the Northern Dynasties, the seat of administration was relocated to the plain. The commandery was abolished at the beginning of the *kai huang* 開皇 reign period (581 – 600) of Sui 隋. Mentioned with 1004.

□ Name of a county. It was established by the Sui 隋. Its seat of administration was located in present-day Ji 薊 county of Tian jin 天津. It was abolished at the beginning of the *hong wu* 洪武 reign period (1368 – 1398) of Ming 明. Mentioned with 23.

Yu zhang 豫章 [7]

Name of a commandery. See → Yu zhang jun 豫章郡. Mentioned with 44, 637, 926, 1412, 1453, 1532.

Yu zhang jun 豫章郡 [1]

Name of a commandery. It was established under Western Han 漢, in 201 BCE. Its seat of administration was at a location east of present-day Nan chang 南昌 city in Jiang xi 江西. During Han times, its administrative territory corresponded to the area of present-day Jiang xi province. After Three Kingdoms' Wei 魏, the territory of administration was made smaller. Under Southern Dynasties' Chen 陳, during the *yong ding* 永定 reign period (557 – 559), the seat of administration was moved to the Hong shi gang 紅石崗 hill, located west of present-day Nan chang city. The administrative area of the commandery comprised present-day Nan chang and Zhang shu 樟樹 and the watershed of the Jin jiang 錦江 in Jiang xi. Under Sui 隋, in 589, the commandery was abolished and Hong zhou

洪州 established instead. In 607, it again became Yu zhang 豫章 commandery. In 622, it again was made Hong zhou, and in 742 Yu zhang commandery again. The seat of administration of the commandery had been moved to within the present-day city of Nan chang. In 758, the area again became Hong zhou. Mentioned with 1516.

Yu zhou 鬱州 [1]

This Yu zhou, or Yu zhou 鬱洲, was originally an island in the ocean. During the reign of the Qing Emperor Kang xi 康熙 (1654 – 1722) it was linked up with the mainland. It is now Yun tai 雲臺 mountain of Lian yun gang 連雲港 city in Jiang su 江蘇. Mentioned with 272, 462, 1443.

Yu zhou 豫州 [1 + 2]

□ Name of a *zhou* 州. [2] It was established by Western Han 漢. Its territory of administration corresponded to an area of Yu dong 豫東 and Wan bei 皖北 extending from the Huai 淮 river toward the North, and from Fu niu 伏牛 mountain toward the East. The administrative seat under Eastern Han was in present-day Bo zhou 亳州 city in An hui 安徽. Three Kingdoms' Wei 魏 moved the seat of administration to the southern bank of the Nan ru 南汝 river northeast of present-day Zheng yang 正陽 county in He nan 河南. Western Jin 晉 moved the seat of administration to present-day Huai yang 淮陽 county in He nan. Later, it was moved frequently and the location was not constant. The administrative area also was reduced in size and also altered without anything being set. During the Sixteen Kingdoms era under Former Zhao 趙, the seat of administration was moved to a location east of present-day Xu chang 許昌 city in He nan. Former Qin 秦 changed Yu zhou to be Dong yu zhou 東豫州. It established another Yu zhou administration northeast of present-day Luo yang 洛陽 city in He nan, the capital from Han to Wei 魏. Northern Wei 魏 changed it to Luo zhou 洛州, and it also changed the Si zhou 司州 of Liu Song 劉宋 to be Yu zhou. Its seat of administration was at present-day Ru nan 汝南 county in He nan. Northern Zhou 周 changed it to be Yu zhou 舒州. At the beginning of Sui 隋, it was again changed to be Yu zhou 豫州. At the beginning of the *da ye* 大業 reign period (605 – 618), it became Cai zhou 蔡州. Another Yu zhou administration was set up at present-day Luo yang city in He nan. In 607, it became He nan commandery. At the beginning of Tang 唐, Yu zhou was reestablished. Its seat of administration was at present-day Ru nan county in He nan. At the beginning of the Tang *bao ying* 寶應 reign period (762-763), the area became Cai zhou. Mentioned with 261.

□ Name of a *zhou*. [2] The area was one of the nine pre-Qin 秦 *zhou*. Mentioned with 423, 536, 1004, 1538.

Yu zhou 渝州 [1]

Name of a *zhou* 州. It was founded under Sui 隋, in 581, by changing Chu zhou 楚州. Its seat of administration was in part of what is present-day Chong qing 重慶 city in Si chuan 四川. In 607, it was changed to be Ba 巴 commandery. Under Tang 唐, in 618, the area again become Yu zhou. In 742, the area was changed to be Nan ping 南平 commandery. It became Yu zhou again in 758. Its territory of administration comprised present-day Chong qing, and the cities and counties of Jiang jin 江津, Bi shan 璧山, and Yong chuan 永川. In 1102, it was changed to Gong zhou 恭州. Mentioned with 1359.

Yu zhou 蔚州 [2]

Name of a *zhou* 州. It was founded under Northern Wei 魏, during the *Yong an* 永安 reign period (528 – 530), from the two garrisons Huai huang 懷荒 and Yu yi 御夷. Its seat of administration was in the region of present-day Zhang bei 張北 and Chi cheng 赤城 in present-day He bei 河北. Later, the seat of administration was moved to within the boundaries of present-day Shan xi 山西. During Tang 唐, at the beginning of the *kai yuan* 開元 reign period (713 – 741), the seat of administration was moved to present-day Yu 蔚 county in He bei. After that time, its administrative area comprised Yang yuan 陽原, Yu county, Lai yuan 淶源 county in present-day He bei, and the counties of Yang gao 陽高, Tian zhen 天鎮, Guang ling 廣靈 and Ling qiu 靈丘 in present-day Shan xi. During Qing 清 times, the *zhou* only controlled the single territory of Yu county. In 1913, the *zhou* was changed to be a county. Mentioned with 122, 595.

Yuan 袁 [1]

Name of a *zhou* 州. See → Yuan zhou 袁州.

Yuan an xian 遠安縣 [1]

Name of a county. It was founded by Northern Zhou 周, in 559. Its seat of administration was in present-day Jiu xian 舊縣 town, located northwest of Yuan an 遠安 county in Hu bei 湖北. Under Ming 明, in 1468, the seat of administration was moved to present-day Yuan an county. During the *chong zhen* 崇禎 reign period (1628 – 1644), it was moved to a location southwest of Yuan an county. Under Qing 清, during the reign of Emperor Kang xi 康熙 (1661 – 1722), the administration was moved backed again to Yuan an county. Mentioned with 381.

Yuan jiang 沅江 [3]

Name of a county. It was founded under Sui 隋, in 598. Its seat of administration was in present-day Yuan jiang city in Hu nan 湖南. During the *qian yuan* 乾元 reign period (758 – 760), the area was named Qiao jiang 橋江 county. Under Northern Song 宋, in 963, it again became Yuan jiang county. It was eliminated under Ming 明, in 1377, but reestablished in 1380. In 1988, in its place Yuan jiang city was established. Mentioned with 87, 664, 726.

Yuan ju 冤句 [34]

This is the name of a county. It was created under Qin 秦. Its seat of administration was at a location northwest of present-day Cao xian 曹縣 in Shan dong 山東. In 1086, it was named Yuan ting 宛亭 county. Under the Jin 金, because the area had been eaten away by the Yellow River, the county was abolished. Mentioned with 31, 53, 126, 233, 258, 369, 381, 437, 462, 525, 623, 677, 722, 740, 771, 787, 839, 911, 916, 975, 980, 1160, 1200, 1218, 1241, 1262, 1321, 1417, 1445, 1491, 1519.

Yuan qiao zhi shan 員嶠之山 [1]

Legendary mountain. Details are lacking. Mentioned with 1325.

Yuan zhou 原州 [1]

Name of a *zhou* 州. It was established under Northern Wei 魏, in 524. Its seat of administration was in Gu yuan 固原 county in present-day Ning Xia 寧夏. Its territory of administration comprised the area from Gu yuan county in present-day Ning xia to Ping liang 平涼 city in Gan su 甘肅. Under Sui 隋, in 607, the *zhou* became Ping liang commandery. At the beginning of Tang 唐, it was changed to be Yuan zhou. In 742, it was changed to be Ping liang commandery. In 758, it was made Yuan zhou again. In 763 the area was conquered by Tibet and, in 803, the seat of administration was moved to Ping liang city in present-day Gan su. In 808, it was moved again to Zhen yuan 鎮原 county in present-day Gan su. In 849, it was administered at Ping gao 平高 county. Later the seat of administration was moved to Zhen yuan county in present-day Gan su. At the beginning of Yuan 元, it became Zhen yuan zhou 鎮原州. Mentioned with 58, 297, 461, 650.

Yuan zhou 袁州 [1]

Name of a *zhou* 州. It was founded under Sui 隋, in 591. Its seat of administration was in present-day Yi chun 宜春 city in Jiang xi 江西. Its territory of administration comprised present-day Ping xiang 萍鄉 city and the watershed of the Yuan shui 袁水 extending from Xin yu 新餘 city toward the West in Jiang xi. At the beginning of the *da ye* 大業 reign period (605 – 618) of Sui 隋, the area became Yi chun commandery. Under Tang 唐, in 621, the area again became Yuan zhou. At the same time, the present-day Yi chun city became the administrative seat of the *zhou*. In 742, the area was changed to be Yi chun commandery. In 758, it again became Yuan zhou. Under the Song 宋, its administrative area, compared to the Tang, in the East it lost Xin yu 新餘, while in the North included present-day Wan zai 萬載. Under Yuan 元, during the *zhi yuan* 至元 reign period (1264 – 1294), the status of the area was raised to be Yuan zhou lu 袁州路. Mentioned with 768, 1051.

Yue 越 [1 + 17 + 9]

□ This is a general designation of the Bai yue 百越 territory, inhabited by the "one hundred Yue tribes" in the Ling nan 嶺南 region during Qin 秦 and Han 漢 times. Mentioned with 1369.

□ This is one of the Spring and Autumn Period feudal states. [17] It was established among the Yue people. The surname of the ruling family was Si 姒. During the initial period, the national capital was located in the Kuai ji 會稽 mountains. During the time of the King of Yue Gou jian 句踐, Yue gradually strengthened itself and flourished. In 490 BCE, during the seventh year of Gou Jian, a capital of Da yue 大越 was established at present-day Shao xing 紹興 city in Zhe jiang 浙江. The territory of administration of the kingdom corresponded to the central and northern part of the present-day province of Zhe jiang. In 472 BCE, under the Zhou Yuan wang 周元王, Gou Jian destroyed Wu 吳 and the capital was moved to present-day Lang ye 琅琊 town, located 46 *li* southwest of Jiao nan 膠南 city in Shan dong 山東. The Yue state then expanded to include the whole present-day province of Jiang su 江蘇 and the southern part of Shan dong. In 379 BCE, under Zhou An wang 周安王, the capital was moved to present-day Su zhou 蘇州 city in Jiang su. In 334 BCE, under Zhou Xian wang 周顯王, Yue was destroyed by Chu 楚. Mentioned with 202, 300, 423, 497, 735, 936, 1064, 1105, 1157, 1162, 1238, 1239, 1419, 1460, 1508.

□ Name of a *zhou* 州. [9] See → Yue zhou 越州. Mentioned with 100, 468, 780, 781, 871, 908, 1324, 1485.

Yue 粵 [8]

Regional name. It was part of the ancient Bai yue 百越/粵, "the hundred Yue 越" and thus the name. It corresponded to the three provinces of present-day Guang dong 廣東, Guang xi 廣西 and Hai nan 海南, and neighboring areas. Mentioned with 139, 537, 763, 1121, 1170, 1272, 1455, 1525.

Yue 岳 [12]

Name of a *zhou* 州. See → Yue zhou 岳州. Mentioned with 644, 1145.

Yue di 越地 [2]

General regional reference to the territory Bai yue 百越, inhabited by the "one hundred Yue tribes" in antiquity. This is the large region of present-day Ling nan 嶺南. Mentioned with 110, 1479.

Yue e 岳鄂 [1]

Name of a regional Defense Command, *fang zhen* 方鎮. Tang 唐, in 751, established a Chief Commissioner for Militiamen, *du tuan lian shou zhuo shi* 都團練守捉使, for the three *zhou* 州 of E 鄂, Yue 岳 and Mian 沔 but in 773 changed this and established an *E yue* 鄂岳 (Yue e 岳鄂) Surveillance Commissioner, *guan cha shi* 觀察使. It was administered from the present-day Wu chang 武昌 district of Wu Han 武漢 city in Hu bei 湖北. Its territory of administration changed over time and for the comparatively longest time it controlled the *zhou* of E, Yue, Qi 蘄, Huang 黃, An 安 and Shen 申. This corresponds to an area extending in Hu bei from the cities and counties of Guang shui 廣水, Ying cheng 應城, Han chuan 漢川 and Pu qi 蒲圻 toward the East, in He nan 河南 the area south of the Huai he 淮河, and in Hu nan 湖南 from Dong ting 洞庭 lake and Mi luo jiang 汨羅江 toward the North. It was once changed to be the Military Commissioner of the Wu chang Army, *Wu chang jun jie du shi* 武昌軍節度使. It was eliminated at the beginning of Northern Song 宋. Mentioned with 270.

Yue jian 越間 [5]

This term is a mistake for Yue sui 越巂. See → Yue sui. Mentioned with 73, 122, 595, 717.

Yue lun si 月輪寺 [1]

Name of a temple. It is in present-day Hang zhou 杭州 city in Zhe jiang 浙江. Mentioned with 1420.

Yue nan 越南 [2]

Regional name. Yue nan originally meant the area to the south of the Bai yue 百越 before it became a county, in 1803. During the Tang 唐 dynasty, the region of Yue nan was the equivalent to Ling nan dao 嶺南道, Ling nan 嶺南 circuit, and some surrounding areas. This included the present-day provinces of Guang dong

廣東, Guang xi 廣西 and Hai nan 海南, and the northern part of the country now called Yue nan, e.g., Vietnam. See → Nan yue. Mentioned with 386, 419.

Yue qing 樂清 [1]
Name of a county. It was established under Five Dynasties' Liang 梁, in 908. Its seat of administration was in present-day Yue qing city in Zhe jiang 浙江. In 1993, it was changed to be Yue qing city. Mentioned with 346.

Yue shan 越山
Name of a mountain. Details are lacking. Mentioned with 31.

Yue sui 越巂 [1]
Name of a commandery. It was established under Western Han 漢, in 111 BCE. Its seat of administration was at a location 5 *li* southeast of present-day Xi chang 西昌 city in Si chuan 四川. Its administrative territory comprised an area in present-day Yun nan 雲南 extending from the Na xi 納西 county of the Li jiang 麗江 toward the East, from the Jin sha jiang 金沙江 toward the West, and from Xiang yun 祥雲 and Da yao 大姚 toward the North, as well as in Si chuan from Mu li 木里, Shi jin 石棉, Gan luo 甘洛 and Lei bo 雷波 toward the South. The administrative area was reduced during the Three Kingdoms period and did not include the southern part of present-day Yun nan. In 239, the seat of administration was returned to Qiong du 邛都 county. Western Jin 晉 moved the seat of administration to present-day Hui li 會理 county in Si chuan. Liu Song 劉宋 re-established Qiong du county. Southern Qi 齊 abolished it. Mentioned with 585.

Yue wen 越轀 [1]
This is an error for the Yue sui 越巂 of the *Tai ping yu lan* 太平御覽, "Collection of the Tai ping 太平 period for the imperial view." See → Yue sui. Mentioned with 1532.

Yue yang 岳陽 [1]
Ancient honorific place name for Yue zhou 岳州 and Ba ling 巴陵. This is present-day Yue yang city in Hu nan 湖南.

Yue zhou 岳州 [2]
Name of a *zhou* 州. It was established under Sui 隋, in 589, by changing Ba zhou 巴州. Its seat of administration was at present-day Yue yang 岳陽 city in Hu nan 湖南. Its administrative territory comprised every county and city on the eastern, southern and northern banks of Dong ting 洞庭 lake in present-day Hu nan. During the *da ye* 大業 (605 – 618) reign period of the Sui, and the *tian bao* 天寶 (742 – 756) and *zhi de* 至德 (756 – 758) reign periods of the Tang 唐, the area periodically became Ba ling 巴陵 commandery. Under Southern Song 宋, in 1155, it was changed to be Chun zhou 純州, but in 1161 it again became Yue zhou. It was changed to be a *lu* 路 under Yuan 元, in 1276. At the beginning of Ming 明, it became a *fu* 府. In 1376, it again became Yue zhou. In 1381, it was changed to be a *fu*. Mentioned with 87, 780.

Yue zhou 越州 [7]
Name of a *zhou* 州. It was established under Sui 隋, in 605. Its seat of administration was in Shao xing 紹興 city in present-day Zhe jiang 浙江. Its territory of

administration comprised the watershed of the Pu yang jiang 浦陽江 (outside of Pu yang 浦陽 county), of the Cao e jiang 曹娥江 and of the Yong jiang 甬江 in Zhe jiang. In 607, it became Kuai ji 會稽 commandery. Under Tang 唐, in 621, it was again changed to be Yue zhou. Later, under Tang, it was changed again to be Kuai ji commandery. In 758, it was again changed to be Yue zhou. Under Southern Song 宋, in 1131, it was changed to be Shao xing fu 紹興府. Mentioned with 382, 499, 668, 741, 948, 991, 1324.

Yue zhou 岳州府 [2]
Name of a *fu* 府. It was established at the beginning of Ming 明. Its seat of administration was at present-day Yue yang 岳陽 city in Hu nan 湖南. Its administrative territory comprised an area on both the Western and Eastern banks of Dong ting 洞庭 lake in the northern section of present-day Hu nan. During the Qing 清, the territory of administration was limited to an area east of Dong ting lake. In 1913 the fu was abolished. Mentioned with 362, 768.

Yun 雲 [2 + 1]
□ Name of a *zhou* 州. [2] It was established under Tang 唐, in 640. Its seat of administration was in present-day Da tong 大同 city in Shan xi 山西. Its territory of administration included an area in present-day Shan xi extending from the Great Wall toward the South and from the Sang gan he 桑干河 toward the North. It was abolished in 682. It was reestablished in 730, with its seat of administration in Da tong city. In 742, it was changed to Yun zhong 雲中 commandery. At the beginning of the *qian yuan* 乾元 reign period (758 – 760), it again became Yun zhou 雲州. Under Liao 遼, in 1044, its status was raised to Da tong fu 大同府. Mentioned with 1037.
□ Abbreviated regional name. [1] See Yun nan 雲南. Mentioned with 157.

Yun an jun 雲安軍 [1]
Name of an army. It was established under Northern Song 宋, in 973. Its seat of administration was in present-day Yun yang 雲陽 town, located east of Yun yang county of Si chuan 四川. Its administrative territory comprised the area of Yun yang county in Si chuan. At the end of Southern Song, it was abolished. It was restored under Yuan 元, in 1278. In 1283, its status was raised to Yun yang zhou 雲陽州. Mentioned with 39.

Yun meng 雲夢 [3]
Regional name. It is a general reference to the hunting areas of the King of Chu 楚 during the Spring and Autumn and Warring States period. By and large this included the entire Yang zi and Han 漢 plateau and a portion of the hilly areas located on the east, west and north sides. In the South, during the Spring and Autumn period, it also included the Jiang nan 江南 area south of Ying du 郢都. During the Warring States period, the area was limited to north of the Yang zi. Mentioned with 1081, 1084, 1400.

Yun meng shan 雲夢山 [1]
Name of a mountain. It is at present-day Yan zhou 兗州 city in Shan dong 山東. Mentioned with 1430.

Yun nan 雲南 [21 + 9 + 3]

□ This is an abbreviation for the Yun nan Provincial Administration Commission, Yun nan *bu zheng shi si* 雲南布政使司. [21] It was established under Ming 明, in 1382, and its seat of administration was in present-day Kun ming 昆明 city in Yun nan 雲南. Its territory of administration comprised Yun nan province as well as parts of present-day Myanmar, Thailand, Laos and Vietnam. The Qing 清 changed it to be Yun nan province. Mentioned with 80, 157, 202, 404, 511, 535, 574, 698, 730, 861, 1057, 1109, 1120, 1139, 1236, 1239, 1248, 1265, 1272, 1369.

□ Regional name. [9] From Tang 唐 times on, this was used as a general designation of the area of Yun nan. It referred generally to Tang era Nan zhao 南詔, the Da li 大理 kingdom of Song 宋 and the province of Yun nan of Yuan 元 times. During the Ming-era, it became the Yun nan Provincial Administration Commission, *Yun nan bu zheng shi si* 雲南布政使司. Mentioned with 14, 80, 404, 535, 664, 943, 1177, 1375.

□ Name of a commandery. [3] It was established under Three Kingdoms Shu 蜀, in 225. Its seat of administration was in Jiu cheng 舊城, located 17 *li* northwest of present-day Yao an 姚安 county in Yun nan. Its administration included the northwest portions of present-day Yun nan, and more or less corresponded to an area extending from Chu xiong 楚雄 city toward the West, from Nan Jian 南澗 county toward the North, from the Lan cang jiang 瀾滄江 toward the East, and from the Jin sha jiang 金沙江 toward the South. Under Western Jin 晉, the seat of administration was within the boundaries of Bin chuan 賓川 county in Yun nan. Eastern Jin moved the seat of administration to a location 34 *li* southeast of Xiang yun 祥雲 county in Yun nan. Its territory of administration comprised a strip of territory reaching from Nan jian county north toward Ning lang 寧蒗 county in Yun nan. Under Southern Qi 齊, it was administered from within the boundaries of present-day Yong sheng 永勝 county in Yun nan. Its administrative area included the present-day counties of Nan jian, Wei shan 巍山, Xiang yun, Bin chuan, Yong sheng and Hua ping 華坪 in Yun nan. It was abolished at the end of Liang 梁. Mentioned with 73, 1369, 1497.

Yun shan 雲山 [2]

Name of a mountain. It is located 15 *li* northwest of Ning yang 寧陽 county in Shan dong 山東. Mentioned with 1344.

Yun tai shu 雲臺戍 [2]

Name of a military area. It was located in the Onon-Kerlen watershed in the eastern part of what is now Mongolia. Further details require additional research. Mentioned with 964, 1433.

Yun yang 雲陽 [1 + 1]

□ The BCGMs reference to the Southern Commandery of Yun yang, Yun nan nan jun 雲陽南郡, is a mistake for Yun nan commandery, Yun nan jun 雲南郡. [1] See → Yun nan 雲南. Mentioned with 1069.

□ Name of a mountain. [1] It is located in the western part of present-day Hu nan 湖南. Further details require additional research. Mentioned with 1069.

Yun yang xian 雲陽縣 [1]

Name of a county. This Yun yang 雲陽 county is an error for Yun nan 雲南 county. It was established under Western Han 漢, in 109 BCE. Its seat of administration was at Guo cheng 果城 which is located northeast of Yun nan yi 雲南驛, which in turn lies 34 *li* southeast of present-day Xiang yun 祥雲 county in Yun nan. It was abolished under Qi and its territory was made part of Yun ping 雲平 county. Mentioned with 1069.

Yun zhong 雲中 [3 + 1]

□ Name of a commandery. [3] It was established during the Warring States Period of Wu ling wang 武靈王 (ca. 340 – 295) of Zhao 趙. During Qin 秦 times, it was administered from Gu cheng 古城 located northeast of Toqto county in present-day Inner Mongolia. Its administrative territory comprised an area in present-day Inner Mongolia extending from the right banner of the Tumed toward the North, from Da qing 大青 mountain toward the South, from Zhuo zi 卓資 county toward the West, as well as from the southern shore of the Yellow River and the Great Wall toward the North. During Western Han 漢, its administrative area was reduced. At the end of Eastern Han the commandery was abolished. Mentioned with 689, 724, 1211.

□ Name of a commandery. [1] It was established under Tang 唐, in 742. Its seat of administration was in present-day Da tong 大同 city in Shan xi 山西. Its territory of administration comprised in present-day Shan xi Da tong city and the counties of Zuo yun 左雲, You yu 右玉, Huai ren 懷仁, Hun yuan 渾源, Da tong and Yang gao 陽高, in Inner Mongolia the forward banner of the right wing of the Chakar, as well as the areas of Xing he 興和 and Feng zhen 豐鎮, and in He bei 河北 parts of the areas of Shang yi 尚義 and Huai an 懷安. In 758, the commandery again became Yun zhou 雲州. Mentioned with 724.

Yun zhou 鄆州 [3]

Name of a *zhou* 州. It was founded under Sui 隋, in 590. Its seat of administration was at a location 16 *li* northeast of present-day Yun cheng 鄆城 county in Shan dong 山東. Its territory of administration corresponded to present-day Dong ping 東平, Liang shan 梁山, Yun cheng and Ju ye 巨野 in Shan dong. At the beginning of the *da ye* 大業 reign period (605 – 618) of the Sui, and during the *tian bao* 天寶 (742 – 756) and *zhi de* 至德 (756 – 758) reign periods of the Tang 唐, the area periodically became Dong ping commandery. Northern Song 宋 moved the seat of administration to present-day Dong ping county and the territory of the *zhou* was reduced. In 1119, its status was raised to Dong ping fu 東平府. Mentioned with 268, 1155, 1573.

-Z-

Zan 贊 [1]
Error made by the BCGM authors. The character should be *fu* 鄜. See → Fu zhou 鄜州. Mentioned with 1462.

Zan zhou 贊州 [1]
Erroneous writing of → Fu zhou 鄜州. Mentioned with 631.

Zang ke 牂牁 [6]
Name of a commandery. It was established under Western Han 漢, in 111 BCE. Its seat of administration was at a location southwest of present-day Huang ping 黄平 county in Gui zhou 貴州. Its territory of administration included most of present-day Gui zhou, the northwestern part of Guang xi 廣西 and the eastern part of Yun nan 雲南. During Western Jin 晉, the seat of administration was moved to a location northeast of present-day Weng an 甕安 county in Gui zhou. The territory of administration was equivalent to the area between Yi jie 畢節, Zun yi 遵義, Ce heng 冊亨, Li bo 荔波 and Huang ping in present-day Gui zhou province, and Nan dan 南丹 county in Guang xi. Southern Qi 齊 changed it to be Nan zhang ke 南牂牁 commandery. Mentioned with 367, 585, 696, 1177, 1395.

Ze 澤 [14]
Name of a *zhou* 州. See → Ze zhou 澤州. Mentioned with 111, 178, 644, 1134, 1178.

Ze zhou 澤州 [10]
Name of a *zhou* 州. It was founded at the beginning of the *kai huang* reign period (581 – 600) of Sui 隋. Its seat of administration was in present-day Gao du 高都 town, located 30 *li* northeast of Jin cheng 晉城 city in Shan xi 山西. Its territory of administration covered Jin cheng 晉城 city in present-day Shan xi along with the counties of Qin shui 沁水, Gao ping 高平, Ling chuan 陵川 and Yang cheng 陽城. Under Tang 唐, in 618, a separate Ze zhou was established. It was administered at present-day Yang cheng county in Shan xi. In 625, the seat of administration was moved to present-day Duan shi 端氏 town, located 60 *li* east of Qin shui county in Shan xi. In 627, it was moved to the present-day Jin cheng city. In 1128, under Jin 金, it was changed to be Nan ze zhou 南澤州, and in 1151 became Ze zhou again. In 1728, its status was raised to Ze zhou fu 澤州府. Mentioned with 47, 698, 748, 931, 1182, 1250, 1383, 1438.

Zeng bin 鋥賓 [1]
Name of an ancient country in what is now Kashmir. Mentioned with 1427.

Zeng cheng 曾城 [1]
This is a mythical city of nine layers said to be on Mount Kun lun 崑崙. Mentioned with 895.

Zhan bei guo 占卑國 [1]
Name of an ancient country at the time of the Tang 唐.era. It was located in the present-day province of Jambi in the southeastern part of the Indonesian island of Sumatra. Mentioned with 842.

Zhan cheng 占城 [5]
Name of an ancient country. See → Zhan cheng guo 占城國. Mentioned with 144, 511, 535, 1139.

Zhan cheng guo 占城國 [3]
This is the name of an ancient country. Also called Zhan po 占婆. The early country was located in the central-eastern part of present-day Vietnam, around Hue. From Han 漢 to Tang 唐, the area was called Lin yi 林邑. From the *zhi de* 至德 reign period (756 – 758) of Tang on, it was called Huan wang 環王. After the 9th century the area became known as Zhan cheng 占城. In 1471, the area was conquered by the Nhà Hậu Lê kingdom. At the end of the 17th century, the area was lost to Qung Nam Nguyn Chúa. Mentioned with 492, 1269.

Zhang 漳 [1]
Name of a *zhou*. See under → Zhang zhou 漳州. Mentioned with 674.

Zhang an 章安 [1]
Name of a county. It was established under Eastern Han 漢. Its seat of administration was in present-day Zhang an town on the northern bank of the Jiao jiang 椒江 at Tai zhou 台州 city in Zhe jiang 浙江. It was eliminated under Sui 隋, in 589, but restored under Tang, in 621. Four years later, in 625, it was abolished. Mentioned with 328.

Zhang de 彰德 [2]
Name of an army. It was founded by Later Jin 晉, in 938. Its seat of administration was in present-day An yang 安陽 city in He nan 河南. Its administrative territory comprised an area extending in present-day He bei 河北 from Lin zhang 臨漳 county toward the South, in He nan from Lin zhou 林州 and Hui xian 輝縣 toward the East, from Fan xian 范縣 county and Qing feng 清豐 county toward the West, and from the Yellow River toward the North. The army was abolished at the beginning of Northern Song 宋. Mentioned with 1051, 1478.

Zhang ming 彰明 [1]
Name of a county. → Zhang ming xian 彰明縣. Mentioned with 322.

Zhang ming xian 彰明縣 [1]
Name of a county. It was established by Five Dynasties' Tang 唐. Its seat of administration was in present-day Zhang ming 彰明 town, located south of Jiang you 江油 city in Si chuan 四川. In 1377, under Ming 明, it was abolished and made part of Mian xian 綿縣 county. In 1380, it was restored. In 1958, it was combined with Jiang you 江油 county. Mentioned with 322.

Zhang shan 鄣山 [1]
This reference is an erroneous reference to Zhang shan 障山, present-day name Zhang shan 章山. It is located 40 *li* east of present-day An lu 安陸 city in Hu bei 湖北. Mentioned with 1435.

Zhang wu 章武 [1]

Name of a county. It was established under Western Han 漢, in 157 BCE, when Dou Guangguo 竇廣國 became the "Lord of Zhang wu", Zhang wu hou 章武侯. In 122 BCE, the area became a county and was administered from present-day Gu xian 古縣 village located southwest of Huang hua 黃驊 city in He bei 河北. Northern Qi 齊 abolished it. Mentioned with 471.

Zhang xian 鄣縣 [1]

Name of a county. It was established by Eastern Han 漢. Its seat of administration was at a location 5 *li* southwest of present-day Zhang xian 鄣縣 county in Gan su 甘肅. It was abolished after the *yong jia* 永嘉 reign period (307 – 313) of Western Jin 晉. When it was reestablished under Northern Wei 魏, in 502, the name was changed to Zhang 彰 county. Sui 隋 changed it to be Zhang xian 障縣 county but ,at the beginning of Tang, the name Zhang xian 鄣縣 county was restored. In 691, it was changed to Wu yang 武陽 county. During the *shen long* 神龍 reign period (705 – 707), it again became Zhang xian 鄣縣 county. During the *guang de* 廣德 reign period (763 – 764), the area was conquered by Tibet. Under Yuan 元, in 1280, it was reestablished at Gu cheng yu 古城峪 where it had been formerly administered. At the beginning of Ming 明, the area was named Zhang xian 漳縣. Mentioned with 471.

Zhang ye 張掖 [3]

Name of a commandery. It was founded under Western Han 漢, in 111 BCE. Its seat of administration was at a location 40 *li* northwest of present-day Zhang ye 張掖 city in Gan su 甘肅. Its territory of administration comprised an area in Gan su extending from Yong chang 永昌 county toward the West and from Gao tai 高台 county toward the East. Sui 隋, in 583, at first eliminated it, but restored it in 607. At the beginning of Tang 唐, the area was changed to be Gan zhou 甘州. In 742, the area again became Zhang ye commandery. In 758, it was changed to Gan zhou again. Mentioned with 1282, 1335.

Zhang zhou 漳州 [1 + 1]

□ Name of a *zhou* 州. [1] It was founded under Tang 唐, in 686. Its seat of administration was in present-day Yun xiao 雲霄 county in Fu jian 福建. In 716, the seat of administration was moved to present-day Zhang pu 漳浦 county. Following the *da li* 大歷 reign period (766 – 779), its administrative area comprised the watershed of the Jiu long jiang 九龍江 and the area southwest of this in Fu jian. During Five Dynasties' Tang, in 945, the area was named Nan zhou 南州. Under Northern Song 宋, in 966, it again became Zhang zhou. Under Yuan 元, in 1279, its status was raised to Zhang zhou lu 漳州路. Mentioned with 674.
□ Name of a *fu* 府. [1] It was established under Ming 明, in 1368, and administered in present-day Zhang zhou city in Fu jian. Its territory of administration comprised the Jiu long jiang watershed and the areas southwest of this. The *fu* was abolished in 1913. Mentioned with 1454.

Zhang zi shan 長子山 [1]

Name of a mountain. It is located southwest of the present Zhang zi 長子 county in Shan xi 山西. Mentioned with 131.

Zhang zi xian 長子縣 [1]

Name of a county. It was established by Qin 秦 and was placed under Shang dang 上黨 commandery. It was administered at a location 8 *li* southwest of the present Zhang zi 長子 county in Shan xi 山西. Mentioned with 131.

Zhao 趙 [3]

Name of an ancient country. See → Zhao guo 趙國. Mentioned with 1110, 1137, 1242.

Zhao guo 趙國 [2]

Name of an ancient country. Mu wang 繆王 (ruled 235 – 228) of Western Zhou 周 enfeoffed Zao Fu 造父 with Zhao cheng 趙城. The ruins are located southwest of present-day Zhao cheng town north of Hong dong 洪洞 county in Shan xi 山西. Under King Wei lie 威烈 of Zhou 周, in 403, Zhao Lie hou 趙烈侯, Han 韓 and Wei 魏 partitioned Jin 晉. The capital was established at a location southwest of present-day Tai yuan 太原 city in Shan xi. In 386, the capital was moved to present-day Han dan 邯鄲 city in He bei 河北. The territory of the county embraced the southwestern part of present-day He bei, the central part of Shan xi and a corner of the northeastern part of Shaan xi 陝西. During the time of King Wu ling 武靈 (ca. 340-295) of Zhao, Yun zhong 雲中, Yan men 雁門 and Dai 代 commandery were established embracing the northern part of present-day Shan xi 山西, the western part of He bei and the Great Bend of the Yellow River. Zhao then formed one of the seven most powerful of the Warring States. In 222 BCE, it was destroyed by Qin 秦. Mentioned with 1389.

Zhao jun 趙郡 [1]

Name of a commandery. It was established by Eastern Han 漢, in 212. Its seat of administration was in present-day Han dan 邯鄲 city in He bei 河北. Its territory of administration corresponded to the present-day counties of Zhao xian 趙縣, Yuan shi 元氏, Gao yi 高邑, Nei qiu 內丘, Lin cheng 臨城, Bai xiang 柏鄉 and Zan huang 贊皇, and portions of the two counties of Ping xiang 平鄉 and Long yao 隆堯 in present-day He bei. Under Three Kingdoms Wei 魏, in 232, the area became Zhao guo 趙國. The seat of administration was moved to a location southwest of present-day Gao yi county. At the end of Western Jin 晉, the area again became Zhao commandery. Northern Wei 魏 moved the seat of administration to Zhao county, and the territory of administration was reduced. It corresponded to the present-day counties of Zhao xian 趙縣, Yuan shi, Gao yi and Bai xiang in He bei. It was abolished at the beginning of Sui 隋. Mentioned with 816.

Zhao ling 召陵 [1]

Name of an ancient city. It was a city of Spring and Autumn period Chu 楚 and located at present-day Zhao ling zhai 召陵寨, 30 *li* east of Yan cheng 郾城 in He nan 河南. Mentioned with

Zhao qing 肇慶 [1]

Name of a *fu*. See → Zhao qing fu. Mentioned with 772.

Zhao qing fu 肇慶府 [1]

Name of a *fu* 府. It was founded under Northern Song 宋, in 1118, by raising the status of Duan zhou 端州. Its seat of administration was in present-day Zhao qing city in Guang dong 廣東. Its territory of administration comprised the three present-day cities of Zhao qing 肇慶, Gao yao 高要, and Si hui 四會 and the area of Guang ning 廣寧 county in Guang dong. Yuan 元 turned it into Zhao qing lu 肇慶路. Early Ming 明 restored it as Zhao qing fu. Its territory extended more or less over the watersheds of the Xi jiang 西江, the Sui jiang 綏江, the Xin xing jiang 新興江 and the Mo yang jiang 漠陽江 and the area of present-day Kai ping 開平 city in Guang dong 廣東. It was abolished in 1911. Mentioned with 972.

Zhao wa 爪哇 [3]

Name of an ancient country. This is present-day Java (Jaba) in Indonesia. Mentioned with 700, 1139, 1236.

Zhe 浙 [15 + 10 + 3 + 2]

□ Administrative unit. [15] This is an abbreviation for the Zhe jiang Provincial Administration Commission, Zhe jiang *cheng xuan bu zheng shi si* 浙江承宣布政使司. See under → Zhe jiang 浙江. Mentioned with 133, 198, 322, 351, 572, 608, 735, 766, 807, 1057, 1149, 1170, 1375, 1485.

□ Abbreviation for the Liang zhe dong lu 兩浙東路 and the Liang zhe xi lu 兩浙西路. [10] The term in general refers to the entire province of Zhe jiang 浙江 and a southern corner of Jiang su 江蘇. Mentioned with 130, 185, 202, 389, 482, 730, 768, 1017, 1036, 1471, 1493.

□ Abbreviation for Zhe jiang 浙江 province. [3] It was established under Yuan 元 by the Ming 明 rebels led by Zhu Yuan zhang 朱元璋, in 1366. Its seat of administration was in present-day Hang zhou 杭州 city in Zhe jiang 浙江. Its territory of administration comprised the whole province of Zhe jiang 浙江 outside of present-day Jia xing 嘉興 city, Hu zhou 湖州 city and Sheng xi 嵊泗 county. In 1376, the area was changed to be the Zhe jiang Provincial Administration Commission. Mentioned with 807, 988, 1067.

□ Name of a river, the present-day Qian tang jiang 錢塘江. [2] Mentioned with 639, 793.

Zhe cheng xian 柘城縣 [2]

Name of a county. It was established under Sui 隋, in 596. Its seat of administration was at a location north of present-day Zhen cheng county in He nan 河南. During the *jia qing* 嘉靖 reign period (1522-1566), the seat of administration was moved to Zhe cheng 柘城 county. Mentioned with 298, 428.

Zhe dong 浙東 [4 + 2]

□ Regional name. [4] It by and large designates the area east and south of the Qian tang 錢塘 river in present-day Zhe jiang 浙江. 597, 606, 1296.

□ This is an abbreviation for Liang zhe dong lu 兩浙東路. [2] It was established under Northern Song 宋, in 1074. Its seat of administration was in Shao xing 紹興 city in Zhe jiang 浙江. Its territory of administration corresponded to a part of present-day Zhe jiang province and included the area east of the Qu jiang 衢江, the Fu chun jiang 富春江, the Qian tang jiang 錢塘江 and Kai hua 開化 county. The *lu* was subsequently abolished but later was reestablished, and soon after abolished again. At the beginning of Southern Song the *lu* was reestablished. It was abolished again at the beginning of Yuan 元. Mentioned with 1167, 1204.

Zhe jiang 浙江 [2]

This is an abbreviation for the Zhe jiang Provincial Administration Commission, Zhe jiang *cheng xuan bu zheng shi si* 浙江承宣布政使司. It was established under Ming 明, in 1376. Its seat of administration was in Hang zhou 杭州 city in Zhe jiang 浙江. Its territory of administration comprised the whole province of Zhe jiang outside of Qu si 嵊泗 county. At the beginning of Qing 清, the area became Zhe jiang province.

Zhe xi 浙西 [1 + 2 + 1]

□ This is the name of a Tang 唐 regional garrison. [1] It is an abbreviation for Zhe jiang xi dao 浙江西道, "Western circuit of Zhe jiang 浙江." It was established in 758 and initially administered at present-day Nan jing 南京 city in Jiang su 江蘇. Subsequently, the seat of administration was moved to present-day Su zhou 蘇州 city in Jiang su. Later, the seat of administration was moved to the Xuan zhou 宣州 district of present-day Xuan cheng 宣城 city in An hui 安徽. Following the *zhen yuan* 貞元 reign period (785 – 805), the administration was established at present-day Zhen jiang 鎮江 city in Jiang su. In 893, it was again moved, this time to present-day Hang zhou 杭州 city. For a long time, its administrative area corresponded to the area south of the Yang zi in present-day Jiang su province, the area east of Mao shan 茅山 mountain and the area north of the Xin an jiang 新安江 in present-day Zhe jiang and the city of Shang hai 上海. It was abolished during the Five Dynasties period. Mentioned with 1057.

□ This is an abbreviation for the Liang zhe xi lu 兩浙西路. [2] The area was established under Northern Song 宋, in 1074. Its seat of administration was in present-day Hang zhou 杭州 city in Zhe jiang 浙江. Its administrative territory corresponded to an area extending in present-day Zhe jiang from the Qu jiang 衢江, the Fu chun jiang 富春江 and the Qian tang jiang 錢塘江 in Kai hua 開化 county toward the North, and in Jiang su from the region of Mao shan 茅山 mountain and Chang dang 長蕩 lake toward the East and toward the South, as well as including the city of Shang hai 上海. The *lu* was subsequently abolished. It was restored in 1076, It was abolished again in 1077. It was reestablished at the beginning of Southern Song, and abolished at the beginning of Yuan 元. Mentioned with 456, 886.

□ Regional name. [1] It more or less corresponds to the area west and north of the Qian tang jiang in present-day Zhe jiang. Mentioned with 1262.

Zhe yang 赭陽 [2]

Name of a county. Also called Du yang 堵陽 county. It was established under Western Han 漢. Its seat of administration was at a location 6 *li* east of present-day Fang cheng 方城 county in He nan 河南. Under Liu Song 劉宋, it was abolished. Mentioned with 474.

Zhe zhou 浙州 [1]
See → Zhe 浙. [1] Mentioned with 730.

Zhen 鎮
See → Zhen ding 鎮定.

Zhen an 鎮安 [1]
Name of a *fu* 府. It was established under Ming 明, in 1369. Its seat of administration was in present-day De bao 德保 county in Guang xi 廣西. Its territory of administration comprised the four counties of Jing xi 靖西, Na po 那坡, De bao 德保 and Tian 天 in present-day Guang xi, and portions of the two counties of Tian yang 田陽 and Tian dong 田東. It was abolished in 1913. Mentioned with 540.

Zhen ding 鎮定 [2]
This is the name of a *zhou* 州. See → Zhen zhou 鎮州. Mentioned with 1109.

Zhen ding 真定 [6 + 5]
▫ Name of a *fu* 府. [6] It was established under Five Dynasties' Tang 唐. Its seat of administration was in present-day Zheng ding 正定 county in He bei 河北. Under Later Jin 晉, in 942, the *fu* was changed to be Heng zhou 恒州. Later Han 漢 changed it to be Zhen zhou 鎮州, and subsequently the area became Zhen ding fu 真定府. The administrative territory of the *fu* corresponded to an area extending in present-day He bei 河北 from the Tang he 唐河 toward the West, and from Gao cheng 藁城 and Yuan shi 元氏 toward the North. Yuan 元 changed the *fu* to be Zhen ding lu 真定路. Ming 明 again created a Zhen ding fu 真定府. The area of administration was expanded and included the counties and cities of present-day Ding zhou 定州, Shen zhou 深州 and Nan gong 南宮. Under Qing 清, in 1723, the area was changed to be Zheng ding fu 正定府. Mentioned with 24, 631.
▫ Name of a county. [5] See Zhen ding xian 真定縣. Mentioned with 99, 145, 631, 1396, 1523.

Zhen ding xian 真定縣 [1]
Name of a county. It was established under Western Han 漢, in 196 BCE. Its seat of administration was at a location northeast of present-day Shi jia zhuang 石家莊 city in He bei 河北. In 113 BCE, under Wu di 武帝, it came under the administration of Zhen ding guo 真定國. Under Tang 唐, in 621, the seat of administration was moved to present-day Zheng ding 正定 county. In 689, its name was changed to be Zhong shan 中山 county. In 705, the name Zhen ding 真定 county was restored. In 1723, under Qing 清, it was changed to be Zheng ding county. Mentioned with 1396.

Zhen jiang 鎮江 [1]
Name of a *fu* 府. It was established under Northern Song 宋, in 1113. Its seat of administration was in present-day Zhen jiang 鎮江 city in Jiang su 江蘇. Its territory of administration comprised the three present-day cities of Zhen jiang, Dan yang 丹陽 and Jin tan 金壇 in Jiang su. Under Yuan 元, in 1276, the area was changed to a *lu*. In early Ming 明, it became Jiang huai fu 江淮府 and, in

1371, it was changed to Zhen jiang fu 鎮江府. The unit was abolished in 1912. Mentioned with 1329.

Zhen kang zhou 鎮康州 [1]

Name of a *zhou* 州. It was founded under Ming 明, in 1384, and shortly thereafter abolished again. In 1409, it was reestablished. Its seat of administration was in present-day Jiu cheng 舊城, located 35 *li* northeast of Yong de 永德 county in Yun nan 雲南. In 1908, the seat of administration was moved to present-day Yong de county. In 1910, the area was changed to Yong kang zhou 永康州. Mentioned with 664.

Zhen la 真臘 [5]

Name of an ancient country. See → Zhen la guo 真臘國. Mentioned with 144, 541, 1139.

Zhen la guo 真臘國 [3]

Name of an ancient country. It appears in Chinese records from the 7th to the 17th century and refers to the Khmer kingdom of the Indo-Chinese peninsula. Mentioned with 256, 1280, 1515.

Zhen yang 真陽 [1]

Name of a county. It was established at the beginning of Liu Song 劉宋. Its seat of administration was north to Jiang kou ji 江口集 in present-day Zheng yang 正陽 county in He nan 河南. Following the *da ming* 大明 reign period (457 – 464), it became Shen yang 慎陽 county. During the *huang xing* 皇興 reign period (467 - 471) of Northern Wei 魏, it again became Zhen yang county. Under Sui 隋, in 591, it was abolished. In 596, a Zhen qiu 真丘 county was established. During the *da ye* 大業 reign period (605 – 618), Zhen qiu 真丘 county was changed to be Zhen yang county. Under Tang 唐, in 689, it was changed to be Huai yang 淮陽, and in 707, it again became Zhen yang county. It was eliminated in 1266, under the early Yuan 元, but later reestablished. In 1371 it was eliminated but reestablished in 1505. Its seat of administration was moved to present-day Zheng yang 正陽 county. In 1723, it was changed to be Zheng yang county. Mentioned with 978.

Zhen yang xian 湞陽縣 [1]

Name of a county. It was established under Western Han 漢. Its seat of administration was at a location north of present-day Weng shui 翁水, east of Ying de 英德 city in Guang dong 廣東. In 467, under Liu Song 劉宋, it was changed to be Zhen yang 貞陽 county. Southern Qi 齊 again called it Zhen yang 湞陽. Under Sui 隋, in 590, it was changed to be Zhen yang 貞陽. In 596, it was abolished and made part of Qu jiang 曲江 county. Under Tang 唐, in 627, it was reestablished and the seat of administration was moved to present-day Ying de city. Northern Song 宋, in 1022, changed it to be Zhen yang 真陽 county. Mentioned with 1532.

Zhen zhou 真州 [1 + 1]

□ This *zhou* 州 was created under Northern Song 宋, in 1013, by raising the status of Jian an 建安 army. [1] It was administered from present-day Yi zheng

儀徵 city in Jiang su 江蘇. Its territory of administration comprised Yi zheng city and the Lu he 六合 district of present-day Nan jing 南京 city in Jiang su. Under Yuan 元, during the *zhi yuan* 至元 reign period (1264 – 1294), its status was raised to Zhen zhou lu 真州路. In 1284, it again became Zhen zhou. It was subordinated to Yang zhou lu 揚州路. It was abolished under Ming 明, in 1369. Mentioned with 26.

□ This *zhou* was created under Tang 唐, in 758, by changing Zhao de 昭德 commandery. [1] It was administered from a location northwest of present-day Mao xian 茂縣 county in Si chuan 四川. Its administrative territory comprised the area northwest of Mao xian county and a region southeast of Hei shui 黑水 county in Si chuan. Later the area was conquered by Tibet. Mentioned with 660.

Zhen zhou 鎮州 [1]

Name of a *zhou* 州. It was founded by Tang 唐, in 820, by changing Heng zhou 恒州 to avoid a taboo on the name of Emperor Mu zong, 穆宗, Li Heng 李恒 (795 – 824). It was administered at present-day Zheng ding 正定 county in He bei 河北. Its territory of administration included Shi jia zhuang 石家莊 city, and the present-day counties of Gao cheng 藁城, Ling shou 靈獸, Xing tang 行唐, Jing xing 井陘, Fu ping 阜平, Luan cheng 欒城 and Ping shan 平山 in He bei. Five Dynasties' Tang changed it to be Zhen ding fu 真定府. Later Jin 晉 changed it to be Heng zhou 恒州. Later Han 漢 restored the name of Zhen zhou 鎮州. Northern Song 宋, in 1048, changed it to be Zhen ding fu 真定府. Mentioned with 675.

Zheng 鄭 [1 + 1]

□ Name of a *zhou* 州. [1] See → Zheng zhou 鄭州. Mentioned with 78.

□ This was a feudal country of Western Zhou 周 times. [1] It had its capital in present-day Hua xian 華縣 county in Shaan xi 陝西. At the end of the reign of King You of Zhou (You wang 幽王, 795-771), the capital was moved to present-day Xin zheng 新鄭 city in He nan 河南. This was during the Spring and Autumn period because the position was in a centralized position. At the beginning of the Warring States period, Zheng was annihilated by Han 韓. Mentioned with 1105.

Zheng shan 鄭山 [1]

Name of a mountain. It is located to the east of present-day Han zhong 漢中 city in Shaan xi 陝西. Mentioned with 1485.

Zheng xian 氶縣

Zheng county was established under Western Han 漢, under Dong hai 東海 commandery. The seat of administration was in present-day Yi cheng 嶧城 town, 10 km south of Zao zhuang 棗莊 city in Shan dong 山東. In 291, it was administered from Lan ling 蘭陵 commandery. Under the Jin 金, in 1195, Zheng county became Lan ling county. Mentioned with 975.

Zheng zhou 鄭州 [2]

Name of a *zhou* 州. It was founded under Sui 隋, in 583. Its seat of administration was in present-day Si shui 汜水 town in Xing yang 滎陽 city in He nan 河南. Its territory of administration comprised the three present-day cities of Zheng zhou 鄭州, Xing yang and Xin zheng 新鄭 along with the counties of Zhong mou 中牟 and Yuan yang 原陽 in He nan. In 606, the seat of administration was moved to the present city of Zheng zhou. In 607, the area was changed to be Xing yang commandery. Under Tang 唐, in 621, it again became Zheng zhou. The seat of administration was moved to present-day Si shui town. In 633, the seat of administration was returned to present-day Zheng zhou city. The *zhou* was abolished in 1072, under Northern Song 宋, but restored in 1085. In 1913, the area was demoted to be Zheng 鄭 county. Mentioned with 733.

Zhi shui 泜水 [1]
Name of a river from the *Shan hai jing* 山海經, "Classic of Mountains and Seas." Further details require additional research. Mentioned with 1466.

Zhi zhi guo 郅支國 [1]
Name of an ancient country. Its capital was located in present-day Schambyl province in Kazakhstan. Mentioned with 731.

Zhong du 中都 [1]
The name of a county. It was established by Tang 唐, in 742. Its seat of administration was in present-day Wen shang 汶上 county in Shan dong 山東. In 1153, it became Wen yang 汶陽 county. Mentioned with 1459.

Zhong guo 中國 [37]
Regional designation. This refers in general terms to the Chinese people in antiquity and the territory occupied by the Han 漢 people. Also it refers to the kingdoms on the central plain. Mentioned with 186, 249, 404, 445, 485, 511, 566, 608, 641, 720, 738, 773, 775, 801, 861, 885, 886, 890, 931, 935, 982, 1009, 1091, 1118, 1124, 1158, 1246, 1252, 1272, 1289, 1296, 1313, 1359, 1406, 1425.

Zhong hua 中華 [3]
Regional name. In the beginning, it designated the middle and lower ranges of the Yellow River. Later, as dynasty borders ebbed and flowed, the term was applied to all the adjoining territories. The term Zhong guo 中國 was also used. Mentioned with 110, 851, 1139.

Zhong jiang xian 中江縣 [1]
Name of a county. It was established by Northern Song 宋, in 1012. Its seat of administration was in present-day Zhong jiang 中江 county in Si chuan 四川. Mentioned with 130.

Zhong li xian 鍾離縣 [1]
Name of a county. It was established by Qin 秦, and made part of Jiu jiang 九江 commandery. Its seat of administration was at a location east of Lin huai 臨淮 pass, northeast of present-day Feng yang 鳳陽 county in An hui 安徽. Tang 唐 moved the seat of administration to present-day Lin huai pass. Jin 金 changed it to Lin huai county, but Yuan 元 restored it as Zhong li 鍾離 county. Ming 明, in 1369, changed it to Zhong li 中立 county. Mentioned with 1037.

Zhong ling shan 冢嶺山 [1]
Name of a mountain. It is located in the northwest of present-day Luo nan 洛南 county in Shaan xi 陝西, in a place abutting Shang zhou 商州 city and Lan tian 藍田 county. Mentioned with 204.

Zhong lu xian 中廬縣 [1]
Name of a county. This is Zhong lu 中盧 county. It was established by Western Han 漢. Its seat of administration was at a location southwest of present-day Xiang yang 襄陽 county in present-day Hu bei 湖北 (one tradition says northeast of Nan zhang 南漳 county). The county was abolished under Southern Liang 梁. Mentioned with 1079.

Zhong mou 中牟 [6]
Name of a county. It was founded by Western Han 漢. Its seat of administration was at a location east of present-day Zhong mou county in He nan 河南. Northern Wei 魏, in 447, combined it with Yang wu 陽武 county. In 500, it was reestablished. Northern Zhou 周, in 565, moved the seat of administration to a location east of present-day Nan zheng zhou 南鄭州 city in He nan. At the beginning of Sui 隋, it was changed to be Nei mou 內牟. At the beginning of Tang 唐, it was again changed to be Zhong mou county. Under Ming 明, during the *tian shun* 天順 reign period (1457 – 1464), the seat of administration was moved to present-day Zhong mou county. Mentioned with 733, 927, 1520.

Zhong nan 終南 [1]
Name of a mountain. See → Zhong nan shan 終南山. Mentioned with 1038.

Zhong nan shan 終南山 [6]
Name of a mountain. This is also called Nan shan 南山, Zhong nan shan 中南山 and Tai yi shan 太一山. This is a branch of the Qin ling 秦嶺 mountain range in present-day Shaan xi 陝西. It runs in an east-west direction and reaches 2000 – 3000 m above sea level. Mentioned with 20, 800, 880, 1210, 1319.

Zhong shan 中山 [5 + 1]
□ Name of a commandery. [5] It was established under Western Han 漢. Its seat of administration was in present-day Ding zhou 定州 city in He bei 河北. Its administrative territory comprised an area extending from Lang ya shan 狼牙山 toward the South, Bao ding 保定 toward the West, from Tang 唐 county toward the East, and north of the Hu tuo 滹沱 river. Emperor Jing 景 of Han (188 – 141) turned the area into Zhong shan country/domain and Later Yan 燕 made its capital in Zhong shan. Northern Wei 魏 turned the area into Zhong shan commandery again. It was abolished at the beginning of the *kai huang* 開皇 reign period (581 – 600) of the Sui 隋. Mentioned with 27, 338, 1022.
□ Name of a *fu* 府. [1] Under Northern Song 宋, in 1113, Ding zhou was promoted to be Zhong shan fu 中山府. Its seat of administration was in present-day Ding zhou city in He bei. Its territory of administration comprised the present-day counties and cities of Ding zhou, Tang xian 唐縣, Xin le 新樂, Shun ping 順平, Wang du 望都, Qu yang 曲陽 and Wu ji 無極. It became Ding zhou again during early Ming. Mentioned with 1430.

Zhong shan 鍾山 [4 + 1]
□ Name of a mountain. [4] The term comes from the *Shan hai jing* 山海經, “Classic of Mountains and Seas.” Further details require additional research. Mentioned with 62, 1406.
□ Name of a mountain. [1] It is located within the boundaries of present-day Lin qu 臨朐 county in Shan dong 山東. Mentioned with 1105.

Zhong shan xian 鍾山縣 [1]
Name of a county. It was established by Sui 隋 at the beginning of the *kai huang* 開皇 reign period (581-600). Its seat of administration was in Zhong shan pu 中山鋪, located northeast of present-day Xin yang 信陽 county in He nan 河南. Under Northern Song 宋, in 976, it was abolished and made part of Yi yang 義陽 county. Mentioned with 1142.

Zhong shui 中水 [1]
Name of a county. See → Zhong shui xian 中水縣. Mentioned with 816.

Zhong shui xian 中水縣 [1]
Name of a county. It was founded under Western Han 漢 when Han Emperor Gao di 漢高帝 (256/247 – 195) enfeoffed meritorious official Lü Matong 呂馬童 (died 170 BCE) to be Lord (*hou* 侯) of Zhong shui 中水. Later, it became a county and was administered from a location 30 *li* northwest of present-day Xian xian 獻縣 county in He bei 河北. The county was abolished under Northern Qi 齊, in 556. Mentioned with 816.

Zhong tai 中臺
See → Zhong tai shan gu 中臺山谷.

Zhong tai shan gu 中臺山谷 [2]
Name of a mountain. It is Wu tai 五台山 in present-day Shan xi 山西. Mentioned with 986, 1124.

Zhong tian zhu guo 中天竺國 [1]
Name of an ancient country. The ancient name of India was Tian zhu. It was divided into an eastern, southern, western, northern and central section and separate names for these five areas exist in the sources. Zhong tian zhu more or less comprised the eastern half of present-day Uttar Pradesh and Rajastan. Mentioned with 1124.

Zhong tiao shan 中條山 [2]
Name of a mountain. It is also called Lei shou shan 雷首山. It is in the southwestern part of present-day Shan xi 山西 between the Yellow River and the rivers Su shui 涑水 and Qin he 沁河. Mentioned with 1014, 1062.

Zhong tu 中土 [4]
Regional name. See → Zhong yuan 中原. Mentioned with 376, 441, 1462, 1500.

Zhong yang 中央 [1]
Positional name referring to a geographical center.

Zhong yuan 中原 [4]

This is a regional name. It is identical with the designations Zhong tu 中土 and Zhong zhou 中州. Already in pre-Qin times a term *tian xia zhi zhong* 天下之中, "Center of the Earth," was in use. Later, when the area inhabited by the Chinese Hua xia 華夏 people expanded, the ancient region of Yu zhou 豫州 came to be seen as the central *zhou* of the so-called nine *zhou* 州. This was called the "central plain." In a narrow sense, the term applied to a region of present-day He nan 河南 province or referred to the entire watershed of the Yellow River. Mentioned with 404, 485, 1109.

Zhong yue 中岳 [3]

Name of a mountain. It was one of the traditional Five Ranges, *wu yue* 五岳. Reference is to Song shan 嵩山 mountain north of present-day Deng feng 登封 city in He nan 河南. Mentioned with 734, 978, 1157.

Zhong zhou 中州 [7]

Regional name; in fact, the area of the central plains; see → Zhong yuan 中原. Mentioned with 330, 794, 954, 1121, 1149, 1274, 1391.

Zhong zhou 忠州 [4]

Name of a *zhou* 州. It was founded under Tang 唐, in 634. Its seat of administration was in present-day Zhong xian 忠縣 county in Chong qing 重慶 city. In 742, it was changed to be Nan bin 南賓 commandery. In 758, it again became Zhong zhou. Its territory of administration comprised the present-day counties of Zhongxian 忠縣, Feng du 豐都, Dian jiang 墊江 and Shi zhu 石柱 in Chong qing municipality. Under Southern Song 宋, in 1265, its status was raised to Xian chun fu 咸淳府. Later, the seat of administration was moved to present-day Huang hua 黃華 city located 20 *li* east of Zhong county. Yuan 元 made it Zhong zhou again. It moved the administration to present-day Zhong county. It was abolished in 1913. Mentioned with 127, 468, 524, 956.

Zhou 周 [6]

Ancient tribal name. Hou ji 后稷 was the ancestor, and the original Zhou seat was present-day Yong an 永安 village, located southwest of Wu gong 武功 county in Shaan xi 陝西. At the time of Duke Liu 劉, it was moved to Bin 彬 county in Shaan xi. At the time of Gu gong dan fu 古公檀父, the Zhou residency was at the present-day location of the Zhou plateau ruins northeast of Qi shan 岐山 county in Shaanxi. During the time of King Wen 文 of Zhou, the capital was moved to the west bank of the Feng he 灃河 river, located northwest of present-day Chang an 長安 county in Shaan xi. In 1066 BCE, King Wu 武 annihilated Shang 商 and established the Zhou Dynasty. Mentioned with 417, 580, 635, 995, 1330, 1380.

Zhu bu guo 竹步國 [1]

Name of an early country. It was located in present-day Somalia along a strip at the mouth of the Jubba River and apparently that is the source of the name. Mentioned with 1196.

Zhu ji 諸暨 [2]

Name of a county. It was established by Qin 秦. Its seat of administration was in present-day Zhu ji city in Zhe jiang 浙江. During the *guang qi* 光啟 reign period (885 – 888) of Tang 唐, the name was changed to Zhu yang 諸陽 county. Under Five Dynasties' Liang 梁, in 908, it again became Zhu ji county. Under Yuan 元, in 1295, its status was raised to Zhu ji zhou 諸暨州. Under the Ming 明 rebels led by Zhu Yuan zhang 朱元璋, in 1366, it became Zhu ji county. In 1989, it became Zhu ji city. Mentioned with 635, 1521.

Zhu ti 朱提 [3]

Name of a county. It was established under Western Han 漢, in 135 BCE. Its seat of administration was in present-day Zhao tong ba zi 昭通垻子 at Zhao tong 昭通 city in Yun nan 雲南. Under Tang 唐, in 618, it was changed to An shang 安上 county. In 624, the old name was restored. During the *tian bao* 天寶 reign period (742 – 756) of Tang, the seat of administration was moved to a location southwest of An bian 安邊 town in Yi bin 宜賓 county in present-day Si chuan 四川. It was abolished at the end of Tang. Mentioned with 82, 311.

Zhu ya 朱 厓 [1]

Name of a commandery. This is Zhu ya 珠崖 commandery. It was established by Western Han 漢, in 111 BCE. Its seat of administration was at a location 30 *li* southeast of present-day Qiong shan 瓊山 city on Hai nan 海南 island. Its territory of administration comprised the northeast part of present-day Hai nan island. In 46 BCE, the commandery was abolished. Under Sui 隋, in 610, it was reestablished. Its seat of administration was at a location southeast of present-day Qiong shan city. Under Tang 唐, in 621, it was changed to be Ya zhou 崖州. In 742, the name was changed to Zhu ya 珠崖 commandery, but it became Ya zhou again in 758. Mentioned with 419.

Zhu ya 朱崖 [6]

Name of a commandery. This is Zhu ya jun 珠崖郡. See → Zhu ya 朱厓 . Mentioned with 82, 828.

Zhuang lang 莊浪 [1]

Name of a guard. See → Zhuang lang wei 莊浪衛. Mentioned with 188.

Zhuang lang wei 莊浪衛 [1]

Name of a guard. It was founded under Ming 明, in 1377. Its seat of administration was in present-day Yong deng 永登 county in Gan su 甘肅. In 1398, it was demoted to be the Zhuang lang Battalion, Zhuang lang *qian hu suo* 莊浪千戶所. In 1403, it was again promoted to be the Zhuang lang wei 莊浪衛. In 1663, it was demoted to be Zhang lang Headquarters, Zhuang lang suo 莊浪所. In 1724, it was changed to be Ping fan 平番 county. Mentioned with 498.

Zi 淄 [6]

Name of a zhou 州. See → Zi zhou 淄州. Mentioned with 208, 359, 644, 980, 1323.

Zi 資 [1]

Name of a zhou 州. See → Zi zhou 資州. Mentioned with 1054.

Zi chuan 淄川 [1]
Name of a county. It was founded under Sui 隋, in 598. Its seat of administration was in present-day Zi chuan cheng 淄川城, located southwest of Zi bo 淄博 city in Shan dong 山東. Ming 明, in 1376, made it part of Zi chuan zhou 淄川州, but in 1379 this was abolished and it again became a county. In 1955, it became a part of Zi bo city. Mentioned with 1317.

Zi chuan 菑川 [1]
This is the name of a feudal state. It was founded under Western Han 漢, in 164 BCE. Its capital was located 30 *li* south of present-day Shou guang 壽光 city in Shan dong 山東. It was rather large as a fief. In the North, it bordered on the gulf of Bo hai 渤海 and in the South went as far as present-day Lin qu 臨朐 county. After the revolt of the Seven Countries, its domain was reduced. During the *yuan yan* 元延 reign period (1314 – 1320), it only comprised the area northeast of Qing zhou 青州 city and Chang le 昌樂 county, and an area west of Shou guang 壽光 city in present-day Shan dong. Under Eastern Han, in 37, it was combined with the Bei hai 北海 country/domain. Mentioned with 619, 1289.

Zi gui 秭歸 [2]
Name of a county. It was established under Western Han 漢. Its seat of administration was in present-day Gui zhou 歸州 town, located northwest of Zi gui county in Hu bei 湖北. Northern Zhou 周 changed it to Chang ning 長寧 county. At the beginning of the *kai huang* 開皇 reign period (581 – 600) of Sui 隋, it was restored as Zi gui county. In 1236, Southern Song 宋 moved the seat of administration to a location southeast of Gui zhou 歸州 town. Ming 明, in 1377, changed it to Chang ning county. In 1380, it was again changed to Gui zhou. In 1912, it was changed to be Gui 歸 county. Mentioned with 462.

Zi tuan 紫團 [1]
Name of a mountain. See → Zi tuan shan 紫團山. Mentioned with 931.

Zi tuan shan 紫團山 [2]
Name of a mountain. It is located southeast of present-day Ping shun 平順 county in Shan xi 山西. Mentioned with 648, 931.

Zi zhou 淄州 [6]
Name of a *zhou* 州. It was founded under Sui 隋, in 596. Its seat of administration was in present-day Zi chuan cheng 淄川城, located southwest of Zi bo 淄博 city in Shan dong 山東. Its territory of administration comprised the cities and counties of Zi bo, Gao qing 高青, Zou ping 鄒平 and Huan tai 桓台 in present-day Shan dong. During the *da ye* 大業 (605 – 618) reign period of the Sui, and the *tian bao* 天寶 (742 – 756) and *zhi de* 至德 (756 – 758) reign periods of the Tang 唐, the area periodically became Zi chuan 淄川 commandery. Under Yuan 元, in 1264, its status was raised to Zi chuan lu 淄川路. Mentioned with 272, 527, 693, 819, 905, 918.

Zi zhou 資州 [4]
Name of a *zhou* 州. It was established under Western Wei 魏. Its seat of administration was at a location northwest of present-day Jian yang 簡陽 city in Si

chuan 四川. Its territory of administration comprised an area of the Tuo jiang 沱江 watershed, extending from Zi yang 資陽 city toward the South and from Nei jiang 内江 city toward the North in present-day Si chuan. Under Northern Zhou 周, in 560, the seat of administration was moved to present-day Zi yang city. Under Sui 隋, in 587, the seat of administration was shifted again to a location 3 *li* north of present-day Zi zhong 資中 county. During the *da ye* 大業 (605 – 618) reign period of the Sui, and the *tian bao* 天寶 (742 – 756) and *zhi de* 至德 (756 – 758) reign periods of the Tang 唐, the area periodically became a commandery. In 865, the seat of administration was moved to a location west of present-day Nei jiang city and the following year it was moved to a location 3 *li* north of the present Zi zhong city. Under Yuan 元, in 1283, it was abolished and combined with Jian zhou 簡州. During the *zhi zheng* 至正 reign period (1341 – 1370), it was reestablished by the peasant rebel Ming Yuzhen 明玉珍 (1331-1366). Its seat of administration was in Zi zhong city in Si chuan. Under Ming 明, in 1371, it was demoted to be Zi xian 資縣 county. In 1728, its status was raised to Zi zhou directly administered *zhou*, *zhi li zhou* 直隸州. In 1913, the *zhou* became Zi zhong 資中 county. Mentioned with 754, 993, 1030, 1468.

Zi zhou 梓州 [6]

Name of a *zhou* 州. It was founded under Sui 隋, in 598. Its seat of administration was in present-day San tai 三台 county in Si chuan 四川. Its territory of administration comprised the present-day counties of San tai, Zhong jiang 中江, Yan ting 鹽亭 and She hong 射洪 in Si chuan. During the *da ye* 大業 (605 – 618) reign period of the Sui, and the *tian bao* 天寶 (742 – 756) and *zhi de* 至德 (756 – 758) reign periods of the Tang 唐, the area periodically became a commandery. Following the *qian yuan* reign period (758 – 760), when Shu 蜀 was divided into Dong chuan 東川 and Xi chuan 西川, Zi zhou was usually administered by the Dong chuan Military Commissioner, Dong chuan *jie du shi* 東川節度使. In 1118, under Northern Song 宋, it was changed to Tong chuan fu 潼川府. Mentioned with 44, 82, 437, 595.

Zou xian 鄒縣 [1]

Name of a county. It was established by Qin 秦. Its seat of administration was at a location 26 *li* southeast of present-day Zou cheng 鄒城 city in Shan dong 山東. Northern Qi 齊 moved the administration to present-day Zou cheng city. In 1992, it was changed to be Zou cheng city. Mentioned with 1444.

Zuo you jiang 左右江 [2]

Regional name. It is a combined designation for the rivers Zuo jiang 左江 and You jiang 右江 that are the upper sources of the Yu jiang 郁江 in present-day Guang xi 廣西. During Song 宋, Zuo jiang dao 左江道 and You jiang dao 右江道 got their names from this. Mentioned with 445, 784, 813.

III. APPENDICES

Appendix A

Chinese Dynasties

Dynasty	Period	Capital
Zhou	1046 - 256 BCE	
↳ Western Zhou	1046 - 771 BCE	Feng jing and Hao jing (in today's Xi an, Shaan xi)
↳ Eastern Zhou	770 - 256 BCE	Luo yi (today's Luo yang)
- Spring and Autumn period	770 - 476 BCE	
- Warring States period	475 - 221 BCE	
Qin	221 - 207 BCE	Xian yang (in today's Xian yang and Xian of Shaan xi)
Han	202 BCE - 220 CE	
↳ Western Han	202 BCE - 9 CE	Chang'an (today's Xi an)
↳ Xin Dynasty	9 - 23	Chang'an (today's Xi an)
↳ Eastern Han	25 - 220	Luo yang

Three Kingdoms	220 - 280	
↳ Kingdom of Wei	220 - 265	Luo yang
↳ Kingdom of Shu	221 - 263	Cheng du
↳ Kingdom of Wu	222 - 280	Jian ye (today's Nan jing, Jiang su)
Jin	265 - 420	
↳ Western Jin	265 - 316	Luo yang
↳ Eastern Jin	317 - 420	Jian kang (Nan jing, Jiang su)
↳ Sixteen Kingdoms	304 - 439	
Southern and Northern Dynasties	420 - 589	
↳ Southern Dynasties	420 - 589	
- Song	420 - 479	Jian kang (today's Nan jing)
- Qi	479 - 502	Jian kang (Nan jing)
- Liang	502 - 557	Jian kang (Nan jing)
- Chen	557 - 589	Jian kang (Nan jing)
↳ Northern Dynasties	386 - 581	
- Northern Wei	386 - 534	Ping cheng (today's Da tong, Shan xi); Luo yang
- Eastern Wei	534 - 550	Ye cheng (in Lin zhang, Handan, He bei)
- Western Wei	535 - 557	Chang'an (today's Xi an)
- Northern Qi	550 - 577	Ye cheng (in Lin zhang, Handan, He bei)
- Northern Zhou	557 - 581	Chang'an (today's Xi an)
Sui	581 - 618	Da xing (in today's Xi an, Shaan xi); Luo yang

Tang	618 - 907	Chang'an (today's Xi an); Luo yang
Five Dynasties and Ten States	907 - 960	Bian liang (Kai feng, He nan); Luo yang
- Later Liang	907 - 923	Bian liang (Kai feng)
- Later Tang	923 - 936	Luo yang
- Later Jin	936 - 946	Bian liang (Kai feng)
- Later Han	947 - 950	Bian liang (Kai feng)
- Later Zhou	951 - 960	Bian liang (Kai feng)
↳ Ten States	902 - 979	
Song	960 - 1279	
↳ Northern Song	960 - 1127	Bian jing (Kai feng)
↳ Southern Song	1127 - 1279	Nan jing (today's Shang qiu, He nan); Lin'an (Hang zhou)
Liao	907 - 1125	Shang jing (Baarin Left Banner, Chi feng, Inner Mongolia)
Western Xia Dynasty	1038 - 1227	Xing qing (today's Yin chuan, Ning xia)
Jin	1115 - 1234	Hui ning (Harbin, Hei long jiang); Zhong du (today's Bei jing); Bian jing (Kai feng)
Yuan	1271 - 1368	Da du (today's Bei jing)
Ming	1368 - 1644	Ying tian (today's Nan jing, Jiang su); Shun tian (today's Bei jing)
Qing	1644 - 1911	Bei jing

Appendix B

Numbers of Pharmaceutically Relevant Substances Mentioned in Connection with Geographic and Administrative Designations

Note: 1. The earlier a text mentioning pharmaceutical substances was compiled, the less certain one can be that today's botanical identification of a substance applies. 2. The botanical species given in the following list may not include all species covered by a Chinese plant name. Here only the most common identifications are provided as a first hint at the nature of a pharmaceutical substance mentioned in connection with a geographic designation or administrative structure. 3. Substances of animal origin are given with their vernacular meaning. 4. Minerals are listed with their English names rather than chemical formulas wherever possible.

Number	Chinese Name	Characters	Preliminary Identification
0001	A le bo	阿勒勃	*Cassia fistula* L.
0002	A fu rong	阿芙蓉	Opium resin
0003	Ai	艾	*Artemisia argyi* Lèvl. et Vant.
0004	Ai na	艾納	Lichen on old pines
0005	Ai na xiang	艾納香	*Blumea balsamifera* (L.) DC.
0006	An lü	庵蕳	*Artemisia keiskeana* Miq.
0007	An luo guo	菴羅果	*Mangifera indica* L.
0008	An mo le	庵摩勒	*Phyllanthus emblica* L
0009	An mo le	菴摩勒	*Phyllanthus emblica* L.
0010	An shi liu	安石榴	*Punica granatum* L.
0011	An xi xiang	安息香	*Styrax benzoin* Dryand.
0012	An zan lu	安咱蘆	Unidentified substance
0013	Ao shu	芺樹	Unidentified evergreen plant

0014	A wei	阿魏	*Ferula assa-foetida* L.
0015	A yue hun zi	阿月渾子	*Pistacia vera* L.
0016	A zhi er	阿只兒	Western regions plant, like → 0612 *Ku shen* 苦參
0017	Ba	魃	Goblin
0018	Ba dan xing	巴旦杏	*Amygdalis communis* L.
0019	Ba dou	巴豆	*Croton tiglium* L.
0020	Bai	柏	*Platycladus orientalis* (L.) Franco
0021	Bai e	白堊	Kaolin
0022	Bai bu	百部	*Stemona sessilifolia* (Miq.) Franch. et Sav."
0023	Bai cao hua	百草花	Unspecified "flowers of a hundred herbs"
0024	Bai ci qi	白瓷器	Porcelain
0025	Bai dou kou	白豆蔻	*Amomum kravanh* Pierre ex Gagnep
0026	Bai fu zi	白附子	*Aconitum coreanum* (Levl.) Rapaics
0027	Bai hao	白蒿	*Artemisia sieversiana* Ehrhart ex Willd.
0028	Bai he	百合	*Lilium brownii* and other *L.* spp
0029	Bai hua she	白花蛇	Embroidered pit viper
0030	Bai hua teng	白花藤	*Trachelospermum jasminoides* (Lindl.) Lem.
0031	Bai ji	白及	*Bletilla striata* (Thunb.) Reichb.f.
0032	Bai ji	白棘	*Zizyphus jujuba* Mill. var. *spinosa*
0033	Bai jiang	敗醬	*Patrinia scabiosaefolia* Fisch. ex Trev.
0034	Bai jie	白芥	*Sinapis alba* L.
0035	Bai ji shi	白肌石	Variety of gypsum
0036	Bai ju	白苣	*Lactuca sativa* L. var. *romana* Hort.
0037	Bai leng teng	百稜藤	Unidentified creeping plant
0038	Bai lian	白斂	*Ampelopsis japonica* (Thunb.) Makino
0039	Bai liang jin	百兩金	*Ardisia crispa* (Thunb.) A. DC.
0040	Bai ma gu	白馬骨	*Serissa serissoides* (DC.) Druce.
0041	Bai mai gen	百脈根	*Lotus corniculatus* L.
0042	Bai mao	白茅	*Imperata cylindrica* (L.) Beauv.
0043	Bai mao xiang	白茅香	*Hierochloa borealis* Roem. et Sch.
0044	Bai qing	白青	Round, light-colored azurite
0045	Bai rui cao	百蕊草	*Thesium chinense* Turcz.

0046	Bai shi hua	白石華	Serpentine
0047	Bai shi ying	白石英	Milky quartz
0048	Bai shi zi shi	白獅子石	Unidentified white stone
0049	Bai shu	白鼠	White, rat-like animal from the Southern Sea
0050	Bai tou weng	白頭翁	*Anemone chinensis* Bunge
0051	Bai tu huo	白兔藿	*Cynanchum caudatum* Maxim.
0052	Bai wei	白微	*Cynanchum atratum* Bunge
0053	Bai xian	白鮮	*Dictamnus angustifolius* G. Don ex Sweet.
0054	Bai xian	白鷴	Silver pheasant
0055	Bai xin	白辛	Poisonous plant with white and fragrant root
0056	Bai yang	白楊	*Populus davidiana* Dode
0057	Bai yang shi	白羊石	Baiyang mountain stone from Shandong 山東
0058	Bai yao zi	白藥子	*Stephania cepharantha* Hayata
0059	Bai yao zu	百藥祖	Unidentified evergreen plant
0060	Bai ying	白英	*Solanum lyratum* Thunb.
0061	Bai yuan zi	白緣子	Tall tree with sweet fruit
0062	Bai yu sui	白玉髓	Chalcedony
0063	Bai zhang qing	百丈青	Vine with opposite leaves
0064	Bai zhi	白芷	*Angelica dahurica* and other *A.* spp.
0065	Ba jiao	芭蕉	→ 0330 *Gan jiao* 甘蕉
0066	Ba ji tian	巴戟天	*Morinda officinalis* How.
0067	Bang	蚌	Clam
0068	Ban mao	斑蝥	Chinese cantharides
0069	Ban tian hui	半天回	Unidentified plant, 2 feet tall, with red spots
0070	Ban xia	半夏	*Pinellia ternata* (Thunb.) Breit.
0071	Bao	鴇	Hailstones
0072	Bao	豹	Eastern bustard
0073	Bao shi	寶石	Differently-colored precious stones
0074	Bao yi shui	胞衣水	Old, liquified placenta
0075	Bao yu	鮑魚	Abalone
0076	Ba qi	菝葜	*Smilax china* L.
0077	Ba zhu	巴朱	Unidentified herbal medicinal
0078	Bei mu	貝母	*Fritillaria unibracteata* Hsiao et K.C. Hsia
0079	Bei shi	椑柹	*Diospyros oleifera* Cheng

0080	Bei zi	貝子	Cowry shells
0081	Ben gui	賁龜	Unidentified "*Ben* tortoise"
0082	Bian qing	扁青	Azurite
0083	Bian shi	砭石	Unidentified stone probes
0084	Bian xu	萹蓄	*Polygonum aviculare* L.
0085	Bi ba	蓽茇	*Piper longum* L.
0086	Bi cheng qie	畢澄茄	*Litsea cubeba* (Lour.)
0087	Bie	鱉	Soft-shelled turtles
0088	Bie ji	别羇	Unidentified plant
0089	Bie qi	䱜齊	Sweet, fragrant juice of unidentified tree
0090	Bi hui lei	辟虺雷	*Aristolochia cinnabarina* C. Y. Cheng et J. L. Wu
0091	Bi li xiang	必栗香	*Platycarya strobilacea* Sieb. et Zucc.
0092	Bi ma	蓖麻	*Ricinus communis* L.
0093	Bi mu yu	比目魚	Flounders
0094	Bing lang	檳榔	*Areca catechu* L.
0095	Bing shu	冰鼠	A thickly furred animal living under the ice in far north
0096	Bi qian	壁錢	A kind of spider
0097	Bi si da	必思荅	*Pistacia vera* L.
0098	Bi si le	必似勒	Unidentified
0099	Bi xie	萆薢	*Dioscorea collettii* Hook f. var. *hypoglauca* (Palibin) Péi et Ting.
0100	Bo he	薄荷	*Mentha canadensis* L.
0101	Bo ji she	簸箕舌	"Tongue," front rim of a traditional dust pan
0102	Bo lao	伯勞	Bull headed shrike
0103	Bo leng	菠薐	*Spinacia oleracea* L.
0104	Bo li	玻璃	Glass
0105	Bo luo hui	博落回	*Macleya cordata* (Willd.) R. Br.
0106	Bo luo mi	波羅蜜	*Artocarpus heterophyllus* Lam.
0107	Bo mu	檗木	*Phellodendron amurense* Ruppr.
0108	Bo si cao	波斯草	*Spinacia oleracea* L.
0109	Bu diao mu	不凋木	*Osteomeles schwerinae* Schneid.
0110	Bu gu zhi	補骨脂	*Psoralea corylifolia* L.
0111	Bu hui mu	不灰木	Asbestos
0112	Bu li cao	布里草	Unidentified herb
0113	Can	蠶	Silkworm
0114	Can dou	蠶豆	*Vicia faba* L.

0115	Cang gua	鶬鴰	Eastern grey crane or grey heron
0116	Cang ji	傖鷄	Three-year-old hawk
0117	Cang ji	鶬鷄	Eastern grey crane or grey heron
0118	Cao chi	草豉	Unidentified
0119	Cao shi can	草石蠶	*Stachys sieboldii* Miq.
0120	Cao wu tou	草烏頭	→ 1253 *Wu tou* 烏頭
0121	Cao xi	草犀	Root of an unidentified plant
0122	Ceng qing	曾青	Malachite
0123	Ce zi	側子	Side roots of *Aconitum carmichaeli* Debx.
0124	Cha	茶	Tea
0125	Chai hu	柴胡	*Bupleurum chinense* D.C.
0126	Chai hu	茈胡	→ 0125 *Chai hu* 柴胡
0127	Chai zi gu	釵子股	*Luisia morsei* Rolfe ex Forbes et Hemsley
0128	Chan chu	蟾蜍	Toad
0129	Chang pu	菖蒲	*Acorus gramineus* Ait. and *A. Calamus* Lour.
0130	Chang shan	常山	*Dichroa febrifuga* Lour.
0131	Chang shi	長石	Felspar
0132	Chang song	長松	*Pinus pumila* (Pall.)Regel
0133	Chang yu	鯧魚	*Pampus argenteus* (Euphrasen)
0134	Chan hua	蟬花	*Cordyceps cicadae* Shing
0135	Chan zi	棎子	A pear
0136	Chan zi	橏子	A pear
0137	Chao	麨	Prepared rice or wheat
0138	Che'ao	車螯	Giant clams
0139	Cheng	蟶	Razor clams
0140	Cheng liu	檉柳	*Tamarix chinensis* Lour.
0141	Chen jia bai yao	陳家白藥	Unidentifed vine
0142	Chen lin mi	陳廩米	Stored rice; *Oryza sativa* L.
0143	Chen si ji	陳思岌	Unidentified vine; acrid, fragrant root and leaf
0144	Chen xiang	沉香	*Aquilaria agallocha* (Lour.) Roxb.
0145	Che qian	車前	*Plantago asiatica* L.
0146	Che qu	車渠	Scallops
0147	Chi	鴟	Sparrow hawk
0148	Chi che shi zhe	赤車使者	*Pellionia radicans* (Sieb. et Zucc.) Wedd.
0149	Chi chi feng	赤翅蜂	Red winged hornet
0150	Chi chong	豉蟲	Gyrinus beetle

0151	Chi de le	池德勒	Root of unidentified plant from West of China
0152	Chi di li	赤地利	*Fagopyrum dibotrys* (D.Don) Hara
0153	Chi he	赤赫	Unidentified
0154	Chi ju	赤舉	Unidentified herb
0155	Chi nie	赤涅	Unidentified herb
0156	Chi shi zhi	赤石脂	Red halloysite
0157	Chi tong	赤銅	Native copper
0158	Chi xiao dou	赤小豆	*Vigna umbellata* (Thunb.) Ohwi et Ohashi
0159	Chi xiu	鴟鵂	Scops owls
0160	Chong bai la	蟲白蠟	Chinese wax
0161	Chong chu tou xi kang	舂杵頭細糠	Ricebran
0162	Chong dong gen	冲洞根	Root of unidentified plant
0163	Chong wei	茺蔚	*Leonurus japonicus* Houtt.
0164	Chu	楮	*Broussonetia papyrifera* (L.) Vent.
0165	Chuan hong	船虹	Unidentified herb
0166	Chui hu gen	捶胡根	Root of unidentified plant
0167	Chu ji	樗鷄	Lantern fly, red cicada
0168	Chun	蒓	*Brasenia schreberi* J. F. Gmel.
0169	Chun	鶉	Quail
0170	Chun chu	椿樗	*Ailanthus altissima* (Mill.) Swingle
0171	Ci gu	慈姑	*Sagittaria trifolia* L. var. *sinensis* (Sims.) Makino
0172	Ci hu	刺虎	*Damnacanthus indicus* (L.) Gaertn. f.
0173	Ci huang	雌黃	Orpiment
0174	Ci mi	刺蜜	*Alhagi Pseudalhagi* Desv.
0175	Ci shi	慈石	Magnetite
0176	Ci wu	慈烏	Crows
0177	Ci yang	牸羊	Unidentified lamb variety from the North-West
0178	Cong	葱	*Allium fistulosum* L.
0179	Cong mu	楤木	Aralia carnescens S. et Z.
0180	Cu	醋	Vinegar from millets, rice, wheat, or barley
0181	Cui feng shi	催風使	Unidentified herbal drug
0182	Cu jiang cao	酢漿草	*Oxalis corniculata* L.
0183	Cu lin zi	醋林子	*Embelia subcoriacea* C. B. Clarke
0184	Cuo shi he cao	撮石合草	*Oxalis corniculata* L.
0185	Da dou	大豆	*Glycine max* (L.) Merr.

0186	Da dou chi	大豆豉	Bean relish
0187	Da fu zi	大腹子	Pericarpium of *Areca catechu* L.
0188	Da huang	大黃	*Rheum palmatum* L.
0189	Da huang feng	大黃蜂	Hornet
0190	Dai mao	瑇瑁	Hawksbill turtle
0191	Dai zhe shi	代赭石	Red haematite
0192	Da ji	大戟	*Euphorbia pekinensis* Rupr.
0193	Da ji	大薊	*Euphorbia pekinensis* Rupr.
0194	Da kong	大空	Unidentified shrub
0195	Da ma	大麻	*Cannabis sativa* L.
0196	Da mai	大麥	*Hordeum vulgare* L.
0197	Dan ba xiang	膽八香	*Canarium strictum* Roxb.
0198	Dan cai	淡菜	Sea mussels
0199	Dang gui	當歸	*Angelica sinensis* (Oliv.) Diels
0200	Dan jian	丹戩	Unidentified bug of the Armadillium type
0201	Dan luo	擔羅	Korean clams
0202	Dan sha	丹砂	Cinnabar
0203	Dan shen	丹參	*Salvia miltiorrhiza* Bunge
0204	Dan yu	丹魚	Gold fish
0205	Dan zhi mu pi	丹桎木皮	Bark of unidentified tree, similar to → 0953 Shan 杉
0206	Dao	稻	*Oryza sativa* L. var. *glutinosa* Matsum.
0207	Dao dou	刀豆	*Canavalia gladiata* (Jacq.) DC.
0208	Da qing	大青	*Clerodendrum cyrtophyllum* Turcz.
0209	Da wei yang	大尾羊	"Fat-tailed" sheep
0210	Da wu gong	大蜈蚣	A centipede
0211	Deng xin cao	燈心草	*Juncus effusus* L.
0212	De qing guo	德慶果	Unidentified evergreen plant with large fruit
0213	Diao	鵰	Eagle
0214	Diao	弔	*Spongilla fragilis* (Leidy)
0215	Diao shu	貂鼠	*Martes zibellina* (Miq.) Miq. ex Havil.
0216	Diao teng	釣藤	*Uncaria rhynchophylla* (Miq.) Miq. ex Havil.
0217	Diao zhang	釣樟	*Lindera erythrocarpa* Makino
0218	Di bai	地柏	*Selaginella Moellendorfii* Hieron.
0219	Di dan	地膽	Oil beetle

0220	Di fang	地防	A cricket-like insect found in loess soil
0221	Di fu	地膚	*Kochia scoparia* (L.) Schrad.
0222	Di huang	地黃	*Rehmannia glutinosa* (Gaertn.) Libosch. ex Fisch et Mey.
0223	Di jiao	地椒	*Thymus mongolicus* Bonn.
0224	Di jin	地錦	*Heteropogon contortus* (L.) Beuav. ex Roem. et Schult.
0225	Di long teng	地龍藤	Unidentified vine
0226	Ding xiang	丁香	*Syzygium aromaticum* (L.) Merr. et Perry
0227	Di pi	狄皮	Bark of an unidentified tree with red-yellow fruit
0228	Di qie zi	地茄子	Unidentified herb
0229	Di sheng yang	地生羊	Western sheep and goats
0230	Di xiu	帝休	Unidentified tree
0231	Di yang mei	地楊梅	*Luzula capitata* (Miq.) ex Kom.
0232	Di ye jia	底野迦	Theriac
0233	Di yu	地榆	*Sanguisorba officinalis* L.
0234	Di zhi	鸐雉	Long-tailed pheasant
0235	Dong bi tu	東壁土	Soil from old-style house's outer wall facing East
0236	Dong feng cai	東風菜	*Doellingeria scaber* (Thunb.) Nees
0237	Dong gua	冬瓜	*Benincasa hispida* (Thunb.) Cogn.
0238	Dong hui	冬灰	Ashes accumulated in a stove during winter
0239	Dong qiang	東廧	*Agriophyllum squarrosum* (L.) Moq.
0240	Dong qing	冬青	*Ilex purpurea* Hask.
0241	Dong yang jiu	東陽酒	Grain alcoholic liquid from Dong yang
0242	Dou fu	豆腐	Soybean curd → 0185 Da dou 大豆
0243	Dou kou	豆蔻	Nutmeg and small cardamoms
0244	Dou mu xiang	兜木香	Spice from a mythical country
0245	Dou na xiang	兜納香	*Platycarya strobilacea* Sieb. et Zucc.
0246	Du guan cao	都管草	*Angelica kiusiana* Maxim.
0247	Du heng	杜衡	*Asarum caulescens* Maxim.
0248	Tu hong shan	土紅山	Unidentified plant
0249	Du huo	獨活	*Angelica biserrata* (Shan et Yuan)
0250	Du jiao feng	獨脚蜂	Horn-tailed wasp
0251	Du jiao xian	獨脚仙	Longicorn beetle
0252	Du jiao zi	都桷子	*Genipa americana* L.

0253	Du jing shan	杜莖山	*Maesa japonica* (Thunb.) Moritzi.
0254	Du juan	杜鵑	Cuckoos
0255	Du nian zi	都念子	*Garcinia mangostana* L.
0256	Du nou xiang	篤耨香	*Shorea robusta* Roth.
0257	Duo jiu	鵽鳩	Pallas' sand grouse
0258	Du ruo	杜若	*Pollia japonica* Hornst.
0259	Du xian zi	都咸子	*Anacardium occidentale* L.
0260	Du yong teng	獨用藤	Unidentified evergreen vine
0261	Du zhong	杜仲	*Eucommia ulmoides* Oliv.
0262	Du zu niao	獨足鳥	A mythological bird with a single leg
0263	E	鵝	Goose
0264	E	鶚	Osprey
0265	E bao	鵝抱	Unidentified vine with roots resembling radish
0266	E yao	䖸藥	Unidentified herb
0267	E gui	鶚龜	Goose tortoise
0268	E jiao	阿膠	Donkey or ass hide gelatin
0269	E jing shui	阿井水	Well water of Dong'e, Shandong 山東
0270	E shi	惡實	*Arctium lappa* L.
0271	Fan bai cao	翻白草	*Potentilla freyniana* Bornm.
0272	Fang feng	防風	*Saposhnikovia divaricata* (Turcz.)
0273	Fang ji	防己	*Aristolochia heterophylla* Hemsl.
0274	Fang jie shi	方解石	Calcite
0275	Fang kui	防葵	*Peucedanum japonicum* Thunb.
0276	Fang mu	方目	Gull-like marsh bird
0277	Fang yu	魴魚	Chinese bream
0278	Fang zhang mu	放杖木	Unidentified tree
0279	Fang zhu	方竹	A bamboo with a rectangular stem
0280	Fan hong hua	番紅花	*Crocus sativus* L.
0281	Fan hun shu	返魂樹	Unidentified tree producing fragrant resin
0282	Fan hun xiang	返魂香	Resins of the → 0281 Fan hun shu 返魂樹
0283	Fan lü	繁縷	*Stellaria media* (L.) Cry.
0284	Fan mu bie	番木鱉	*Strychnos nux vomica* L.
0285	Fan shi	礬石	Potash
0286	Fan xiao	番消	Imported salt petre
0287	Fei cui	翡翠	Halcyon, usually a Kingfisher

0288	Fei fei	狒狒	Moupin langur
0289	Fei lian	飛廉	*Carduus crispus* L.
0290	Fei lian	蜚蠊	Cockroach
0291	Fei meng	蜚虻	Gadfly
0292	Fei shi	榧實	*Toreya grandis* Fort. ex Lindl.
0293	Feng	封	Peculiar organism with a slimy composite body
0294	Feng huang	鳳凰	Phoenixes
0295	Feng lan	糞藍	Unidentified herb
0296	Feng li	風狸	Sloth monkey
0297	Feng liu	楓柳	*Pterocaya stenoptera* DC.
0298	Feng mi	蜂蜜	Honey
0299	Feng shi	封石	Copper ore
0300	Feng xiang zhi	楓香脂	*Liquidambar formosana* Hance.
0301	Feng yang	封羊	A humped sheep of Gansu 甘肅
0302	Feng yan mu	風延母	Unidentified vine from the Southern Sea
0303	Fen xi	粉錫	White lead
0304	Fo jia cao	佛甲草	*Sedum lineare* Thunb.
0305	Fu	鳧	Duck
0306	Fu bi	腐婢	Flower of → 0158 Chi xiao dou 赤小豆
0307	Fu bian zi	夫編子	Fruit of unidentified tree
0308	Fu fang teng	扶芳藤	*Euonymus fortunei* (Turcz.) Hand.-Mazz.
0309	Fu ji zi gen	伏雞子根	Unidentified vine with thin, round leaves
0310	Fu lan luo le	浮爛羅勒	*Magnolia hypoleuca* Sieb. et Zucc.
0311	Fu ling	茯苓	*Poria cocos* (Schw.) Wolf
0312	Fu long gan	伏龍肝	Furnace earth
0313	Fu niu hua	伏牛花	*Damnacanthus indicus* (L.) Gaertn. f.
0314	Fu pen zi	覆盆子	*Rubus chingii* Hu
0315	Fu ren yue shui	婦人月水	Menstrual liquid
0316	Fu sang	扶桑	*Hibiscus rosa-sinensis* L.
0317	Fu she	蝮蛇	Pallas pit viper
0318	Fu shi	浮石	Porous lava
0319	Fu yi	扶移	*Populus cathayana* Rehd.
0320	Fu yi	伏翼	Bat
0321	Fu zhong	𠂤螽	Locust
0322	Fu zi	附子	*Aconitum carmichaeli* Debx.

0323	Gan	柑	*Citrus chachiensis* Hort.
0324	Gan cao	甘草	*Glycyrrhiza uralensis* Fisch
0325	Gang tie	鋼鐵	Steel
0326	Gan guo	甘鍋	Crucible used for melting metal utensils
0327	Gan jia bai yao	甘家白藥	Unidentified herb
0328	Gan jiang	乾薑	*Zingiber officinale* Rosc.
0329	Gan jian zi	甘劍子	*Aleurites moluccana* (L.) Willd.
0330	Gan jiao	甘蕉	*Musa sapientum* L.
0331	Gan lan	甘藍	*Brassica oleracea* L var. *capitata* L.
0332	Gan lan	橄欖	*Canarium album* (Lour.) Raeusch.
0333	Gan lu	甘露	"Sweet dew" exudation of an unidentified plant
0334	Gan lu mi	甘露蜜	"Sweet dew honey" exudation of an unidentified plant
0335	Gan lu teng	甘露藤	Unidentified climbing plant with sweet flavor
0336	Gan shu	甘薯	*Dioscorea esculenta* (Lour.) Burkhill
0337	Gan song xiang	甘松香	*Nardostachys chinensis* Batal.
0338	Gan sui	甘遂	*Euphorbia kansui* T. N. Liou ex T. P. Wang
0339	Gan tai	乾苔	*Enteromorpha prolifera* (Muell.) AG.
0340	Gan teng	甘藤	Unidentified creeper
0341	Gan tu	甘土	Bentonite
0342	Gan tuo mu pi	乾陀木皮	Unidentified tree bark
0343	Gan yu	鱤魚	False salmon
0344	Gan zhe	甘蔗	*Saccharum sinensis* Roxb.
0345	Gao ben	藁本	*Ligusticum sinense* Oliv.
0346	Gao liang jiang	高良薑	*Alpinia conchigera* Griff. .
0347	Gao lu	皋蘆	*Camellia sinensis* (L.) O. Kuntze f. *Macrophylla* (Sieb.) Kitamura
0348	Ge [gen]	葛[根]	*Pueraria lobata* (Willd.) Ohwi
0349	Ge hua cai	葛花菜	*Balanophora japonica* Makino
0350	Ge jie	蛤蚧	Gecko
0351	Ge li	蛤蜊	Clams
0352	Geng xiang	耕香	Unidentified
0353	Ge shang ting zhang	葛上亭長	Blister beetles, unidentified plant
0354	Ge shan xiao	隔山消	*Cynanchum auriculatum* Royle ex Wight
0355	Ge zhu cao	格注草	*Psoralea corylifolia* L.

0356	Gou	狗	Dog
0357	Gou bao	狗寶	Dog bezoar
0358	Gou gu	枸骨	*Ilex cornuta* Lindl. *ex* paxt.
0359	Gou ji	狗脊	*Cimbotium barometz* (L.) J. Smith
0360	Gou li	鈎栗	*Castanopsis tibetana* Hance.
0361	Gou qi	枸杞	*Lycium barbarum* L. and *Lycium chinense* Mill.
0362	Gou wen	鈎吻	*Gelsemium elegans* (Gardn.et Champ.) Benth.
0363	Gou yin	苟印	Unidentified scaly animal
0364	Gu	菰	*Zizania caduciflora* (Turcz. ex Trin.) Hand.-Mazz.
0365	Gua lou	栝樓	*Trichosanthes kirilowii* Maxim.
0366	Gua lu	瓜蘆	*Camellia sinensis* (L.) O.Kuntze f. *macrophylla* (Sieb.) Kitamura
0367	Guang lang zi	桄榔子	*Arenga pinnata* (Wurmb.) Merr.
0368	Guang ming yan	光明鹽	Crystal salt
0369	Guan zhong	貫衆	*Dryopteris crassirhizoma* Nakai
0370	Gua teng	瓜藤	Unidentified evergreen vine
0371	Hu chao	鶻嘲	Loochoo green pidgeon
0372	Gu chong	蠱蟲	*Gu* poison
0373	Gu du zi	古度子	Unidentified figlike plant
0374	Gu huo	姑活	Unidentified herb
0375	Gu huo niao	姑獲鳥	Goatsucker
0376	Gui	桂	*Cinnamomum cassia* Presl.
0377	Gui bo teng	鬼膊藤	Unidentified vine with pear-like leaves
0378	Gui che niao	鬼車鳥	Goatsucker
0379	Gui dan	鬼彈	Mythological animal living in waters, believed to cause putrescence in the skin of humans
0380	Gui du chong	桂蠹蟲	Cinnamon tree grub
0381	Gui jiu	鬼臼	*Dysosma versipellis* (Hance) M. Cheng ex Ying
0382	Gui yu	鱖魚	Mandarin fish
0383	Gui zao jia	鬼皂莢	Unidentified small plant like → 1444 Zao jia 皂莢
0384	Gu jing	古鏡	Old copper mirrors
0385	Gu jing cao	穀精草	*Eriocaulon buergerianum* Koern.
0386	Gu lu zhi	骨路支	Unidentified plant

0387	Gu mi	菰米	*Zizania caduciflora* (Turcz. ex Trin.) Hand.-Mazz.
0388	Guo ran	果然	Proboscis monkey
0389	Gu sui bu	骨碎補	*Drynaria fortunei* (Kunze) J. Smith
0390	Gu tuo qin	骨托禽	The ostrich
0391	Gu wen qian	古文錢	Old copper coins
0392	Hai dai	海帶	*Laminaria japonica* Areschoug
0393	Hai ge	海蛤	Clam
0394	Hai gen	根	*Polygonum virginicum* L. var. *filiforme* Nakai.
0395	Hai hong	海紅	*Malus micromalus* Makino
0396	Hai hong dou	海紅豆	*Adenanthera pavonina* L. var. *microsperma* (Teijsm. et Binnend.) Nielsen
0397	Hai huan pi	海獾皮	Skin of the badger
0398	Hai jing	海鏡	Scallop
0399	Hai jin sha	海金沙	*Lygodium japonicum* (Thunb.) Sw.
0400	Hai luo	海螺	Sea snail
0401	Hai ma	海馬	Sea horses
0402	Hai man li	海鰻鱺	Marine eels
0403	Hai niu	海牛	Sea cow
0404	Hai song zi	海松子	*Pinus koraiensis* Sieb. et Zucc.
0405	Hai tong	海桐	*Erythrina variegata* L.
0406	Hai wu zi	海梧子	Fruit of unidentified tree
0407	Hai xia	海蝦	Chinese shrimp
0408	Hai yan	海燕	Starfish
0409	Hai yao yu	海鷂魚	Stingray
0410	Hai yu	海芋	*Alocasia macrorrhiza* (L.) Schott.
0411	Hai yue	海月	Windowpane oyster
0412	Hai zao	海藻	*Sargassum fusiforme* (Harv.) Setch.
0413	Hai zhe	海蛇	*Ropilema esculenta* Kishinouye
0414	Ha ma	蛤蟆	Small toad
0415	Han cai	蔊菜	*Rorippa indica* (L.) Hiern.
0416	Han chun teng	含春藤	Unidentified evergreen climbing plant
0417	Han hao chong	寒號蟲	Feces of *Trogopterus xanthipes* Milne-Edwards
0418	Han huo	寒火	A "cold-type" fire burning from phosphorus, human bones, etc.
0419	Han shui teng	含水藤	*Gnetum parvifolium* (Warb.) C.Y. Cheng ex Chun

0420	Hao que	蒿雀	Buntings
0421	Hao zhu	豪猪	Porcupine
0422	He	貉	Racoon dog
0423	He huan	合歡	*Albizzia julibrissin* Durazz.
0424	Hai can	海蠶	Sea-worms found on hilly rocks in the South Seas shaped like a silkworm as big as the thumb
0425	Hei shi hua	黑石華	Unidentified mineral
0426	He ji	鶡鷄	Manchurian snow pheasant
0427	He li le	訶黎勒	*Terminalia chebula* Retz., myrobalans
0428	He shou wu	何首烏	*Polygonum multiflorum* Thunb.
0429	He tun	河豚	*Fugu* puffer
0430	He xin mu	合新木	Unidentified tree
0431	He yu shi	合玉石	Sand for cutting and polishing nephrite
0432	Shi er shi chong	十二時蟲	*Calotes alticristatus* Schmidt
0433	Hong bai lian hua	紅白蓮花	*Nymphaea alba* L.
0434	Hong lan hua	紅藍花	*Carthamus tinctorius* L.
0435	Hong mao cao	紅茂草	*Dianthus caryophyllum* L.
0436	Hong pu cao	紅蒲根	*Sparganium stoloniferum* Buch.-Ham.
0437	Hou po	厚朴	*Magnolia officinalis* Rehd. et Wils.
0438	Hou yu	鱟魚	Horse-shoe or king crabs
0439	Hu	鵠	Swans
0440	Hu	狐	Foxes
0441	Hu	葫	*Allium sativum* L.
0442	Hu	虎	Tiger
0443	Huai	槐	*Sophora japonica* L.
0444	Huai mu	淮木	Timber found as relics from ancient city dwellings
0445	Huai xiang	蘹香	*Platycarya strobilacea* Sieb. et Zucc.; fennel
0446	Hua mao	花貓	Cat with a coat of multiple colors
0447	Hua mu	樺木	*Betula platyphylla* Suk.
0448	Huan	貛	The common badger
0449	Huang fan	黃礬	Yellow iron alum
0450	Huang gu yu	黃鯝魚	False culter
0451	Huang han she	黃頷蛇	Chicken snakes
0452	Huang hua liao	黃花了	Unidentified plant

0453	Huang huan	黃環	A leguminous plant; possibly *Wisteria chinensis*, DC
0454	Huang hu cao	黃護草	Unidentified herb
0455	Huang jing	黃精	*Polygonatum sibiricum* Delar. ex Redoute
0456	Huang lian	黃連	*Coptis chinensis* Franch.
0457	Huang liang	黃粱	→ 0639 Liang 粱
0458	Huang liao lang	黃寮郎	Unidentified herb
0459	Huang lu	黃櫨	*Cotinus coggygria* Scop. var. *cinerea* Engl.
0460	Huang pi guo	黃皮果	*Clausena lansium* (Lour.) Skeels
0461	Huang qi	黃耆	*Astragalus membranaceus* Bunge var. *mongolicus* (Bunge) P. K. Hsiao
0462	Huang qin	黃芩	*Scutellaria baicalensis* Georgi
0463	Huang shi hua	黃石華	Unidentified mineral
0464	Huangs hu	黃鼠	Sand rat
0465	Huang teng	黃藤	*Fibraurea cisa* Pierre
0466	Huang xie	黃屑	Unidentified tree producing a yellow dye
0467	Huang yang	黃羊	Goitered antelope
0468	Huang yao zi	黃藥子	*Clematis terniflora* D.C.
0469	Huang yin	黃銀	Brass
0470	Huang zheng	黃蒸	Yellow or green mould growing on rice and wheat congee
0471	Huan jun	雚菌	Unidentified fungi
0472	Huan yu	鯇魚	Carp
0473	Hua ru shi	花乳石	Dolomite
0474	Hua shi	滑石	Soapstone
0475	Hu cao	蔛草	*Monochoria vaginalis* (Burm. f.) Presl.
0476	Hu cong	胡葱	*Allium cepa* L., but also a shallot *A. Ascalonicum*
0477	Hu gua	胡瓜	*Cucumis sativus* L., cucumber
0478	Hu huang lian	胡黃連	*Picrorhiza scrophulariiflora* Pennell.
0479	Hui yao	灰藥	Unidentified substance resembling black ash powder
0480	Hu jiao	胡椒	*Piper nigrum* L., black pepper
0481	Hu jin cao	胡堇草	Unidentified herb
0482	Hu lu	壺盧	*Lagenaria siceraria* (Molina) Standl.

0483	Hu lu ba	胡蘆巴	*Trigonella foenum-graecum* L.
0484	Hu luo bo	胡蘿蔔	*Daucus carota* L. var. *sativa* Hoffm.
0485	Hu ma	胡麻	*Sesamum indicum* L.
0486	Hu mian mang	胡面莽	Unidentified plant from the Southeast. Leaf similar to that of → 0222 Di huang 地黄.
0487	Huo shu	火鼠	Supposed large rat from Xin jiang 新疆 and the South Sea
0488	Huo tan mu cao	火炭母草	*Polygonum chinense* L.
0489	Huo xiang	藿香	*Agastache rugosa* (Fisch. et Mey.) O. Kuntze
0490	Huo yao	火藥	Gunpowder
0491	Huo zhen	火針	Heated iron needle
0492	Huo zhu	火珠	Crystal burning glass
0493	Hu po	琥珀	Amber
0494	Hu sui	胡荽	*Coriandrum sativum* L.
0495	Hu tao	胡桃	*Juglans regia* L., walnut
0496	Hu tong lei	胡桐淚	Resin of *Populus euphratica* Oliv.
0497	Hu tui zi	胡頹子	*Elaeagnus pungens* Thunb.
0498	Hu yang	胡羊	Arabian sheep, over three feet high
0499	Hu zhang	虎杖	*Polygonum cuspidatum* Sieb.et Zucc..
0500	Jingtian	景天	*Hylotelephium erythrostictum* (Miq.) H. Ohba
0501	Ji	雞(鶏)	Chicken
0502	Ji	蕺	*Houttuynia cordata* Thunb.
0503	Ji	麂	Chinese deer
0504	Ji	稷	*Panicum miliaceum* L., millet
0505	Ji	薊	Fowls
0506	Jia die	蛺蝶	Butterflies
0507	Jia mi	莢蒾	*Grevia biloba* G. Don.
0508	Jian cao	剪草	*Chloranthus fortunei* (A. Gray) Solms-Lamb.
0509	Jiang huang	薑黃	*Curcuma longa* L.
0510	Jiang shi	薑石	Gravel
0511	Jiang zhen xiang	降真香	*Dalbergia odorifera* T. Chen, rose-wood
0512	Jian shui cao	建水草	Unidentified herb
0513	Jian zhong xiao	見腫消	*Gynura segetum* (Lour.) Merr.
0514	Jian zi	蕑子	Unidentified vine, with pear-like fruit

0515	Jiao jing	鵁鶄	Chinese Squacco Heron
0516	Jiao long	蛟龍	Crocodiles
0517	Jiao tu	狡兔	A rabbit-like animal
0518	Jiao yu	鮫魚	A houndshark
0519	Jia su	假蘇	*Schizonepeta multifida* (L.) Briq.
0520	Jia yu	嘉魚	Char
0521	Ji ding chong	吉丁蟲	*Chalcophora japonica* (Gory)
0522	Jie	芥	*Brassica juncea* (L.) Czern.et Coss.
0523	Jie che xiang	藒車香	Unidentified fragrant plant
0524	Jie du zi	解毒子	*Stephania epigaea* H. S. Lo.
0525	Jie geng	桔梗	*Platycodon grandiflorus* (Jacq.) A. DC
0526	Jie sha	結殺	Flowers of unidentified tree from the West
0527	Jie xin cao	芥心草	Unidentified plant
0528	Jie yu	鮆魚	False carp
0529	Ji hou cai	鷄侯菜	Unidentified edible plant
0530	Ji jiu	鵋鶀	Eurasian hoopoe
0531	Ji ju chong	寄居蟲	*Diogenes edwardsii* de Haan
0532	Ji li	蒺藜	*Tribulus terrestris* R.
0533	Ji li cao	吉利草	Unidentified plant
0534	Ji mu	麂目	Fruit of unidentified tree
0535	Jin	金	Native gold
0536	Jin	錦	Brocade
0537	Jin can	金蠶	Tapestry moth
0538	Jin cao	藎草	*Arthraxon hispidus* (Thunb.) Makino
0539	Jin chuang xiao cao	金瘡小草	*Ajuga pygmaea* A. Gr.
0540	Jin di luo	錦地羅	*Drosera Burmanni* Vahl.
0541	Jing	粳	*Oryza sativa* L.
0542	Jin gang shi	金剛石	Diamond
0543	Jing ji	麖麂	Chinese deer, big muntjac
0544	Jing quan shi	井泉石	"Stones from wells and springs"
0545	Jing san leng	京三棱	*Scirpus Yagara* Ohwi
0546	Jing san leng	荊三棱	*Scirpus Yagara* Ohwi
0547	Jin gui zi	金龜子	Golden chafer
0548	Jing yan	井鹽	Salt produced from the brine of inland wells
0549	Ji nie	鷄涅	Unidentified plant
0550	Jin ju	金橘	*Fortunella margarita* (Lour.) Swingle

0551	Jin leng teng	金稜藤	Unidentified evergreen with no flowers
0552	Jin she	金蛇	Unidentified "Golden snakes"
0553	Jin shi	金石	Brown mica
0554	Jin si cao	金絲草	*Pogonatherum crinitum* (Thunb.) Kunth
0555	Jin xing cao	金星草	*Phymatopsis griffithiana* (Hook.) J. Smith
0556	Jin xing shi	金星石	Biotite
0557	Jin ya shi	金牙石	Iron pyrites
0558	Jin ying zi	金櫻子	*Rosa laevigata* Michx.
0559	Jin yu	金魚	Gold fish
0560	Jin zhan cao	金盞草	*Calendula arvensis* L.
0561	Jin zi gen	筋子根	Unidentified herb
0562	Ji shi	芰實	*Trapa bispinosa* Roxb.
0563	Ji su	鷄蘇	Alternative name for → 1087 Shui su 水蘇
0564	Ji tong	鷄桐	Unidentified plant
0565	Jiu	韭	*Allium tuberosum* Rottl. ex Spreng.
0566	Jiu	酒	Liquor
0567	Jiu bei teng zi	酒杯藤子	Unidentified vine with stems as thick as an upper arm, and fruits like a finger
0568	Jiu niu cao	九牛草	*Chrysanthemum decaisneanum* Matsum.
0569	Jiu xiang chong	九香蟲	Stink-bug
0570	Jiu xian zi	九仙子	Unidentified vine with egg-sized root tubers
0571	Ji weng teng	鷄翁藤	Unidentified vine
0572	Ji xue cao	積雪草	*Centella asiatica* (L.) Urban
0573	Ji yu	鯽魚	Golden carp
0574	Ji zong	鷄㙡	*Termiotomyces albuminosus* (Berk.) Heim
0575	Ju	菊	*Dendranthema morifolium* (Ramat) Tzvel., chrysanthemum
0576	Ju	櫸	*Zelkova schneideriana* Hand.-Mazz.
0577	Ju	豦	Unidentified monkey-like animal
0578	Ju	橘	*Citrus reticulata* Blanco
0579	Juan bai	卷柏	*Selaginella involvens* Spr.
0580	Jue	蕨	*Pteridium aquilinum* (L.) Kuhn var. *Latiusculum* (Desv.) Underw.

0581	Jue	玃	Large apes
0582	Jue chang	爵牀	*Rostellularis procumbens* (L.) Nees
0583	Jue ming	決明	*Cassia tora* L.
0584	Jue shu	鱖鼠	Jumping hare
0585	Ju jiang	蒟醬	*Piper betle* L.
0586	Jun gui	箘桂	*Cinnamomum cassia* Presl.
0587	Jun qian zi	君遷子	*Diospyros lotus* L.
0588	Ju ruo	蒟蒻	*Amorphallus revieri* Durieu
0589	Ju you	橘柚	Tangelo, hybrid of tangerines and grapefruits
0590	Ju yuan	枸櫞	*Citrus medica* L.
0591	Ke	珂	Inferior type of jade
0592	Ke shu	柯樹	*Lithocarpus glaber* (Thunb.) Nakai
0593	Ke teng zi	榼藤子	*Entada phaseoloides* (L.) Merr.
0594	Kong gong nie	孔公孽	Middle part of a stalactite with hole in the center
0595	Kong qing	空青	Malachite, large hollow variety
0596	Kong que	孔雀	Malayan Peacock
0597	Ku ao	苦芙	*Lactuca tartarica* (L.) C. A. Mey.
0598	Kuai can yu	鱠殘魚	Silver fish or ice fish
0599	Kuan dong hua	款冬花	*Tussilago farfara* L.
0600	Kuang mai	穬麥	*Hordeum vulgare* var. *nudum* Hook. f.
0601	Kuang shi	曠石	Unidentified herb
0602	Ku cai	苦菜	*Sonchus oleraceus* L.
0603	Ku gua	苦瓜	*Momordica charantia* L.
0604	Ku hu	苦瓠	*Lagenaria siceraria* (Molina) Standl. var. *microcarpa* (Naud.) Hara
0605	Kui	葵	*Malva verticillata* L.
0606	Kui ge	魁蛤	*Scapharca inflata* (Reeve) clam
0607	Ku jie zi	苦芥子	Unidentified herb
0608	Kun bu	昆布	*Laminaria japonica* Aresch.
0609	Kuo yu	蛞蝓	Slug
0610	Ku qiao mai	苦蕎麥	*Fagopyrum tartaricum* Gaertn.
0611	Ku qie	苦茄	*Solanum dulcamara* L.
0612	Ku shen	苦參	*Sophora flavescens* Ait.
0613	Ku sun	苦筍	Bamboo shoots
0614	Lai fu	萊菔	*Raphanus sativus* L.
0615	Lan	藍	Plants used to produce indigo dye
0616	Lan cao	蘭草	*Eupatorium fortunei* Turcz.
0617	Lan dian	藍澱	Indigo dye

0618	Lang	狼	Wolf
0619	Lang dang	莨菪	*Hyoscyamus niger* F.W.Schmidt
0620	Lang du	狼毒	*Stellaria chamaejasme* L.; *Euphorbia fischeriana* St.
0621	Lang jun zi	郎君子	Opercula of top shells
0622	Lang mei	榔梅	Fruit of legendary tree
0623	Lang ya	狼牙	*Agrimonia pilosa* Ledeb.
0624	Lan she	藍蛇	Unidentified "blue snake"
0625	Lan teng	藍藤	Unidentified creeping plant
0626	Lao	酪	Cream from cow, sheep, buffalo, camel or horse milk
0627	Lei mo	雷墨	Meteorites
0628	Lei shu	鸓鼠	Flying squirrel
0629	Lei wan	雷丸	*Omphalia lapidescens* Schroet.
0630	Le yu	勒魚	Long-finned herring
0631	Li	梨	*Pyrus bretschneideri* Rehd.; pear
0632	Li	狸	Wild cat
0633	Li	藜	*Chenopodium album* L.
0634	Li	李	*Prunus salicina* Lindl., plum
0635	Li	栗	*Castanea molissima* L., chestnut
0636	Lian	楝	*Melia azedarach* L.
0637	Lian ou	蓮藕	*Nelumbo nucifera* Gaertn., lotus
0638	Lian bo	簾箔	Thin bamboo or reed curtain
0639	Liang	粱	*Setaria italica* (L.) Beauv.
0640	Liang da	良達	Unidentified plant
0641	Liang tou she	兩頭蛇	"Two headed snake"
0642	Lian jiang	廉薑	*Alpinia chinensis* (Retz.) Rosc.
0643	Lian qian cao	連錢草	*Centella asiatica* (L.) Urban.
0644	Lian qiao	連翹	*Forsythia suspensa* (Thunb.) Vahl.
0645	Liao	蓼	*Polygonum hydropiper* L.
0646	Liao luo	蓼螺	Seasnails, whelks
0647	Li chang	鱧腸	*Eclipta prostrata* L.
0648	Li chun cao	麗春草	*Papaver rhoeas* L.
0649	Li dou	黎豆	*Stizolobium capitatum* (Sweet) O.Kuntze
0650	Lie dang	列當	*Orobanche coerulescens* Steph.
0651	Li ge cao	離鬲草	Unidentified herb
0652	Li lou cao	離樓草	Unidentified herb
0653	Li lu	藜蘆	*Veratrum nigrum* L.
0654	Ling li	鯪鯉	Pangolin
0655	Ling ling xiang	零陵香	*Ocimum basilicum* L.

0656	Ling mao	靈猫	The civet
0657	Ling shi	陵石	Unidentified mineral
0658	Ling shou mu	靈壽木	Unidentified tree
0659	Ling yang	羚羊	Mythological animal
0660	Ling yang	麢羊	Antilope
0661	Ling zhi	靈芝	→ 1469 Zhi 芝
0662	Lin mu	橉木	*Laurocerasus spinulosa* Sieb. et Zucc. Schneid.
0663	Lin qin	林檎	*Malus asiatica* Nakai
0664	Lin she	鱗蛇	Python
0665	Li shi	蠡實	*Iris lactea* Pall. var. *chinensis* (Fisch.) Koidz.
0666	Li shi	理石	Alabaster
0667	Liu	柳	*Salix babylonica* L.
0668	Liu ji nu cao	劉寄奴草	*Artemisia anomala* S.Moore.
0669	Liu jun dai	留軍待	Unidentified plant
0670	Liu li	琉璃	Lapis lazuli
0671	Liu lian	榴蓮	Durian tree
0672	Li yu	鯉魚	Serpent-head
0673	Li yu	鱧魚	Serpent-head
0674	Li zhi	荔枝	*Litchi chinensis* Sonn.
0675	Long	龍	"Dragon," fossil bones and teeth
0676	Long chang cao	龍常草	*Diarrhena manshurica* Maxim.
0677	Long dan	龍膽	*Gentiana scabra* Bunge
0678	Long kui	龍葵	*Solanum nigrum* L.
0679	Long li	龍荔	Unidentified plant
0680	Long nao xiang	龍腦香	Borneo campher
0681	Long she cao	龍舌草	*Ottelia alismoides* (L.) Pers.
0682	Long shou teng	龍手藤	Unidentified vine
0683	Long xian shi	龍涎石>	Unidentified mineral
0684	Long xu cai	龍鬚菜	*Gracilaria asiatica* C. F. Chang et B. M. Xia
0685	Long yan	龍眼	*Dimocarpus longan* Lour.
0686	Lou lan zi	漏籃子	*Aconitum carmichaeli* Debx.
0687	Lou lu	漏盧	*Stemmacantha uniflorum* (L.) Dittrich
0688	Lu	蘆	*Phragmites communis* Trin.
0689	Lu	鹿	Deer
0690	Lu	鷺	Bundles of green ginseng foliage
0691	Lü	驢	The ass
0692	Luan hua	欒華	*Koelreuteria paniculata* Laxm.

0693	Luan jing	欒荊	A member of genus *Vitex*
0694	Lu ci	鸕鷀	The Chinese cormorant
0695	Lü fan	緑礬	Green vitriol
0696	Lu feng fang	露蜂房	Hornets' and wasps' nests
0697	Lü fu qing	緑膚青	Azurite
0698	Lu gan shi	爐甘石	Zincspar
0699	Lu gu zi	橹罟子	Fruit of *Pandanus tectorius* Soland
0700	Lu hui	盧會	*Aloe vera* L.
0701	Lu huo	鹿藿	*Rhynchosia volubilis* Lour.
0702	Lu jian	鹵碱	Native lake salt
0703	Lu jiao cai	鹿角菜	Red algae
0704	Lu jin cao	露筋草	Unidentified herb
0705	Lu jing	盧精	Unidentified herb
0706	Lu li	鹿梨	*Pyrus calleryana* Decne.
0707	Lü mao gui	緑毛龜	Tortoises with algae growth on head
0708	Lü mu	櫚木	*Ormosia henryi* Prain
0709	Luo	騾	The mule
0710	Luo huang zi	羅晃子	*Sterculia nobilis* Smith
0711	Luo kui	落葵	*Basella alba* L.
0712	Luo le	羅勒	*Ocimum basilicum* L.
0713	Luo mo	蘿摩	*Metaplexis japonica* (Thunb.) Makino
0714	Luo shi	絡石	*Trachelospermum jasminoides* (Lindl.) Lem.
0715	Luo wang zi	羅望子	Fruit of *Tamarindus indica* L.
0716	Luo yan mu	落雁木	Unidentified herb
0717	Lü qing	緑青	Malachite
0718	Lü ru	藺茹	*Euphorbia ebracteolata* Hayata
0719	Lu ti cao	鹿蹄草	*Pyrola decorata* H. Andr.
0720	Lü yan	緑鹽	Persian zingar, green verdigris
0721	Lu yao	鹿藥	*Smilacina japonica* A. Gray
0722	Lu ying	陸英	*Sambucus chinensis* Lindl.
0723	Lu yu	鱸魚	Japanese Sea Bass
0724	Ma	馬	The horse
0725	Ma bian cao	馬鞭草	*Verbena officinalis* L.
0726	Ma bing lang	馬檳榔	*Capparis masaikai* Lévl.
0727	Ma chang gen	馬腸根	Unidentified herb
0728	Ma chi xian	馬齒莧	*Portulaca oleracea* L.
0729	Ma dao	馬刀	Giant mussels
0730	Ma dou ling	馬兜鈴	*Aristolochia contorta* Bunge

0731	Ma gan shi	馬肝石	A bluish-black stone said to be magical
0732	Ma gu jiu	麻姑酒	Yellow liquor from Ma gu shan 麻姑山
0733	Ma huang	麻黃	*Ephedra sinica* Stapf
0734	Mai fan shi	麥飯石	Porphyry
0735	Mai men dong	麥門冬	*Ophiopogon japonicus* (L.f.) Ker-Gawl.
0736	Mai zi mu	賣子木	*Ixora chinensis* Lam.
0737	Ma lu	馬陸	Centipedes
0738	Ma nao	馬腦	Agate
0739	Mang	芒	*Miscanthus sinensis* Anders.
0740	Mang cao	莽草	*Illiceum lanceolatum* A. C. Smith
0741	Man jing	蔓荊	*Vitex trifolia* L. var. *simplicifolia* Cham.
0742	Man li yu	鰻鱺魚	Eels
0743	Man to luo hua	曼陀羅花	*Datura metel* L.
0744	Man yu teng	曼游藤	Unidentified vine
0745	Mao gen	毛茛	*Ranunculus japonicus* Thunb.
0746	Mao niu	犛牛	The hairy yak
0747	Mao niu	牦牛	The hairy yak
0748	Mao xiang	茅香	*Cymbopogon citratus* (D C.) Stapf.
0749	Mao zhi han	茆質汗	Unidentified plant
0750	Ma xian hao	馬先蒿	*Pedicularis resupinata* L.
0751	Ma yang mu	馬瘍木	Unidentified tree
0752	Mei	梅	*Armeniaca mume* Sieb.
0753	Mei die	媚蝶	Variety of grasshopper
0754	Mei shi wang mu	每始王木	Unidentified vine
0755	Meng chong	虻蟲	Horsefly
0756	Meng niang cai	孟娘菜	Unidentified edible evergreen plant
0757	Meng shi	礞石	Micacous earth
0758	Meng song	蒙頌	A small proboscis monkey
0759	Meng tong	鳥十蒙, 鳥十童	*Antherococeros coronatus albirostris* Saw et Nodder
0760	Mi	麋	Elk, moose
0761	Mi cu	米醋	Vinegar made from rice
0762	Mi feng	蜜蜂	Honey bee
0763	Mi hou	獼猴	Macaca monkeys
0764	Mi hou tao	獼猴桃	Kiwi fruit
0765	Mi la	蜜蠟	Beeswax

0766	Mi li zi	蜜栗子	Variety of limestone
0767	Mi meng hua	密蒙花	*Buddleia officinalis* Maxim.
0768	Ming	茗	*Camellia sinensis* L.
0769	Ming zha	榠楂	*Cydonia sinensis* (Thouin] Koehne
0770	Mi tuo seng	密陀僧	Litharge
0771	Mi wu	蘼蕪	Young leaves of → 1308 Xiong qiong 芎藭
0772	Mi xiang	蜜香	*Aquilaria agallocha* (Lour.) Roxb.
0773	Mo	墨	Soot from burning pine wood
0774	Mo	貘	The Malaya tapir
0775	Mo chu zi	摩厨子	*Styrax japonicum* Sieb. et Zucc.
0776	Mo gu xun	蘑菰蕈	Focally *Agaricus bisporus* (Lange) Sing. In North China: *Tricholoma mongolicum* Imai
0777	Mo li	茉莉	*Jasminum sambac* (L.) Ait.
0778	Mo tou yu	墨頭魚	Black-headed maigre
0779	Mo yao	沒藥	Resin of *Commiphora myrrha* Engl.
0780	Mu bie zi	木鱉子	*Momordica cochinchinensis* (Lour.) Spreng.
0781	Mu dan	牡丹	*Paeonia suffruticosa* Andr.
0782	Mu er	木耳	*Auricularia auricula* (L. ex Hook.) Underw.
0783	Mu fu rong	木芙蓉	*Hibiscus mutabilis* L.
0784	Mu gou	木狗	Silver fox
0785	Mu gua	木瓜	*Chaenomeles speciosa* (Sweet) Nakai
0786	Mu jin	木槿	*Hibiscus syriacus* L.
0787	Mu jing	牡荊	*Vitex negundo* L. var. *cannabifolia* (Sieb. et Zucc.) Hand.-Mazz.
0788	Mu ke niao	木客鳥	Mythological bird
0789	Mu lan	木蘭	*Magnolia* L.
0790	Mu li	牡蠣	Oysters
0791	Mu lian	木蓮	*Ficus pumila* L.
0792	Mu ma	木麻	Unidentified plant
0793	Mu meng	木虻	Snipe-fly
0794	Mu mian	木綿	*Bombax malabaricum* DC. Kapok
0795	Mu mi cao	牧靡草	Unidentified poisonous herb
0796	Mu nai yi	木乃伊	*Mummia*, Human mummy confection
0797	Mu tian liao	木天蓼	*Actinidia polygama* (Sieb. et Zucc.) Maxim.

0798	Mu wei zi	木威子	*Canarium pimela* Leenh.
0799	Mu xiang	木香	*Aucklandia lappa* Decne
0800	Mu xi xin	木細辛	Unidentifiable plant similar to → 1311 Xi xin 細辛
0801	Mu xu	苜蓿	*Medicago hispida* Gaertn.
0802	Mu zei	木賊	*Hippochaete hiemale* (L.) Borher
0803	Mu zhu zi	木竹子	*Garcinia multiflora* Champ, ex Benth.
0804	Nai	柰	*Malus pumila* Mill.
0805	Neng bie	能鱉	Mythological three footed turtle
0806	Nan	楠	*Phoebe zhennan* S.Lee et F. N. Wei .
0807	Nan gua	南瓜	*Cucurbita moschata* (Duch. ex Lam.) Duch. ex Poir.
0808	Nan huo lan	難火蘭	Unidentified plant
0809	Nan teng	南藤	*Piper wallichii* (Miq.) Hand.-Mazz. var. *hupehense* (C. DC.) Hand.-Mazz.
0810	Nan zhu	南燭	*Vaccineum bracteatum* Thunb.
0811	Nao sha	硇砂	Sal ammoniac
0812	Na qi xi	那耆悉	Unidentified tree growing in Southwest China
0813	Niao feng	鳥鳳	*Psittacula longicauda* Boddaert
0814	Nie tie	嚙鐵	Southern tapir, said to be the size of a water buffalo
0815	Ni luo	泥螺	Seasnails
0816	Ning shui shi	凝水石	Calcareous spar; gypsum
0817	Niu	牛	Ox; cow
0818	Niu bian	牛扁	*Aconitum barbatum* Pers. var. *puberulum* Ledeb.
0819	Niu huang	牛黃	Cow bezoar
0820	Niu jiao zhi	牛角芝	A mythological plant
0821	Niu ling teng	牛領藤	Unidentified vine
0822	Niu she shi	牛舌實	Unidentified “cattle-tongue fruit“
0823	Niu xi	牛膝	*Achyranthes bidentata* Bl.
0824	Niu yu	牛魚	*Dugong dugan* Müller
0825	Ni yu	鯢魚	Giant salamander
0826	Nu ge sa er	奴哥撒兒	Unidentified herb
0827	Nu hui zi	奴會子	Unidentified plant
0828	Nü qing	女青	*Cynanchum thesinides* (Freyn) K. Schum.

0829	Nü wan	女菀	*Turczaninowia fastigiata* (Fisch.) DC.
0830	Nü wei	女萎	*Clematis apiifolia* DC.
0831	Nu zhe	奴柘	*Maclura cochinchinensis* (Lour.) Corher
0832	Nü zhen	女貞	*Ligustrum lucidum* Ait.
0833	Ou	鷗	Gulls
0834	Pai cao xiang	排草香	*Anisochilus carnosus* (L.) Wall.
0835	Pan dao zeng	攀倒甑	Unidentified plant
0836	Pang jiang	龐降	Cicada sloughs
0837	Peng cao zi	蓬草子	*Artemisia* spp.
0838	Peng e zhu	蓬莪术	*Curcuma aeruginosa* Roxb.
0839	Peng lei	蓬虆	*Rubus buergeri* Miq.
0840	Peng sha	蓬砂	Borax
0841	Pi	羆	The brown bear
0842	Pian tao ren	偏桃仁	Unidentified tree
0843	Pi li le	毗梨勒	*Terminalia belerica* (Gaertn.) Roxb.
0844	Pi li zhen	霹靂砧	Meteorites
0845	Ping	蘋	*Marsilea quadrifolia* L.
0846	Ping peng cao	萍蓬草	*Nuphar pumilum* (Hoffm.) DC.
0847	Ping xiang	瓶香	Unidentified plant from the Southern Seas
0848	Pi pa	枇杷	*Eriobotrya japonica* (Thunb.) Lindl.
0849	Pi shi	砒石	Arsenic trioxide
0850	Pi ti	鷿鷉	Chinese little grebe
0851	Po luo de	婆羅得	*Semecarpus anacardium* L.
0852	Po luo men bai yao	婆羅門白藥	Unidentified herb
0853	Po luo men shen	婆羅門參	→ 1279 Xian mao 仙茅
0854	Po luo men zao jia	婆羅門皂莢	→ A le bo阿勒勃
0855	Po suo shi	婆娑石	Unidentified green pebbles of foreign origin
0856	Po xiao	朴消	Crude Glauber's salt
0857	Pu gong ying	蒲公英	*Taraxacum mongolicum* Hand-Mazz.
0858	Pu sa cao	菩薩草	Unidentified plant
0859	Pu sa shi	菩薩石	Quartz
0860	Pu shan	蒲扇	Old, rotten fans prepared from cattail and reed
0861	Pu tao	葡萄	*Vitis vinifera* L.

0862	Pu tao jiu	葡萄酒	Grape wine
0863	Pu xi	蒲席	Old, rotten sleeping mats prepared from cattail and reed
0864	Qi	漆	*Toxicodendrum verniciflauum* (Stokes) F. A. Barkl.
0865	Qi ai	蘄艾	→ 0003 Ai 艾 collected in Hu bei 湖北 province
0866	Qian	鉛	Lead
0867	Qian cao	茜草	*Rubia cordifolia* L.
0868	Qian dan	鉛丹	Minium
0869	Qiang lang	蜣螂	Dung beetle
0870	Qiang wei lu	薔薇露	Volatile rose oil
0871	Qian hu	前胡	*Peucedanum praeruptorum* Dunn.
0872	Qian jin e cao	千金鎘草	Unidentified herb
0873	Qian jin teng	千金藤	*Stephania japonica* (Thunb.) Miers
0874	Qian li ji	千里及	*Senecio scandens* Ham. (Ch. HC.)
0875	Qian ma	蕁麻	*Urtica laetevirens* Maxim.
0876	Qian nian ai	千年艾	*Crossostephium chinense* (L.) Makino ex Cham. et Schltr.
0877	Qian shi	芡實	*Euryale ferox* Salisb.
0878	Qian sui zi	千歲子	Unidentified vine
0879	Qian sui fu	千歲蝮	A viper much like the ordinary *agkistrodon*
0880	Qian sui lei	千歲虆	*Vitis flexuosa* Thunb.
0881	Qiao fu niao	巧婦鳥	Local bird called wren
0882	Qiao mai	蕎麥	*Fagopyrum esculentum* Moench
0883	Qiao yao	翹摇	*Vicia hirsuta* (L.) S.F.Gray
0884	Qi cao	蠐螬	Dung beetle larva
0885	Qi dun guo	齊墩果	*Olea europaea* L., olive
0886	Qie	茄	*Solanum melongena* L.
0887	Qi lin jie	騏驎竭	*Daemonorops draco* Bl.
0888	Qin di li	秦荻藜	A kind of → 0633 *Li* 藜
0889	Qing ci	青雌	Unidentified plant
0890	Qing dai	青黛	Indigo
0891	Qing feng teng	清風藤	*Sabia japonica* Maxim.
0892	Qing fu	青蚨	Cicada sloughs
0893	Qing hao	青蒿	*Artemisia carvifolia* Buch.-Ham. ex Roxb.
0894	Qing jing gan shi xin fan	青精乾飿石飯	Dried black rice

0895	Qing lang gan	青琅玕	From the sea: coral; from the mountains: malachite
0896	Qing ling	蜻蛉	A kind of dragonfly
0897	Qing tian he	青田核	A mythological plant with huge and heavy seed kernels
0898	Qing tong	青銅	Bronze
0899	Qin gui	秦龜	The Shensi tortoise
0900	Qing xiang	青葙	*Celosia argentea* L.
0901	Qing yu	青鱼	Black carp
0902	Qing yu	青玉	Sapphire
0903	Qing zhou da shi bing	青州大柹餅	Biscuits prepared with persimmon from Qing zhou
0904	Qing zhou zao	青州棗	Large dates/jujubes from Qing zhou
0905	Qi ni	薺苨	*Adenophora trachelioides* Maxim.
0906	Qi ning	薺薴	*Mosla grosserrata* Maxim.
0907	Qin jiao	秦艽	*Gentiana macrophylla* Pall.
0908	Qin jiao	秦椒	*Zanthoxylum* spp
0909	Qin ji liao	秦吉了	A grackle or hill mynah
0910	Qin mu	梫木	*Pieris japonica* (Thunb.) D. Don. ex G. Don.
0911	Qin pi	秦皮	*Fraxinus rhynchophylla* Hance
0912	Qi po teng	祁婆藤	Unidentified evergreen climbing plant
913	Qiu	楸	*Catalpa bungei* C. A. Mey.
0914	Qiu yin	蚯蚓	Earthworm
0915	Qiu yu	鰌魚	Loaches
0916	Qi zi	柒紫	Unidentified herb
0917	Qu cao	屈草	Possibly *Polygonym palmatum* Dunn
0918	Quan shen	拳參	*Polygonum bistorta* L.
0919	Que	雀	The tree sparrow
0920	Que weng	雀甕	Cocoon of the slug-caterpillar
0921	Qu jie cao	曲節草	*Peristrophe japonica* (Thunb.) Bremek.
0922	Qu mai	瞿麥	*Dianthus superbus* S.
0923	Qu sou	渠搜	Tiger from Turkestan
0924	Rang he	蘘荷	*Zingiber mioga* (Thunb.) Rosc.
0925	Ran she	蚺蛇	The python
0926	Ran shi	然石	Flint

0927	Rao hua	蕘花	*Wikstroemia canescens* (Wall.) Meissn.
0928	Ren dong	忍冬	*Lonicera japonica* Thunb.
0929	Ren gan teng	人肝藤	Unidentified vine with split leaves in three sections and purple flowers
0930	Ren mian zi	人面子	*Dracontomelon duperreanum* Pierre
0931	Ren shen	人參	*Panax ginseng* C. A. Meyer
0932	Ren yu	人魚	Giant salamander
0933	Rong	狨	The gibbons
0934	Rou cong rong	肉蓯蓉	*Cistanche deserticola* Y. C. Ma.
0935	Rou dou kou	肉豆蔻	*Myristica fragrans* Houtt., nutmeg
0936	Rou yu	柔魚	Cuttle fish
0937	Rou zhi niu	月支牛	Ox from Western Mongolia and Xinjiang 新疆
0938	Ruan shi	碝石	Variety of opaque, whitish quartz
0939	Ru chong	乳蟲	Cultivated dung beetle larva
0940	Ru gan	乳柑	→ 0323 Gan 柑; mandarin orange
0941	Rui he	蕤核	*Prinsepia uniflora* Batal.
0942	Rui xiang	瑞香	*Daphne acutiloba* Rehd.
0943	Rui zi	蚋子	Gnat
0944	Ruo	箬	*Indocalamus tesselatus* (Munro) Keng
0945	Ru xiang	乳香	Frankincense, resin of *Boswellia carteri* Birdw. and other *B.* spp
0946	Sa ba er	撒八兒	Mythical sperm liquid secreted by the hawksbill turtle
0947	San bai cao	三白草	*Saururus chinensis* (Lour.) Baill.
0948	Sang	桑	*Morus alba* L.
0949	Sang shang ji sheng	桑上寄生	"Mulberry epiphyte", *Taxillus chinensis* (DC) Danser
0950	San leng	三稜	*Scirpus Yagara* Ohwi
0951	San qi	三七	*Panax notoginseng* (Burk.) F. H. Chen ex C. Chow
0952	Sha la chong	唼臘蟲	An ancient beetle said to eat human corpses by preference
0953	Shan	杉	*Cunninghamia lanceoloata* (Lambt.) Hook
0954	Shan cha	山茶	*Camellia japonica* L.
0955	Shan dan	山丹	*Lilium concolor* Salisb.
0956	Shan dou gen	山豆根	*Sophora tonkinensis* Gagnep.
0957	Shan du	山都	A human-like spirit

0958	Shan fan	山礬	*Symplocos chinensis* (Lour.) Druce
0959	Shang lu	商陸	*Phytolacca acinosa* Roxb.
0960	Shan yang	山羊	The wild sheep or argali
0961	Shan hu	珊瑚	Coral
0962	Shan ji	杉鷄	Long tailed pheasan
0963	Shan jiang	山薑	*Alpinia japonica* (Thunb.)
0964	Shan jiu	山韭	*Allium thunbergii* G. Don
0965	Shan jun	杉菌	Fungi growing on Chinese cedar
0966	Shan lü	山驢	"Mountain" donkey
0967	Shan nai	山柰	*Kaempferia galanga* L.
0968	Shan sao	山猱	The moupin langur
0969	Shan suan	山蒜	*Allium nipponicum* Fr. et Sav.
0970	Shan ta	山獺	Chinese otter
0971	Shan yu	鱔魚	Mud eels
0972	Shan zao	山棗	*Zizyphus jujuba* Mill. var. *spinosa* (Bunge) Hu ex H.F.Chow.
0973	Shan zha	山楂	Fruit of *Crataegus pinnatifada* Bunge var. *major* N. F. Br., hawthorne
0974	Shan zhi zhu	山躑躅	*Rhododendron simsii* Planch.
0975	Shan zhu yu	山茱萸	*Cornus officinalis* Sieb. et Zucc.
0976	Shan zi	穇子	*Eleucine corocana* (L.) Gaertn.
0977	Shao jiu	燒酒	Brandy, distilled liquor
0978	Shao yao	芍藥	*Paeonia lactiflora* Pall.
0979	Shao zi	韶子	*Nephelium chryseum* Bl.
0980	Sha shen	沙參	*Adenophora stricta* Miq.
0981	Sha shi	沙蝨	Unidentified "sandlouse"
0982	Sha tang	沙糖	*Saccharum sinensis* Roxb.
0983	Sha tang guo	沙棠果	Unidentified wild pear
0984	Sha yu	鯊魚	Sharks
0985	She	蛇	Snake
0986	She	麝	Musk deer, moschus
0987	She chuang	蛇牀	*Cnidium monnieri* (L.) Cuss.
0988	She gan	射干	*Belamcanda chinensis* (L.) DC.
0989	She gui	攝龜	Mythical snake-eating tortoise
0990	She han	蛇含	*Potentilla kleiniana* Wight et Arn.
0991	She huang	蛇黄	Nodular iron pyrates
0992	She jiao	蛇角	The rhinoceros viper
0993	Sheng gua cai	生瓜菜	*Trigonotis peduncularis* Bth.
0994	Sheng jiang	生薑	*Zingiber officinale* Rosc., unprocessed ginger

0995	Sheng ma	升麻	*Cimicifuga foetida* L.
0996	Sheng teng	省藤	*Daemonorops margaritae* (Hance) Becc.
0997	Shen hu cao	神護草	Unidentified plant
0998	She po	蛇婆	Seasnakes
0999	She she	蛇舌	"Snake tongue," unidentified plant
1000	She tui	蛇蜕	Snake sloughs
1001	She wang cao	蛇網草	→ 0152 Chi di li 赤地利
1002	Shi	獅	Lion
1003	Shi	蓍	*Achillea alpine* L.
1004	Shi	豕	Pig
1005	Shi	柹	*Diospyros kaki* Thunb.
1006	Shi ban yu	石斑魚	Bass
1007	Shi bi yu	石鮅魚	*Barilius* spp
1008	Shi can	石蠶	"Stone silkworms"; dragonfly larvae?
1009	Shi cao	蒒草	*Carex kobomugi* Ohwi
1010	Shi chang sheng	石長生	*Adiantum monochlamys* Eaton
1011	Shi chui	石垂	Unidentified plant
1012	Shi chun	石蓴	*Ulva lactuca* L.
1013	Shi ci mu	石刺木	Unidentified woody epiphyte of trees
1014	Shi dan	石膽	Chalcanthite
1015	Shi er	石耳	*Umbilicaria esculenta* (Miyoshi) Minks
1016	Shi gan	石肝	"Stone liver," unidentified
1017	Shi gao	石膏	*Gypsum fibrosum*
1018	Shi gua	石瓜	*Carica papaya* L.
1019	Shi he cao	石合草	Unidentified herb
1020	Shi hu	石斛	*Dendrobium nobile* Lindl.
1021	Shi hua cai	石花菜	*Euchema gelatinae* (Esp.) J. Ag.
1022	Shi hui	石灰	Limestone
1023	Shi jian	石鹼	Soda
1024	Shi jie	石蜐	Sea anemones
1025	Shi jing	石荆	Unidentified plant
1026	Shi jiu	鳲鳩	The Eastern cuckoo
1027	Shi jue ming	石决明	Abalone, sea ear
1028	Shi jun zi	使君子	*Quisqualis indica* L.
1029	Shi liu chi	石硫赤	Sulphur, amorphous red
1030	Shi liu huang	石硫黃	Sulphur

1031	Shi liu qing	石硫青	Sulphur, amorphous black
1032	Shi long chu	石龍芻	*Juncus setchuensis* L.
1033	Shi long rui	石龍芮	*Ranunculus sceleratus* L.
1034	Shi long zi	石龍子	Lizards
1035	Shi luo	蒔蘿	*Anethum graveolans* L.
1036	Shi mi	石蜜	*Saccharum sinensis* Roxb.
1037	Shi mian	石麪	"Stone flour", powder of Dolomite
1038	Shi nan	石南	*Photinia serrulata* Lindl
1039	Shi nao	石腦	Geodes
1040	Shi nao you	石腦油	Petroleum
1041	Shi nu	石砮	Unidentified stone probes
1042	Shi pi	石脾	"Stone spleen," a feldspathic rock
1043	Shi rui	石蕊	*Cladonia rangiferina* (L.) Web.
1044	Shi she	石蛇	Ammonite
1045	Shi she shu	食蛇鼠	Mongoose
1046	Shi shou yu	石首魚	Croaker
1047	Shi shu	鼫鼠	Squirrels
1048	Shi song	石松	*Lycopodium clavatum* L.
1049	Shi suan	石蒜	*Lycoris radiata* (L'Herit.)
1050	Shi sui	石髓	"Stone marrow," a kind of stalactite
1051	Shi tan	石炭	Coal
1052	Shi wei	石韋	*Pyrrosia lingua* (Thunb.) Farw.
1053	Shi xian	石莧	*Lippia nodifera* Rich.
1054	Shi xiang ru	石香葇	*Mosla chinensis* Maxim.
1055	Shi xiao yao cao	石逍遙草	Unidentified herb
1056	Shi xie	石蟹	"Stone crabs," fossil crabs
1057	Shi yan	食鹽	Cooking salt
1058	Shi yan	石燕	"Stone swallows," fossil shells
1059	Shi yao	石藥	Unidentified mineral
1060	Shi yu	鰣魚	Hilsa herring
1061	Shi zhi	石芝	Mythical „stone fungi"
1062	Shi zhong huang zi	石中黃子	Conglomerate masses of → 1438 Yu yu liang 禹余粮
1063	Shi zhong ru	石鍾乳	Stalactites
1064	Shi zhu yu	食茱萸	*Zanthoxylum ailanthoides* Sieb. et Zucc.
1065	Shou gong	守宮	Geckos
1066	Shu	秫	*Setaria italica* (L.) Beauv.
1067	Shu	黍	*Panicum miliaceum* L. var. *glutinosa* Bretschn.
1068	Shu	鼠	Mice; rats

1069	Shuang tou lu	雙頭鹿	"Two headed deer"
1070	Shu di	數伭	Seeds similar to → 1035 *Shi luo* 蒔蘿
1071	Shu fu	鼠婦	Armadillidium, pill bug
1072	Shu ge	蜀格	Unidentified fungi
1073	Shu gu	鼠姑	Armadillidium, pill bug
1074	Shu hu lan	蜀胡爛	Seeds similar to → 1035 *Shi luo* 蒔蘿
1075	Shui bai dou	水白豆	*Vigna unguiculata* (L.) Walp. var. *cylindrica* (L.) Ohashi
1076	Shui cai	睡菜	*Menyanthes trifoliata* L.
1077	Shui gan cao	水甘草	*Amsonia sinensis* Tsiang et P. T .Li.
1078	Shui gui	水龜	Terrapin
1079	Shui hu	水虎	Mythical scaly animal living in water
1080	Shui jing	水精	Rock-crystal
1081	Shui jue	水蕨	*Ceratopteris thalictroides* (L.) Brongn.
1082	Shui ku mai	水苦蕒	*Veronica anagallis-aquatica* L.
1083	Shui ping	水萍	*Spirodela polyrhiza* (L.) Schleid.
1084	Shui qin	水靳	*Oenanthe javanica* (Bl.) DC.
1085	Shui she	水蛇	A water snake
1086	Shui song	水松	*Codium fragile* (Sur.) Har.
1087	Shui su	水蘇	*Stachys japonica* Miq.
1088	Shui ta	水獺	Fresh water otter
1089	Shui xian	水仙	*Narcissus tacetta* L. var. *chinensis* Roem.
1090	Shui yang	水楊	*Salix sinopurpurea* C.Wang et Ch.Y. Yang
1091	Shui yin	水銀	Quicksilver
1092	Shui ying	水英	1. Plant of unclear identity, 2. → 1084 Shui qin水靳
1093	Shui zao	水藻	*Myriophyllum spicatum* L.
1094	Shui zhi	水蛭	Leeches
1095	Shui zhong bai shi	水中白石	Riverbed pebbles
1096	Shu jiao	蜀椒	*Zanthoxylum bungeanum* Maxim, Chinese pepper
1097	Shu kui	蜀葵	*Althaea rosea* (L.) Cav.
1098	Shu li	鼠李	*Rhamnus utilis* Decne
1099	Shu qu cao	鼠麴草	*Gnaphalium affine* D. Don
1100	Shu shu	蜀黍	*Sorghum vulgare* Pers.; great millet

1101	Shu teng	鼠藤	Unidentified vine mice like to eat.
1102	Shu tou jiu	樹頭酒	Wine prepared from unidentified fruit resembling coconuts
1103	Shu wei cao	鼠尾草	*Salvia japonica* Th.
1104	Shu yang quan	蜀羊泉	*Sagina japonica* (Sw.) Ohwi
1105	Shu yu	薯蕷	*Dioscorea opposita* Thunb.
1106	Si gua	絲瓜	*Luffa cylindrica* (L.) Roem.
1107	Si ji liu	四季榴	A pomegranate, *Punica granatum* L., flowering all year
1108	Si wei guo	四味果	*Elaeagnus angustifolia* L., oleaster
1109	Song	松	*Pinus armandi* Franch.
1110	Song	菘	*Brassica campestris* L.
1111	Song luo	松蘿	*Usnea longissima* Ach.
1112	Song shi	松石	Seeds of *Pinus koraienis* Sieb. et Zucc.
1113	Song yang	松楊	*Swida macrophylla* (Wall.)
1114	Sou shu	溲疏	*Deutzia scabra* Thunb.
1115	Su	酥	Butter made from milk of cow, buffalo or sheep
1116	Su	蘇	*Perilla frutescens* (L.) Britt. var. *arguta* (Benth.) Hand.-Mazz.
1117	Su	粟	*Setaria italica* (L.) Beauv. , short millet
1118	Suan	蒜	*Allium sativum* L., garlic
1119	Suan jiang	酸漿	*Physalis alkekengi* L. var. *franchetii* (Mast.) Makino
1120	Suan jiao	酸角	*Tamarindus indica* L.
1121	Suan sun	酸筍	Seasoned shoots of *Phyllostachys nigra* (Lodd. ex Lindl.) Munro var. *henonis* (Mitf.) Stapf
1122	Suan zao	酸棗	*Zizyphus jujuba* Mill. var. *spinosa* (Bunge) Hu ex H. F.Chow
1123	Su fang mu	蘇方木	*Cesalpinia sappan* L.
1124	Su he xiang	蘇合香	Resin of *Liquidambar orientalis* Mill.
1125	Sui shi	遂石	Flint
1126	Suo cao	莎草	*Cyperus rotundus* L.
1127	Suo mu mian	莎木麪	*Metroxylon sagu* Rottb.
1128	Suo mu mian	莏木麪	*Metroxylon sagu* Rottb.
1129	Suo sha mi	縮砂蔤	*Amomum villosum* Lour. and *A. xanthioides* (Wall. ex Baker)
1130	Suo yang	鎖陽	*Cynomorium songaricum* Rupr.

1131	Su xin	素馨	*Jasminum grandiflorum* L.
1132	Su you	酥油	Butter made from milk of cow, buffalo or sheep
1133	Da feng zi	大風子	*Hydnocarpus anthelmintica* Pierre, chaulmoogra
1134	Tai yi yu liang	太一餘糧	Brown haematite occuring in ravines
1135	Tan	檀	*Dalbergia hupeana* Hance
1136	Tang	螗	*Cordyceps cicadae* Shing; fungus sclerotium
1137	Tang lang	螳螂	Mantis
1138	Tang niu	犛牛	Unidentified kind of buffalo
1139	Tan xiang	檀香	*Santalum album* L.
1140	Tao	桃	*Amygdalus persica* L.; peach
1141	Tao fu	桃符	A charm made from peachwood
1142	Tao hua shi	桃花石	Marmor (white and red)
1143	Tao yang	洮羊	Sheep from Gan su 甘肅
1144	Teng yu	騰魚	Rock fish
1145	Teng huang	藤黃	*Garcinia morella* Desv. (M. J.)
1146	Te peng sha	特蓬殺	Borax
1147	Te sheng yu shi	特生礜石	Colored arsenolite
1148	Tian cai	菾菜	*Beta vulgaris* L. var. *cicla* L.
1149	Tian gua	甜瓜	*Cucumis melo* L.
1150	Tian hua xun	天花蕈	*Pleurotus ostreatus* (Jacq. ex Fr.) Quél.
1151	Tian ke chong	腆顆蟲	A ground beetle
1152	Tian ling cao	天靈草	Unidentified plant
1153	Tian luo	田螺	→ 1106 Si gua 丝瓜
1154	Tian luo le	天羅勒	A plant resembling → 1106 Si gua 丝瓜
1155	Tian ma	天麻	*Gastrodia elata* BL.
1156	Tian ma	田麻	*Gastrodia elata* BL.
1157	Tian men dong	天門冬	*Asparagus cochinchinensis* (Lour.) Merr.
1158	Tian ming jing	天名精	*Carpesium abrotanoides* L.
1159	Tian mu cao	田母草	Unidentified plant
1160	Tian nan xing	天南星	*Arisaema heterophyllum* Bl.
1161	Tian niu	天牛	Longicorn beetle
1162	Tian she	天蛇	Unidentified snake
1163	Tian shi li	天師栗	*Aesculus chinensis* Bunge
1164	Tian shou gen	天壽根	Unidentified plant
1165	Tian teng	甜藤	Unidentified vine

1166	Tian xian guo	天仙果	*Ficus erecta* Thunb. var. *beecheyana* (Hook. et Arn.) King
1167	Tian xian teng	天仙藤	*Aristolochia debilis* Sieb. et Zucc.
1168	Tian xiong	天雄	*Aconitum carmichaeli* Debx.
1169	Tian zhu gan jiang	天竺乾薑	*Zingiber officinale* Rosc.
1170	Tian zhu gui	天竺桂	*Cinnamomum japonicum* Sieb.
1171	Tie	鐵	Iron
1172	Tie ge	鐵葛	Unidentified creeping plant
1173	Tie xian cao	鐵綫草	*Adiantum flabellatum* L.
1174	Ti hu	鵜鶘	Pelicans
1175	Ting li	葶藶	*Lepidium apetalum* Willd.
1176	Ti yu	鮧魚	Sheat-fish
1177	Tong	桐	*Paulownia fortunei* (Seem.) Hemsl.
1178	Tong cao	通草	*Akebia quinata* (Thunb.) Decne
1179	Tong gu cao	銅鼓草	Unidentified plant
1180	Tong kuang shi	銅礦石	Copper ore
1181	Tong tuo mu	通脱木	*Tetrapanax papyriferus* (Hook.) K. Koch
1182	Tou shan gen	透山根	Unidentified plant, very poisonous
1183	Tu bo shu	土撥鼠	The marmot
1184	Tu feng	土蜂	Bumble bee
1185	Tu fu ling	土茯苓	*Smilax glabra* Roxb.
1186	Tu jue bai	突厥白	Unidentified substance
1187	Tu jue que	突厥雀	Pallas' sand grouse
1188	Tu jun	土菌	*Sarcodon fuligineo-albus* (Fr.) Quél.
1189	Tu kui	菟葵	*Malva parviflora* L.
1190	Tu luo cao	土落草	Unidentified herb
1191	Tu ma zong	土馬騣	*Polytrichum commune* L. ex Hedw.
1192	Tuo	駝	The Bactrian camel
1193	Tuo de hua	陀得花	Unidentified herb
1194	Tuo long	鼉龍	Alligators
1195	Tuo lu	駝鹿	Unidentified deer with a very large body
1196	Tuo niao	駝鳥	"Camel bird," the ostrich
1197	Tu qiu	鵚鶖	The adjutant bird
1198	Tu shou ji	吐綬鷄	The medallion pheasant
1199	Tu shu	鼵鼠	A variety of rat
1200	Tu si zi	菟絲子	*Cuscuta chinensis* Lam.
1201	Tu yin nie	土殷孽	Variety of stalactite, gained from earth caves

1202	Tu yu	土芋	*Dioscorea sativa* L.
1203	Tu zao	兔棗	Unidentified herb
1204	Wa	蛙	Frogs
1205	Wa na shou	膃肭獸	Testes and penises of seal and beaver
1206	Wan dou	豌豆	*Pisum sativum* L.
1207	Wang bu liu xing	王不留行	*Vaccaria segetalis* (Neck.) Garcke
1208	Wang gua	王瓜	*Thladiantha dubia* Bunge
1209	Wang liang	罔兩	A sprite
1210	Wang sun	王孫	*Paris bashanensis* Wang et Tang
1211	Wan jiao	蔓椒	*Zanthoxylum nitidum* (Roxb.) DC.
1212	Wan yi teng	萬一藤	Unidentified vine
1213	Wei	薇	*Vicia sativa* L.
1214	Wei	蝟	The hedgehog
1215	Wei ling xian	威靈仙	*Clematis chinensis* Osbeck.
1216	Wei mao	衛矛	*Euonimus alatus* (Thunb.) Sieb.
1217	Wei rui	萎蕤	*Polygonatum odoratum* (Mill.) Druce
1218	Wei xian	薇銜	*Senecio nikaensis* Miq.
1219	Wei yu	鮠魚	Catfish
1220	Wei zhi	隈支	*Maclura tricuspidata* Carr.
1221	Wen bo	榅桲	*Cydonia oblonga* Mill.
1222	Weng cai	蕹菜	*Ipomea aquatica* Forsk.
1223	Wen ge	文蛤	Venus shells, salt water clams
1224	Wen guang guo	文光果	*Xanthoceras sorbifolia* Bge.
1225	Wen jing	問荆	*Equisetum arvense* L.
1226	Wen mu niao	蚊母鳥	Goatsucker
1227	Wen shi	文石	Agate
1228	Wen tang	温湯	Water from a warm puddle
1229	Wen teng	温藤	Unidentified plant
1230	Wen yao yu	文鰩魚	Flying fish
1231	Wen zi	蚊子	Mosquito
1232	Wo ju	萵苣	*Lactuca sativa* L.
1233	Wo luo	蝸螺	Watersnails
1234	Wo xue yu shi	握雪礜石	Yellowish-white arsenolite
1235	Wu bei zi	五倍子	Galls produced on *Rhus chinensis*
1236	Wu die ni	烏爹泥	*Acacia catechu* Willd.
1237	Wu feng du yao cao	無風獨搖草	*Desmodium gyrans* (L. f.)
1238	Wu gong	蜈蚣	A centipede
1239	Wu hua guo	無花果	*Ficus carica* L.
1240	Wu huan zi	無患子	*Sapindus mukorossi* Gaertn.

1241	Wu jia	五加	*Acanthopanax gracilistylus* W. W. Smith
1242	Wu jing	蕪菁	*Brassica rapa* L.
1243	Wu jiu mu	烏桕木	*Sapium sebiferum* (L.) Roxb.
1244	Wu lian mei	烏蘞苺	*Cayratiajaponica*(Thunb.)Gagnep..
1245	Wu lian zi	五斂子	*Averrhoa carambola* L.
1246	Wu lou zi	無漏子	*Phoenix dactylifera* L.
1247	Wu ming yi	無名異	Pyrolusite
1248	Wu mu	烏木	*Diospyros ebenum* Koen.
1249	Wu se fu	五色符	Unidentified plant: blue, yellow, black, white varieties
1250	Wu se shi zhi	五色石脂	Siliceous clays: blue, yellow, black, white, red varieties
1251	Wu she	烏蛇	Black grass snake
1252	Wu shi zi	無食子	Oak galls from *Quercus infectoria* Oliv. with *Cynips gallae-tinctoria* Oliv.
1253	Wu tou	烏頭	Tuber of *Aconitum carmichaelii* Debeaux
1254	Wu wei zi	五味子	*Schisandra chinensis* Turcz. Baill.
1255	Wu xin cao	無心草	1. → Shu qu cao 鼠麴草; 2. unidentified plant
1256	Wu ya	烏鴉	Thick-billed crows
1257	Wu yao	烏藥	*Lindera aggregata* (Sims.) Kosterm.
1258	Wu yi	蕪荑	*Ulmus macrocarpa* Hance
1259	Wu yu	烏芋	*Eleocharis dulcis* (Burm. f.) Trin. ex Henschel
1260	Wu yu shi	五羽石	Unidentified yellowish stone
1261	Wu zei yu	烏賊魚	Cuttle fish
1262	Wu zhu yu	吴茱萸	*Evodia rutaecarpa* (Juss.) Benth.
1263	Wu zi shi	五子實	Unidentified plant with fruit like pears
1264	Xi	犀	The Indian rhinoceros
1265	Xi	錫	Tin
1266	Xi er	枲耳	*Xanthium sibiricum* Patrin ex Widder
1267	Xia	蝦	Crabs
1268	Xia ku cao	夏枯草	*Prunella vulgaris* L.
1269	Xian	秈	*Oryza sativa* L. var.
1270	Xian	莧	*Amaranthus tricolor* L.
1271	Xian cao	鹹草	Unidentified plant tasting salty

1272	Xiang	象	The Indian elephant
1273	Xiang pu	香蒲	*Typha angustifolia* L.
1274	Xiang ru	香薷	*Elsholtzia ciliata* (Thunb.) Hyland.
1275	Xiang shi	橡實	*Quercus acutissima* Carr.
1276	Xiang si zi	相思子	*Abrus precatorius* L.
1277	Xiang xun	香蕈	*Lentinus edodes* (Berk.) Sing.
1278	Xian jin	蝛蜼	Fan mussel
1279	Xian mao	仙茅	*Curculigo orchioides* Baertn.
1280	Xian ping shu	鹹平樹	Acid condiment used in Cambodia
1281	Xian ren zhang cao	仙人掌草	Possibly cactus or fern species
1282	Xian ren zhang cao	仙人杖草	*Lactuca laciniata* Mak. *forma indivisa* Mak.
1283	Xiao	鴞	Owls
1284	Xiao er qun	小兒群	Unidentified herb
1285	Xiao bai	小檗	*Berberis silva-taroucana* Schneid.
1286	Xiao ji	小薊	*Cirsium setosum* (Willd.) MB.
1287	Xiao mai	小麥	*Triticum aestivum* L.
1288	Xiao qing	小青	*Ardisia pusilla* A. DC.
1289	Xiao shi	消石	Salpetre
1290	Xiao wen jiu	孝文韭	*Allium ledebourianum* Schult.
1291	Xi chi	鸂鶒	The tufted duck
1292	Xie	蝎（蠍）	Scorpions
1293	Xie	薤	*Allium macrostemon* Bunge
1294	Xie	蟹	Crabs
1295	Xi gou	溪狗	Newts
1296	Xi gua	西瓜	*Citrullus lanatus* (Thunb.) Matsum. et Nakai
1297	Xi gui	蠵龜	Asiatic loggerhead turtle
1298	Xi gui chong	溪鬼蟲	Unidentified bug living in water
1299	Xi lin zhi	錫吝脂	Stibnite
1300	Xi ming	菥蓂	*Thlaspi arvense* L.
1301	Xing	杏	*Armeniaca vulgaris* Lam., apricot
1302	Xing cai	莕菜	*Nymphoides peltatum* (Gmel.) O. Kuntze
1303	Xing xing	猩猩	Orangoutang
1304	Xing ye	行夜	Ground beetle
1305	Xin yi	辛夷	*Magnolia biondii* Pamp.
1306	Xiong	熊	Bear
1307	Xiong huang	雄黃	Realgar
1308	Xiong qiong	芎藭	*Ligusticum chuanxiong* Hort.
1309	Xiwang teng	息王藤	Unidentified evergreen vine

1310	Xi xian	豨薟	*Siegesbeckia orientalis* L.
1311	Xi xin	細辛	*Asarum heteropoides* Fr. Schmidt var. *manshuricum* (Maxim.) Kitag.
1312	Xuan cao	萱草	*Hemerocallis citrina* Baroni
1313	Xuan fu hua	旋覆花	*Inula japonica* Thunb.
1314	Xuan gou zi	懸鈎子	*Rubus palmatus* Th.
1315	Xuan gui	旋龜	Unidentified "revolving tortoise"
1316	Xuan hua	旋花	*Calystegia sepium* (L.) R. Br.
1317	Xuan huang shi	玄黃石	Possibly an iron oxide
1318	Xuan jing shi	玄精石	Selenite
1319	Xuan ming fen	玄明粉	Sodium sulfate
1320	Xuan mu	旋目	Unidentified Hubei 湖北 waterbird
1321	Xuan shen	玄蔘	*Scrophularia ningpoensis* Hemsl.
1322	Xuan shi	玄石	Nonmagnetic iron oxide
1323	Xu chang qing	徐長卿	*Cynanchum paniculatum* (Bunge) Kitag.
1324	Xu duan	續斷	*Dipsacus asperoides* C.Y.Cheng et T.M. Ai.
1325	Xue can	雪蠶	"Snow worms."
1326	Xue jie	血竭	Resin of *Daemonorops draco* Bl.
1327	Xue teng	血藤	*Sargentodoxa cuneata* (Oliv.) Rehd. et Wils.
1328	Xu li	徐李	A kind of → 0634 Li 李, having no kernel
1329	Xun cao	薰草	*Ocimum basilicum* L.
1330	Xun yu	鱘魚	A sturgeon variety
1331	Xu sui zi	續隨子	*Euphorbia lathyris* L.
1332	Ya bu lu	押不蘆	Unspecified Mandrake or *Datura* ssp.
1333	Yai jiao	崖椒	*Zanthoxylum simulans* Hance.
1334	Ya ma	亞麻	*Linum usitatissimum* L.
1335	Yan	鹽	Cooking salt
1336	Yan	雁	Wild goose
1337	Yan	燕	Eastern house swallow
1338	Yan	鷃	Quail
1339	Yan fu zi	鹽麩子	*Rhus chinensis* Mill.
1340	Yang	羊	Sheep
1341	Yang huo Yin huo	陽火陰火	"Yang fire; Yin fire"
1342	Yang mei	楊梅	*Myrica rubra* (Lour.) Sieb. et Zucc.
1343	Yang pen	仰盆	Unidentified vine

1344	Yang qi shi	陽起石	Asbestos
1345	Yang shi	羊實	Unidentified herb
1346	Yang ti	羊蹄	*Rumex japonicus* Houtt.
1347	Yang ti gen	羊蹄根	Root of → 1346 Yang ti 羊蹄
1348	Yang wu	陽烏	Black stork
1349	Yang yao zi	楊摇子	Unidentified tree with fruit growing from the bark
1350	Yang zhi zhu	羊躑躅	*Rhododendron molle* (Bl.) G. Don
1351	Yan hu suo	延胡索	*Corydalis yanhusuo* W. T. Wang
1352	Yan lai hong	雁來紅	Unidentified plant resembling *Celosia cristata* L.
1353	Yan long	鹽龍	Monitor
1354	Yan shu	鼹鼠	Mole
1355	Yan shu jiu	嚴樹酒	Alcoholic beverage produced from the bark and leafs of unidentified Yan shu tree
1356	Yan yao	研藥	Unidentified small tree
1357	Yan yao	鹽藥	Glauber's salt
1358	Yan zhi	燕脂	Rouge
1359	Yao shi gen	藥實根	Seed of an unidentified plant
1360	Ya zhi cao	鴨跖草	*Commelina communis* L.
1361	Ya zong	崖椶	*Carex siderosticta* Hance
1362	Ye lan gen	野蘭根	A kind of thistle
1363	Ye lü	野驢	The ass
1364	Ye ma	野馬	Wild horse
1365	Ye mao	野貓	Wild cat
1366	Ye nü	野女	Orangoutang
1367	Ye zhu	野猪	Wild boar
1368	Ye zhu wei	野猪尾	Unidentified evergreen vine without visible flowers
1369	Ye zi	椰子	*Cocos nucifera* L.
1370	Yi	瑿	Black amber
1371	Yi	蟻	Ant
1372	Yi dai cao	倚待草	Unidentified herb
1373	Yi gong	弋共	Unidentified herb
1374	Yi jue cao	益决草	Unidentified herb
1375	Yin	銀	Silver
1376	Yi nai cao	益奶草	Unidentified plant with leaves similar to → 1446 Ze lan 澤蘭

1377	Yi nan cao	宜南草	*Oroxylum indicum* (L.) Vent.
1378	Yin chen hao	茵陳蒿	*Artemisia scoparia* Waldst. et Kit.
1379	Yin di jue	陰地厥	*Scerpteridium ternatum* (Thunb.) Lyon
1380	Ying	鶯	Black-naped oriole
1381	Ying	鷹	Hawks
1382	Ying huo	螢火	Firefly
1383	Ying ji	英鷄	Unidentified bird, possibly the chukar
1384	Ying shi	營實	*Rosa multiflora* Thunb.
1385	Ying tao	櫻桃	*Cerasus pseudocerasus* (Lindl.) G. Don.
1386	Ying wu	鸚鴞	Parrots
1387	Ying yu	蘡薁	*Vitis adstricta* Hance
1388	Ying zi tong	罌子桐	*Vermicia fordii* (Hemsl.) Airy-Shaw
1389	Yin nie	殷櫱	Stalactite
1390	Yin shu	隱鼠	The tapir-mole
1391	Yin xing	銀杏	*Ginkgo biloba* L.
1392	Yin yang huo	淫羊藿	*Epimedium brevicornum* Maxim.
1393	Yin yu	茵芋	*Skimmia reevesiana* Fort.
1394	Yi tang	飴糖	Rice candy from *Oryza sativa* L.
1395	Yi weng	蠮螉	Solitary wasps
1396	Yi yi	薏苡	*Coix lacryma-jovi* L. var. *ma-yuen* (Romanet) Stapf
1397	Yi yu	衣魚	Silverfish
1398	Yi yu	鮧魚	Sheat-fish (Chinese welsh)
1399	Yi zhi zi	益智子	*Alpinia oxyphylla* Miq.
1400	You	柚	*Citrus grandis* (L.) Osbeck
1401	You	蕕	*Digitaria sanguinalis* (L.) Scop.
1402	You ba	由跋	*Pinellia pedatisecta* Schott
1403	You dian	優殿	Unidentified vegetable
1404	You shu	鼬鼠	Siberian weasel
1405	Yu	榆	*Ulmus pumila* L.
1406	Yu	玉	Nephrite
1407	Yu	芋	*Colocasia esculenta* (L.) Schott
1408	Yuan	猿	The gibbons
1409	Yuan	黿	Bamboo snakes
1410	Yuan can	原蠶	Silkworm
1411	Yuan ci le	元慈勒	Unidentifiable substance (resin ?) from the Persian Empire
1412	Yuan hua	芫花	*Daphne Genkwa* Sieb. et Zucc.

1413	Yuan qing	芫青	Blister fly
1414	Yuan wei	鳶尾	*Iris tectorum* Maxim.
1415	Yuan yang	鴛鴦	Mandarin duck
1416	Yuan yi	垣衣	*Weisia controversa* Hedw.
1417	Yuan zhi	遠志	*Polygala tenuifolia* Willd.
1418	Yue di	越砥	Minerals used to produce wet-stones
1419	Yue gua	越瓜	*Cucumis melo* L. var. *conomon* (Thunb.) Makino
1420	Yue gui	月桂	*Laurus nobilis* L.
1421	Yue wang yu suan	越王餘筭	*Junceella juncea* (Pallas)
1422	Yu hu	魚虎	Porcupine fish
1423	Yu hu	雨虎	A kind of caddis fly
1424	Yu huo shi	玉火石	Variety of Gypsum
1425	Yu jin	鬱金	*Curcuma longa* L, turmeric
1426	Yu jing shui	玉井水	Jade well water
1427	Yu jin xiang	鬱金香	*Tulipa gesneriana* L.
1428	Yu li	郁李	*Cerasus japonica* (Thunb.) Lois
1429	Yun dang zhu	篔簹竹	A kind of bamboo
1430	Yun mu	雲母	Mica
1431	Yun shi	雲師	*Cesalpinia decapetala* (Roth) Alston
1432	Yun shi	暈石	Pumice stone
1433	Yun tai	芸薹	*Brassica campestris* L.
1434	Yu shi	魚師	Amberjack
1435	Yu shi	礜石	Arsenolite
1436	Yu shu shu	玉蜀黍	*Zea mays* L.
1437	Yu yu	鱊魚	Unidentified very small fish
1438	Yu yu liang	禹餘糧	1. Limonite 2. *Carex kobomugi* Ohwi
1439	Yu zha	魚鮓	Fish condiment
1440	Yu zhi	魚脂	Fish oil
1441	Yu zhi zi	預知子	*Trichosanthes cucumeroides* (Ser.) Maxim.
1442	Zan cai	鏨菜	*Leonurus pseudomacranthus* Kitag.
1443	Zao	棗	*Zizyphus jujuba* Mill., Jujube
1444	Zao jia	皂莢	*Gleditsia sinensis* Lam.
1445	Zao xiu	蚤休	*Paris polyphylla* Smith var. *chinensis* (Franch.) Hara
1446	Ze lan	澤蘭	*Lycopus lucidus* Turcz.

1447	Zeng	甑	An ancient earthen utensil for steaming rice
1448	Ze qi	澤漆	*Euphorbia helioscopia* L.
1449	Ze xie	澤瀉	*Alisma orientale* (Sam.) Juz.
1450	Zha da	鮓答	Bezoar stones
1451	Zha mu pi	柵木皮	Unidentified plant resembling the mulberry
1452	Zhan	氈	Felt
1453	Zhang	樟	*Cinnamomum camphora* (L.) Presl.
1454	Zhang nao	樟腦	Camphora
1455	Zhang yu	章魚	Octopus
1456	Zhan si	占斯	*Taxillus nigrans* (Hance) Danser
1457	Zhan tang xiang	詹糖香	*Lindera erythrocarpa* Makino
1458	Zhan yu	鱣魚	Sturgeons
1459	Zha zi	楂子	*Chaenomeles cathayensis* (Hemsl) Schneid.
1460	Zhe gu	鷓鴣	Francolins
1461	Zhe kui	赭魁	*Dioscorea cirrhosa* Lour.
1462	Zhen	榛	*Corylus heterophylla* Fisch ex Bess., hazelnut
1463	Zhen	鴆	A big hawk
1464	Zhen cha	真茶	*Camellia sinensis* L., tea
1465	Zhen wu jiang	鴆鳥漿	Urine of → 1463 Zhen bird
1466	Zhen yu	鱵魚	Gar-Fish
1467	Zhen zhu	真珠	Genuine pearl
1468	Zhe shang mu	折傷木	*Viburnum opulus* L.
1469	Zhi	芝	*Ganoderma* ssp, Fungi
1470	Zhi	枳	*Citrus aurantium* L.
1471	Zhi	紙	Paper
1472	Zhi	雉	Ring-necked-pheasants
1473	Zhi dang	蛭蟷	→ 1480 Zhi zhu 蜘蛛
1474	Zhi han	質汗	A medication produced from various herbal substances boiled with blood
1475	Zhi ju	枳椇	*Hovenia dulcis* Th.
1476	Zhi ke	枳殼	Fruit of *Citrus aurantium* L.
1477	Zhi li	陟釐	*Spirogyra nitida* (Dillw.) Link
1478	Zhi mu	知母	*Anemarrhena asphodeloides* Bunge
1479	Zhi niao	治鳥	Mythical bird
1480	Zhi zhu	蜘蛛	Unidentified spider
1481	Zhi zhu xiang	蜘蛛香	*Valeriana jatamansii* Jones

1482	Zhi zi	卮子	*Gardenia jasminoides* Ellis
1483	Zhong shi	終石	Unidentified mineral
1484	Zhong si zao	仲思棗	A kind of → 1443 Zao 棗
1485	Zhu	术 (朮)	*Atractylodes macrocephala* Koidz.
1486	Zhu	竹	*Phyllostachys nigra* (Lodd. *ex* Lindl.) Munro var. *henonis* (Mitf.) Stapf ex Rendle.
1487	Zhu	猪	Pig
1488	Zhu feng	竹蜂	Mason bee
1489	Zhu huang	竹黃	Sclerotium of fungus infested bamboo
1490	Zhu ji	竹鷄	*Bambusicola thoracica* (Temminck)
1491	Zhu ling	猪苓	*Polyporus umbellatus* (Pers.) Fr.
1492	Zhu liu	竹鼺	The bamboo rat
1493	Zhu ma	苧麻	*Boehmeria nivea* (L.) Gaud.
1494	Zhuo mu niao	啄木鳥	Woodpecker
1495	Zhu ru	竹蓐	*Shiraia bambusicola* P.Henn.
1496	Zhu sha gen	硃砂根	*Ardisia crenata* Sims
1497	Zhu she	諸蛇	Snakes
1498	Zhu shi	竹蝨	Whitefly
1499	Zhu sun	竹筍	Bamboo shoots
1500	Zhu yao zi	猪腰子	*Whitfordiodendron filipes* (Dunn)
1501	Zhu ya shi	猪牙石	Unidentified ivory-like stone
1502	Zhu yu	鸀瑦	The egret
1503	Zhu yu	竹魚	"Bamboo Fish", goby
1504	Zhu zi	櫧子	*Castanopsis sclerophylla* (Lindl.) Schott., Acorns
1505	Zi	梓	*Catalpa ovata* G. Don.
1506	Zi bei	紫貝	Purple cowries
1507	Zi bei jin pan cao	紫背金盤草	*Ajuga nipponensis* Makino
1508	Zi cai	紫菜	*Porphyra haitanensis* T. J. Chang et B. F. Zheng
1509	Zi cao	紫草	*Arnebia euchroma* (Royle) Johnst.
1510	Zi ge	紫葛	*Ampelopsis delavayana* (Franch.) Planch.
1511	Zi jia shi	紫佳石	Unidentified purple colored mineral
1512	Zi jing	紫荆	*Cercis chinensis* Bunge
1513	Zi jin niu	紫金牛	*Ardisia japonica* Bl. [(M. J. G.)
1514	Zi jin teng	紫金藤	*Kadsura longipedunculata* Finet et Gagnep.

1515	Zi kuang	紫鉚	Shellac
1516	Zi qin	紫堇	*Corydalis edulis* Maxim.
1517	Zi ran hui	自然灰	Unidentifiable plant ash
1518	Zi ran tong	自然銅	Copper pyrites
1519	Zi shen	紫參	*Polygonum bistorta* L.
1520	Zi shi hua	紫石華	Amethyst
1521	Zi shi ying	紫石英	Amethyst
1522	Zi teng	紫藤	*Wisteria sinensis* Sweet.
1523	Zi wan	紫菀	*Aster tataricus* L. f.
1524	Zi wei	紫葳	*Campsis grandiflora* (Thunb.) Loisel ex K. Schum.
1525	Zi yu	鯔魚	Grey mullet
1526	Zong lü	椶櫚	*Trachycarpus fortunei* (Hook) H.Endl.
1527	Zui xing cao	醉醒草	Unidentified herb
1528	Zui yu cao	醉魚草	*Buddleya lindleyana* Fort.
1529	Zuo mu	柞木	*Xylosma congestum* (Lour.) Merr.
1530	Zuo na cao	坐拿草	Unidentified plant
1531	Zuo ye he cao	昨葉何草	*Orostachys fimbriatus* (Turcz.) Breger
1532	Ren gui	人傀	Human monstrosities
1533	Shan gui	山龜	The Shensi tortoise, → 0899 Qin gui 秦龜
1534	An xi you	安息油	A tree resin
1535	Ren bao	人胞	Human placenta
1536	Ren dan	人膽	Human gallbladder
1537	Niao bai yin	溺白垽	Urine sediments
1538	Fang min	方民	Different human beings because of environmental influences
1539	Xiang fu zi	香附子	→ 1126 Suo cao 莎草
1540	Pi shi	癖石	Arsenic trioxide
1541	Shui yi niang jiu	水宜釀酒	Water suitable for brewing
1542	Yu kuai	魚鱠	Fish hash
1543	Chuan jin pi	川槿皮	→ 0786 Mu jin木槿
1544	Zhu tie qi	諸鐵器	Various iron utensils
1545	Ren gu	人骨	Human bones
1546	Zao	糟	Fermented grain
1547	Jiang gan ji zu	箭笴及鏃	Arrow shaft and arrow-head
1548	Bao han cao	抱罕草	Unidentified plant used for → 0324 Gan cao 甘草
1549	Bai shui qi	白水耆	A kind of → Huang qi 黄芪

1550	Han dao	旱稻	Dry rice
1551	Jing quan shui	井泉水	Water from wells and springs
1552	Hui hui cong	回回葱	→ c476 Hu cong 胡葱
1553	Ji ti bi sheng	屐屜鼻繩	Rotten shoestrings and upper parts of old shoes
1554	Tie ruo	鐵爇	Residue produced by heating bamboo or peach stones on an ax blade
1555	Lu shui	露水	Dew water
1556	Rou xing	肉杏	Apricot pulp
1557	Ren shi	人屎	Human feces
1558	Li quan	醴泉	Spring water as sweet as wine.
1559	Wu tong	梧桐	*Firmiana platanifolia* (L.f.) Marsili
1560	Gou ying	狗蠅	Dog louse fly
1561	Ren shi	人蝨	Human louse
1562	Zhe chong	䗪蟲	Ground beetle
1563	Ren shi	人勢	Human penis
1564	Zi jing si sheng	自經死繩	Rope used to commit suicide
1565	Jiao jiao bu	繳脚布	Cloth formerly used for binding the feet of a woman
1566	Ai huo	艾火	Fire generated from Artermisia herb by means of reflecting sun light with a shiny bronze mirror
1567	Ru zhi	乳汁	Human milk
1568	Ren niao	人尿	Human urine
1569	Ren qi	人氣	Congenital fire as source of life
1570	Shan yan quan shui	山巖泉水	Mountain cliff spring water
1571	Tao tu	騊駼.	Wild horse
1572	Mian huang qi	綿黃耆	A kind of → 0461 Huang qi 黃耆
1573	Chi jian	赤箭	*Gastrodia elata* Bl.
1574	Zhu bie	珠鱉	Variety of turtle
1575	Fan luo	飯籮	Bamboo basket for food
1576	Zhu bie	朱鱉	Variety of turtle
1577	Kou jin tuo	口津唾	Human saliva
1578	Che zhi	車脂	Axle grease
1579	Shan hui	山渾	Dog-like animal with human face

Appendix C

Index of Entries of Geographic and Administrative Designations

Bao qing 寶慶
Bao shan 爆山
Bao xie dao 褒斜道
Bei 北
Bei 貝
Bei bian 北邊
Bei dai shan 北代山
Bei dao 北道
Bei di 北狄
Bei di 北地
Bei ding shan 北定山
Bei du 北都
Bei fan 北番
Bei fang 北方
Bei gan shan 北甘山
Bei guo 北國
Bei hai 北海
Bei hu 北胡
Bei huang 北荒
Bei jian 北間
Bei jie 北界
Bei lu 北虜
Bei lan ling 北蘭陵
Bei ma dao 北馬道
Bei ren 北人
Bei shan 北山
Bei tian zhu 北天竺
Bei tian zhu guo 北天竺國
Bei ting 北庭
Bei ting shan 北庭山
Bei tu 北土
Bei yan 北燕
Bei yi shan 北邑山
Bei yuan 北苑 [2]
Bei yue 北岳
Bei zhan guo 卑占國
Beng cheng 祊城
Bi 壁
Bian 汴
Bian dong 汴東
Bian du 汴都
Bian jing 汴京
Bian liang 汴梁
Bian luo 汴洛
Bian xi 汴西
Bian zhong 汴中
Bian zhou 汴州
Bin 賓
Bin zhou 賓州
Bin zhou 濱州
Bin zhou 豳州
Bin zhou 邠州
Bing 并
Bing xue 丙穴
Bing zhou 并州
Bo 亳
Bo dao 僰道
Bo hai 渤海
Bo lü guo 波律國
Bo ni 渤泥
Bo ping jun 博平郡
Bo si 波斯
Bo si guo 波斯國
Bo zhou 亳州
Bu shan xian 布山縣

Cai 蔡
Cai zhou 蔡州
Can ling 蠶陵
Cang 滄
Cang di 傖地
Cang Wu 蒼梧
Cang zhou 滄州
Cao 曹
Cao zhou 曹州
Cen zhou 岑州
Cha ling 茶陵
Chai sang 柴桑
Chan yu 單于
Chang an 長安
Chang hua 昌化
Chang le zhen 長樂鎮
Chang li xian 昌黎縣
Chang ming 昌明
Chang ning 長寧
Chang sha 長沙
Chang shan 長山
Chang shan 常山

Chang shan jun 常山郡
Chang yang shan 昌陽山
Chang yue 常岳
Chang zhou 昌州
Chang zhou 常州
Chao 潮
Chao ge 朝歌
Chao xian 朝鮮
Chao zhou 潮州
Che shi guo 車師國
Chen 郴
Chen 辰
Chen 陳
Chen cang 陳倉
Chen liu 陳留
Chen zhou 郴州
Chen zhou 辰州
Chen zhou 陳州
Cheng 成
Cheng 澄
Cheng du 成都
Cheng du fu 成都府
Cheng gao zhu shan 成皋諸山
Cheng xian 承縣
Cheng zhou 成州
Cheng zhou 澄州
Chi 池
Chi mu er cheng 赤木兒城
Chi shan 赤山
Chi shui 赤水
Chi shui he 赤水河
Chi zhou 池州
Chong qing 重慶
Chong shan 崇山
Chong wu zhi shan 崇吾之山
Chu 滁
Chu 楚
Chu 處
Chu di 楚地
Chu guo 楚國
Chu shan 楚山
Chu zhong 楚中
Chu zhou 滁州
Chu zhou 楚州
Chu zhou 處州
Chuan 川
Chuan dong 川東
Chuan guang 川廣
Chuan nan 川南
Chuan qian 川黔
Chuan shaan 川陝
Chuan shu 川蜀
Chuan xi 川西
Chuan xia 川峽
Chuan zhong 川中
Chun zhou 春州
Chun zhou 淳州
Ci shan 慈山
Ci yang 慈陽
Ci xi 慈谿
Ci zhou 慈州
Cong long zhi shan 蔥聾之山
Cong shui 從水

Da bie shan 大別山
Da bin xian 大賓縣
Da ci zhi shan 大次之山
Da da 韃靼
Da heng shan 大橫山
Da li fu 大理府
Da niao shan 大鳥山
Da qin 大秦
Da qin guo 大秦國
Da rou zhi 大月氏
Da rou zhi guo 大月氏國
Da shi 大食
Da shi guo 大食國
Da shi zhu fan 大食諸番
Da shi zhu guo 大食諸國
Da tong 大同
Da tong fu 大同府
Da wan 大宛
Da wu 大吳
Da xian 大峴
Da ya shan 大牙山
Da yi 大邑
Da yu ling 大庾嶺
Da yue shi 大月氏

Da yue shi guo　大月氏國
Dai　代
Dai bei　代北
Dai jun　代郡
Dai zhou　代州
Dan　丹
Dan er　儋耳
Dan shan zhi nan　丹山之南
Dan shui　丹水
Dan tu　丹徒
Dan xi　丹溪
Dan xue zhi shan　丹穴之山
Dan yang　丹陽
Dan yuan　亶爰
Dan yuan zhi shan　亶爰之山
Dan zhou　丹州
Dang chang　宕昌
Dang shan　碭山
Dang yang　當陽
Dang yang xian　當陽縣
Dang zhou　當州
Dao　道
Dao zhou　道州
De qing zhou　德慶州
De shun jun　德順軍
Deng　鄧
Deng　登
Deng zhou　登州
Deng zhou　鄧州
Deng zhou dao　登州島
Di　氐
Di hu　氐胡
Di qiang　氐羌
Dian　滇
Dian cang shan　點蒼山
Dian guang　滇廣
Dian nan　滇南
Ding　鼎
Ding hai　定海
Ding ling guo　丁零國
Ding zhou　鼎州
Ding zhou　定州
Dong　東
Dong bei　東北
Dong bei hu　東北胡
Dong bei yi　東北夷
Dong chuan　東川
Dong dao　東道
Dong du　東都
Dong e　東阿
Dong e xian　東阿縣
Dong fang　東方
Dong guan xian　東莞縣
Dong hai　東海
Dong hai dao　東海島
Dong hai jun　東海郡
Dong hai zhu dao　東海諸島
Dong hu　東胡
Dong jian　東間
Dong jing　東京
Dong jing　東境
Dong jun　東郡
Dong lai　東萊
Dong nan　東南
Dong nan hai　東南海
Dong nan hai wai　東南海外
Dong nan zhou jun　東南州郡
Dong nan zhu jun　東南諸郡
Dong ping　東平
Dong ping jun　東平郡
Dong shan　東山
Dong ting　洞庭
Dong ting shan　洞庭山
Dong tu　東土
Dong wu　東吳
Dong wu　東武
Dong wu cheng　東武城
Dong xi jing　東西京
Dong yang　東陽
Dong yi　東夷
Dong yue　東嶽
Dou　竇
Dou cheng　都城
Dou guang　都廣
Dou kun guo　都昆國
Dou liang　都梁
Dou liang shan　都梁山
Dou qu guo　兜渠國

Dou xia 都下
Dou xiang 都鄉
Du shuo shan 度朔山
Duan zhou 端州
Dun huang 敦煌
Dun huang shan 敦煌山
Dun xun guo 頓遜國

E 阿
E 鄂
E jing 阿井
E mei 峨眉
E mei 峨嵋
E mei shan 峨眉山
E mei shan 峨嵋山
E xian cheng 阿縣城
E zhou 鄂州
E zhu 鄂渚
En zhou 恩州
Er chuan 二川
Er guang 二廣
Er mao shan 二茅山
Er zhe 二浙

Fa xing si 法性寺
Fan 番
Fan 梵
Fan dong 番峒
Fan gong quan 范公泉
Fan guo 番國
Fan he xian 番禾縣
Fan shan 樊山
Fan shan 礬山
Fan shui 泛水
Fan yang 范陽
Fan zhong 番中
Fang 坊
Fang 房
Fang lin yuan 芳林苑
Fang ling 房陵
Fang ling xian 房陵縣
Fang shan 方山
Fang tai shan 方臺山
Fang zhou 房州
Fei niao shan 飛鳥山
Fen 汾
Fen liu shan 分流山
Fen zhou 汾州
Feng 鳳
Feng 風
Feng cheng 豐城
Feng gao 奉高
Feng hua xian 奉化縣
Feng pei 豐沛
Feng shan 豐山
Feng xi xian 封溪縣
Feng xiang 鳳翔
Feng zhou 封州
Feng zhou 澧州
Feng zhou 鳳州
Fo lin 佛林
Fo shi guo 佛誓國
Fu 鄜
Fu 福
Fu 撫
Fu du 涪都
Fu feng 夫風
Fu feng jun 扶風郡
Fu gao shan gu 傅高山谷
Fu gou 扶溝
Fu hai zhou 扶海洲
Fu han 枹罕
Fu jian 福建
Fu jian zhou 福建州
Fu lang 富浪
Fu li zhi shan 鳧麗之山
Fu liang 浮梁
Fu lin 拂林
Fu lin guo 拂林國
Fu ling 符陵
Fu ling jun 涪陵郡
Fu lu cheng 福祿城
Fu lu xian 福祿縣
Fu nan 扶南
Fu nan guo 扶南國
Fu qi 弗其
Fu sang 扶桑
Fu shan 服山

Guang nan 廣南
Guang xi 廣西
Guang zhe 廣浙
Guang zhong 廣中
Guang zhou 廣州
Guang zhou 光州
Gui 歸
Gui 貴
Gui 桂
Gui ci guo 龜茲國
Gui fang 鬼方
Gui fu 桂府
Gui fu cun 桂府村
Gui guang 桂廣
Gui hai 桂海
Gui lin 桂林
Gui ling 桂嶺
Gui shun 歸順
Gui yang 桂陽
Gui yang xian 桂陽縣
Gui zhou 桂州
Gui zhou 貴州
Gui zhou 媯州
Gui zhou 歸州
Guo 虢
Guo guo 咼國
Guo zhou 虢州
Guo zhou 果州

Ha la huo 哈喇火
Ha mi 哈密
Ha mi wei 哈密衛
Hai 海
Hai bei 海北
Hai bian guo 海邊國
Hai bin 海濱
Hai dong 海東
Hai feng 海豐
Hai guo 海國
Hai kang 海康
Hai ling 海陵
Hai nan 海南
Hai ning 海寧
Hai xi 海西
Hai xi nan 海西南
Hai ya guo 海牙國
Hai yan 海鹽
Hai yang 海陽
Hai zhou 海州
Han 漢
Han cheng 韓城
Han chuan 漢川
Han dan 邯鄲
Han di 漢地
Han gu 函谷
Han guo 韓國
Han jiang 漢江
Han mian 漢沔
Han nan 漢南
Han shang 漢上
Han shi shan 寒石山
Han yang 漢陽
Han zhong 漢中
Hang 杭
Hang zhou 杭州
Hang yue jian 杭越間
Hao 濠
Hao zhou 濠州
He 河
He 合
He 賀
He bei 河北
He dong 河東
He ji 河濟
He jian 河間
He ling guo 訶陵國
He luo 河洛
He ming 鶴鳴
He nan 河南
He nan bei 河南北
He nei 河內
He pu 合浦
He pu xian 合浦縣
He shaan 河陝
He shang 河上
He shui 涸水
He shuo 河朔
He xi 河西

He xi shan 河西山
He yang 河陽
He yuan 河源
He zhong 河中
He zhong fu 河中府
He zhou 河州
He zhou 河洲
He zhou 合州
He zhou 和州
He zhou 賀州
Hei 黑
Hei kun lun 黑崑崙
Hei qi dan 黑契丹
Hei shui 黑水
Heng 衡
Heng gao 衡皋
Heng he 恒河
Heng jing 橫涇
Heng shan 佷山
Heng shan 衡山
Heng shan 恒山
Heng shan ceng qing gang 衡山層青岡
Heng yang 衡陽
Heng zhou 衡州
Heng zhou 橫州
Hong 洪
Hong nong 弘農
Hong nong jun 弘農郡
Hong zhou 洪州
Hu 胡
Hu 湖
Hu bei 湖北
Hu di 胡地
Hu guang 湖廣
Hu guo 胡國
Hu ling 湖嶺
Hu mian 湖沔
Hu nan 湖南
Hu nan bei 湖南北
Hu shan 壺山
Hu shou shan 虎壽山
Hu wei zhi shan 虎尾之山
Hu xian 鄠縣
Hu xiang 湖湘
Hu zhong 胡中
Hu zhou 湖州
Hua 滑
Hua 華
Hua 化
Hua gai shan 華蓋山
Hua guo 滑國
Hua rong 華容
Hua shan 華山
Hua tai 滑臺
Hua xia 華夏
Hua yang 華陽
Hua yin 華陰
Hua yuan 華原
Hua zhou 華州
Huai 懷
Huai 淮
Huai an 懷安
Huai bei 淮北
Huai dian 淮甸
Huai hai 淮海
Huai li 槐里
Huai ling 淮嶺
Huai nan 淮南
Huai qing 懷慶
Huai shui 淮水
Huai xi 淮西
Huai yang 淮揚
Huai yang 淮陽
Huai yang jun 淮陽郡
Huai yi 淮夷
Huai you 淮右
Huai yuan 淮源
Huai zhe 淮浙
Huai zhou 懷州
Huang 黃
Huang he 黃河
Huang ling 黃陵
Huang mei shan 黃梅山
Huang shan 黃山
Huang shui 黃水
Huang zhou 黃州
Huang zhou 晃州

Huang zhou fu 黃州府
Hui 徽
Hui chang 會昌
Hui he 回紇
Hui hu 回鶻
Hui hu guo 回鶻國
Hui hui 回回
Hui hui guo 回回國
Hui shui 徽水
Hui shui wan 會水灣
Hui zhou 徽州
Hun tong jiang 混同江
Hun xi zhi shan 渾夕之山
Huo shan 霍山
Huo shan jun 火山軍
Huo yan shan 火焰山
Huo zhou 火州
Huo zhou 火洲

Ji 吉
Ji 冀
Ji bin guo 罽賓國
Ji cui chi 積翠池
Ji jun 汲郡
Ji men 薊門
Ji nan 濟南
Ji nan jun 濟南郡
Ji ning 濟寧
Ji ning 冀寧
Ji sha shan 積沙山
Ji shan 箕山
Ji shan 雞山
Ji shi shan 積石山
Ji shui 濟水
Ji tou shan 雞頭山
Ji yang jun 濟陽郡
Ji yin 濟陰
Ji yin jun 濟陰郡
Ji yuan 濟源
Ji yun guo 吉雲國
Ji ze 稷澤
Ji zhou 薊州
Ji zhou 冀州
Ji zhou 吉州
Ji zhou 箕州
Jia 嘉
Jia ding 嘉定
Jia qing fang 嘉慶坊
Jia xing 嘉興
Jia xing xian 嘉興縣
Jia zhou 嘉州
Jian 建
Jian an jun 建安郡
Jian chang 建昌
Jian jin shan 揀金山
Jian kang 建康
Jian nan 劍南
Jian ning 建寧
Jian ning jun 建寧郡
Jian ping 建平
Jian ping jun 建平郡
Jian wei 犍為
Jian yang 建陽
Jian zhou 劍州
Jian zhou 建州
Jian zhou 簡州
Jiang 江
Jiang 絳
Jiang bei 江北
Jiang biao 江表
Jiang dong 江東
Jiang guang 江廣
Jiang han 江漢
Jiang he 江河
Jiang hu 江湖
Jiang hu nan bei 江湖南北
Jiang hua xian 江華縣
Jiang huai 江淮
Jiang lai zhi xu 姜賴之墟（虛)
Jiang lin shan 江林山
Jiang ling 江陵
Jiang ling 江嶺
Jiang ling fu 江陵府
Jiang nan 江南
Jiang nan bei 江南北
Jiang nan zhu dao 江南諸道
Jiang ning 江寧
Jiang ning fu 江寧府

Jiang pu 江浦
Jiang shan 江山
Jiang shan 蔣山
Jiang wai 江外
Jiang xi 江西
Jiang xia 江夏
Jiang yang 江陽
Jiang yang shan 江陽山
Jiang yin 江陰
Jiang yuan 江源
Jiang zhe 江浙
Jiang zhou 江州
Jiang zhou 絳州
Jiang zuo 江左
Jiao 交
Jiao dong 膠東
Jiao guang 交廣
Jiao he 交河
Jiao ling 交嶺
Jiao zhi 交趾
Jiao zhou 膠州
Jiao zhou 交州
Jie 階
Jie di 階地
Jie gu guo 結骨國
Jie qiao 橋
Jie yu 揭雩
Jie zhou 階州
Jin 金
Jin 錦
Jin 晉
Jin an 晉安
Jin bian bei di 近汴北地
Jin cheng 金城
Jin chi 金齒
Jin di 晉地
Jin hua 金華
Jin kang 晉康
Jin ling 金陵
Jin ling 晉陵
Jin ling jun 晉陵郡
Jin ning xian 晉寧縣
Jin xi zhu man 晉溪諸蠻
Jin xing xian 晉興縣
Jin ya tuan 金牙湍
Jin yang 晉陽
Jin yang xiang 晉陽鄉
Jin yun 縉雲
Jin zhou 金州
Jin zhou 錦州
Jin zhou 晉州
Jin zhou 靳州
Jing 荊
Jing 京
Jing chu 荊楚
Jing de zhen 景德鎮
Jing dong 京東
Jing du 京都
Jing fu 荊府
Jing hu 荊湖
Jing kou 京口
Jing le xian 靜樂縣
Jing lu 京陸
Jing luo 京洛
Jing man 荊蠻
Jing men jun 荊門軍
Jing nan 荊南
Jing shan 荊山
Jing shan 景山
Jing shan xian 荊山縣
Jing shi 京師
Jing xi 京西
Jing xia 京下
Jing xiang 荊湘
Jing xiang 荊襄
Jing yang 荊揚
Jing yang 涇陽
Jing ying 荊郢
Jing yuan 涇原
Jing zhao 京兆
Jing zhou 景州
Jing zhou 涇州
Jing zhou 荊州
Jiu he 九河
Jiu hua 九華
Jiu jiang 九江
Jiu keng 鳩坑
Jiu ling 鷲嶺

Jiu quan 酒泉
Jiu xian shan 九仙山
Jiu yi shan 九疑山
Jiu yuan 九原
Jiu zhen 九真
Jiu zhou 九州
Ju jia cun 劇家村
Ju ku zhou 聚窟州
Ju lu 鉅鹿
Ju luo shan 拘羅山
Ju qing shan 句青山
Ju qu shan 句曲山
Ju yan 舉巖
Ju ye 鉅野
Juan shan 卷山
Juan xian 卷縣
Jue shui 決水
Jun 均
Jun shan 君山
Jun shui 均水
Jun zhou 筠州
Jun zhou 均州

Kai ming shan 開明山
Kai yuan si 開元寺
Kai zhou 開州
Kang qian he 康乾河
Kang guo 康國
Kang zhou 康州
Ke shan 騍山
Kuang lu 匡廬
Kuang shui 狂水
Kuai ji 會稽
Kui 夔
Kui chuan 夔川
Kui lu 夔路
Kui zhou 夔州
Kun lun 昆侖
Kun lun guo 崑崙國
Kun lun pan pan guo 崑崙盤盤國
Kun lun shan 崑崙山
Kun lun xu 崑崙墟
Kun ming chi 昆明池
Kun shan 崑山
Kun wu shan 昆吾山
Kuo 括
Kuo cang 括蒼
Kuo zhou 廓州

Lai 萊
Lai zhou 萊州
Lan cang 瀾滄
Lan ling 蘭陵
Lan tian 藍田
Lan ting 蘭亭
Lan xian 蘭縣
Lan zhou 蘭州
Lang 朗
Lang ling 朗陵
Lang ya 琅邪
Lang ya 琅琊
Lang zhong 閬中
Lang zhou 閬州
Lang zhou 朗州
Lao 佬
Lao shan 牢山
Lao shan 勞山
Lao shui 澇水
Lao wo 老撾
Le bi guo 勒畢國
Le lang 樂浪
Le ping 樂平
Le ping jun 樂平郡
Le you yuan 樂游苑
Le zhou 勒州
Lei 雷
Lei chi 雷池
Lei yang 耒陽
Lei zhou 雷州
Lei ze 雷澤
Li 澧
Li 漓
Li 利
Li cheng 歷城
Li dong 黎峒
Li guo zhi shui 歷虢之水
Li jiang 麗江
Li mu shan 黎母山

Li pu 荔浦
Li shan 歷山
Li shan 黎山
Li shan 驪山
Li shui 澧水
Li xia 歷下
Li xian 酈縣
Li yang 歷陽
Li zhou 利州
Li zhou 黎州
Li zhou 澧州
Lian 連
Lian 廉
Lian shui 廉水
Lian zhou 廉州
Liang 梁
Liang 涼
Liang chuan 兩川
Liang guang 兩廣
Liang guo 梁國
Liang han 梁漢
Liang huai 兩淮
Liang jiang 兩江
Liang jing 兩京
Liang shan 梁山
Liang yi 梁益
Liang zhe 兩浙
Liang zhou 涼州
Liang zhou 梁州
Liao 僚
Liao 獠
Liao 遼
Liao 蓼
Liao ban shan 遼坂山
Liao cheng xian 膋城縣
Liao dong 遼東
Liao hai 遼海
Liao she 聊攝
Liao xi 遼西
Liao yang 遼陽
Liao zhou 遼州
Lin an 臨安
Lin chuan 臨川
Lin feng zhou 麟鳳洲
Lin hai 臨海
Lin he 臨賀
Lin huai 臨淮
Lin jiang jun 臨江軍
Lin ju 臨沮
Lin lü shan 林慮山
Lin ping 臨平
Lin qiong 臨邛
Lin qu 臨朐
Lin ren xian 林任縣
Lin ru 臨汝
Lin tao 臨洮
Lin ting 臨汀
Lin tong 臨潼
Lin wu 臨武
Lin yi 林邑
Lin yi 臨沂
Lin yi zhu guo 林邑諸國
Lin yuan xian 臨沅縣
Lin zhang 臨漳
Lin zi 臨淄
Lin zi jun 臨淄郡
Lin zi xian 臨淄縣
Ling 陵
Ling 嶺
Ling bei 嶺北
Ling biao 嶺表
Ling chuan xian 陵川縣
Ling ling 零陵
Ling ling xian 零陵縣
Ling nan 嶺南
Ling nan xi dong 嶺南溪峒
Ling qiao 嶺嶠
Ling qiu 靈丘
Ling shan xiang 靈山鄉
Ling wai 嶺外
Ling wai zhou jun 嶺外州郡
Ling yin 陵陰
Ling yin si 靈隱寺
Ling zhou 靈州
Liu 柳
Liu cheng jun 柳城郡
Liu qiu 琉球
Liu qiu guo 琉球國

Liu sha 流沙
Liu zhou 柳州
Long 龍
Long 隴
Long an 龍安
Long cheng 龍城
Long chuan xian 龍川縣
Long dong 龍洞
Long ji shan 龍濟山
Long men 龍門
Long men shan 龍門山
Long nao gang 龍腦岡
Long shan 壟山
Long shan 龍山
Long shang 隴上
Long shu 隴蜀
Long xi 隴西
Long zhou 隴州
Long zhou 龍州
Lu 廬
Lu 瀘
Lu 魯
Lu 潞
Lu an 六安
Lu di 魯地
Lu guo 魯國
Lu jiang 廬江
Lu ling 廬陵
Lu ling jun 廬陵郡
Lu meng shan 魯蒙山
Lu rong 盧容
Lu shan 盧山
Lu shan 廬山
Lu shan 魯山
Lu shi 盧氏
Lu shi xian 盧氏縣
Lu tai 鹿臺
Lu zhong 虜中
Lu zhou 潞州
Lu zhou 瀘州
Lu zhou 廬州
Lü yu he 綠玉河
Lü xiang xian 呂鄉縣
Lü xiang xian 呂香縣
Luo 羅
Luo 洛
Luo cha guo 羅刹國
Luo cheng xian 羅城縣
Luo fu shan 羅浮山
Luo gu 駱谷
Luo jiang 羅江
Luo shui 洛水
Luo xi 洛西
Luo yang 洛陽
Luo zhong 洛中
Luo zhou 洛州
Luo zhou 羅州

Ma cheng 麻城
Ma Dao 馬道
Ma Gu 麻姑
Ma hu 馬湖
Ma ling shan 馬嶺山
Ma yang 麻陽
Man gu 滿谷
Man jie 蠻界
Man la jia guo 滿剌加國
Man yi 蠻夷
Mang bu 芒部
Mao 茂
Mao ling 茂陵
Mao luo dao 毛羅島
Mao shan 茅山
Mao zhou 茂州
Mei 眉
Mei ling 梅嶺
Mei shan 禖山
Mei shan 眉山
Mei xian 郿縣
Mei zhou 眉州
Meng 蒙
Meng 孟
Meng shan 蒙山
Meng xi 孟溪
Meng xi 夢溪
Meng xian 鄳縣
Meng yang 孟養
Meng zhou 孟州

Mi 密
Mi shan 密山
Mi yun 密雲
Mi zhou 密州
Mian dian 緬甸
Mian shang 綿上
Mian shui 沔[水]
Mian xian 沔縣
Mian zhou 沔州
Mian zhou 綿州
Miao 苗
Min 岷
Min 閩
Min guang 閩廣
Min ling 閩嶺
Min shan 岷山
Min yue 閩越
Min yue 閩粵
Min zhong 閩中
Min zhou 岷州
Ming 明
Ming sha xian 鳴沙縣
Ming shan 明山
Ming shan xian 茗山縣
Mo bei 漠北
Mo luo duan chi guo 抹羅短叱國
Mo qie tuo guo 摩伽陀國
Mu 睦
Mu fu shan 幕阜山
Mu lan zhou 木蘭洲
Mu men 木門
Mu yang 牧羊
Mu yang shan 牧羊山
Mu yun chang 暮雲場
Mu zhou 睦州

Nan 南
Nan an 南安
Nan bang zhu guo 南邦諸國
Nan cheng 南城
Nan chu 南楚
Nan dan 南丹
Nan dan zhou 南丹州
Nan di 南地
Nan en zhou 南恩州
Nan fan 南番
Nan fan zhu guo 南番諸國
Nan fang 南方
Nan guang 南廣
Nan hai 南海
Nan hai huo zhou 南海火洲
Nan hai zhu guo 南海諸國
Nan he xian 南河縣
Nan huang 南荒
Nan jian 南劍
Nan jiang 南江
Nan jing 南京
Nan jun 南郡
Nan kang 南康
Nan kang jun 南康軍
Nan kang jun 南康郡
Nan liang jun 南涼郡
Nan man 南蠻
Nan ping cheng 南平城
Nan pu 南浦
Nan qiu cun 南丘村
Nan shan 南山
Nan tian zhu 南天竺
Nan tu 南土
Nan xi 南息
Nan xiong 南雄
Nan yang 南陽
Nan ye xi 南野溪
Nan yi 南夷
Nan yin du 南印度
Nan yin du jing 南印度境
Nan yue 南越
Nan yue 南粵
Nan yue 南岳
Nan yue 南嶽
Nan yue shan 南越山
Nan zhao 南詔
Nan zheng 南鄭
Nan zhong 南中
Nan zhong ba jun 南中八郡
Nan zhong zhou jun 南中州郡
Nan zhou 南州
Nei huang 內黃

Nei xiang 內鄉
Ni bo luo guo 尼波羅國
Ni shan 泥山
Ning 寧
Ning bo 寧波
Ning guo 寧國
Ning pu 寧浦
Ning xia 寧夏
Ning xiang 寧鄉
Ning zhou 寧州
Niu tou shan 牛頭山
Niu yang zhi shan 杻陽之山
Niu zhu ji 牛渚磯
Nü chuang zhi shan 女床之山
Nü gua 女瓜
Nü guo 女國
Nü ji zhi shan 女幾之山
Nü zhen 女真
Nü zhen di mian 女真地面
Nü zhi 女直

Ou yue 甌越

Pan hou zhi shan 潘侯之山
Pan pan guo 盤盤國
Pan yu 番禺
Pan zhou 潘州
Pei 沛
Pei guo 沛國
Peng cheng 彭城
Peng jia shan 蓬葭山
Peng lai 蓬萊
Peng lai shan 蓬萊山
Peng lai xian 蓬萊縣
Peng xi 蓬溪
Peng xian 彭縣
Piao guo 剽國
Ping gu 平谷
Ping jiang 平江
Ping mian 平緬
Ping nan xian 平南縣
Ping quan 平泉
Ping shi 平氏
Ping shou 平壽
Ping xian 平縣
Ping yang 平陽
Ping yi 馮翊
Ping yi jun 馮翊郡
Ping zhou 平州
Po li 頗黎
Po ling guo 頗陵國
Po lü guo 婆律國
Po luo men 婆羅門
Po luo men guo 婆羅門國
Po yang 鄱陽
Pu 蒲
Pu ban xian 蒲坂縣
Pu ding fen si 普定分司
Pu man 蒲蠻
Pu tian 莆田
Pu yang 濮陽
Pu yang xian 濮陽縣
Pu zhou 蒲州

Qi 岐
Qi 齊
Qi 蘄
Qi an 齊安
Qi dan 契丹
Qi di 齊地
Qi di 蘄池
Qi dong 齊東
Qi fu lu 乞弗虜
Qi ge shan 祈閣山
Qi gui 齊歸
Qi guo 齊國
Qi jun 齊郡
Qi li zhou 七里洲
Qi lian shan 祁連山
Qi lu 齊魯
Qi men 祁門
Qi men 蘄門
Qi shan 齊山
Qi shui 淒水
Qi shui 蘄水
Qi ting 岐亭
Qi xian 蘄縣
Qi xu 齊徐

Qi yan　齊兗
Qi yang　蘄陽
Qi yang xian　祁陽縣
Qi yun　齊鄆
Qi zhou　岐州
Qi zhou　齊州
Qi zhou　蘄州
Qi zhou wei　蘄州衛
Qian　虔
Qian　黔
Qian ling　乾陵
Qian nan　黔南
Qian shan　前山
Qian shan　鉛山
Qian shan xian　鉛山縣
Qian tang　錢塘
Qian tang xian　錢塘縣
Qian wei　犍為
Qian yang　黔陽
Qian yang xian　汧陽縣
Qian zhong　黔中
Qian zhong jun　黔中郡
Qian zhou　乾州
Qian zhou　黔州
Qiang　羌
Qiang dao　羌道
Qiang di　羌地
Qiang li　羌里
Qiang long　羌隴
Qiang zhong　羌中
Qiao　譙
Qiao jun　譙郡
Qiao nan　嶠南
Qiao shan　喬山
Qie mi shan　且彌山
Qin　秦
Qin di　秦地
Qin guan　秦關
Qin jin　秦晉
Qin ling　秦嶺
Qin long　秦隴
Qin ning xian　秦寧縣
Qin shan　秦山
Qin shui　沁水
Qin ting　秦亭
Qin zhong　秦中
Qin zhou　欽州
Qin zhou　沁州
Qin zhou　秦州
Qin zhou　勤州
Qing　青
Qing cheng shan　青城山
Qing dui　青堆
Qing he　清河
Qing liang si　清涼寺
Qing lin hu　青林湖
Qing liu　清流
Qing qi　青齊
Qing qiu zhi shan　青丘之山
Qing xi　青溪
Qing yang　慶陽
Qing yi　青衣
Qing yi xian　青衣縣
Qing yuan. 慶遠
Qing zhou　青州
Qiong　瓊
Qiong po sai jiang　邛婆塞江
Qiong zhou　瓊州
Qiong zhou　邛州
Qiu chi　仇池
Qiu ci guo　龜茲國
Qu　衢
Qu jiang　曲江
Qu ren xian　朐肕縣
Qu shan　朐山
Qu shan　區山
Qu tan　曲灘
Qu zhou　衢州
Qu zhou　渠州
Quan　全
Quan　泉
Quan zhou　泉州
Quan zhou　全州
Que shan　鵲山

Ran mang yi　冉駹夷
Rang cheng　穰城
Rao　饒

Shang zhou 商州
Shao 韶
Shao 邵
Shao ling 邵陵
Shao shi 少室
Shao shi shan 少室山
Shao shi zhi shan 少室之山
Shao wu 紹武
Shao wu 邵武
Shao wu jun 邵武軍
Shao xing 紹興
Shao yang 韶陽
Shao yang shan 燒羊山
Shao yang zhi shan 少陽之山
Shao zhou 韶州
She 歙
She yang 射陽
She zhou 歙州
Shen 申
Shen mu xian 神木縣
Shen zhou 申州
Shen zhou 深州
Sheng nan 勝南
Shi 施
Shi an 始安
Shi cheng 石城
Shi cui zhi shan 石脆之山
Shi cui zhi shan 石翠之山
Shi feng 始豐
Shi men 石門
Shi mo shan 石墨山
Shi xing 始興
Shi zhou 十洲
Shi zhou 石州
Shi zhou 施州
Shi zi guo 師子國
Shou 壽
Shou chun 壽春
Shou yang 壽陽
Shou yang 首陽
Shou yang shan 首陽山
Shou zhou 壽州
Shu 舒
Shu 蜀
Shu bei 蜀北
Shu chuan 蜀川
Shu dao 蜀道
Shu di 蜀地
Shu du 蜀都
Shu han 蜀漢
Shu jiang 蜀江
Shu jiao 蜀徼
Shu jun 蜀郡
Shu kui 蜀夔
Shu le 疏勒
Shu shan 蜀山
Shu tu 蜀土
Shu xi 蜀西
Shu xi jiao wai 蜀西徼外
Shu xiang 蜀鄉
Shu you 蜀右
Shu zhong 蜀中
Shu zhou 蜀州
Shu zhou 舒州
Shuang jing 雙井
Shuang shui 瀧水
Shuang zhou 瀧州
Shun an jun 順安軍
Shun chang 順昌
Shun qing 順慶
Shun tian fu 順天府
Shun yang xian 順陽縣
Shun zheng 順政
Shun zheng jun 順政郡
Shun zhou 順州
Si 泗
Si an 思安
Si chuan 四川
Si diao 斯調
Si diao guo 斯調國
Si hui xian 四會縣
Si ming 四明
Si ming shan 四明山
Si yang 四陽
Si zhou 泗州
Si zhou 司州
Song 淞
Song 宋

Song gao　嵩高
Song gao shan　嵩高山
Song jiang　淞江
Song li shan　宋里山
Song pan　松潘
Song shan　嵩山
Song yang　松陽
Song yang　嵩陽
Song yang xian　松楊縣
Song yue　嵩岳
Song zhou　松州
Su　蘇
Su fang guo　蘇方國
Su he guo　蘇合國
Su men da la guo　蘇門答剌國
Su shen guo　肅慎國
Su shui　涑水
Su zhou　肅州
Su zhou　宿州
Su zhou　蘇州
Suan zao xian　酸棗縣
Sui　綏
Sui　隨
Sui　遂
Sui ding xian　綏定縣
Sui jun　隨郡
Sui ning　遂寧
Sui yang　睢陽
Sui zhou　隨州

Tai　台
Tai bai shan　太白山
Tai cang　太倉
Tai gu　太谷
Tai hang　太行
Tai hang shan　太行山
Tai he　太和
Tai he shan　太和山
Tai hu　太湖
Tai hua　太華
Tai hua shan　太華山
Tai ning xian　泰寧縣
Tai qing gong　太清宮
Tai shan　太山
Tai shan　泰山
Tai wu　太吳
Tai ye chi　太液池
Tai yuan　太原
Tai zhou　泰州
Tai zhou　台州
Tan　潭
Tan chang　宕昌
Tan ya　檀崖
Tan yu shan　檀嵎山
Tan zhou　宕州
Tan zhou　檀州
Tan zhou　潭州
Tang　唐
Tang luo　溏濼
Tang luo jie he　塘濼界河
Tang shan xian　唐山縣
Tang shao shan　堂少山
Tang xian　唐縣
Tang yin　湯陰
Tao yang　洮陽
Teng zhou　藤州
Tian di zhi shan　天帝之山
Tian fang guo　天方國
Tian lou shan　天婁山
Tian mu shan　天目山
Tian shui　天水
Tian tai　天台
Tian tai shan　天台山
Tian zhu　天竺
Tian zhu guo　天竺國
Tian zhu zhu guo　天竺諸國
Ting shan　亭山
Tong　通
Tong　同
Tong an　同安
Tong bai　桐柏
Tong bai shan　桐柏山
Tong cheng xian　通城縣
Tong chuan　潼川
Tong guan　銅官
Tong ling xian　銅陵縣
Tong lu　桐廬
Tong shan　銅山

Tong zhou 同州
Tong zhou 通州
Tu bo 吐番
Tu fan 土番
Tu huo luo 吐火羅
Tu jue 突厥
Tu jue guo 突厥國
Tu ling 荼陵
Tu yu hun 吐谷渾
Tuo 沱
Tuo shan 槖山

Wai fan 外番
Wai guo 外國
Wan an 萬安
Wan zhou 萬州
Wang chu shan 望楚山
Wang wu 王屋
Wang wu shan 王屋山
Wei 威
Wei 衛
Wei 魏
Wei cheng 渭城
Wei di 魏地
Wei guo 魏國
Wei jun 魏郡
Wei qiang shan 韋羌山
Wei sheng jun 威勝軍
Wei shui 渭水
Wei xing 魏興
Wei zhou 渭州
Wei zhou 衛州
Wei zhou 維州
Wei zhou 威州
Wen 溫
Wen 汶
Wen quan xian 溫泉縣
Wen shan 汶山
Wen shan jun 汶山郡
Wen xiang 閿鄉
Wen zhou 汶州
Wen zhou 文州
Wen zhou 溫州
Wo 倭
Wo guo 倭國
Wu 婺
Wu 吳
Wu chang 武昌
Wu chang guo 烏場國
Wu cheng 武城
Wu cheng xian 烏程縣
Wu chu 吳楚
Wu dang 武當
Wu dang shan 武當山
Wu di 吳地
Wu du 武都
Wu du 吳都
Wu gang zhou 武岡州
Wu gong 武功
Wu gou shan 烏勾山
Wu ji guo 勿吉國
Wu jiang 吳江
Wu jun 吳郡
Wu kuai 吳會
Wu lao xian 無勞縣
Wu ling 武陵
Wu ling 吳陵
Wu ling 五嶺
Wu ling jun 武陵郡
Wu ling zhou 武陵洲
Wu meng shan 烏蒙山
Wu meng xia 烏蒙峽
Wu ping 武平
Wu shan 巫山
Wu sun guo 烏孫國
Wu tai 五臺
Wu tai shan 五臺山
Wu tai zhu shan 五臺諸山
Wu tao shan 無桃山
Wu wan 烏丸
Wu wei 武威
Wu wei zhou 無為州
Wu xi 五溪
Wu xi shi ku 舞磎石窟
Wu xian 巫縣
Wu xing 吳興
Wu xing jun 吳興郡
Wu xu guo 烏許國

Wu yang 武陽
Wu yang 吳揚
Wu yang 巫陽
Wu yu he 烏玉河
Wu yu zhi shan 務隅之山
Wu yuan 五原
Wu yuan cheng 五原城
Wu yue 五岳
Wu yue 吳越
Wu yue 吳粵
Wu zhong 吳中
Wu zhou 婺州
Wu zhou 梧州

Xi 西
Xi 奚
Xi an 西安
Xi an zhu jun 熙安諸郡
Xi bei 西北
Xi bei fan jie 西北番界
Xi bei fang 西北方
Xi bei zhou jun 西北州郡
Xi bian 西邊
Xi cheng 析城
Xi chuan 西川
Xi dong 溪峒
Xi fan 西番
Xi fang 西方
Xi guo 西國
Xi guo zhu fan 西國諸番
Xi guo zhu rong 西國諸戎
Xi hai 西海
Xi he 西河
Xi hu 西胡
Xi hu 西湖
Xi jian 西間
Xi jiao zhu zhou 西徼諸州
Xi jing 西京
Xi liang 西涼
Xi liao ban 西遼坂
Xi lu 西路 [1]
Xi luo 西洛
Xi nan 西南
Xi nan fan 西南番
Xi nan guo ming 西南國名
Xi nan hai 西南海
Xi nan hai yang 西南海洋
Xi nan jiao wai 西南徼外
Xi nan wai 西南外
Xi nan yi 西南夷
Xi nan zhang hai 西南瘴海
Xi nan zhu fan 西南諸番
Xi nan zhu guo 西南諸國
Xi ping shan 西平山
Xi qi dan 奚契丹
Xi qiang 西羌
Xi qiang bei di 西羌北地
Xi rong 西戎
Xi rong jie 西戎界
Xi shan 錫山
Xi shan 西山
Xi shu 西蜀
Xi shu zhou jun 西蜀州郡
Xi tu 西土
Xi xi si 西溪寺
Xi xia 西夏
Xi yang 西洋
Xi yang 西陽
Xi yi 西夷
Xi yu 西域
Xi yue 西岳
Xi zhou 溪州
Xi zhou 溪州
Xi zhou 西州
Xi zhou 巂州
Xia 峽
Xia guo 夏國
Xia pi 下邳
Xia shan 峽山
Xia zhong 峽中
Xia zhou 硤州
Xia zhou 峽州
Xian ju 仙居
Xian luo 暹羅
Xian luo guo 暹羅國
Xian shan 峴山
Xian yang 咸陽
Xian zhou 憲州

Xiang 湘
Xiang 襄
Xiang dong 湘東
Xiang guo si 相國寺
Xiang han 襄漢
Xiang lin 象林
Xiang ling 襄陵
Xiang mian 襄沔
Xiang nan 湘南
Xiang ning xian 鄉寧縣
Xiang shan 象山
Xiang shan si 湘山寺
Xiang shan xian 象山縣
Xiang shan xian 湘山縣
Xiang shui 湘水
Xiang xiang xian 襄鄉縣
Xiang yang 襄陽
Xiang zhou 象州
Xiang zhou 襄州
Xiang zhou 湘州
Xiang zhou 相州
Xiao 蕭
Xiao gui xian 小桂縣
Xiao huo shan 小霍山
Xiao ping 小坪
Xiao qiu 蕭丘
Xiao shan 蕭山
Xie 解
Xie chi 解池
Xie gu 斜谷
Xie gu xi li 斜谷西嶺
Xie zhou 解州
Xin 信
Xin an 新安
Xin cai 新蔡
Xin cheng jun 新城郡
Xin du 信都
Xin du jun 信都郡
Xin gan 新淦
Xin luo 新羅
Xin luo guo 新羅國
Xin ning 新寧
Xin ping xian 新平縣
Xin xing xian 新興縣
Xin yang 信陽
Xin yang zhou 信陽州
Xin ye 新野
Xin zhou 新洲
Xin zhou 信州
Xing gu 興古
Xing guo 興國
Xing guo zhou 興國州
Xing hua 興化
Xing hua jun 興化軍
Xing nan 滎南
Xing qing chi 興慶池
Xing yang 滎陽
Xing yuan 興元
Xing yuan fu 興元府
Xing zhou 興州
Xing zhou 邢州
Xiong 雄
Xiong er 熊耳
Xiong er shan 熊耳山
Xiong she xhan 熊舍山
Xiu 秀
Xiu chuan 秀川
Xiu jiang 修江
Xiu ren 修仁
Xiu shui 休水
Xu 徐
Xu jiang 盱江
Xu pu 溆浦
Xu shan 續山
Xu shan 徐善亭
Xu wen xian 徐聞縣
Xu wu shan 徐無山
Xu yi xian 盱眙縣
Xu zhou 敘州
Xu zhou 徐州
Xuan 宣
Xuan cheng 宣城
Xuan cheng 宣城
Xuan cheng jun 宣城郡
Xuan shan 玄山
Xuan tu 玄菟
Xuan weng zhi shan 懸甕之山
Xuan zhou 宣州

Xue shan 雪山
Xun 潯
Xun 循
Xun yang 潯陽
Xun yang jiang 潯陽江
Xun zhou 循州
Xun zhou 潯州

Ya 崖
Ya men shan 牙門山
Ya shan 丫山
Ya zhou 崖州
Ya zhou 雅州
Yan 延
Yan 兗
Yan 燕
Yan an fu 延安府
Yan bei 燕北
Yan chang 延長
Yan cheng 鹽城
Yan dao 嚴道
Yan dao xian 嚴道縣
Yan jing 燕京
Yan ling 嚴陵
Yan ling 延陵
Yan men 雁門
Yan qi guo 焉耆國
Yan shan 鹽山
Yan shan 弇山
Yan shan 鉛山
Yan shan xian 鉛山縣
Yan shou xian 延壽縣
Yan sui 延綏
Yan yu 兗豫
Yan zhou 弇州
Yan zhou 兗州
Yan zhou 嚴州
Yan zhou 鹽州
Yan zhou 延州
Yan zhou fu 兗州府
Yang 揚
Yang cheng 陽城
Yang di 陽翟
Yang gu xian 陽谷縣
Yang gu xian 陽穀縣
Yang jiang xian 陽江縣
Yang keng 陽坑
Yang po 陽坡
Yang pu 楊樸
Yang qi shan 陽起山
Yang shan 陽山
Yang shan xian 陽山縣
Yang xian 陽羨
Yang xian xian 陽羨縣
Yang zhou 洋州
Yang zhou 揚州
Yang zi 揚子
Yao 瑤
Yao 耀
Yao dong 瑤峒
Yao shan 堯山
Yao shan 搖山
Yao zhou 耀州
Ye 冶
Ye bei bai shan 掖北白山
Ye bei shan 液北山
Ye bei xiang 液北鄉
Ye du 鄴都
Ye huo luo 葉火羅
Ye jun 鄴郡
Ye xi 耶溪
Ye xian 掖縣
Ye zhong 鄴中
Yi 沂
Yi 宜
Yi 益
Yi bin 宜賓
Yi chang 益昌
Yi chun jun 宜春郡
Yi du 益都
Yi du 宜都
Yi feng xian 移風縣
Yi ling 夷陵
Yi lou 挹婁
Yi luo 伊洛
Yi men 夷門
Yi qing shan 義情山
Yi shi xian 猗氏縣

Yi shui 伊水
Yi wu 義烏
Yi yang 義陽
Yi yang 易陽
Yi yang xian 宜陽縣
Yi yang xian 伊陽縣
Yi zhou 翼州
Yi zhou 益州
Yi zhou 易州
Yi zhou 儀州
Yi zhou 宜州
Yi zhou 沂州
Yin 鄞
Yin fan shan 隱蕃山
Yin ping 陰平
Yin shan 陰山
Yin xian 鄞縣
Yin zhou 鄞州
Ying 英
Ying 郢
Ying cheng 郢城
Ying chuan 潁川
Ying chuan jun 潁川郡
Ying dao 營道
Ying hou zhi shan 嬰侯之山
Ying shan 英山
Ying tian fu 應天府
Ying yang 潁陽
Ying zhou 郢州
Ying zhou 營州
Ying zhou 瀛洲
Ying zhou 英州
Yong 邕
Yong 雍
Yong 永
Yong chang 永昌
Yong chang jun 永昌郡
Yong ji 雍冀
Yong jia 永嘉
Yong kang 永康
Yong ning wei 永寧衛
Yong shun 永順
Yong xing 永興
Yong xing jun 永興軍
Yong yang 永陽
Yong zhou 雍州
Yong zhou 邕州
Yong zhou 永州
You 幽
You jiang 右江
You xi zhi shan 遊戲之山
You yan 幽燕
You yang 酉陽
You zhou 幽州
Yu 虞
Yu 渝
Yu 豫
Yu 蔚
Yu ci 榆次
Yu ci zhi shan 羭次之山
Yu er 語兒
Yu er 御兒
Yu gan 餘干
Yu hang 餘杭
Yu hang shan 餘杭山
Yu he 玉河
Yu hua tai 雨花臺
Yu lei 玉壘
Yu lin 鬱林
Yu lin gang 榆林港
Yu lin jun 鬱林郡
Yu lin zhou 鬱林州
Yu men 玉門
Yu qian 於潛
Yu qing xian 虞卿縣
Yu shan 玉山
Yu shan 羽山
Yu shan xian 玉山縣
Yu tian 玉田
Yu tian 於闐
Yu tian 于闐
Yu tian guo 于闐國
Yu tian xian 玉田縣
Yu yang 漁陽
Yu zhang 豫章
Yu zhang jun 豫章郡
Yu zhou 鬱州
Yu zhou 豫州

Yu zhou 渝州
Yu zhou 蔚州
Yuan 袁
Yuan an xian 遠安縣
Yuan jiang 沅江
Yuan ju 冤句
Yuan qiao zhi shan 員嶠之山
Yuan zhou 原州
Yuan zhou 袁州
Yue 越
Yue 粵
Yue 岳
Yue di 越地
Yue e 岳鄂
Yue jian 越間
Yue lun xi 月輪寺
Yue nan 越南
Yue qing 樂清
Yue shan 越山
Yue sui 越巂
Yue wen 越韞
Yue yang 岳陽
Yue zhou 岳州
Yue zhou 越州
Yue zhou fu 岳州府
Yun 雲
Yun an jun 雲安軍
Yun meng 雲夢
Yun meng shan 雲夢山
Yun nan 雲南
Yun shan 雲山
Yun tai shu 雲臺戍
Yun yang 雲陽
Yun yang xian 雲陽縣
Yun zhong 雲中
Yun zhou 鄆州

Zan 贊
Zan zhou 贊州
Zang ke 牂牁
Ze 澤
Ze zhou 澤州
Zeng bin 鋥賓
Zeng Cheng 曾城
Zhan bei guo 占卑國
Zhan cheng 占城
Zhan cheng guo 占城國
Zhang 漳
Zhang an 章安
Zhang de 彰德
Zhang ming 彰明
Zhang ming xian 彰明縣
Zhang shan 鄣山
Zhang wu 章武
Zhang xian 鄣縣
Zhang ye 張掖
Zhang zhou 漳州
Zhang zi shan 長子山
Zhang zi xian 長子縣
Zhao 趙
Zhao guo 趙國
Zhao jun 趙郡
Zhao ling 召陵
Zhao qing 肇慶
Zhao qing fu 肇慶府
Zhao wa 爪哇
Zhe 浙
Zhe cheng xian 柘城縣
Zhe dong 浙東
Zhe jiang 浙江
Zhe xi 浙西
Zhe yang 赭陽
Zhe zhou 浙州
Zhen 鎮
Zhen an 鎮安
Zhen ding 鎮定
Zhen ding 真定
Zhen ding xian 真定縣
Zhen jiang 鎮江
Zhen kang zhou 鎮康州
Zhen la 真臘
Zhen la guo 真臘國
Zhen yang 真陽
Zhen yang xian 湞陽縣
Zhen zhou 真州
Zhen zhou 鎮州
Zheng 鄭
Zheng shan 鄭山

Zheng xian 烝縣
Zheng zhou 鄭州
Zhi shui 泜水
Zhi zhi guo 郅支國
Zhong du 中都
Zhong guo 中國
Zhong hua 中華
Zhong jiang xian 中江縣
Zhong li xian 鍾離縣
Zhong ling shan 冢嶺山
Zhong lu xian 中廬縣
Zhong mou 中牟
Zhong nan 終南
Zhong nan shan 終南山
Zhong shan 中山
Zhong shan 鍾山
Zhong shan xian 鍾山縣
Zhong shui 中水
Zhong shui xian 中水縣
Zhong tai 中臺
Zhong tai shan gu 中臺山谷
Zhong tian zhu guo 中天竺國
Zhong tiao shan 中條山
Zhong tu 中土
Zhong yang 中央
Zhong yuan 中原
Zhong yue 中岳
Zhong zhou 中州
Zhong zhou 忠州
Zhou 周
Zhu bu guo 竹步國
Zhu ji 諸暨
Zhu ti 朱提
Zhu ya 朱厓
Zhu ya 朱崖
Zhuang lang 莊浪
Zhuang lang wei 莊浪衛
Zi 淄
Zi 資
Zi chuan 淄川
Zi chuan 菑川
Zi gui 秭歸
Zi tuan 紫團
Zi tuan shan 紫團山
Zi zhou 淄州
Zi zhou 資州
Zi zhou 梓州
Zou xian 鄒縣
Zuo you jiang 左右江